Recent Advances in Assistive Technologies to Support Children with Developmental Disorders

Nava R. Silton
Marymount Manhattan College, USA

A volume in the Advances in Medical Technologies and Clinical Practice (AMTCP) Book Series

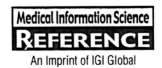

Medical Information Science
REFERENCE
An Imprint of IGI Global

Managing Director:	Lindsay Johnston
Managing Editor:	Austin DeMarco
Director of Intellectual Property & Contracts:	Jan Travers
Acquisitions Editor:	Kayla Wolfe
Production Editor:	Christina Henning
Development Editor:	Caitlyn Martin
Typesetter:	Michael Brehm & Tucker Knerr
Cover Design:	Jason Mull

Published in the United States of America by
Medical Information Science Reference (an imprint of IGI Global)
701 E. Chocolate Avenue
Hershey PA, USA 17033
Tel: 717-533-8845
Fax: 717-533-8661
E-mail: cust@igi-global.com
Web site: http://www.igi-global.com

Library of Congress Cataloging-in-Publication Data

Recent advances in assistive technologies to support children with developmental disorders / Nava R. Silton, editor.
     pages cm
  Includes bibliographical references and index.
  Summary: "This book raises awareness of disabled children and what can be done to help them grow and develop alongside their peers by bringing together personal experiences with academic investigation"-- Provided by publisher.
  ISBN 978-1-4666-8395-2 (hardcover) -- ISBN 978-1-4666-8396-9 (ebook) 1. Children with disabilities--Services for. 2. Self-help devices for people with disabilities. 3. Children with disabilities--Education. 4. Assistive computer technology. I. Silton, Nava R., 1981-
  HV1569.5.R43 2015
  362.3--dc23
                                        2015008002

This book is published in the IGI Global book series Advances in Medical Technologies and Clinical Practice (AMTCP) (ISSN: 2327-9354; eISSN: 2327-9370)

British Cataloguing in Publication Data
A Cataloguing in Publication record for this book is available from the British Library.

For electronic access to this publication, please contact: eresources@igi-global.com.

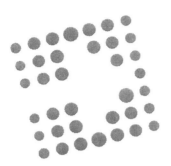

Advances in Medical Technologies and Clinical Practice (AMTCP) Book Series

Srikanta Patnaik
SOA University, India
Priti Das
S.C.B. Medical College, India

ISSN: 2327-9354
EISSN: 2327-9370

MISSION

Medical technological innovation continues to provide avenues of research for faster and safer diagnosis and treatments for patients. Practitioners must stay up to date with these latest advancements to provide the best care for nursing and clinical practices.

The **Advances in Medical Technologies and Clinical Practice (AMTCP) Book Series** brings together the most recent research on the latest technology used in areas of nursing informatics, clinical technology, biomedicine, diagnostic technologies, and more. Researchers, students, and practitioners in this field will benefit from this fundamental coverage on the use of technology in clinical practices.

COVERAGE

- Biometrics
- Nutrition
- Telemedicine
- Nursing Informatics
- Patient-Centered Care
- Neural Engineering
- Medical Imaging
- E-health
- Clinical Nutrition
- Diagnostic Technologies

IGI Global is currently accepting manuscripts for publication within this series. To submit a proposal for a volume in this series, please contact our Acquisition Editors at Acquisitions@igi-global.com or visit: http://www.igi-global.com/publish/.

Titles in this Series

For a list of additional titles in this series, please visit: www.igi-global.com

Advanced Technological Solutions for E-Health and Dementia Patient Monitoring
Fatos Xhafa (Universitat Politècnica de Catalunya, Spain) Philip Moore (School of Information Science and Engineering, Lanzhou University, China) and George Tadros (University of Warwick, UK)
Medical Information Science Reference • copyright 2015 • 389pp • H/C (ISBN: 9781466674813) • US $215.00 (our price)

Assistive Technologies for Physical and Cognitive Disabilities
Lau Bee Theng (Swinburne University of Technology, Malaysia)
Medical Information Science Reference • copyright 2015 • 321pp • H/C (ISBN: 9781466673731) • US $205.00 (our price)

Fuzzy Expert Systems for Disease Diagnosis
A.V. Senthil Kumar (Hindusthan College of Arts and Science, India)
Medical Information Science Reference • copyright 2015 • 401pp • H/C (ISBN: 9781466672406) • US $265.00 (our price)

Handbook of Research on Computerized Occlusal Analysis Technology Applications in Dental Medicine
Robert B. Kerstein, DMD (Former clinical professor at Tufts University School of Dental Medicine, USA & Private Dental Practice Limited to Prosthodontics and Computerized Occlusal Analysis, USA)
Medical Information Science Reference • copyright 2015 • 1093pp • H/C (ISBN: 9781466665873) • US $475.00 (our price)

Enhancing the Human Experience through Assistive Technologies and E-Accessibility
Christos Kouroupetroglou (Caretta-Net Technologies, Greece)
Medical Information Science Reference • copyright 2014 • 345pp • H/C (ISBN: 9781466661301) • US $265.00 (our price)

Applications, Challenges, and Advancements in Electromyography Signal Processing
Ganesh R. Naik (University of Technology Sydney (UTS), Australia)
Medical Information Science Reference • copyright 2014 • 404pp • H/C (ISBN: 9781466660908) • US $235.00 (our price)

Innovative Technologies to Benefit Children on the Autism Spectrum
Nava R. Silton (Marymount Manhattan College, USA)
Medical Information Science Reference • copyright 2014 • 343pp • H/C (ISBN: 9781466657922) • US $195.00 (our price)

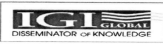

DISSEMINATOR OF KNOWLEDGE

www.igi-global.com

701 E. Chocolate Ave., Hershey, PA 17033
Order online at www.igi-global.com or call 717-533-8845 x100
To place a standing order for titles released in this series, contact: cust@igi-global.com
Mon-Fri 8:00 am - 5:00 pm (est) or fax 24 hours a day 717-533-8661

Editorial Advisory Board

Table of Contents

Detailed Table of Contents

Chapter 1
Larah van der Meer, Victoria University of Wellington, New Zealand

The Apple iPod Touch™ and iPad™ are increasingly used as augmentative and alternative communication (AAC) devices. This chapter discusses the use of iPods™/iPads™ loaded with software applications that enable speech output and thereby transform them into speech-generating devices (SGD). While a popular mode of communication for children with developmental disorders (DD) who have little or no spoken language, assessment of the effectiveness of such new technology to enhance communicative functioning is necessary. Research on the use of iPods™/iPads™ was evaluated to assess whether they are (a) effective as AAC devices, (b) at least as effective as other AAC interventions, and (c) effective at the individual level of implementation. Findings suggested that the use of iPods™/iPads™ as AAC devices is promising, also in comparison to other AAC systems. Children typically preferred using iPods™/iPads™. Selection of an AAC system based on the child's preference coupled with appropriate instructional strategies may lead to the enhancement of communicative functioning for children with DD.

Chapter 2
Cathi Draper Rodríguez, California State University – Monterey Bay, USA
Iva Strnadová, University of New South Wales, Australia
Therese M Cumming, University of New South Wales, Australia

This book chapter describes implementation implications of using the iPad and other mobile technologies with students (birth to adult) with intellectual disabilities. iPad and other mobile technologies offer many built-in features which facilitate their use for students with disabilities, particularly students with Intellectual Disabilities (ID). This chapter details ways that mobile technology can be used to make school and other environments (e.g., home, social) more accessible to students with ID. The theoretical framework underpinning this chapter is Universal Design for Learning (UDL), and it is applied to research-based practices for students with ID. This forms a solid base from which to examine: (a) available mobile applications (apps), (b) how apps can be used to support students with ID in accessing the curriculum, and (c) how teachers can use a framework to review and choose apps for their students.

Chapter 3

Using iPads and Mobile Technology for Children with Developmental Disabilities: Facilitating
Language and Literacy Development 45

Lisa A. Proctor, Missouri State University, USA
Ye Wang, Teachers College, Columbia University, USA

With increasing access to iPads and mobile technology in both home and school settings, evidence regarding how best to use this technology to enhance language and literacy learning is lacking, particularly for children with developmental disabilities. As a comprehensive review, this chapter discusses the use of iPads and mobile technology in the language and literacy development of this population. It concludes that while iPads and mobile technology provide opportunities for language and literacy development, the inherent challenges and limitations of this technology warrant attention from parents, educators and speech-language pathologists. iPads and mobile technology may be a valuable accelerator for the language and literacy development of children with developmental disabilities if used properly; however, improper or careless usage can become a distraction that further delays the communication development of this population.

Chapter 4

Early Literacy and AAC for Learners with Complex Communication Needs 79

Janis Doneski-Nicol, Northern Arizona University, USA
Jody Marie Bartz, Northern Arizona University, USA

Augmentative and Alternative Communication (AAC) systems are a common assistive technology (AT) intervention for learners with complex communication needs (CCN) – those learners who are unable to use speech and language as a primary mode of communication. AAC systems can be a powerful intervention; however, these systems must be integrated with strong, early and conventional literacy instructional opportunities. In this chapter, we provide parents, educators, researchers, academics, and other professionals with the most up to date and innovative information as well as practical resources regarding early literacy and AAC for learners with CCN. Emphasis will be on young children with CCN in preschool and early elementary school settings. Features of AAC systems and evidence-based literacy assessment and intervention, as well as the benefits and challenges, are presented to provide the reader with information on the current state of the field. The chapter concludes with directions for future research and provides a comprehensive list of resources and organizations.

Chapter 5

The Use of Mobile Technologies for Students At-Risk or Identified with Behavioral Disorders
within School-Based Contexts 114

Frank J. Sansosti, Kent State University, USA
Peña L. Bedesem, Kent State University, USA

Students at-risk or identified with behavioral disorders often present complex challenges to educators. The purpose of this chapter is to: (a) highlight the benefits and challenges of using mobile technologies within school-based contexts; (b) provide a brief overview of the contemporary research regarding the use of mobile devices for improving the outcomes of students with behavioral disorders within schools; and (c) offer essential techniques, methods, and ideas for improving instruction and management for students with behavioral difficulties via mobile technologies. Taken together, the intent is to call attention to the evidence that supports the use of mobile technologies for students who are at-risk or identified with behavioral disorders in schools, raise awareness of those strategies that appear to be the most effective for such students and assist service providers in providing accountable education.

Chapter 6

With the increased development of mobile technologies, such as smartphones and tablets (i.e. iPhone, iPad), the field of augmentative and alternative communication (AAC) has changed rapidly over the last few years. Recent advances in technology have introduced applications (apps) for AAC purposes. These novel technologies could provide numerous benefits to individuals with complex communication needs. Nevertheless, introducing mobile technology apps is not without risk. Since these apps can be purchased and retrieved with relative ease, AAC assessments and collaborative evaluations have been circumvented in favor of the "quick fix"-simply ordering a random app for a potential user, without fully assessing the individual's needs and abilities. There is a paucity of research pertaining to mobile technology use in AAC. Therapists, parents and developers of AAC applications must work collaboratively to expand the research pertaining to the assessment and treatment of children who utilize AAC mobile technologies for communication purposes.

Chapter 7

This chapter is designed to provide parents, professionals, and individuals with Autism Spectrum Disorder (ASD) with tools to help them evaluate the effectiveness of computer-mediated interventions to support the social and emotional development of individuals with ASD. Starting with guidelines for selecting computer-mediated interventions, we highlight the importance of identifying target skills for intervention that match an individual's needs and interests. We describe how readers can assess the degree to which an intervention is evidence-based, and include an overview of different types of experiments and statistical methods. We examine a variety of computer-mediated interventions and the evidence base for each: computer-delivered instruction (including games), iPad-type apps, virtual environments, and robots. We describe websites that provide additional resources for finding educational games and apps. We conclude by emphasizing the uniqueness of each individual with ASD and the importance of selecting interventions that are well-matched to the specific needs of each individual.

Chapter 8

In recent years, there has been a burgeoning field of research on the applications of virtual reality and
robots for children, adolescents, and adults with a wide range of developmental disabilities. The influx
of multidisciplinary collaborations among developmental psychologists and computer scientists, as well
as the increasing accessibility of interactive technologies, has created a need to equip potential users
with the information they need to make informed decisions about using virtual reality and robots. This
chapter aims to 1) provide parents, professionals, and individuals with developmental disabilities with
an overview of the literature on virtual reality and robot interventions in childhood, adolescence, and
adulthood; and to 2) address overarching questions pertaining to utilizing virtual reality and robots. This
chapter will shed light on the far-reaching potential for interactive technologies to transform therapeutic,
educational, and assessment contexts, while also highlighting limitations and suggesting directions for
future research.

This chapter provides a literature overview concerning microswitch-based programs (MBP) to promote
communication, occupation and leisure skills for children with multiple disabilities. The first aim of
the chapter is to present an overview of the empirical studies about the use of MBP, published in the
last decade (i.e. period from 2004 to 2014) to emphasize the most recent strategies for children with
developmental disabilities, providing a general picture of the different options available. The second goal
is to underline strengths and weaknesses of the various studies included in the overview. Finally, the third
purpose is to outline issues and questions to be addressed in the future and discuss their implications
for research and practice.

Chapter 10

Conventional methods of addressing the needs of students with print disabilities include text-to-speech
services. One major drawback of text-to-speech technologies is that computerized speech simply
articulates the same words in a text whereas human voice can convey emotions such as excitement,
sadness, fear, or joy. Audiobooks have human narration, but are designed for entertainment and not for
teaching word identification, fluency, vocabulary, and comprehension to students. This chapter focuses
on the 3-year pilot of CRISKids; all CRIS recordings feature human narration. The pilot demonstrated
that students who feel competent in their reading and class work tend to be more engaged in classroom
routines, spend more time on task and demonstrate greater comprehension of written materials. When

more demonstrate these behaviors and skills, teachers are better able to provide meaningful instruction, since less time is spent on issues of classroom management and redirection. Thus, CRISKids impacts not only the students with print disabilities, but all of the students in the classroom.

Chapter 11

Video modeling is an evidence-based practice for learners with autism spectrum disorders (ASD). However, the use of video modeling interventions for learners with other developmental disabilities has received less applied attention in home, community, and classroom settings. This is unfortunate since the research literature supports the use of video modeling interventions for all learners with developmental disabilities. The purpose of this chapter is to introduce the research literature and make suggestions for implementing video modeling with learners who have developmental disabilities other than autism.

Chapter 12

About two million individuals in the United States use augmentative and alternative communication (AAC) devices with text-to-speech (TTS) synthesis to speak on their behalf. In this chapter, two specific systems are introduced and evaluated as potentially significant emerging tools for children with communication disorders. The VocalIDTM project was developed to provide unique voices for children who otherwise speak through standard adult voices. Free SpeechTM is an image-based system designed to address grammatical concepts perceived as abstract by children with language disorders. This chapter also reviews the latest developments in electropalatography (EPG): biofeedback technology, which enables the visualization of tongue to palate contact during speech production. SmartPalateTM has developed cutting-edge hardware and software technology to make EPG more intuitive and more accessible in the therapy room and at home.

Chapter 13

Ongoing advances in technology have provided a platform to extend the accessibility of services for children with developmental disabilities across locations, languages and the socioeconomic continuum. Teletherapy, the use of video-conferencing technology to deliver therapy services, is changing the face of healthcare by providing face-to-face interactions among specialists, parents and children. The current literature has demonstrated success in utilizing teletherapy as a modality for speech-language intervention and for social-behavioral management, while research on feeding therapy remains scarce. The current chapter discusses the prevalence of feeding disorders among infants, toddlers and children with developmental disorders. Using evidence from the current literature, a rationale for the utilization of teletherapy as a means of feeding therapy is presented.

The following chapter presents a compilation of research about various types of technology that are employed by music therapists to benefit children with developmental delays. Music therapy can be an effective way to meet the goals of the individual. Music can also be a very powerful motivator. Previous musical skill or experience is not required for music therapy to be effective for clients with developmental disabilities or for clients more generally. Many music-based technologies are designed to create a positive, successful, and enjoyable experience for all users. Music therapy can provide a safe and confidence building environment where children are able to feel in control of a situation, possibly for the first time in their lives.

Over the last decade, vast research has been conducted on assistive technology devices and the potential implementation of these devices in the daily lives of individuals with disabilities. Many devices are new to the public and may require further development, but it is important to disseminate information about these useful technologies, which often afford users more independence with their activities of daily living. Unfortunately individuals with disabilities often encounter stigma; research suggests that assistive technology devices may at times contribute to this ostracism. This chapter reviews a variety of technologies that have been used to improve the quality of life of individuals with varying disabilities. These devices are presented in the context of introducing a new children's television show, Realabilities, a pro-social and stop-bullying children's television program that seeks to enhance the social interaction and initiation of typical children towards children with disabilities. Directions for future research and implementation of these devices are also discussed.

Chapter 16

Social competence includes a complex set of skills that impacts quality of life across all environments: home, school, employment, and the community. Elements that impact social competence, such as theory of mind, weak central coherence, regulation and relationship building, must be taught to individuals with disabilities, including those with autism spectrum disorder. Evidence-based interventions that incorporate low, medium and high technology have the potential to support skill development in social competence in a meaningful manner. This chapter reviews the concept known as social competence and offers a variety of practices to support its development.

Foreword

As an educator, an academic, a researcher, a TV & film producer, an educational technologist, a consultant and parent, I have witnessed the immense benefits of assistive technology from a variety of vantage points. The two dramatic examples below further attest to the incredible potential of assistive technology to improve the daily life functioning of individuals with disabilities:

Video Technology via iPad

When Addy came to the Jenny Clarkson School, she was an awkward girl who had a lot of trouble with personal interactions. Addy worked with her clinician intensely to improve her social-emotional skills, including her body language, appropriate voice, her distance away from a person during a conversation, appropriate hugging, shaking hands, making eye contact and making good decisions. These behaviors were all extremely challenging for her and interfered with her making friends, relating to adults and making informed decisions, which would have impacted her transition to college. With the help of her clinician and using the iPad, Addy created a series of public service videos, on how to meet and greet someone, start a conversation, end a conversation and make a friend. She actually asked to have another girl participate in the video with her, who became her friend as a result. Addy also created a video on how to make wise decisions, gather information, evaluate the pros and cons and then act upon this information. This helped her apply to college, choose a course of study and remain in a class she did not really like. She is now able to function well within the college setting. Addy reflects upon the videos she made to reinforce the skills she has learned, and refers to them on an on-going basis. After all, they were life-changing for this young woman, as none of this would have been possible before the advent of this technology.

Interactive E-Text

As a researcher for the University of Oregon at the Center for Advanced Technology in Education I created an interactive e-text version of a specific science text to help secondary students with learning disabilities better access the information they needed to pass the New York State Regents Exam. Following the principles of Universal Design for Learning, we created context-specific definitions, phrases and the use of the Paraphrasing Strategy from University of Kansas Center for Learning. The results were so positive that students, who were previously failing, were able to understand the text, test for their own meaning, self-pace, learn paraphrasing skills and actually got excited about learning these difficult concepts. At the end of the study, the students asked me to please make all of their textbooks and content areas in this format to help them better learn and be more successful in school. Unfortunately my time with them ended, but they did have the program in this subject on their computers. I only wish I could have stayed and done more with them.

The remarkable examples above further attest to the incredible potential of technology to accommodate the interests and functioning of individuals with developmental disabilities.

In the past, I have worked with computer programming companies to plan computer simulation environments to instruct teachers on how to manage students in classrooms, and I am currently working with clinicians to develop technology tools and clinical approaches to assist children with autism transition into successful adults. When Dr. Nava Silton asked me to write the Foreword, I was excited to read about the latest findings using assistive technology to help individuals with a variety of disabilities. My areas of interest range from language and literacy, transitional skills, social emotional, behavioral, and cognitive issues to music. This edition is of great interest to me and to the people with whom I currently work.

As I read the authors in this volume, I respond to their findings under the following specific topics: language and literacy, communication, social emotional, behavioral and life skills, executive function, language and speech, health challenges, best practices and educational outreach. Several examples under these topics include language and literacy which is addressed in the chapter by Ben-Avie et al. (Chapter 10) examining how to improve students' academic learning by helping students access text. Rodriguez, Strnadova & Cumming (Chapter 2) examine best practices using the Universal Design for Learning principles to help all students with disabilities access the curriculum when using mobile devices.

Van Der Meer (Chapter 1) explores how children with developmental disabilities can learn how to use iPods and iPads in addition to other AAC devices for functional communication, showing positive outcomes. Ancelle (Chapter 12) explores the use of VocalIDTM, Free SpeechTM, and SmartPalateTM, assistive technologies for children with communication disorders. Doneski –Nicol & Bartz (Chapter 4) research early literacy and AAC for children with complex communication needs. Social, emotional, behavioral and life skills are addressed by Gillespie et al. (Chapter 7) in using interactive technology for social-emotional development in children with autism. Mass communication, information dissemination, sensitivity and educational outreach are explored in the chapter by Arucevic (Chapter 15) by looking at the television show and comic book series, REALABILITIES.

Discussions about how to best help children with a variety of disabilities and provide individualized services exist in many different formats over a long period of time. With the fast-paced invention and use of technology and its enhanced applications, keeping up can be a daunting task for even the savviest professional. While I have read many books on the use of assistive technology for children with disabilities, there is a great need for a book like this to inform not just academics, but parents, educators, special educators, therapists and anyone involved in the field of disabilities. These varied chapters highlight the newest, cutting edge technology available in terms that everyone can understand. Silton consolidates these new ideas and interventions into one seminal publication, rather than relying on isolated journals that may be inaccessible to the public to convey this important information. These selected chapters highlight methodologies that are peer reviewed, research-based and are applicable to real life settings. This book also addresses different categories of disabilities in terms of assistive technology, including cognitive, social-emotional and physical disabilities proposing avant-garde, multi-purpose interventions that may be used across populations, and importantly, across platforms.

Various media and emerging technologies including avatars, e-text, video modeling, iPads, iPods and smart technology, communication devices, robots, Telehealth technology and television programming are examined in terms of usefulness and real-world application. These specific interventions are used in a variety of settings: school, home, the clinic- where these individuals can benefit from assistive technology. I also found it extremely useful that the needs of different age groups-early childhood onward through transition to adulthood are included rather than narrowing it to one population.

Dr. Silton and her authors have illustrated very relevant key issues facing individuals, particularly children and youth with disabilities, and the ongoing progressive use of assistive technology. Evaluation of the efficacy of these emerging technologies contributes to the field and informs decisions made by families, practitioners, clinicians and the end-users of these aids and interventions. It is equally important to disseminate information and encourage the acceptance of persons with disabilities, as well. While the conversation continues about the usefulness, appropriateness and purpose of these technologies, this scholarly but eminently readable book illustrates some of the most recent findings and best practices available at this time and advances the field in contemporary assistive technology for individuals with developmental disabilities.

Carol Kahan Kennedy
Fordham University, USA

Carol Kahan Kennedy, *Ph.D., Doctor of Philosophy from New York University, The Steinhardt School of Education Program in Educational Communication and Technology; Specialty in Special Education. She is a professional development coach for Fordham University Graduate School of Education doing staff development in NYC schools. Dr. Kennedy is a published, author, presenter, technology consultant, and a member of the UN NGO Committee for Education. Previously she was Assistant Professor, Director of Educational Technology, Program Director Special Education, LIU Hudson Rockland Graduate Campus. She is the Educational Technology Consultant at Jenny Clarkson/REACH school in Valhalla New York, working with clinicians, faculty and residential staff to integrate technology into the residential and academic life of adolescents with Autism Spectrum Disorder. Dr. Kennedy helps clinicians work with clients to create social story videos as part of clinical practice to improve life skills. She is affiliated with the American Association for the Advancement of Science and the University of Oregon at the Center for Advanced Technology in Education.*

Preface

Background

In a 2012 review of Andrew Solomon's *Far From the Tree*, Emma Brockes noted in The *Guardian*, "The Internet has changed the fortunes of many millennial children who might otherwise have grown up feeling isolated and, along with their parents, [it has] given them communities." Early in 2014 our first volume of well researched studies—*Innovative Technologies to Benefit Children on the Autism Spectrum*—appeared. It described dramatic breakthroughs in assistive technology that promised to radically improve the training, progress and communication of children and adults on the autism spectrum. Various forms of hand-held technology were featured in this previous collection. These devices comprised perhaps the most wonderful invention ever for children on the autism spectrum. Their affordability, portability, ease of use and acceptability in a society saturated with such devices meant that individuals on the spectrum could privately, repeatedly and comfortably practice anything that could be "inputted" to suit their individual needs and their social-emotional and cognitive development.

This present volume, *Recent Advances in Assistive Technology to Support Individuals with Developmental Disabilities*, features numerous authors, who, driven with a passion fired by personal and familial encounters with affected children or by the charisma of mentors in their institutions and fields, are refining their evaluations of previous findings and assessing the true efficacy of apps on iPads and iPods, avatars, gaming, microswitch-based (MSB) programs, music technology, robots, text to speech services, speech therapy devices, tele-rehabilitation, video modeling, virtual reality, and websites.

They insist that we must carefully customize programs and technology to ensure a perfect fit. But there is more. Here we branch out to consider advances in help for developmental disorders of all types: accessing texts, pediatric feeding disorders, help for children who live far from urban, well equipped health centers, how to use music to mitigate the effect of severe developmental disabilities and even comic books and films to convey to young, typical peers, exactly how significant and beneficial some of these assistive devices are for the characters depicted.

Thankfully, the astounding proliferation of technological advances also allows for the fruitful collaboration of the researchers, themselves. They can work in settings thousands of miles from each other and merge or challenge their respective ideas and studies of how the most recent advances in assistive technology can serve individuals with developmental disabilities of very diverse kinds. They have toiled to collaborate on a text that will be useful to parents, physicians, pre- and primary school teachers, special educators, research scientists and technologists, who are working to enhance the impact of assistive technology on the social, cognitive and physical functioning of individuals with developmental disorders.

Chapters

In Chapter 1 (iPods and iPads as AAC Devices for Children with Developmental Disorders),

Larah van der Meer of Victoria University of Wellington, New Zealand, considers the seemingly magical but altogether popular capability of iPods/iPads, loaded with software, that virtually create speech generating devices. She questions whether they are truly as effective as older AAC devices and customizable for each individual application. The children definitely prefer the use of the iPod/iPad technology; if the software and devices are carefully calibrated for their use and if the children are well trained, these devices hold great promise for them.

In Chapter 2 (Implementing iPad and Mobile Technology for Children with Developmental Disabilities: Facilitating Language and Literacy Development), Cathi Draper Rodriguez, Iva Strndova and Terry Cummings join forces to detail ways mobile technology can be harnessed to make school, home and social environments more accessible to students with intellectual disabilities (ID). Underpinning the chapter is the UDL (Universal Design for Learning) which comprises a solid base from which to examine apps that are available, how students can access curriculum using these apps and how teachers can select the best apps for each student. Cathi Draper Rodriguez, based in the United States, researches technologies to teach English to individuals with and without disabilities and offers early intervention to young Latina mothers. Iva Strndova of New South Wales specializes in understanding the life experience of women with intellectual disabilities, and Terry Cummings researches students with emotional and behavioral disorders.

In Chapter 3 (Using iPads and Mobile Technology for Children with Developmental Disabilities: Facilitating Language and Literacy Development), Lisa Proctor and Ye Wang posit that though mobile technology provides ample opportunity for language and literacy development, parents, educators and speech-language pathologists need to be vigilant about their use. Improper use, they caution, could actually serve as an impediment or as a distraction in this population's communication development. Proctor and Wang's chapter focuses on home and school settings, and no wonder. Already in graduate school, Lisa Proctor observed a young girl with a severe communication disorder who was empowered and given a voice through technology. Proctor has continued to work in this area for the last thirty years. Ye Wang's awareness of the struggles of deaf individuals in her family- Chinese deaf individuals- was realized early on. Her parents, both deaf, had different trajectories: her father never attended school, while at age 40 her mother was the first deaf individual to receive a college degree in her hometown. Wang's great passion to study the field of deaf education and Special Education with a special emphasis on technology clearly derives from these salient experiences back home.

In Chapter 4 (Early Literacy and AAC for Learners with Complex Communication Needs), Janis Doneski-Nicol and Jody Marie Bartz offer the most up-to-date information and practical resources for early (pre-school and elementary) students with complex learning needs and assess benefits, challenges and ideas for future research. Janis Doneski-Nicol, a speech-language pathologist and special education teacher has provided Assistive Technology (AT) for over 20 years, and Jody Marie Bartz, who has been in the field of developmental disabilities since her nephews were diagnosed with autism, combine forces to take readers up to the front lines. Bartz's own research includes studying the impact of educational, communal, familial and medical collaboration on outcomes for children with disabilities

In Chapter 5, The Use of Mobile Technologies for Students At-Risk or Identified with Behavioral Disorders within School-Based Contexts, is the particular passion of Frank J. Sansosti and Peña L. Bedesem, both of Kent State University. Fully cognizant of how powerful these devices can be in regulating behavior, stimulating motivation and learning new skills, they worry that educational service providers do not collect enough data to demonstrate their impact on student outcomes. The team checks for technological know-how among school personnel, and the ideal training for educators that would afford the finest outcomes in embracing the latest technologies. As such, this chapter offers recommendations (and the research to support them) for parents teachers and aids in terms of becoming familiar with the generally available technologies for these at-risk students or for those diagnosed with behavioral disorders.

In Chapter 6 (Recent Advances in Augmentative and Alternative Communication: The Advantages and Challenges of Technology Applications for Communicative Purposes), Toby Mehl, a speech-language pathologist from the City University of New York, cautions that despite the benefits of the latest, novel and easily accessible techniques of technology applications for communication, detailed assessments and collaborative evaluations concerning individual needs and abilities have been lacking. She insists that therapists, parents and developers of AAC applications must work together to ensure success and a "good fit" for children who utilize these devices.

In Chapter 7 (Selecting Computer-Mediated Interventions to Support the Social and Emotional Development of Individuals with Autism Spectrum Disorder), a super research troop from the College of Staten Island, City University aims to delve deeply into the importance of developing target skills and matching the individual's needs and interests to the technology available. The reader is invited to sample various experiments using iPad type apps, virtual environments, even robots, and consult websites that offer additional resources. The ultimate goal: to be able to select interventions which are good fits for individuals with ASDs. This impressive research team is led by Kristen Gillespie-Lynch who was originally inspired to work with technology and children with ASDs by reading a dissertation about how computers might be to autism what sign language is for the Deaf; she then designed a survey to assess computer mediated communication for people with ASD. All of the team members, Gillepsie, Brooks, Gaggi, Sturm and Ploog, have interests ranging from the design and development of apps and gaming, social networking for entertainment and educational purposes – to college age kids with autism and the study of abnormal attention patterns.

In Chapter 8 (Avatars, Humanoids, and the Changing Landscape of Assessment and Intervention for Individuals with Disabilities across the Lifespan), Emily Hotez offers parents, professionals and individuals with disabilities a glimpse into the literature about virtual reality and robot-based interventions with children, adolescents and adults. She then delves into directions for future research. Hotez, a student at Hunter College/City University, believes her interest in autism was inspired by her sister, Rachel, whose strengths and challenges have motivated her study of family engagement in interventions. Hotez currently investigates factors that predict the efficacy of parent-mediated interaction for children with ASD and works to improve developmental screening practices in NYC pediatric offices.

In Chapter 9 (Microswitch-Based Programs (MBP) to Promote Communication, Occupation and Leisure Skills for Children with Multiple Disabilities: A Literature Overview), Fabrizio Stasolla and Viviana Perilli offer an overview of microswitch-based (MSB) programs to improve communication, occupation and leisure skills for children with multiple disabilities. They begin with studies published from 2004 -2014; next they consider the strengths and weaknesses of these studies and conclude with a number of issues to be addressed in the future. From Italy we are gifted with the research of Fabrizio Stasolla – whose interest in children with severe to profound developmental disabilities was inspired by Professor Giulio Lancioni's work at the University of Bari. She studies how to provide cognitive/behavior interventional assistive technology for children with multiple disabilities, developmental disabilities, Autism and Rett and Down syndromes. Viviana Perilli is the first researcher to study the cognitive rehabilitation of dementia with a special interest in supporting the residual abilities of individuals with Alzheimer's disease using assistive technology.

In Chapter 10 (Improving Student's Academic Learning by Helping them Access Text), Michael Ben Avie, Regine Randall, Diane Weaver Dunne and Chris Kelly, focus this chapter on CRISKids recordings – text to speech services that can express human emotions. Since children who can read and understand text are more on task and engaged in classroom routines, teachers can spend far less time redirecting them. So everyone wins: students with print disabilities and the rest of the class. CRISKids for Schools is the brainchild of Diane Weaver Dunne whose father unknowingly suffered from dyslexia and dropped out of school at age 14, still unable to read. Now an avid reader at age 70, he discovered that two of his nephews and one great nephew were diagnosed with dyslexia, the disability that he and his own brothers had shared.

In Chapter 11 (Video Modeling for Learners with Developmental Disabilities), Peggy Whitby, Christine Ogilvie and Krista Garland introduce research literature on video modeling and offer practical suggestions on how to implement video modeling with individuals on the spectrum and with other developmental disorders. Already early in her teaching career, Christine Ogilvie found that she could reach more of her students while employing assistive technologies focused both on communication and academics. Once she tried the devices out with children on the spectrum, she found her calling. Peggy Whitby of the University of Arkansas and Krista Vince Garland from Buffalo State University, join her in demonstrating how video modeling can successfully be used by learners with varying developmental disabilities.

In Chapter 12 (Assistive Technologies at the Edge of Language and Speech Science for Children with Communication Disorders: VocalID™, Free Speech™, and SmartPalate ™), Josephine Ancelle of Teacher's College, Columbia University, offers a fascinating glimpse into the development and use of Free Speech™ – an app developed to transform disorganized single concept images into meaningful sentences. Smart Palate™, which makes EPG (Electropalatography – which enables visualization of tongue to palate contact during speech production) more accessible in therapy and at home, and VocalID™ are additional topics that are introduced and expertly evaluated in this chapter.

In Chapter 13 (Telehealth Technology and Pediatric Feeding Disorders), Taylor Luke and Rebecca Ruchlin describe the benefits of utilizing Telehealth Technology for Pediatric Feeding Disorders. Telehealth Technology is alive and well in a large variety of health services throughout the country. It utilizes video conferencing technology to deliver various health therapy services, offering face-to-face interactions among specialists, parents and children. For some time, teletherapy has offered help for speech-language intervention and social behavior management. Luke, whose passion to find solutions is driven by the overwhelming number of children who need services but cannot, for reasons of geographic, language, and socioeconomic barriers, access adequate care, looks to technology for powerful answers. Ruchlin, who has witnessed therapists work tirelessly with Matthew, her brother with autism, wants very much to help, especially in the area of feeding and swallowing disorders. With the authors' special interest in the pediatric population and familial sources of inspiration, Luke and Ruchlin combine talents and the notion of teletherapy to remedy feeding disorders in infants, toddlers and children with developmental disorders world-wide.

In Chapter 14 (Music and Developmental Disorders), Michelle Blumstein, who has loved music from a very early age, presents a survey of research about the types of technology that music therapists use to aid children with developmental delays. Music is a powerful motivator, since it provides an enjoyable experience and allows children to feel a sense of control that too often eludes them.

In Chapter 15 (Dissemination of Assistive Technology Devices for Children with Disabilities through *Realabilities)*, Senada Arucevic, of Long Island University in Brooklyn, NY creatively contextualizes her discussion of various forms of assistive technology on the characters with disabilities who are portrayed in the TV Show and Comic Book Series, *Realabilities.*

Realabilties, a series of animated episodes and comic books created and tested by Silton, Arucevic, Ruchlin and Norkus, found that typical children who watched and read about these spirited and capable children with disabilities, demonstrated enhanced cognitive attitudes and behavioral intentions towards individuals with disabilities. After all, these exciting episodes feature young people with disabilities who utilize assistive devices in clever ways, reducing the stigma that wheelchairs, hearing aids, etc. often elicit. In this way, the team is working from the outside in: the robust world can learn and appreciate a thing or two about the benefits and significance of the devices and much more about the stuff these heroes with differences are made of. Read this chapter and cheer. Then go out and find the comic books!

In Chapter 16 (Using Technology to Support Social Competence), our collection closes with a wonderful team composed of researchers, occupational therapists and special educators who deal directly with how to impart social competence which comprises a complex set of skills that affects quality of life across all environments: home, school, employment and the community. Theory of Mind, relationship building and self-regulation must be learned by individuals with ASD and all kinds of disabilities. The team, led by Brenda Myles, who has been acknowledged by the University of Texas as the second most productive researcher of ASD in the world, and Jan Rogers, Director of The Ohio Center for Autism and Low Incidence Assistive Technology, Amy Bixler Coffin, a special educator for 24 years, Wendy Szakacs and Theresa Vollrath, review this area of study and suggest a variety of practices to support its development.

Adaptive and Assistive devices have existed from time immemorial. Canes and crutches, for example, are used as often today as they ever were for basic mobility, but they don't go so far as to bolster self-esteem, self-actualization and social acceptability. All the studies we've included, indeed all work with developing ever more refined models of technological modalities to empower and socialize individuals with disabilities. These chapters largely focus on inclusion or, at least, a path to social inclusion, away from the margins of society from which so many individuals with disabilities watch the robust world go by. The stunning gains achieved with the devices described in the following pages are breathtaking and humbling. May the work of these authors be blessed and then undertaken by many of you who can see the critical need and new opportunities all around.

Nava R. Silton
Marymount Manhattan College, USA

Acknowledgment

This text would not have been possible without a brilliant meeting of gifted minds. First and foremost, I want to thank all of the talented and esteemed authors who shared their latest engrossing findings in the area of assistive technologies to support individuals with a variety of developmental disabilities. I look forward to our future correspondence and collaboration. Secondly, I'd like to graciously thank the peer reviewers who meticulously evaluated the relevance of content, syntax and empirical rigor of each chapter. Thank you Dr. Michael Ben-Avie (Yale University), Tamara Balaban, MSOTR/L (Support by Design), Dr. Jody Marie Bartz (Northern Arizona University), Dr. Ariel Brandwein (Long Island Jewish Medical Center), Dr. Cathi Draper Rodriguez (California State University), Dr. Kristen Gillepsie (CUNY Graduate Center, College of Staten Island), Emily Hotez, M.A. (CUNY Graduate Center, Hunter College), Toby Mehl, M.S., CCC-SLP (CUNY Graduate Center, Brooklyn College), Dr. Brenda Myles (Ohio Center for Autism and Low Incidence), Christina Shane-Simpson (CUNY Graduate Center, College of Staten Island), Shira Silton, LMSW (Montefiore Medical Center), Dr. Linda Solomon (Marymount Manhattan College), and Dr. Peggy Whitby (University of Arkansas).

Marymount Manhattan College (MMC) students Senada Arucevic '14, Alicia Ferris '16, Jaromir Myszczynski '14, Rebecca Ruchlin '14, and Yolianda Zackschewski '15 graciously offered their assistance in the early stages of this project. It did not take long before they were genuinely moved and inspired by the innovative research in this area. I thank Dr. Benedetta Sampoli Benitez, a wonderful Divisional Chair at MMC, for her constant guidance and encouragement and the administration, psychology faculty and general faculty at Marymount Manhattan College for their continuous support and appreciation for this important field.

Additionally, I am grateful to Allyson Gard, Rachel Ginder, Caitlyn Martin, Jan Travers, and Kayla Wolfe for their invaluable guidance during the editing process. They were always prompt, comprehensive, patient and gracious in their responses.

Moreover, I would like to thank my dedicated husband, Ariel Brandwein and my charming little men, Judah Lior and Jonah Gabriel Brandwein, for their good nature, humor, inspiration and patience throughout this endeavor. I want to acknowledge my father, Rabbi Paul Silton and my wonderful siblings, Elana, Michal, Akiva, Tamar, Aviva, and my twin sister Shira for their constant encouragement and support. Finally, I owe a huge debt of gratitude to a consummate renaissance woman and to one of my greatest heroines, my mother, Faye Silton. Her creativity, eloquence, wisdom, patience and love know no bounds. I will cherish this text all the more since her brilliant mind and loving hands painstakingly reviewed its contents.

Acknowledgment

I want to extend a final note of gratitude to all of the incredible parents, teachers, special educators, technology specialists, researchers, siblings, family members and peers of children with developmental disabilities. Each of you works tirelessly to creatively endow your loved ones and students with the very best technologies, tools and instruction to best support and enhance their development and potential. I hope that this text will further broaden their opportunities and enhance their level of comfort in accessing technologies that are best suited for them. Finally, I would like to thank our exceptional children with differences, who have inspired the advancement of these technologies and continue to challenge our traditional approaches in favor of divergent thinking and creative problem-solving. It is these glorious minds who will inspire a true "community," which is sensitive to diverse needs, learning styles and capabilities and will pioneer these new, cutting edge technologies.

Chapter 1
iPods and iPads as AAC Devices for Children with Developmental Disorders

Larah van der Meer
Victoria University of Wellington, New Zealand

ABSTRACT

The Apple iPod Touch™ and iPad™ are increasingly used as augmentative and alternative communication (AAC) devices. This chapter discusses the use of iPods™/iPads™ loaded with software applications that enable speech output and thereby transform them into speech-generating devices (SGD). While a popular mode of communication for children with developmental disorders (DD) who have little or no spoken language, assessment of the effectiveness of such new technology to enhance communicative functioning is necessary. Research on the use of iPods™/iPads™ was evaluated to assess whether they are (a) effective as AAC devices, (b) at least as effective as other AAC interventions, and (c) effective at the individual level of implementation. Findings suggested that the use of iPods™/iPads™ as AAC devices is promising, also in comparison to other AAC systems. Children typically preferred using iPods™/iPads™. Selection of an AAC system based on the child's preference coupled with appropriate instructional strategies may lead to the enhancement of communicative functioning for children with DD.

INTRODUCTION

A defining feature of developmental disorders (DD) is a delay and/or impairment in the development of speech, language, and communication skills (Centers for Disease Control and Prevention, 2011; Odom, Horner, Snell, & Blacher, 2007). Since communication can involve both speech and language, as well as other components, this broader term will be used to describe speech, language, and communication impairments. Such communication impairments are heterogeneous across children with different DD. For example, at least 25% of individuals with autism spectrum disorder (ASD) do not develop any spoken language (Osterling, Dawson, & McPartland, 2001), while others exhibit only subtle difficulties in the use of spoken language. For children who do not develop speech or have failed to develop sufficient

DOI: 10.4018/978-1-4666-8395-2.ch001

speech to meet their everyday communication needs, non-oral communication systems (e.g., picture boards and manual signs) might be utilized. These modes of communication are often referred to as types of augmentative and alternative communication (AAC; Beukelman & Mirenda, 2013).

This chapter will provide a brief overview of AAC, narrowing to the use of speech-generating devices (SGD). The chapter will then discuss the introduction of general purpose hardware, such as the iPod Touch™ and iPad™ produced by Apple Corporation (http://www.apple.com/ipod/; http://www.apple.com/ipad/) loaded with software applications, such as Proloquo2Go™ produced by Assistiveware (http://www.assistiveware.com/product/Proloquo2Go/) to serve as SGD. The use of iPods™/iPads™ as SGD is seemingly leading to a paradigm shift in AAC interventions towards the use of low cost, easy to obtain and transport, readily available, and socially acceptable devices (Shane et al., 2012).

Despite these potential benefits of general purpose hardware devices, there remain a number of significant challenges in the adoption of these new technologies (McNaughton & Light, 2013). The mere provision of the new technology is not enough to enhance the communication skills of children with DD. The focus must remain on appropriate assessment and intervention to support a wide variety of communicative functions. Since there is a risk of adopting new technologies without evaluating the evidence of their effectiveness, three criteria of evidence (Detrich, 2013) will be used to assess the research base on implementing iPods™/iPads™ as AAC devices for children with DD. These criteria include evaluating whether the new technologies (iPods™/iPads™) are (a) effective as AAC devices, (b) at least as effective when compared to other AAC interventions (e.g., picture exchange systems), and (c) effective at the individual level of implementation.

BACKGROUND

Augmentative and Alternative Communication

AAC is an area of research and clinical practice that focuses on supplementing (augmentative) or replacing (alternative) natural speech and/or handwriting. It is typically considered for individuals who have failed to acquire, or who have temporarily impaired speech or handwriting such that their everyday communication needs are not met (Beukelman & Mirenda, 2013). AAC systems have been classified as either unaided or aided. Unaided AAC does not rely on external equipment, instead utilizing the individual's own body as the mode of communication. It generally comprises the use of body movements or sequences of coordinated body movements to represent an object, idea, action, or relationship. Examples include eye gaze, pointing, physically leading a communication partner's hand to an object, conventional body language (e.g., head nodding), gestures, finger spelling, and manual signing (MS). MS comprises the use of natural sign language (e.g., American Sign Language) to the production of manual signs as a code for a spoken language (Blischak, Lloyd, & Fuller, 1997).

Aided AAC involves the use of external equipment to communicate messages. This includes the use of graphics (traditional orthography/printed words, photographs, line drawings, or other pictographic symbols) ranging from low-tech nonelectronic picture communication boards and picture exchange (PE) systems to high-tech portable electronic devices with speech output. The use of portable electronic SGD, otherwise referred to as voice-output communication aids (VOCA; Schlosser, 2003a; Schlosser & Blischak, 2001), are becoming increasingly widespread. The screen of the device is displayed with graphic symbols that represent a word or phrase. Touching or pressing the symbols activates the word or phrase, which results in speech output.

Speech-Generating Devices

A defining feature of SGD is the speech output, and consideration of the type of speech used (digitized versus synthesized) is a potentially important variable to consider when designing interventions (Schlosser, 2003a; Schlosser & Blischak, 2001). Prerecorded digitized speech is typically used in less complex AAC devices for beginning communicators and is presumed to be close to, or as intelligible as, natural (nonrecorded) speech. Complex, high-tech AAC devices utilize synthetic speech, which allow for a text-to-speech conversion, or the conversion of selected input to auditory output. A variety of SGD can be selected and customized for intervention. SGD can vary in design including graphic symbols used, permanence of the display (static or dynamic), number and size of graphic symbols on the display, shape, and size of the device (Drager et al., 2004; Drager, Light, & Finke, 2009).

SGD can be described as either dedicated or nondedicated (Johnston & Feeley, 2012). Dedicated SGD are developed and used solely for communication purposes (e.g., DynaVox Maestro [http://www.dynavoxtech.com/products/maestro/interaact/] and GoTalk 32+ produced by Mayer-Johnson [http://www.mayer-johnson.com/gotalk-32/]). Nondedicated SGD include laptop/desktop computers, tablet computers, personal digital assistants, and cell phones. Special-purpose software can be downloaded onto these nondedicated devices for use as AAC systems. Dedicated AAC devices have, in the past, been viewed as expensive, cumbersome, time consuming to program and personalise, and often stigmatising to the user. As a result, developments in mobile technology, and particularly the introduction of the iPod™/iPad™, have provided important new tools for communication. An increased interest in the use of nondedicated, general-purpose hardware (e.g., iPods™/iPads™) is seemingly leading to a paradigm shift in AAC intervention (Shane et al., 2012). This shift is toward devices that are commercially available and therefore easier to obtain. They are low cost, smaller, and transportable. This "mobile technology revolution" (McNaughton & Light, 2013, p.107) has also improved social awareness and acceptance of AAC and attitudinal barriers to the use of AAC have decreased. Since these devices are "cool", individuals requiring AAC are also more likely to use them to enhance communicative competence (Light & McNaughton, 2014).

iPods™ and iPads™ as AAC Devices

Since the inception of iPods™/iPads™ as communication tools, the development of software applications ("apps") to serve as full AAC systems has been rapid with literally hundreds of apps available, many of which are free (Bradshaw, 2013). An example of an app that has maintained popularity since it was developed in 2008 is Proloquo2Go™ (Sennott & Bowker, 2009). It runs on iPods™/iPads™ and can be programmed to serve as an AAC system. Several potential advantages of this system include (a) the large set (14,000) of colour graphic symbols, (b) the high quality of synthesized speech output, (c) the relatively low cost, and (d) the small size and light weight (Mirenda, 2009). It can be programmed to meet each child's needs and abilities (see Figures 1 and 2). Other apps (e.g., First/Then, MyChoiceBoard available from https://www.apple.com/itunes/) allow iPods™/iPads™ to serve a range of functions such as organisation and choice making. In addition to their low cost, apps are typically customizable and user-friendly (Shane et al., 2012). These advantages, paired with the idea that many children with DD appear to have an interest in technology and find computer activities to be reinforcing (Stromer, Kimball, Kinney, & Taylor, 2006), make the use of iPods™/iPads™ well suited to children with DD who require alternative forms of communication.

Figure 1. Photograph of an iPod Touch™ produced by Apple Corporation (http://www.apple.com/ipod/) configured with the Proloquo2Go™ software application produced by Assistiveware (http://www.assistiveware.com/product/Proloquo2Go/) to serve as an SGD. The visual display contains graphic symbols for snacks, toys, and social interaction taken from the existing Proloquo2Go™ symbol set. Touching a symbol produces corresponding speech output (e.g., I want a snack please). The iPod is placed inside an iMainGo2™ speaker case produced by Portable Sound Laboratories (http://www.portablesoundlabs.com) to improve sound amplification.

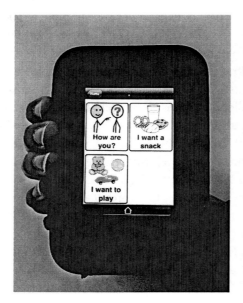

EVALUATION OF IPODS™ AND IPADS™ AS AAC DEVICES

Issues, Controversies, Problems

There are also a number of significant challenges in the adoption of high-technology AAC devices. The mere use of technology is not enough to bring about change in communicative competence for children with DD (Passerino & Santarosa, 2008). The strategies for teaching children to use the device are equally, if not more, important than the device itself. It is well documented in the AAC field that individuals require concerted intervention to learn to use alternative communication systems for a range of communicative functions (Beukelman & Mirenda, 2013). Because iPods™/iPads™ and other high-tech AAC devices are readily available to the consumer, there is a risk that devices will be purchased for children without a clear idea of how the technology will be used to support communication development. Appropriate assessment and intervention based on individual skills and needs is required to support a wide variety of communicative functions (McNaughton & Light, 2013).

Several other factors have been identified as influencing implementation of high technology AAC. These include ease of use of the device, reliability, and availability of technical support (Baxter, Enderby, Evans, & Judge, 2012a). It has been suggested that some of these issues may be addressed by the introduction of the iPod™/iPad™ (Bradshaw, 2013). For example, the technology is known to be intuitive and reliable. However, they are prone to being dropped and to water damage, which can lead to extended

Figure 2. Photograph of an iPad™ produced by Apple Corporation (http://www.apple.com/ipad/) config-ured with the Proloquo2Go™ software application produced by Assistiveware (http://www.assistiveware. com/product/Proloquo2Go/) to serve as an SGD. The visual display contains imported photographs for snacks. Touching a photograph produces corresponding speech output (e.g., I want a pretzel please).

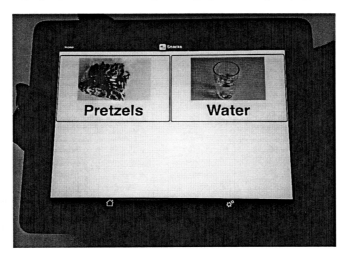

lengths of time without the device while it is being repaired or replaced. Similarly, in the past, dedicated AAC technology manufacturers provided technical support in the cost of the device, including repair services, equipment demonstrations, set-up, and training. Such support is not provided upon purchase of nondedicated hardware (iPods™/iPads™) and AAC apps (McNaughton & Light, 2013). This might explain the difference in cost between dedicated and nondedicated SGD. It is therefore imperative for parents, teachers, and practitioners to gain confidence in programming and maintaining the hardware and software to meet each individual's communication needs. This remains a challenge for intervention planning, with limited practitioner expertise in SGD practice (Anderson, Balandin, & Stancliffe, 2014). The remainder of the chapter will use the three evaluation criteria (Detrich, 2013) to assess whether iPods™/iPads™ can effectively be used as AAC devices for children with DD. Findings will be used to support intervention planning.

Is The New Technology Effective?

Regardless of any such advantages and disadvantages, there is no doubt that iPods™/iPads™ are increasingly being used as AAC devices for children with DD. As a result, there have been calls for empirical research to evaluate the impact of iPods™/iPads™ as SGD on the communication develop-ment of individuals requiring AAC. An increasing number of recent studies have been identified as using single-case experimental designs (Kennedy, 2005) to demonstrate whether or not the interven-tion procedures (i.e., independent variable) were responsible for increased correct use of the iPod™/iPad™ SGD (i.e., dependent variable; Sigafoos, O'Reilly, Lancioni, & Sutherland, 2014). Table 1 provides an overview of 12 such studies that investigated the effectiveness of using iPod™/iPad™ SGD for children with DD.

Table 1. The Use of iPods™ and iPads™ as SGD in Communication Interventions for Children with DD.

Study	Participants	Device and Application	Target Skills	Research Design	Intervention Procedures	Results
(Achmadi et al., 2012)	2 (13 & 17; ASD, ID, OCD, ADHD)	iPod Touch™, Proloquo2Go™	Request; turn on device, unlock screen, navigate to application	Multiple-probe across participants	Cue, 10 s time delay, least-most prompting, differential reinforcement, backward chaining	Acquisition of behavioral chain and request for each participant
(Dundon, McLaughlin, Neyman, & Clark, 2013)	1 (5; DD, ASD)	iPad™, My Choice Board, Go Talk Now Free	Request	Multiple-baseline across applications	Model, lead, test prompting procedure	Acquisition of request for each application
(Ganz, Hong, Goodwyn, Kite, & Gilliland, 2013)	1 (4; ASD)	iPad™, PECS Phase III™	Receptive identification of photos of objects	Multiple-baseline across vocabulary words	Four-step error correction (modified PECS protocol; Frost & Bondy, 2002)	Mild improvement for two of three vocabulary words
(Kagohara et al., 2012)	2 (13 & 17; ASD, ID, OCD, ADHD)	iPod Touch™, Proloquo2Go™	Label (picture naming)	Multiple-probe across participants	Cue, 10 s time delay, least-most prompting, differential reinforcement	Acquisition of labels in response to open- and closed-ended questions for each participant
(Kagohara et al., 2010)	1 (17, ASD, OCD, ADHD)	iPod Touch™, Proloquo2Go™	Request	Reversal (ABAB)	Delayed prompting (0 s, 5 s, 10 s), differential reinforcement	Acquisition of request
(King et al., 2014)	3 (3-5; ASD)	iPad™, Proloquo2Go™	Request	Multiple-probe across participants	Most-least prompting within modified PECS protocol (Frost & Bondy, 2002)	Acquisition of Phases 1-3a for each participant; acquisition of Phase 3b for two participants. Increase in vocal requests for each participant
(Lorah, Crouser, Gilroy, Tincani, & Hantula, 2014)	4 (4-6; ASD)	iPad™, Proloquo2Go™	Request (discriminating between picture symbols)	Multiple-probe across participants changing criterion	Within stimulus prompting and stimulus fading, differential reinforcement	Acquisition of request, while discriminating between increasing picture-symbols for each participant
(Sigafoos et al., 2013)	2 (4 & 5; ASD)	iPad™, Proloquo2Go™	Request continuation of play	Multiple-baseline across participants	Cue, 10 s delay, graduated guidance, differential reinforcement	Acquisition of request for each participant; maintenance and generalization

continued on following page

This research has assessed the use of iPod™/iPad™ SGD in a relatively small sample of children (aged three to 23 years) with a range of DD, but most commonly ASD. Only one of the 21 participants did not acquire use of the iPod™/iPad™ SGD for the targeted communication skills. All 12 studies reviewed focused on teaching initial requesting functions (e.g., requesting preferred toys and snacks) and five of those also targeted teaching a considerable range of communicative functions. These included answering questions, labeling items, receptive understanding of vocabulary, greetings, and etiquette as

Table 1. Continued

Study	Participants	Device and Application	Target Skills	Research Design	Intervention Procedures	Results
(Strasberger & Ferreri, 2013)	4 (5-2; ASD)	iPod Touch™, Proloquo2Go™	Request, answer questions	Multiple-baseline across participants	Cue/question, 2-5 s time delay, graduated guidance, differential reinforcement, peer assisted communication training (PACA); modified PECS protocol (Frost & Bondy, 2002)	Acquisition of request for each participant; answering: *What do you want?* for three; answering: *What is your name?* for two
(van der Meer, Kagohara, et al., 2011)	3 (13-23; ASD, ID, Klinefelter syndrome, seizure disorder)	iPod Touch™, Proloquo2Go™	Request	Delayed multiple-probe across participants	Cue, 0 s (for the first three discrete trials) and 10 s time delay, physical prompting, differential reinforcement	Acquisition of request for two participants. One participant did not learn after 40 training trials
(van der Meer, Sigafoos, et al., 2013)	1 (10; ASD, ID, developmental coordination disorder, epilepsy). Previously participated in van der Meer, Sutherland et al. (2012) and van der Meer, Kagohara et al. (2013)	iPad™, Proloquo2Go™	Request, label (people, actions, emotions), answer questions, greetings, etiquette	ABC single-case	10 s time delay before verbal cue then 10 s time delay before least-most prompting, differential reinforcement	Acquisition of communicative interactions across categories after verbal cue in intervention. Independent/spontaneous communication by long-term follow-up
(Ward, McLaughlin, & Neyman, 2013)	1 (5; ASD)	iPad™, Go Talk Now Free	Request	ABC single-case	Model, lead, test prompting procedure	Acquisition of request

well as turning on and navigating the iPad™. This is in line with previous research assessing the use of dedicated SGD, where the majority of studies targeted requesting functions only (Rispoli, Franco, van der Meer, Lang, & Carmargo, 2010). Overall results of the 12 studies suggest that the use of well-established instructional strategies, including one-on-one instruction, time delay, response prompting, and differential reinforcement (Duker, Didden, & Sigafoos, 2004) were effective in teaching children to use these devices for basic communication.

It has been suggested that such structured, trial-based training may be more practical and appropriate when teaching early communication skills (requesting), while a naturalistic approach might be appropriate when targeting more complex communication that is social in nature (Drager et al., 2009). However, little research to date has evaluated naturalistic approaches to promote social interactions for children with DD who use AAC. Indeed a recent review of published interventions using high-technology AAC devices found that although improvements in communicative ability were indicated, there was considerable variation in the outcomes of published research and a lack of high-quality research designs to evaluate the utility of the intervention procedures and AAC technology (Baxter, Enderby, Evans, & Judge, 2012b). In response to such promising, but limited data on the effectiveness of high technology SGD for children with DD, Kasari and colleagues (2014) utilized a randomized control-trial design to compare two naturalistic developmental behaviorally based interventions that focused on communication development – JASPER (joint attention symbolic play engagement and regulation) and EMT (enhanced milieu teaching) with and without the use of SGD. Results for 61 minimally verbal children (aged five to eight years) with ASD indicated that the interventions paired with the use of the SGD were more effective in supporting the development of spontaneous communicative utterances than without the SGD or with delayed introduction of the SGD. The study utilized DynaVox Maestro and iPad™ SGD, but did not provide any further information about the devices (e.g., type of app used on the iPad™). Full evaluation of the effectiveness of the iPad™ as an SGD in this study is therefore not possible. However, the study is one of the first to demonstrate increases in minimally verbal children's spontaneous communication beyond requesting, including different types of words and functions.

Is The New Technology at Least as Effective when Compared to Other Interventions?

The aforementioned research provides initial evidence of the potential positive impact of iPods™/iPads™ to serve as communication systems. Similarly, widespread research and reviews synthesizing findings from the existing body of literature suggest dedicated SGD (e.g., Rispoli et al., 2010), PE, and MS (e.g., Schlosser & Wendt, 2008a; Wendt, 2009) are all viable AAC options for children with DD. With evidence to support the use of each of these three common AAC systems there has been a long-standing debate regarding which option is best suited to meet the communication needs of individuals with DD (Mirenda, 2003; Schlosser & Sigafoos, 2006).

Schlosser (2003b) indicated that once an individual intervention approach has been demonstrated to be efficacious, it is important to know whether another approach might be more efficacious. Efficacy studies have used controlled experimental research methods to compare acquisition of dedicated SGD to PE or MS (e.g., Bock, Stoner, Beck, Hanley, & Prochnow, 2005; Boesch, Wendt, Subramanian, & Hsu, 2013; Iacono & Duncum, 1995; Tincani, 2004) for early functional communication skills (e.g., requesting preferred items). However, with a lack of any major difference in acquisition rates between these AAC systems, it has been suggested that there does not seem to be one option that is appropriate for all beginning communicators (Sigafoos & Drasgow, 2001). Furthermore these studies did not compare the acquisition of all three AAC systems (SGD, PE, and MS) or compare the use of nondedicated SGD (e.g., iPods™/iPads™) to other AAC systems. In order to further evaluate the effectiveness of iPods™/iPads™ as AAC devices, a direct comparison between the new technology (iPods™/iPads™) and alternative AAC interventions is needed, where the iPod™/iPad™ SGD need to be at least as effective as PE and MS AAC systems.

Table 2 provides an overview of ten studies that assessed the comparative efficacy of the three commonly used AAC systems for children with DD. Specifically each study evaluated iPod™/iPad™ SGD in comparison with a low technology PE system and/or MS. Again, all studies utilized a single-case experimental design; typically an alternating treatments design to compare how efficiently and effectively participants learned the targeted communication skills across each AAC system. These studies represent a larger sample size with 40 participants (aged three to 13 years) also most commonly diagnosed with ASD. Eleven of the studies targeted requesting communicative skills only, while one also involved intervention to teach question answering and etiquette (e.g., please and thank you). Twenty-five participants reached acquisition criterion with each AAC system (iPod™/iPad™ SGD, PE, and/or MS) for the targeted communication skills. While the remaining participants learned to use the SGD and PE to varying levels of proficiency, eight participants did not demonstrate any, or only little, learning of MS ($\leq 20\%$ accuracy).

Through analysis of these findings it has been hypothesized that difficulty in learning to use MS might be related to (a) increased demands on working memory compared to SGD and PE (selecting graphic symbols for SGD and PE involves recognition memory, while producing correct signs for MS requires recall memory), (b) MS requires more complex motor skills, (c) children may prefer and enjoy using other communication systems, and (d) MS might be more difficult for instructors to teach (van der Meer, Sutherland, O'Reilly, Lancioni, & Sigafoos, 2012). Overall though, results of these comparative studies suggest that while some participants learned to use one AAC system more quickly or easily than others, the extent of difference in performance between systems was not large, and most children learned to use each system within comparable time periods.

Is the New Technology Effective at the Individual Level of Implementation?

The lack of any major differences in the comparison studies suggests that how quickly an individual acquires the use of an AAC option may not be the most critical variable to consider when selecting an AAC option for any given child. Each of the aforementioned ten studies also assessed participants' preference for using one AAC system over the others. With the exception of Flores et al. (2012), participants were given structured, choice-making opportunities across various stages of the study to assess which AAC system was preferred. When participants consistently selected one AAC system above the others, it was considered preferred. Flores et al. (2012), on the other hand, always had each system available to the participant and preference was assessed by the frequency with which participants used the AAC systems as well as anecdotal information from observation of behaviors. The idea of assessing the child's preference for using one AAC system over another allows for evaluation of evidence for effectiveness of the new technology (iPod™/iPad™) at the individual level of implementation. Results indicate that the majority of participants in the research to date have exhibited a preference for using the iPod™/iPad™ SGD. Indeed, 68% (27/40) of participants indicated a preference for using the iPod™/iPad™ SGD. Participants were also often better able to use their preferred communication system. This suggests that the child's preference for using one AAC system over another is an important variable to consider when selecting an AAC system. However, Sigafoos and colleagues (2014) stress that there is not yet enough data to make the claim that using a preferred AAC system improves outcomes for AAC interventions.

SOLUTIONS AND RECOMMENDATIONS

Preference-Enhanced Communication Intervention

Findings from the comparison studies (Table 2) provide a potential new approach to selecting suitable AAC options for children with DD (Sigafoos, et al., 2014). The approach involves a three-stage process: (a) teaching the child to use various AAC systems, (b) providing choice-making opportunities to assess

Table 2. Comparison of iPods™ and iPads™ as SGD to other AAC Systems in Communication Interventions for Children with DD.

Study	Participants	AAC Systems	Target Skills	Research Design	Intervention Procedures	Results
(Achmadi et al., 2014)	4 (4-5; DD, ASD)	SGD (iPod Touch™, Proloquo2Go™), PE, MS	Request	Alternating treatment with initial baseline and long-term follow-up	Cue, 0, 3, 5, 10 s time delay schedule, graduated guidance, differential reinforcement	Acquisition to criterion with each AAC system for three participants; acquisition to criterion with PE only for one. Three participants preferred SGD (during follow-up); one preferred PE
(Couper et al., 2014)	9 (4-8; ASD)	SGD (iPod Touch™, iPad™, Proloquo2Go™), PE, MS	Request	Alternating treatments, nonconcurrent multiple-baseline across participants	Cue, 10 s delay, graduated guidance, differential reinforcement	Acquisition to criterion with each AAC system for five participants; one learned each system to varying levels; two acquired PE and SGD only; one did not acquire any AAC system. Eight participants preferred SGD; one didn't demonstrate a preference
(Flores et al., 2012)	5 (8-11; ASD, multiple disabilities, ID)	SGD (iPad™, Pick a Word), PE	Request	Reversal (ABABA)	SGD training: Cue, 5 s time delay, verbal prompt, 5 s time delay, physical prompt. Intervention: differential reinforcement	Three participants demonstrated higher frequency of communication with the SGD; mixed results for two. Two participants appeared to prefer the SGD
(Ganz, Hong, & Goodwyn, 2013)	3 (3-4; ASD, PDD-NOS)	SGD (iPad™, PECS Phase III™), PE	Request	Multiple-baseline across participants with concurrent baseline	Four-step error correction (modified PECS protocol; Frost & Bondy, 2002)	PE mastered prior to study; acquisition of SGD for each participant. Two participants preferred SGD; one preferred PE
(Lorah et al., 2013)	5 (3-5; ASD)	SGD (iPad™, Proloquo2Go™), PE	Request	Alternating treatment with initial baseline	Cue, 5 s time delay, physical prompt, differential reinforcement	Acquisition to criterion with SGD and PE for each participant. Four participants preferred SGD; one preferred PE
(Roche et al., 2014)	2 (9 & 11; ASD)	Direct select (iPad™, six cartoon videos), tangible system, PE	Request	Alternating treatments, multiple-baseline across participants	Cue, 10 s time delay, least-most prompting, differential reinforcement	Acquisition to criterion with each AAC system for both participants. Both preferred tangible symbols
(van der Meer, Didden, et al., 2012)	4 (6-13; ASD, childhood disintegrative disorder, ID, Angelman syndrome, DD)	SGD (iPod Touch™, Proloquo2Go™), PE, MS	Request	Alternating treatments, multiple-probe across participants	Cue, 10 s time delay, graduated guidance, differential reinforcement	Acquisition to criterion with each AAC system for two participants; acquisition with SGD and PE only for two. Three participants preferred SGD; one preferred PE

continued on following page

Table 2. Continued

Study	Participants	AAC Systems	Target Skills	Research Design	Intervention Procedures	Results
(van der Meer, Kagohara, et al., 2012)	4 (5-10; ASD, multi-system developmental disorder, Down syndrome, congenital myotonic dystrophy)	SGD (iPod Touch™, Proloquo2Go™), MS	Request	Alternating treatments, multiple-probe across participants	Cue, 10 s time delay, graduated guidance, differential reinforcement	Acquisition to criterion with both AAC systems for three participants; acquisition to criterion with SGD only for one. Three participants preferred SGD; one preferred MS
(van der Meer, Kagohara, et al., 2013)	2 (10 & 11; ASD). Previously participated in van der Meer, Sutherland et al. (2012)	SGD (iPod Touch™, iPad™, Proloquo2Go™), PE, MS	Request, answer questions, etiquette	Alternating treatments with initial baseline	Cue, 10 s time delay, correspondence training, least-most prompting, differential reinforcement	Acquisition of communication interaction across categories with each AAC system for one participant; continued preference for SGD. Moderate proficiency for two-step request only with each AAC system for one participant; continued preference for PE
(van der Meer, Sutherland, et al., 2012)	4 (4-11; ASD)	SGD (iPod Touch™, iPad™, Proloquo2Go™), PE, MS	Request	Alternating treatments, non-concurrent multiple-baseline across participants	Cue, 10 s delay, graduated guidance, differential reinforcement	Acquisition to criterion with each AAC system for two participants; moderate proficiency with each AAC system for one; acquisition for SGD and PE only with one. Two participants preferred SGD, two preferred PE

which option the child prefers to use, and (c) continuing intervention with the most preferred option. For example Ian, a 10-year-old boy diagnosed with various developmental disabilities, participated in three studies by van der Meer and colleagues (van der Meer, Kagohara, et al., 2013; van der Meer, Sigafoos, et al., 2013; van der Meer, Sutherland, et al., 2012). He learned to use an iPod™ and iPad™ SGD, PE, and MS for basic communicative functions, such as requesting preferred games as well as some more social communicative functions, such as greetings. During this initial intervention with each AAC system a structured choice-making protocol (Sigafoos, 1998) was implemented to assess preference for using one AAC system over another (Table 3). Ian consistently chose and was better able to use the iPad™ SGD. Subsequently, further intervention was implemented with his preferred AAC system only (the iPad™). Results suggested that the approach facilitated the development of spontaneous and socially oriented communication (van der Meer, Sigafoos, et al., 2013).

Table 3. Structured choice-making protocol

1. **Offer:** Offer the child two or more items spaced some distance apart
2. **Ask:** While making an offer, ask the child which item he/she wants to use
3. **Wait:** Wait a reasonable amount of time (e.g., 10 s) for the child to make a choice
4. **Response:** A choice occurs when the child makes any voluntary motion toward one of the items (e.g., points, reaches), maintains physical contact, or looks at one item for at least three seconds
5. **Reinforce:** When a choice occurs, give the child the selected item

This "preference-enhanced communication intervention" (van der Meer, Sigafoos, et al., 2013; p.282) shows promise to improve communicative outcomes for children with DD. It can be seen as one way of incorporating aspects of self-determination into AAC interventions (Wehmeyer, Palmer, Agran, Mithaug, & Martin, 2000; Wehmeyer, Sands, Doll, & Palmer, 1997). While self-determination can be viewed as important in its own right, providing children with opportunities for choice and control in the interventions they receive may be one way to enhance the success of the intervention (van der Meer, Sigafoos, O'Reilly, & Lancioni, 2011). This reinforces the notion that the child's preference for using a particular AAC system should be considered. For the majority of children it appears this might involve the use of iPods™/iPads™ as AAC devices. In order to implement a preference-enhanced communication intervention there are several components that might be considered. This includes decisions with regards to (a) selecting appropriate AAC systems, (b) using effective instructional strategies to teach the child to use the AAC systems, and (c) identifying a range of communicative functions in order to facilitate communicative competence and long-term use of AAC.

Selecting AAC systems

The initial stage of the preference-enhanced communication intervention involves teaching the use of a range of AAC systems. While considerations surrounding the selection of low-tech unaided and aided AAC systems (e.g., PE, MS) are beyond the scope of this chapter, several recommendations might be given for the selection of high-tech AAC software and hardware. With this said the research base for selecting appropriate AAC apps for iPods™/iPads™ is still limited. Table 1 and 2 provide an overview of a total of 22 studies that have evaluated the effectiveness of using iPods™/iPads™ as AAC devices. Sixteen (73%) of these used the Proloquo2Go™ app. While this provides evidence for the utility of Proloquo2Go™ as an AAC system, it also suggests a practice of fitting the child to the device and app, rather than the device and app to the particular abilities and needs of the child (Bradshaw, 2013; Gosnell, Costello, & Shane, 2011a). Although hundreds of communication apps are available, only four other apps (Pick a Word, Go Talk Now Free, PECS Phase III™, My Choice Board all available from https://www.apple.com/itunes/) were evaluated in the studies reviewed. With little research evidence to support the selection of appropriate AAC apps, knowledge from clinical practice might be used. For example, feature matching is a systematic process by which a child's strengths, abilities, and needs are matched to available tools and strategies (Shane & Costello, 1994). This includes selecting an SGD that can be easily operated given the cognitive, behavioral, sensory, and physical capabilities of the child with DD (Beukelman & Mirenda, 2013). Several feature matching rubrics and matrices have been developed to assist iPod™/iPad™ app selection (e.g., Gosnell, Costello, & Shane, 2014b). Table 4 provides an overview of some of the features that might be considered when selecting AAC apps.

As well as individual assessment of appropriate software apps, careful selection of the hardware itself is required. For example, the iPad™ has a larger screen than the iPod™ and since its release in 2010 the majority of research reviewed (see Tables 1 and 2) has selected the iPad™ as the mode of AAC hardware. This might be since earlier research using the iPod™ suggested that some children had difficulty activating the iPod™ SGD (e.g., Kagohara et al., 2010). Follow-up studies found that the larger-sized icons, the ability to allow more icons on the screen to improve navigation, and the increased sensitivity of the screen on the iPad™ led to increased accuracy in communicative responding (van der Meer, Kagohara, et al., 2013; van der Meer, Sigafoos, et al., 2013; van der Meer, Sutherland, et al., 2012). Nonetheless, the small size of the iPod™ means that it is portable and therefore easily used across communicative environments.

Table 4. Features to Consider when Selecting AAC Apps

Category	Example
Speech Output	• Digitized/synthesized speech • Male/female/child voice • Volume, pitch, rate of speech • When the device speaks out loud (e.g., speech after each word or speech after message selection) • Availability of multiple languages
Representation	• Icon/symbol options within the app (e.g., Symbolstix, photographs) • Ability to import and modify icons
Display	• Layouts (e.g., choice boards or scene-based displays) • Dynamic/static features • Ability to change size of icons, font, color, borders
Feedback and Enhancement	• Input when an icon is presented (e.g., highlight/zoom/enlargement of an icon) • Input when an icon is selected (e.g., tactile/vibration feedback) • Strategies to increase efficiency of communication output (e.g., word prediction, abbreviation expansion, recently used lists, grammar prediction)
Access	• How the user interacts with the device (e.g., direct selection, pointer, scanning) • Required motor skills (e.g., pinch or swipe)

Effective Instructional Strategies

In order to teach children to use the selected AAC systems careful selection of instructional strategies is required. As identified in the reviewed literature, the majority of studies successfully used systematic and explicit instructional strategies (Duker et al., 2004) to teach iPod™/iPad™ use for specific communicative purposes. Table 5 provides an overview of this approach which utilizes one-on-one instruction to create structured opportunities for communication using the AAC system. Specific strategies include cues, time delay, response prompting, prompt fading, error correction, and differential reinforcement. Although the research base to support its use is limited, a naturalistic approach to teach AAC use for a wider range of communicative skills might be recommended (Drager et al., 2009; Kasari et al., 2014). This approach typically (a) involves family and other caregivers, (b) takes place in the natural environment, (c) is embedded into functional and meaningful contexts, and (d) is reciprocal in nature. A defining feature of naturalistic AAC instructional strategies is the use of modeling (Drager et al., 2009). Two common components include augmenting the message and providing a model of expansion. For example, an instructor might verbally say *Hello,* while simultaneously selecting the icon for *HELLO* on the screen of the SGD (also resulting in the speech output *"Hello"*). In turn the AAC user would use the SGD to say *"Hello"*. The instructor might build on this by verbally asking *How are you?*, while simultaneously modeling the question using the SGD. Importantly, the idea of engaging in motivating activities that are meaningful to the child is critical in order to encourage language and communication development in children with DD. For example, in the preference-enhanced communication intervention example (van der Meer et al., 2013), opportunities for communicative interactions (greetings, requesting, commenting, answering questions) were set up within Ian's preferred DVD watching activity.

Table 5. Systematic instructional strategies

Strategy	Example
Cue	Instructor holds up a preferred snack, such as a chip
Time delay	Instructor waits several seconds for child to make request for that item using the iPod™/iPad™ SGD (or other AAC system).
Response prompting/ error correction	If the child does not respond or makes an incorrect request, the instructor might take the child's hand and physically help him/her to touch the icon on the screen of the SGD corresponding to the item on offer to activate speech output (e.g., *"I would like a chip, please"*).
Differential reinforcement	Upon a correct request using the SGD the item it is given to the child
Prompt fading	Physical guidance is faded until the child is able to independently and correctly request using the SGD

Identifying Communicative Functions

It is evident from the research reviewed on the use of iPods™/iPads™ as AAC devices (Tables 1 and 2) that teaching children with DD an initial requesting repertoire appears to be a successful place to commence communication intervention. While the literature provides effective strategies for teaching these basic communication skills (including also labeling pictures, answering questions etc), best practices for advancing social communication skills remain an obvious area for future research. Using a preference-enhanced communication intervention it is imperative that continued intervention with the child's preferred AAC system advances communicative competence. This involves not only thinking about expressive and receptive vocabulary (core and fringe) expansion, but all aspects of language (phonology, semantics, syntax, morphology, and pragmatics) learning and development (Beukelman & Mirenda, 2013). Table 6 provides an overview of some communicative functions that might be taught in AAC interventions for children with DD.

Table 6. Overview of communicative functions that can be supported in communication interventions for children with DD.

Category	Example
1. Requesting	• Desired activities, objects, people o Includes expression of preferences, choices • Help, attention, people o Includes expression of negotiation
2. Rejecting	• Negation, rejection, protest
3. Naming, describing, elaborating	• Labeling • Share, tell, comment • Asking and answering questions
4. Social interaction	• Greeting/leave-taking • Small talk • Compliments, etiquette • Reciprocal exchanges/turn-taking • Initiating, maintaining, redirecting, terminating conversation

Finally, in order to assess the effects of the intervention on communicative functioning, it is important to regularly collect learner-generated performance data (Sigafoos, Drasgow, & Schlosser, 2003). This data (e.g., frequency of use and for which communicative function) will give an indication of the child's progress. Based upon these findings modifications to the intervention can be made as required to ensure continued development of communication skills. This ongoing evaluation and individual level of analysis will support successful and effective use of AAC.

FURTHER RESEARCH DIRECTIONS

Communication delay is a common parental concern and is often the initial reason for parents to seek a referral and possible diagnosis of a DD (Horovitz & Matson, 2010). While this chapter suggests the research findings for new technologies, such as iPods™/iPads™ as AAC devices are promising, potentially misleading media anecdotes can have the effect of it leading to unrealistic, miraculous expectations. The impact of such claims on parental expectations and stress remains unknown. For example, Shane and Allen (2014) warn that this might give parents the idea that high-technology mobile devices, such as iPod™/iPad™ SGD, will enable their children to speak. Although reviews of the research suggest that the introduction of AAC does not inhibit the development of speech production, only modest increases in spoken language have been indicated (Schlosser & Wendt, 2008b). Of the research on iPod™/iPad™ SGD interventions, primarily there have only been anecdotal reports of increased spoken language (e.g., Couper et al., 2014; Flores et al., 2012; see Tables 1 and 2), with one study collecting data on frequency of vocal requests with an increase for each participant (King et al., 2014). Research is yet to systematically assess the effects of iPod™/iPad™ SGD intervention on the development of speech production.

The reviewed research suggests assessing the child's preference for using one AAC system over another might support selection of an AAC system to best suit each individual's needs. However, even if the iPod™/iPad™ SGD is indicated as preferred and the child has demonstrated an ability to use it, successful communicative interactions are dependent on the communication partner, typically the parents. It would therefore seem imperative to assess parent/caregiver and key stakeholders' perceptions of the AAC system (i.e., social validity) as well as the child's preference for using it. This level of social acceptance is important since although the intervention may be proven objectively effective, if stakeholders (e.g., parents) do not believe that the intervention can bring a significant positive change, then the intervention is less likely to be implemented (McNaughton et al., 2008; Schlosser, 1999). Few studies have assessed the social validity of AAC systems (e.g., Boesch et al., 2013; Flores et al., 2012; Tincani, 2004). If a preference-enhanced approach to intervention is to be implemented, it will be important to assess parent, teacher, and practitioner perceptions of the usefulness of the AAC intervention, whether the child's communicative interactions improved with intervention, the utility of the preference assessment, and their own preference for one AAC system over the others. In the study by Flores et al. (2012), staff reported that students appeared to enjoy using the iPad™, that it resulted in faster communication, and that it was easier for students to manipulate than the PE system. Furthermore, staff reported that the iPad™ was easier for them as teachers to implement and that they preferred the iPad™ over PE. While three of the five participants used the iPad™ more frequently than PE, anecdotal information suggested two participants preferred the iPad™. This indicates that parent, teacher, and practitioner preferences for an AAC system might not always match that of the child. Research is needed to assess how this could be resolved. For instance, this might involve multimodal AAC use (Sigafoos & Drasgow, 2001), in which the child's preferred AAC option could be incorporated into certain communicative exchanges and conditional use of other AAC options (that the child has already learned to use) could be taught depending on the context.

If children are to successfully integrate iPod™/iPad™ SGD as their primary mode of communication for a range of communicative functions across environments, considerations surrounding access need to be made. For example, there are ethical issues associated with the provision of new technologies in intervention research for child participants (van der Meer & Weijers, 2013). Namely, it seems negligent and unfair to withdraw expensive new technology (e.g., iPod™/iPad™ SGD) from a child with DD at the end of the study if the child made considerable progress with the device and wouldn't be supplied with a replacement technology. Ideally, money should be allocated in the research proposal to fund the new technology for each participant to keep personally (if the intervention is successful for that child). Outside of the research environment cost should also be considered, especially because availability of funding has been identified as a barrier to the implementation and use of high technology AAC devices (McNaughton & Bryen, 2007). While teaching the use of, and assessing preferences for, a range of AAC systems is intensive initially, it has been proposed that long-term maintenance of communication skills with the child's preferred AAC system could reduce the continued time and cost associated with implementing communication interventions (Achmadi et al., 2014). Furthermore, because device abandonment is a common issue at the conclusion of initial interventions (Abbott, Brown, Evett, Standen, & Wright, 2011; Johnson, Inglebret, Jones, & Ray, 2006), it is anticipated that using the child's preferred AAC system will reduce this risk.

While promising, the research on the use of iPods™/iPads™ as AAC devices for children with DD published to date (reviewed in Tables 1 and 2) involved relatively small sample sizes (one to nine participants), with broad age ranges (three to 23 years). Furthermore, although participants represented various DD, the majority were diagnosed ASD which might limit the generalizability of results to other disorders. Although the reviewed research compared iPods™/iPads™ as SGD to PE and MS AAC systems, no research to date has compared them to dedicated SGD (e.g., GoTalk 32+, DynaVox Maestro) or to other tablet technologies (e.g., Android tablets that can also be loaded with AAC apps). Such research is needed to better inform the comparative efficacy of these systems. One study (Dundon et al., 2013; see Table 1) demonstrated the participant learned to use two different AAC apps (My Choice Board and Go Talk Now Free). However, further research is required to assess the relative efficacy of the multitude of AAC apps available. It would be worthwhile to assess whether participants within studies respond differently to the same apps to ascertain what individual characteristics might be considered when selecting an app (Baxter et al., 2012b).

However, with the focus on intervention to teach skills to individuals in need of AAC, little research has investigated improving the design of these AAC systems. Light and McNaughton (2014) stress that it is the design of the AAC device that significantly impacts learning. They have made a call for research to investigate the visual, cognitive, linguistic, and motor processing demands of AAC systems. There is a need to define basic design features that will support use across apps. With too much change to these design features, individuals with DD might struggle to keep up and learn the new operational requirements of emerging technologies. In response to such calls, manufacturers have developed accessibility features for individuals with disabilities. iPods™/iPads™ now come with built-in assistive hearing, vision, physical and motor, and learning and literacy features. For example, the guided access feature helps individuals with ASD and other sensory and attention challenges to stay focused on the task, by disabling the home button and restricting touch input on certain areas of the screen. This is particularly useful when iPods™/iPads™ are used as AAC devices in order to restrict use to the communication app (e.g., Proloquo2Go™) and maintain focus on communication skills.

CONCLUSION

The literature suggests there is emerging evidence for the use of iPods™/iPads™ as AAC devices to support the development of functional communication for children with DD. Furthermore, comparative efficacy research suggests the iPod™/iPad™ SGD can be as efficacious as other AAC systems. Importantly, the use of iPods™/iPads™ is preferred by many of the children themselves. This chapter therefore emphasizes the use of a preference-enhanced approach to communication intervention. This involves systematic selection of an AAC device based on the child's preference combined with individual analysis of the child's abilities and needs as well as the use of suitable instructional strategies to allow for the development of a range of communicative functions.

REFERENCES

Abbott, C., Brown, D., Evett, L., Standen, P., & Wright, J. (2011). *Learning difference and digital technologies: A literature review of research involving children and young people using assistive technologies 2007-2010*. Retrieved from www.kcl.ac.uk/sspp/departments/education/research/crestem/steg/recentproj/assistivetech.aspx

Achmadi, D., Kagohara, D., van der Meer, L., O'Reilly, M. F., Lancioni, G. E., Sutherland, D., & Sigafoos, J. et al. (2012). Teaching advanced operation of an iPod-based speech-generating device to two students with autism spectrum disorders. *Research in Autism Spectrum Disorders*, *6*(4), 1258–1264. doi:10.1016/j.rasd.2012.05.005

Achmadi, D., Sigafoos, J., van der Meer, L., Sutherland, D., Lancioni, G. E., O'Reilly, M. F., & Marschik, P. B. et al. (2014). Acquisition, preference, and follow-up data on the use of three AAC options by four boys with developmental disability/delay. *Journal of Developmental and Physical Disabilities*, *26*(5), 565–583. doi:10.1007/s10882-014-9379-z

Allen, A. A., & Shane, H. (2014). Autism spectrum disorders in the era of mobile technologies: Impact on caregivers. *Developmental Neurorehabilitation*, *17*(2), 110–114. doi:10.3109/17518423.2014.8824 25 PMID:24694311

Anderson, K., Balandin, S., & Stancliffe, R. (2014). Australian parents' experiences of speech generating device (SGD) service delivery. *Developmental Neurorehabilitation*, *17*(2), 75–83. doi:10.3109/175 18423.2013.857735 PMID:24304229

Baxter, S., Enderby, P., Evans, P., & Judge, S. (2012a). Barriers and facilitators to the use of high-technology augmentative and alternative communication devices: A systematic review and qualitative synthesis. *International Journal of Communication Disorders*, *47*(2), 115–129. doi:10.1111/j.1460-6984.2011.00090.x PMID:22369053

Baxter, S., Enderby, P., Evans, P., & Judge, S. (2012b). Interventions using high-technology communication devices: A state of the art review. *Folia Phoniatrica et Logopaedica*, *64*(3), 137–144. doi:10.1159/000338250 PMID:22653226

Beukelman, D., & Mirenda, P. (2013). *Augmentative and alternative communication: Supporting children and adults with complex communication needs* (4th ed.). Baltimore: Paul H. Brookes Publishing Co.

Blischak, D., Lloyd, L., & Fuller, D. (1997). Terminology issues. In L. Lloyd, D. Fuller, & H. Arvidson (Eds.), *Augmentative and alternative communication: A handbook of principles and practices* (pp. 38–42). Boston: Allyn & Bacon.

Bock, S. J., Stoner, J. B., Beck, A. R., Hanley, L., & Prochnow, J. (2005). Increasing functional communication in nonspeaking preschool children: Comparison of PECS and VOCA. *Education and Training in Developmental Disabilities, 40*(3), 268–278.

Boesch, M. C., Wendt, O., Subramanian, A., & Hsu, N. (2013). Comparative efficacy of the Picture Exchange Communication System (PECS) versus a speech-generating device: Effects on requesting skills. *Research in Autism Spectrum Disorders, 7*(3), 480–493. doi:10.1016/j.rasd.2012.12.002

Bradshaw, J. (2013). The use of augmentative and alternative communication apps for the iPad, iPod, and iPhone: An overview of recent developments. *Tizard Learning Disability Review, 18*(1), 31–37. doi:10.1108/13595471311295996

Centers for Disease Control and Prevention. (2011). *Developmental disabilities*. Retrieved February 7, 2012, from http://www.cdc.gov/ncbddd/dd/default.htm

Couper, L., van der Meer, L., Schafer, M. C. M., McKenzie, E., McLay, L., O'Reilly, M. F., & Sutherland, D. et al. (2014). Comparing acquisition of and preference for manual signs, picture exchange, and speech-generating devices in nine children with autism spectrum disorder. *Developmental Neurorehabilitation, 17*(2), 99–109. doi:10.3109/17518423.2013.870244 PMID:24392652

Detrich, R. (2013, November). *Evidence or infomercial: The necessity of evaluating technological innovations*. Paper presented at the ABAI 2nd Education Conference. Innovations in Education: Apps, Games Technology & the Science of Behavior, Chicago, IL.

Drager, K. D. R., Light, J. C., Carlson, R., D'Silva, K., Larsson, B., Pitkin, L., & Stopper, G. (2004). Learning of dynamic display AAC technologies by typically developing 3-year olds: Effect of different layouts and menu approaches. *Journal of Speech, Language, and Hearing Research: JSLHR, 47*(5), 1133–1148. doi:10.1044/1092-4388(2004/084) PMID:15603467

Drager, K. D. R., Light, J. C., & Finke, E. (2009). Using AAC technologies to build social interaction with young children with autism spectrum disorders. In P. Mirenda & T. Iacono (Eds.), *Autism spectrum disorders and AAC* (pp. 247–278). Baltimore: Paul H. Brookes Publishing Co.

Duker, P., Didden, R., & Sigafoos, J. (2004). *One-to-one training: Instructional procedures for learners with developmental disabilities*. Austin, TX: Pro-Ed.

Dundon, M., McLaughlin, T. F., Neyman, J., & Clark, A. (2013). The effects of a model, lead, and test procedure to teach correct requesting using two apps on an iPad with a 5 year old student with autism spectrum disorder. *Education Research International, 1*(3), 1–10.

Flores, M., Musgrove, K., Renner, S., Hinton, V., Strozier, S., Franklin, S., & Hil, D. (2012). A comparison of communication using the Apple iPad and a picture-based system. *Augmentative and Alternative Communication, 28*(2), 74–84. doi:10.3109/07434618.2011.644579 PMID:22263895

Frost, L., & Bondy, A. (2002). *Picture Exchange Communication System training manual* (2nd ed.). Newark, DE: Pyramid Education Products.

Ganz, J. B., Hong, E. R., Goodwyn, F., Kite, E., & Gilliland, W. (2013). Impact of PECS tablet computer app on receptive indentification of pictures given a verbal stimulus. *Developmental Neurorehabilitation, 18*(2), 82–87. doi:10.3109/17518423.2013.821539 PMID:23957298

Ganz, L. B., Hong, E. R., & Goodwyn, F. D. (2013). Effectiveness of the PECS Phase III app and choice between the app and traditional PECS among preschoolers with ASD. *Research in Autism Spectrum Disorders, 7*(8), 973–983. doi:10.1016/j.rasd.2013.04.003

Gosnell, J., Costello, J., & Shane, H. (2011a). There isn't always an app for that! *Perspectives on Augmentative and Alternative Communication, 20*(1), 7–8. doi:10.1044/aac20.1.7

Gosnell, J., Costello, J., & Shane, H. (2011b). Using a clinical approach to answer 'what communication apps should we use?'. *Perspectives on Augmentative and Alternative Communication, 20*(3), 87–96. doi:10.1044/aac20.3.87

Horovitz, M., & Matson, J. L. (2010). Communication deficits in babies and infants with autism and pervasive developmental disorder-not otherwise specified (PDD-NOS). *Developmental Neurorehabilitation, 13*(6), 390–398. doi:10.3109/17518423.2010.501431 PMID:20887201

Iacono, T., & Duncum, J. (1995). Comparison of sign alone and in combination with an electronic communication device in early language intervention: Case study. *Augmentative and Alternative Communication, 11*(4), 249–259. doi:10.1080/07434619512331277389

Johnson, J. M., Inglebret, E., Jones, C., & Ray, J. (2006). Perspectives of speech language pathologists regarding success versus abandonment of AAC. *Augmentative and Alternative Communication, 22*(2), 85–99. doi:10.1080/07434610500483588 PMID:17114167

Johnston, S., & Feeley, K. (2012). AAC system features. In S. Johnston, J. Reichle, K. Feeley, & E. Jones (Eds.), *AAC strategies for individuals with moderate to severe disabilities* (pp. 51–80). Baltimore: Paul H. Brookes Publishing Co.

Kagohara, D., van der Meer, L., Achmadi, D., Green, V. A., O'Reilly, M. F., Lancioni, G. E., & Sigafoos, J. et al. (2012). Teaching picture naming to two adolescents with autism spectrum disorders using systematic instruction and speech-generating devices. *Research in Autism Spectrum Disorders, 6*(3), 1224–1233. doi:10.1016/j.rasd.2012.04.001

Kagohara, D., van der Meer, L., Achmadi, D., Green, V. A., O'Reilly, M. F., Mulloy, A., & Sigafoos, J. et al. (2010). Behavioral intervention promotes successful use of an iPod-based communication device by an adolescent with autism. *Clinical Case Studies, 9*(5), 328–338. doi:10.1177/1534650110379633

Kasari, C., Kaiser, A., Goods, K., Nietfeld, J., Mathy, P., Landa, R., & Almirall, D. et al. (2014). Communication interventions for minimally verbal children with autism: A sequetional multiple assignment randomized trial. *Journal of the American Academy of Child and Adolescent Psychiatry, 53*(6), 635–646. doi:10.1016/j.jaac.2014.01.019 PMID:24839882

Kennedy, C. (2005). *Single-case designs for educational research.* Boston: Pearson Education Inc.

King, M. L., Takeguchi, K., Barry, S. E., Rehfeldt, R. A., Boyer, V. E., & Matthews, T. L. (2014). Evaluation of the iPad in the acquisition of requesting skills for children with autism spectrum disorder. *Research in Autism Spectrum Disorders, 8*(9), 1107–1120. doi:10.1016/j.rasd.2014.05.011

Light, J. C., & McNaughton, D. (2014). Communicative competence for individuals who require augmentative and alternative communication: A new definition for a new era of communication? *Augmentative and Alternative Communication, 30*(1), 1–18. doi:10.3109/07434618.2014.885080

Lorah, E. R., Crouser, J., Gilroy, S. P., Tincani, M., & Hantula, D. (2014). Within stimulus prompting to teach symbol discrimination using an iPad® speech generating device. *Journal of Developmental and Physical Disabilities, 26*(3), 335–346. doi:10.1007/s10882-014-9369-1

Lorah, E. R., Tincani, M., Dodge, J., Gilroy, S. P., Hickey, A., & Hantula, D. (2013). Evaluating picture exchange and the iPad as a speech generating device to teach communication to young children with autism. *Journal of Developmental and Physical Disabilities, 25*(6), 637–649. doi:10.1007/s10882-013-9337-1

McNaughton, D., & Bryen, D. N. (2007). AAC technologies to enhance participation and meaningful societal roles for adolescents and adults with developmental disabilities who require AAC. *Augmentative and Alternative Communication, 23*(3), 217–229. doi:10.1080/07434610701573856 PMID:17701741

McNaughton, D., & Light, J. C. (2013). The iPad and mobile technology revolution: Benefits and challenges for individuals who require augmentative and alternative communication. *Augmentative and Alternative Communication, 29*(2), 107–116. doi:10.3109/07434618.2013.784930 PMID:23705813

McNaughton, D., Rackensperger, T., Benedek-Wood, E., Krezman, C., Williams, M. B., & Light, J. C. (2008). "A child needs to be given a chance to succeed": Parents of individuals who use AAC describe the benefits and challenges of learning AAC technologies. *Augmentative and Alternative Communication, 24*(1), 43–55. doi:10.1080/07434610701421007 PMID:18256963

Mirenda, P. (2003). Toward functional augmentative and alternative communication for students with autism: Manual signs, graphic symbols, and voice output communication aids. *Language, Speech, and Hearing Services in Schools, 34*(3), 203–216. doi:10.1044/0161-1461(2003/017)

Mirenda, P. (2009). Introduction to AAC for individuals with autism spectrum disorders. In P. Mirenda & T. Iacono (Eds.), *Autsim spectrum disorders and AAC* (pp. 3–22). Baltimore: Paul H. Brookes Publishing Co.

Odom, S., Horner, R., Snell, M., & Blacher, J. (2007). The construct of developmental disbilities. In S. Odom, R. Horner, M. Snell, & J. Blacher (Eds.), *Handbook of developmental disabilities* (pp. 3–14). New York: The Guilford Press.

Osterling, J., Dawson, G., & McPartland, J. (2001). Autism. In C. Walker & M. Roberts (Eds.), *Handbook of clinical child psychology* (3rd ed., pp. 432–452). New York: John Wiley & Sons.

Passerino, L. M., & Santarosa, L. M. C. (2008). Autism and digital learning environments: Processes of interaction and mediation. *Computers & Education, 51*(1), 385–402. doi:10.1016/j.compedu.2007.05.015

Rispoli, M. J., Franco, J. H., van der Meer, L., Lang, R., & Carmargo, S. P. H. (2010). The use of speech generating devices in communication interventions for individuals with developmental disabilities: A review of the literature. *Developmental Neurorehabilitation, 13*(4), 276–293. doi:10.3109/17518421003636794 PMID:20629594

Roche, L., Sigafoos, J., Lancioni, G. E., O'Reilly, M. F., van der Meer, L., Achmadi, D., & Marschik, P. B. et al. (2014). Comparing tangible symbols, picture exchange, and a direct selection response for enabling two boys with developmental disabilities to access preferred stimuli. *Journal of Developmental and Physical Disabilities, 26*, 249–261. doi:10.1007/s10882-013-9361-1

Schlosser, R. (1999). Social validation of interventions in augmentative and alternative communication. *Augmentative and Alternative Communication, 15*(4), 234–247. doi:10.1080/07434619912331278775

Schlosser, R. (2003a). Roles of speech output in augmentative and alternative communication: Narrative review. *AAC: Augmentative & Alternative Communication, 19*, 5–27.

Schlosser, R. (2003b). Comparative efficacy studies using single-subject experimental designs: How can they inform evidence-based practice? In R. Schlosser (Ed.), *The efficacy of augmentative and alternative communication: Toward evidence-based practice* (Vol. 553-595). San Diego: Academic Press.

Schlosser, R., & Blischak, D. (2001). Is there a role for speech output in interventions for persons with autism? *Focus on Autism and Other Developmental Disabilities, 16*(3), 170–178. doi:10.1177/108835760101600305

Schlosser, R., & Sigafoos, J. (2006). Augmentative and alternative communication interventions for persons with developmental disabilities: Narrative review of comparative single-subject experimental studies. *Research in Developmental Disabilities, 27*(1), 1–29. doi:10.1016/j.ridd.2004.04.004 PMID:16360073

Schlosser, R., & Wendt, O. (2008a). Augmentative and alternative communication intervention for children with autism. In J. Luiselli, D. Russo, W. Christian, & S. Wilczynski (Eds.), *Effective practices for children with autism: Educational and behavioral support interventions that work* (pp. 325–389). Oxford: Oxford University Press.

Schlosser, R., & Wendt, O. (2008b). Effects of augmentative and alternative communication intervention on speech production in children with autism: A systematic review. *American Journal of Speech-Language Pathology, 17*(3), 212–230. doi:10.1044/1058-0360(2008/021) PMID:18663107

Sennott, S., & Bowker, A. (2009). Autism, AAC, and Proloquo2Go. *Perspectives on Augmentative and Alternative Communication, 18*(4), 137–145. doi:10.1044/aac18.4.137

Shane, H., & Costello, J. (1994, November). *Augmentative communication assessment and the feature matching process*. Mini-seminar presented at the annual convention of the American Speech-Language-Hearing Association, New Orleans, LA.

Shane, H., Laubscher, E., Schlosser, R., Flynn, S., Sorce, J., & Abramson, J. (2012). Applying technology to visually support language and communication in individuals with autism spectrum disorders. *Journal of Autism and Developmental Disorders*, *42*(6), 1228–1235. doi:10.1007/s10803-011-1304-z PMID:21691867

Sigafoos, J. (1998). Choice making and personal selection strategies. In J. Luiselli & M. Cameron (Eds.), *Antecedent control: Innovative approaches to behavioral support* (pp. 187–221). Baltimore: Paul H. Brookes Publishing Co.

Sigafoos, J., & Drasgow, E. (2001). Conditional use of aided and unaided AAC: A review and clinical case demonstration. *Focus on Autism and Other Developmental Disabilities*, *16*(3), 152–161. doi:10.1177/108835760101600303

Sigafoos, J., Drasgow, E., & Schlosser, R. (2003). Strategies for beginning communicators. In R. Schlosser (Ed.), *The efficacy of augmentative and alternative communication: Toward evidence-based practice* (pp. 323–346). San Diego: Academic Press.

Sigafoos, J., Lancioni, G. E., O'Reilly, M. F., Achmadi, D., Stevens, M., Roche, L., & Green, V. A. et al. (2013). Teaching two boys with autism spectrum disorders to request the continuation of toy play using an iPad-based speech-generating device. *Research in Autism Spectrum Disorders*, *7*(8), 923–930. doi:10.1016/j.rasd.2013.04.002

Sigafoos, J., O'Reilly, M. F., Lancioni, G. E., & Sutherland, D. (2014). Augmentative and alternative communication for individuals with autism spectrum disorder and intellectual disability. *Current Developmental Disorders Reports*, *1*(2), 51–57. doi:10.1007/s40474-013-0007-x

Strasberger, S. K., & Ferreri, S. J. (2013). The effects of peer assisted communication application training on the communicative and social behaviors of children with autism. *Journal of Developmental and Physical Disabilities*, *26*(5), 513–526. doi:10.1007/s10882-013-9358-9

Stromer, R., Kimball, J. W., Kinney, E. M., & Taylor, B. A. (2006). Activity schedules, computer technology, and teaching children with autism spectrum disorders. *Focus on Autism and Other Developmental Disabilities*, *21*(1), 14–24. doi:10.1177/10883576060210010301

Tincani, M. (2004). Comparing the Picture Exchange Communication System and sign language training for children with autism. *Focus on Autism and Other Developmental Disabilities*, *19*(3), 152–163. doi:10.1177/10883576040190030301

van der Meer, L., Didden, R., Sutherland, D., O'Reilly, M. F., Lancioni, G. E., & Sigafoos, J. (2012). Comparing three augmentative and alternative communication modes for children with developmental disabilities. *Journal of Developmental and Physical Disabilities*, *24*(5), 451–468. doi:10.1007/s10882-012-9283-3

van der Meer, L., Kagohara, D., Achmadi, D., Green, V., Herrington, C., Sigafoos, J., & Rispoli, M. et al. (2011). Teaching functional use of an iPod-based speech-generating device to students with developmental disabilities. *Journal of Special Education Technology*, *26*(3), 1–12.

van der Meer, L., Kagohara, D., Achmadi, D., O'Reilly, M. F., Lancioni, G. E., Sutherland, D., & Sigafoos, J. (2012). Speech-generating devices versus manual signing for children with developmental disabilities. *Research in Developmental Disabilities*, *33*(5), 1658–1669. doi:10.1016/j.ridd.2012.04.004 PMID:22554812

van der Meer, L., Kagohara, D., Roche, L., Sutherland, D., Balandin, S., Green, V., & Sigafoos, J. et al. (2013). Teaching multi-step requesting and social communication to two children with autism spectrum disorders with three AAC options. *Augmentative and Alternative Communication*, *29*(3), 222–234. doi:10.3109/07434618.2013.815801 PMID:23879660

van der Meer, L., Sigafoos, J., O'Reilly, M. F., & Lancioni, G. E. (2011). Assessing preferences for AAC options in communication interventions for individuals with developmental disabilities: A review of the literature. *Research in Developmental Disabilities*, *32*(5), 1422–1431. doi:10.1016/j.ridd.2011.02.003 PMID:21377833

van der Meer, L., Sigafoos, J., Sutherland, D., McLay, L., Lang, R., Lancioni, G. E., & Marschik, P. B. et al. (2013). Preference-enhanced communication intervention and development of social communicative functions in a child with autism spectrum disorder. *Clinical Case Studies*, *13*(3), 282–295. doi:10.1177/1534650113508221

van der Meer, L., Sutherland, D., O'Reilly, M. F., Lancioni, G. E., & Sigafoos, J. (2012). A further comparison of manual signing, picture exchange, and speech-generating devices as communication modes for children with autism spectrum disorders. *Research in Autism Spectrum Disorders*, *6*(4), 1247–1257. doi:10.1016/j.rasd.2012.04.005

van der Meer, L., & Weijers, D. (2013). Educational psychology research on children with developmental disabilities using expensive ICT devices. *Observatory for Responsible Research and Innovation in ICT*. Retrieved from http://responsible-innovation.org.uk/torrii/resource-detail/1182

Ward, M., McLaughlin, T. F., & Neyman, J. (2013). Use of an iPad application as functional communication for a five-year-old preschool student with autism spectrum disorder. *International Journal of Engineering Education*, *2*(4), 231–238.

Wehmeyer, M. L., Palmer, S. B., Agran, M., Mithaug, D. E., & Martin, J. E. (2000). Promoting causal agency: The self-determined learning model of instruction. *Exceptional Children*, *66*, 439–453.

Wehmeyer, M. L., Sands, D. J., Doll, B., & Palmer, S. (1997). The development of self-determination and implications for educational interventions with students with disabilities. *International Journal of Disability Development and Education*, *44*(4), 305–328. doi:10.1080/0156655970440403

Wendt, O. (2009). Research on the use of manual signs and graphic symbols in autism spectrum disorders: A systematic review. In P. Mirenda & T. Iacono (Eds.), *Autism spectrum disorders and AAC* (pp. 83–140). Baltimore: Paul H. Brookes Publishing Co.

ADDITIONAL READING

Alexander, J. L., Ayres, K. M., Smith, K. A., Shepley, S. B., & Mataras, T. K. (2013). Using video modeling on an iPad to teach generalized matching on a sorting mail task to adolescents with autism. *Research in Autism Spectrum Disorders*, *7*(11), 1346–1357. doi:10.1016/j.rasd.2013.07.021

Boesch, M. C., Wendt, O., Subramanian, A., & Hsu, N. (2013). Comparative efficacy of the picture exchange communication system (PECS) versus a speech-generating device: Effects on social-communicative skills and speech development. *Augmentative and Alternative Communication*, *29*(3), 197–209. doi:10.3109/07434618.2013.818059 PMID:23952565

Cihak, D., Fahrenkrog, C., Ayres, K., & Smith, C. (2010). The use of video modeling via a video iPod and a system of least prompts to improve transitional behaviors for students with autism spectrum disorders in the general education classroom. *Journal of Positive Behavior Interventions*, *12*(2), 103–111. doi:10.1177/1098300709332346

Crowley, K., McLaughlin, T., & Kahn, T. (2013). Using direct instruction flashcards and reading racetracks to improve sight word recognition of two elementary students with autism. *Journal of Developmental and Physical Disabilities*, *25*(3), 297–311. doi:10.1007/s10882-012-9307-z

Ganz, J. B., Earles-Vollrath, T. I., Heath, A. K., Parker, R. I., Rispoli, M. J., & Duran, J. B. (2012). A meta-analysis of single-case research studies on aided augmentative and alternative communication systems with individuals with autism spectrum disorders. *Journal of Autism and Developmental Disorders*, *42*(1), 60–74. doi:10.1007/s10803-011-1212-2 PMID:21380612

Hart, J. E., & Whalon, K. J. (2012). Using video self-modeling via iPads to increase academic responding of an adolescent with autism spectrum disorder and intellectual disability. *Education and Training in Autism and Developmental Disabilities*, *47*(4), 438–446.

Howlin, P., Gordon, R. K., Pasco, G., Wade, A., & Charman, T. (2007). The effectiveness of Picture Exchange Communication System (PECS) training for teachers of children with autism: A pragmatic, group randomised controlled trial. *Journal of Child Psychology and Psychiatry, and Allied Disciplines*, *48*(5), 473–481. doi:10.1111/j.1469-7610.2006.01707.x PMID:17501728

Johnston, S., Reichle, R., Feeley, K., & Jones, E. (2012). *AAC strategies for individuals with moderate to severe disabilities*. Baltimore: Paul H. Brookes Publishing Co.

Jowett, E. L., Moore, D. W., & Anderson, A. (2012). Using an iPad-based video modelling package to teach numeracy skills to a child with an autism spectrum disorder. *Developmental Neurorehabilitation*, *15*(4), 304–312. doi:10.3109/17518423.2012.682168 PMID:22690736

Kagohara, D., Achmadi, D., van der Meer, L., Lancioni, G. E., O'Reilly, M. F., Lang, R., & Sigafoos, J. et al. (2013). Teaching two students with asperger syndrome to greet adults using social stories and video modeling. *Journal of Developmental and Physical Disabilities*, *25*(2), 241–251. doi:10.1007/s10882-012-9300-6

Kagohara, D., Sigafoos, J., Achmadi, D., O'Reilly, M. F., & Lancioni, G. E. (2012). Teaching children with autism spectrum disorders to check the spelling of words. *Research in Autism Spectrum Disorders*, *6*(1), 304–310. doi:10.1016/j.rasd.2011.05.012

Kagohara, D., Sigafoos, J., Achmadi, D., van der Meer, L., O'Reilly, M. F., & Lancioni, G. E. (2011). Teaching students with developmental disabilities to operate an iPod Touch to listen to music. *Research in Developmental Disabilities, 32*(6), 2987–2992. doi:10.1016/j.ridd.2011.04.010 PMID:21645989

Kagohara, D., van der Meer, L., Ramdoss, S., O'Reilly, M. F., Lancioni, G. E., Davis, T. N., & Sigafoos, J. et al. (2013). Using iPods and iPads in teaching programs for individuals with developmental disabilities: A systematic review. *Research in Developmental Disabilities, 34*(1), 147–156. doi:10.1016/j.ridd.2012.07.027 PMID:22940168

Knight, V., McKissick, B. R., & Saunders, A. (2013). A review of technology-based interventions to teach academic skills to students with autism spectrum disorder. *Journal of Autism and Developmental Disorders, 43*(11), 2628–2648. doi:10.1007/s10803-013-1814-y PMID:23543292

Lancioni, G. E., O'Reilly, M. F., Cuvo, A. J., Singh, N. N., Sigafoos, J., & Didden, R. (2007). PECS and VOCAs to enable students with developmental disabilities to make requests: An overview of the literature. *Research in Developmental Disabilities, 28*(5), 468–488. doi:10.1016/j.ridd.2006.06.003 PMID:16887326

Lancioni, G. E., Sigafoos, J., O'Reilly, M. F., & Singh, N. N. (2013). *Assistive technology interventions for individuals with severe/profound and multiple disabilities*. New York: Springer.

Lee, A., Lang, R., Davenport, K., Moore, M., Rispoli, M., van der Meer, L., & Chung, C. et al. (2013). Comparison of therapist implemented and iPad-assisted interventions for children with autism. *Developmental Neurorehabilitation, 18*(2), 97–103. doi:10.3109/17518423.2013.830231 PMID:24088050

Mirenda, P., & Iacono, T. (2009). *Autism spectrum disorders and AAC*. Baltimore: Paul H. Brookes Publishing Co.

Murdock, L. C., Ganz, J., & Crittendon, J. (2013). Use of an iPad play story to increase play dialogue of preschoolers with autism spectrum disorders. *Journal of Autism and Developmental Disorders, 43*(9), 2174–2189. doi:10.1007/s10803-013-1770-6 PMID:23371509

Neely, L., Rispoli, M., Camargo, S., Davis, H., & Boles, M. (2013). The effect of instructional use of an iPad on challenging behavior and academic engagement for two students with autism. *Research in Autism Spectrum Disorders, 7*(4), 509–516. doi:10.1016/j.rasd.2012.12.004

O'Malley, P., Lewis, M. E. B., Donehower, C., & Stone, D. (2014). Effectiveness of using iPads to increase academic task completion by students with autism. *Universal Journal of Educational Research, 2*, 90–97. doi:10.13189/ujer.2014.020111

Schlosser, R. (2003). *The efficacy of augmentative and alternative communication: Toward evidence-based practice*. San Diego: Academic Press.

Sigafoos, J., & Iacono, T. (1993). Selecting augmentative communication devices for persons with severe disabilities: Some factors for educational teams to consider. *Australia and New Zealand Journal of Developmental Disabilities, 18*, 133–146.

Stephenson, J., & Limbrick, L. (2013). A review of the use of touch-screen mobile devices by people with developmental disabilities. *Journal of Autism and Developmental Disorders*. doi:10.1007/s10803-013-1878-8 PMID:23888356

Vandermeer, J., Beamish, W., Milford, T., & Lang, W. (2013). iPad-presented social stories for young children with autism. *Developmental Neurorehabilitation*, *18*(2), 75–81. doi:10.3109/17518423.2013.809811 PMID:23815083

KEY TERMS AND DEFINITIONS

Applications (Apps): A software program. While apps can refer to a program for any hardware platform, they are typically used to describe programs for mobile devices such as tablets (see iPod™/iPad™).

Augmentative and Alternative Communication (AAC): The supplementation (i.e., augmentation) or replacement (i.e., alternative) of natural speech and/or handwriting. Unaided AAC refers to using the individual's own body as the mode of communication (e.g., gestures). Aided AAC refers to using supplementary equipment to communicate messages (e.g., pictures).

Communication Impairment: Encompassing deficits in speech, language, and communication. For children with DD this typically involves either highly unintelligible speech or a failure to develop sufficient spoken language to meet everyday communication needs, such that there is the need for non-oral communication systems (see augmentative and alternative communication).

iPod™/iPad™: Hardware known as a mobile device or tablet designed, developed, and marketed by the Apple Corporation. A tablet is a portable computer that has a touch screen interface, which is used to control the device.

Preference-Enhanced Intervention: (a) Teaching the use of multiple AAC systems, (b) providing choice making opportunities to assess which system the child prefers, and (c) continuing intervention with the preferred AAC system.

Proloquo2Go™: An application run only on Apple Corporation products (iPod™/iPad™) that serves as a full AAC system. It comes with two default vocabulary options, thousands of color symbols, and it is fully customizable with the ability to import your own images. Symbols are presented within grid systems on the screen, with each symbol activating a spoken word or phrase. It uses high-quality speech output. A keyboard can be used to type for text-to-speech (text is converted to speech output).

Self-Determination: Acting as the causal agent whereby one has autonomy and control in determining his/her course of action. Self-determined behavior is based on one's own choices, preferences, and interests as opposed to behavior that is caused by someone or something else.

Speech-Generating Device (SGD): Portable electronic devices that produce digitized or synthesized speech output. The screen is displayed with graphic symbols that represent a word or phrase. Touching or pressing the symbols activates the word or phrase, which results in speech output.

Chapter 2
Implementing iPad and Mobile Technologies for Students with Intellectual Disabilities

Cathi Draper Rodríguez
California State University – Monterey Bay, USA

Iva Strnadová
University of New South Wales, Australia

Therese M Cumming
University of New South Wales, Australia

ABSTRACT

This book chapter describes implementation implications of using the iPad and other mobile technologies with students (birth to adult) with intellectual disabilities. iPad and other mobile technologies offer many built-in features which facilitate their use for students with disabilities, particularly students with Intellectual Disabilities (ID). This chapter details ways that mobile technology can be used to make school and other environments (e.g., home, social) more accessible to students with ID. The theoretical framework underpinning this chapter is Universal Design for Learning (UDL), and it is applied to research-based practices for students with ID. This forms a solid base from which to examine: (a) available mobile applications (apps), (b) how apps can be used to support students with ID in accessing the curriculum, and (c) how teachers can use a framework to review and choose apps for their students.

INTRODUCTION

Students with Intellectual Disabilities (ID; formerly mental retardation; in UK also referred to as learning disabilities) are identified by significant delays in cognitive functioning and adaptive behaviour (IDEA, 2004), with the adaptive deficits limiting functioning in one or more activities of daily life, across multiple environments (American Psychiatric Association, 2013). There are three main domains of adaptive

DOI: 10.4018/978-1-4666-8395-2.ch002

functioning: (a) conceptual (academic), (b) social, and (c) practical (American Psychiatric Association, 2013). The conceptual domain includes academic skills, such as reading, math reasoning, problem solving, judgement in novel situations, etc. The social domain covers friendship abilities, social judgement, and for example awareness of other people's thoughts and feelings. The practical domain contains skills like learning and self-management across life settings, money management, and self-management of behaviour (American Psychiatric Association, 2013).

As with all disability classifications, the range of abilities among students identified with ID varies greatly. The extent of needed support exists on a continuum, ranging from intermittent to pervasive (American Psychiatric Association, 2013). Educators need to be aware of the individual needs of their students, since many students with ID require extra supports in order to make educational and social advances. For example, some students with intellectual disabilities may require support in the areas of reading, counting, note-taking, communication, and memory (Glidden, 2008). Students with the most severe intellectual disabilities, who are often referred to as 'students with high support needs' (Lyons & Cassebohm, 2012) or 'students with profound multiple disabilities' (Arthur-Kelly et al., 2008), constitute a specific group of learners. These students need extensive support in all areas of life (including eating, dressing or hygiene), and are dependent on others. Some of these students develop challenging self-stimulatory behaviours (Beirne-Smith, Patton, & Kim, 2006). Self-stimulatory behaviours are repetitive and appear to observers to serve no function. These behaviours become challenging when they are injurious, impede the learning of the student or the learning of others. Furthermore, severe intellectual disabilities are often combined with other disabilities, such as sensory impairments or physical disabilities (Heward, 2013).

The use of technology is one of the ways that supports can be provided to students of all ages with disabilities. Mobile technology has built in accessibility features that allow the user to change font, listen to text spoken out loud, and alter the motor demands of using the device; these features allow teachers to support students in learning through modalities that suit each individual best (Cumming, et al., 2014). However, Wehmeyer et al (2008) found that students with intellectual disabilities have limited access to technology and that technology is generally underused by this population. Palmer et al (2012) conducted a study and found that technology use among students with ID had remained steady or only slightly increased from a study conducted from 1999 to 2012. Part of the reason for this trend may be that educators do not have the knowledge base necessary to implement technology with their students (Aslan & Reigeluth, 2011). Educators may be given iPads for use in their classrooms, but are unsure how to integrate iPad applications into their curriculum.

The chapter will introduce Universal Design for Learning as the underpinning theoretical framework for using mobile technologies for students of all ages with ID. The existing evidence-based learning and teaching practices recommended for students with intellectual disabilities will be described and then the authors will identify how mobile technologies can enhance the education of people with disabilities. The authors will present findings of preliminary studies which demonstrate why incorporating mobile learning into the daily lives of students with ID is important. Finally, these practices will be aligned with recommendations of how to effectively incorporate mobile technology into the learning and teaching of this population.

INCLUSIVE CLASSROOMS AND THE UNIVERSAL DESIGN FOR LEARNING MODEL

Over the last several decades, there has been substantial momentum towards the inclusion of students with disabilities in the general education classroom. The theoretical framework that best supports the delivery of the standard curriculum to all students is Universal Design for Learning. Universal Design for Learning (UDL) is an educational framework based on research in the learning sciences that guides the development of flexible learning environments (CAST, 2011). It is defined as:

"A set of principles for curriculum development that give all individuals equal opportunities to learn. UDL provides a blueprint for creating instructional goals, methods, materials, and assessments that work for everyone--not a single, one-size-fits-all solution but rather flexible approaches that can be customized and adjusted for individual needs."

CAST (2011b) describes the three principles that guide implementation of UDL: (a) Provide Multiple Means of Representation; (b) Provide Multiple Means of Action and Expression; and (c) Provide Multiple Means of Engagement. These three principles, and the Universal Design for Learning Model are now widely accepted and recommended as part of different teaching models, including the popular Differentiated Instruction Model (Tomlinson, 2008). The Differentiated Instruction Model refers to modifying instruction to meet the individual needs of all students in a classroom. Mobile technology, such as iPods or iPads, allow for multiple means of representation that can accommodate individual students' needs. For example, the size, colour and font of the text can be easily altered; students can read ibooks or listen to audio books. In other words, students with intellectual disabilities can access any text in a manner that is the most suitable for them in terms of their individual learning styles, learning needs and preferences (Cumming et al., 2014).

In terms of the second UDL principle, providing multiple means of action and expression, mobile technology provides a myriad of opportunities. For example, students with intellectual disabilities can learn not only by following a teacher's presentation, but also by using specific apps to acquire taught skills and knowledge, such as *Pancake Maker, Cupcakes and Fruits and Vegetables* apps for cooking; *Spelling Cat/ Spelling Magic* and *Language Builder/ Story Builder* for literacy. Students can also combine different iPhone/ iPad tools and apps, for example they can use the built-in camera, and use the pictures taken to create their own recipe book with *My recipe book* (Cumming et al., 2014). Virtual experiences provide students with practice before they enter the real environment, other tools allow students to practice skills to aid in fluency, and still others allow them to demonstrate what they have learned in ways that don't involve taking a test or writing an essay.

The third principle of UDL, providing multiple means of engagement, also fits very well with specific mobile technologies. Students with intellectual disabilities can use diverse ways to demonstrate what they learned; for example, instead of using traditional ways of demonstrating knowledge, such as writing essays, students can prepare PowerPoint presentations including photos taken by the built-in camera. Students with intellectual disabilities who have speech impairments or who have only a limited use of verbal language can use apps such as *Proloque2Go,* which can provide speech for the students, to present what they learned.

BEST PRACTICES FOR TEACHING STUDENTS WITH INTELLECTUAL DISABILITY

The movement in education is for students with intellectual disabilities to have greater access to the general education curriculum. Students with ID are a very heterogeneous group of students (Heward, 2013). Research indicates that the majority of students with ID are supported through task analysis, time delay, and scaffolding, all widely used and accepted educational interventions (Heward, 2013). In addition, research has shown that students with ID are able to learn and progress successfully through the general education curriculum in math (Browder et al., 2008), literacy (Browder et al., 2009), and science (Courtade, Spooner, & Browder, 2007). Thoroughly understanding this research and the most effective teaching practices is important in order to appropriately identify mobile applications, which utilize them.

One of the issues related to lower levels of cognitive ability is difficulty with abstract thinking (Parmenter, 2011). In other words, students with intellectual disabilities are concrete learners, and thus benefit from teachers using specific, concrete examples of a subject content that is taught, as well as benefitting from having an opportunity to practice newly acquired skills in a real life setting. Multiple and complex instructions, with multiple steps might be overwhelming and/or confusing to the student, thus using one or two-step instructions is preferable. Being explicit is important when teaching students with intellectual disabilities, whether it comes to academic, social skills and expected behaviour.

Another problematic area might be their short attention span, and therefore longer explanations need to be broken into smaller chunks of information (Bowman & Plourde, 2012). Breaking down a task into step-by-step instruction is often called Task Analysis or Task Analytic Instruction. This process allows the teacher to break down a task (e.g., cleaning eyeglasses) into smaller activities (e.g., wiping the lenses). The teacher is able to identify where in the chain of activities the student does not have the necessary skills. The instruction can then focus on the activity or set of activities, which the student does not yet possess. Task analytic instruction has been proven to be an effective strategy for teaching academic skills including literacy (Jimenez, Browder, & Courtade, 2008; Mechling, 2004), math (Hansen & Morgan, 2008; Jimenez et al., 2008), and science (Courtade, Browder, Spooner, & DiBiase, 2010) to students with ID. An iPod/iPad application that has a task analysis piece to it is: *MyLifeSkillsBox*. This application uses visual aids to break down tasks (mostly independent living type skills) for students to complete them and cross them off upon completion.

Students with intellectual disabilities might also have problems with memory retention (Schuchardt, Gebhardt, & Maehler, 2010); therefore employing repetition throughout learning (e.g., flashcards, repeated readings) is crucial. Time Delay Instruction is an instructional strategy during which the goal is to decrease the number of prompts necessary for the student to complete the skill (Neitzel, & Wolery, (2009). This method gradually increases the time between the instruction and the prompt. Time delay procedures have been effectively used to increase the literacy skills of students with developmental disabilities (Collins et al., 2007; Mechling, 2004; Mechling et al., 2007, Tucker Cohen et al., 2008). They have also been used to positively impact math and other daily living skills (Bozart & Gursel, 2005; DiPipi-Hoy & Jitendra, 2004; Jameson et al., 2008). Time delay could be implemented through the use of an iPod timer application. Additionally, educators should look for iPod applications, which allow them to manipulate the time between the instruction and the prompt.

Scaffolding is another commonly used teaching strategy when educating students with intellectual disabilities. Bowman and Plourde (2012) mention four types of scaffolds, which include (a) written scaffolds, (b) visual scaffolds, (c) oral scaffolds, and (d) decision-making scaffolds. Written scaffolds can include filling in the blanks or providing students with sentence starters. A number of apps utilise these, which makes learning more accessible for the student. Providing information to students with visual aids and using visual scaffolds is also important (Heward, 2013). The *Photomind app* allows students with ID to attach a photo of their choice to a task or a reminder. The *Visual Schedule Planner* app assists with providing different learning modalities, as it includes very useful options, such as recording one's own voice and adding it to an event, or different formats, in which a student can view his/her calendar.

Use of Technology with Students with ID

There is an increasing number of software and computer applications purported to provide educational experiences for students with developmental disabilities, including ID (Ramdoss, et al., 2011; Ramdoss, Lang, et al., 2012; Ramdoss, Machalicek, et al., 2012; Ramdoss, Mulloy, et al. 2011). As the use of mobile technologies with students with ID grows, it is important to understand the evidence-base behind this practice. Many studies both research and anecdotal have described how these technologies can be used with students with ID (Friedlander & Besko-Maughan, 2012; Hager, 2010; Seeton, 2009).

Flores et al. (2012) conducted a comparison study between the iPad and PECS augmentative and alternative communication systems. The participants in this study were five elementary age children with autism and developmental delays. Students used the iPad with the *Pick a Word* application. Results of this study were mixed, meaning the students either performed as well as PECS or better when using the iPad application. It does not appear that the iPad stifled their communication in any way.

Burke, et al. (2010) conducted a study with six individuals with autism spectrum disorder. The purpose of this study was to determine if an iPhone application could be used to teach specific vocational skills (i.e., fire safety training) to the individuals. Burke et al. were evaluating the use of the iPhone application as compared to behavioural skills training only. Five of the six participants acquired the skills necessary when using the behavioural training and the iPhone application while only one student was able to obtain the skills with the behaviour training only. These findings indicate that mobile technology in conjunction with teacher training may increase retention of skills.

Cihak, et al. (2010) examined the use of mobile technology (iPod) on the transitioning skills of four students with autism. The students in this study learned how to effectively use the mobile device. Using an ABAB withdrawal design, the authors determine that the participants were more independent during transition while using the iPod and independence decreased when the mobile technology intervention was removed.

Studies have been conducted to understand the impact of mobile technology on a variety of aspects of life for students with ID. Research has shown that mobile technology can increase the quality of life and independence of students with ID (Brown, et al., 2011; Gentry et al., 2010). One study found that the use of iPads can increased academic skills, specifically through the use of the spell check function by students with Asperger's Syndrome and ADHD (Gentry et al., 2010). Similarly, the majority of research done with this population has been conducted in relation to communication skills. Kagohara et al., (2013) conducted a meta-analysis of eight studies that explored the use of mobile technology to impact communication skills of students with ID. Their findings suggest generally positive outcomes (e.g., increased communication, increased ability to use the mobile devices) for students with developmental disabilities. Kagohara et al. also looked at the use of mobile devices, including the areas of academics, communication, leisure skills, employment, and transitioning. Their findings indicate largely positive impacts from the use of iPods, iPads, and similar devices, which improved academic, communication, leisure, employment, and transition skills for students with developmental disabilities.

In recent years, few studies have studied the impact of mobile technologies for students with ID. However, there are generally positive findings. The increase in technology for use with students in special education means that educators must be ever more vigilant to ensure that they are choosing technologies and programs which are both available for purchase, affordable, and educationally sound.

Necessary Features for Effective Educational Applications

Mobile technology is a recent addition to the traditional learning tools that teachers have at their disposal. Choosing applications that are both effective and engaging can be a daunting task for teachers, since there is very little information on evidence-based practices in this area. To overcome this obstacle, the framework for reviewing computer learning games suggested by Su and Draper Rodriguez (2012) has been adapted for use with an iPad apps. This framework advises that educators look at the following features of educational games for their use with students: a) scaffolding, b) interaction patterns, c) digitized speech, d) colourful graphics, e) interactive tasks, f) clear instructions, g) practice tasks, h) intervals of time, i) encouragement, reinforcement, and modelling, j) feedback, and k) age and developmental appropriateness.

Understanding the features that are necessary in order for the applications to be effective is essential when deciding which ones to incorporate into classroom teaching and learning. There are two main requirements that application developers need to consider (Gredler, 1996). The first is that the simulation will meet the desired outcomes for the type of exercise (symbolic or experiential). The second requisite is that the simulation must ensure that students acquire the desired knowledge, since the purpose of the game is content learning. The main advantage of using these applications is that, like their computer software counterparts, they have the unique ability to engage children and enhance their learning through the use of age-appropriate, interactive color, sound, animation, audio and visual feedback (Chute & Miksad, 1997; Kirchner, 2002).

Studies have shown that student engagement, student motivation, digitized speech, colorful graphics, clear instructions, and audio feedback are important to the educational impact for students (Blok et al., 2002; Chute & Midsad, 1997; Levy, 2009; Lonigan, et al., 2003; Nikolopoulou, 2007; Shahrimin & Butterworth, 2001). Student engagement and motivation resulted in an increase in literacy skills and influenced their perceptions of reading (Mioduser, Tur-Kaspa, & Leitner, 2000). Lonigan, et al. (2003) examined the effects of Computer Aided Instruction (CAI) on the phonological skills of pre-school age children who were considered at-risk in their reading skills. Among the software's features were highly digitized speech and colorful graphic images which kept the student's attention while they completed a series of interactive tasks. Throughout the game, children heard auditory content using headphones. The game provided clear, comprehensible instructions for the students to follow, thus requiring an active response from the child. Another finding was that the students were able to review the instructions at any time during game play. This allowed students to remind themselves what they were supposed to be doing.

Audio feedback for educational software is necessary to provide encouragement, reinforcement and modeling (Chute & Miksad, 1997). Nikolopoulou (2007) noted that feedback to "right" and "wrong" responses should be provided in a pedagogically and developmentally appropriate way so students are encouraged to continue working. In addition, age appropriateness is as important as feedback and it should apply to the skills to be developed, the concepts to be learned, and the attitudes to be cultivated (Nikolopoulou, 2007).

In this culture of videogames and computers as compared to past generations, more stimuli to keep students involved in the learning process is required (Gredler, 1996). Keeping this in mind, making an effective learning software can be a difficult task, but knowing what features to implement and what features to look for in software is a significant step. Well-designed software requires effective use of color, sound, animation, gender preference, and audio- visual feedback that is age appropriate, and uses sound pedagogical scaffolding is. Well-made software allows children to learn through active exploration and interaction (Lonigan et al., 2003).

EDUCATIONAL APPLICATIONS FOR STUDENTS WITH INTELLECTUAL DISABILITIES

Kagohara et al. (2013) conducted a systematic review of research related to the use of mobile technologies (most commonly, the iPod or iPad) and found an overall positive impact on the skills of students with developmental disabilities. They concluded that these technologies are workable options in improving the academic, communication, employment, and transitioning skills of students with developmental disabilities. The text that follows focuses on the following topics: Communication, Behavior, Academics, Social skills, Self-determination, and Adult education. For each topic, examples of how to integrate the iPod/ iPad, a subsection of sample apps, and an explanation as to how these apps fit into the framework will be provided. The authors also suggest ways to support home-school collaboration when implementing and using iPads across environments.

Communication

Communication is an important aspect of daily life. Communication occurs when two or more people engage in language and behaviour which is comprehended by all involved (Cogher, 2005). The majority of individuals identified with ID will exhibit some difficulty in the area of communication (Lacono & Johnson, 2004). There are typically speech and language deficits present in students with ID that have high support needs. Students with the most severe intellectual disabilities are commonly non-verbal or use only a couple of words. Therefore Augmentative and Alternative Communication (AAC) is of crucial importance for this population. AAC refers to methods and technologies used to assist people who have difficulty using or understanding language. Mobile technology allows for easy portability and comfortable use across environments. There is a myriad of apps allowing for alternative communication, such as *Proloquo2Go*, *Voice4u*, *Look2Learn*, and *Tap to Talk*. Brown, Prendergast and Woodfin (2011) piloted these apps with a group of their students with severe intellectual disabilities, and concluded that *Proloquo2Go* was the most frequently used app because it allowed for the greatest customization in order to address students' individual needs. Indeed, *Proloquo2Go* is the most widely used AAC mobile application. This application has been successfully used with students with ID, autism, cerebral palsy and other disabilities to support student communication. *Proloquo2go* allows students to communicate using pictures, pre-programmed or programmable buttons, send emails and texts, edit the devices and use a variety of dialects. However, this application is currently only available on Apple devices.

Voice4u is an AAC application that is available through Google Play. This application allows students to express their emotions to others, request items, create visual schedules and explain situations. This app includes pre-programmed icons as well as allows the student or teacher to create their own icons.

Look2Learn is an AAC application that allows students and educators to use photographs to communicate. Students can use a pre-programmed voice or record their own messages. This application is programmable to fit the individual needs of the students. *Tap to Talk* provides similar supports to students with ID like the AAC applications mentioned already. It is recommended that educators find the application that will best fit the needs of their students.

Behaviour

Intellectual disabilities, especially in the moderate to severe range, can often cause deficits in students' adaptive behaviours, including those required to successfully function socially (Cohen & Spenciner, 2005). Contrary to popular belief, students with intellectual disabilities are also at risk for emotional disorders, which can manifest themselves in a variety of behaviours that are not always appropriate in classroom settings (Henley, Ramsey, Algozzine, 2009). As classrooms become increasingly more inclusive, there is a growing need to identify emotional and behavioral disorders in the classroom. Teachers have an arsenal of evidence-based strategies, which can be used to support student behaviour. These strategies can focus on incorporating mobile technology, which does not yet have a strong research base, into evidence-based practices (Cumming, 2013).

Having clear, well-defined classroom expectations is one of the first steps to maximizing engagement and instructional time by minimizing off-task and disruptive behaviors. Mobile technology can be employed to support students with intellectual disabilities in understanding and remembering these expectations. iPods, iPads, or iPhones can be used to take a picture of the posted classroom expectations so students can refer to them frequently. Student engagement in learning and following the expectations can be maximized by allowing them to use the built-in cameras in their devices to take pictures demonstrating what the expectations look like when they are being carried out. The photos could then be imported into a presentation app such as *Keynote* or a book-authoring app such as *Creative Book Builder* to create books that students can refer to themselves or share with others in class or in the school. If the students' mobile devices are equipped with video recorders, they can record the expectations being met in different situations. The videos can then be edited using a movie editing app (*iMovie, Magisto,* or *Pinnacle Studio*) in order to create short "public service announcements" or video models. The resulting photo books or videos will provide students with conveniently accessible models that can be shared with the class or even others in the school.

Keeping students actively engaged in instruction will minimize their participation in unwanted behaviors such as talking out or leaving their seats (Ornelles, 2007). Providing students with increased opportunities to respond will provide them with the opportunity to be more actively engaged during academic instruction (Simonsen, Fairbanks, Briesch, & Myers, 2008). According to Simonsen, et al. (2008), response cards are one proven way to accomplish this, and there are several electronic audience response systems that allow students to respond to the teacher's questions via their mobile devices through a Bluetooth or an Internet connection. Several different apps with different features are available (*SocrativeTeacher/ Socrative Student, iResponse, eClicker,* and *Responseware)* and they accommodate short answers, true/false, multiple choice, quizzes, tests, and contests.

Alberto and Troutman (2009) recommend the use of the following classroom management strategies: (a) specific and/or contingent praise, (b) class-wide group contingencies, (c) behavioral contracting, and (d) token economies. There are mobile apps that support each of these strategies. *iPraiseU* is an app that provides 100 positive praise statements that can be used as a lead-in to specific praise. For example, if a student has remained on task during a period of seatwork, rather than continuously using the phrase, "Good job staying on task!" the teacher can shake the device and the app will provide another statement, such as, "You have outdone yourself staying on task today!" The app also includes animation that the student can watch while the statement is being presented. However, this app may be more motivating and appropriate for younger students, particularly those in elementary school.

Simonsen, et al. (2008) recommend using token economies, which are a symbolic reinforcement system based on a monetary system. There are several token economy/contingency contract applications commercially available that can be used to support the use of token economies. *Goal Tracker* and *iReward* are customizable reinforcement systems that allow the user to add their own tasks, pictures, audio and video to personalize the token economy and make it more reinforcing. Additionally, they can be modified to provide visual reinforcement for class-wide group contingencies. *Class Dojo* is another electronic option, since it provides teachers with a fully customizable way to reward both individual students and the whole class with a click of their mobile phone or other device. The app also collects behavioral data and generates reports that can be shared with students, parents, and administrators. Behavioral contracting is similar to a token economy, but is more specific to a particular behavior and time frame. A written contract between a student and a teacher is developed, focusing on the performance of specific target behaviors in exchange for specific consequences (Zirpoli & Melloy, 2007). Apps such as *Rich Kids Behavior Contract* and *Canvas Behavior Contract* can assist teachers in the creation of electronic contracts. One advantage to electronic contracts is that the electronic format is easier to share with all involved. A student can store the contract on his or her mobile device, and have the ability to view and review the contract whenever necessary.

Academics

There are a number of apps that can be used in order to support the development of conceptual adaptive skills. These include shapes and colour apps, such as *DTT Shapes*, *Slide & Spin* and *Timor Shapes*. The *DTT Shapes* application uses the Discrete Trial Training (DTT) in order to assist students with learning basic shapes. The *TriZen* app is a challenging app, which allows a student to practice shapes in the format of a puzzle. Its track function enables students, their teachers, and/ or parents to observe their development. Other available puzzle apps are *Trainyard* and *Puzzles 'n' Colouring – Sea Life*. The latter one allows for three levels of difficulty, ranging from "easy" (6 pieces), "medium" (12 pieces) to "hard" (20 pieces). A development of matching skills (e.g., matching by colour, shape, size) is an important area that is often one of the foci of literacy and numeracy curricula for students with high support needs. The *Memory Matcher* app allows for learning shapes, numbers and letters. However many of the apps previously mentioned were developed for toddlers or pre-school children, which creates an issue with age-appropriateness. In other words, while skills developed by these apps are crucial for students with high support needs throughout their schooling years, their design does not fit well especially with those students who are already at the secondary level. Similar issues are also true for literacy and numeracy apps, such as *Little Matchups ABC, ABC Alphabet Phonics, Letter Quiz Free, Little Speller – Three*

Letter Words, Play 123 for iPhone and *My First Numbers*, to name a few. Cameras on iPods/ iPads can be used by teachers, and/or parents to take photos of real objects and used in a way that students with high support needs choose a concrete object from a choice of two.

As mentioned in the Introduction, students and adults with intellectual disabilities often struggle with fine motor skills. The *Dexteria – Fine Motor Skills Development* is an app designed for both children and adults. It is not a game-based app, but rather a set of therapeutic hand and finger exercises and activities. The *Fish School* app is an engaging application including activities such as touching fish to create letters and numbers, matching, and differences. The *Interactive Alphabet - ABC Flash Cards* allows students with ID not only to develop their fine motor skills, but also to acquire a better understanding of cause and effect.

Social Skills

The importance of students' social skills cannot be overstated in today's inclusive learning environments. Students with intellectual disabilities are required to interact with a wide variety of peers and adults both during the school day and outside of school, with family and community members. Social skills instruction has long been an accepted practice in both special and general education environments (Zirpoli & Melloy, 2007). Two of the traditional challenges of social skills instruction are motivating students to participate in and learn from the lesson, and that the skills learned in the classroom are not generalised to other settings (Gresham, 2002). Research over the last decade has suggested that incorporating technology into social skills instruction has the potential to meet both of these challenges (Fitzgerald, 2005). Several types of technology have an evidence base to support their use in assisting students with intellectual disabilities to improve their social skills.

It has been suggested that virtual reality may be a powerful tool to ameliorate the issues with generalizing what is learned during classroom social skills lessons to the real world (Cumming, 2007; Parsons & Mitchell, 2002). *If You Can* is an app that uses virtual reality to provide students with the opportunity to role play and problem solve in real life relevant situations, in order to improve their social emotional learning. Other forms of virtual reality accessible through mobile technology include video modeling and video self-modeling. Most mobile devices have a built in video recorder that can be used to create films of students or others using appropriate social skills. This may require some expertise in the area of movie editing, so for those with less confidence in their technological skills, an app may be the answer. *My Pictures Talk* is a video modeling app that allows the user to create his or her own social skill videos, social stories, and talking photo albums. Another option is to purchase apps that contain pre-recorded social skills lessons, videos and social stories, which allows for more immediate use as compared to making videos with the student being taught. An example of this would be the *Functional Skills System*, a series of apps that cover a variety of social skills in various settings, such as school, home and the community.

Students with intellectual disabilities often struggle to understand the "hidden curriculum" of social interactions and relationships. The term "hidden curriculum" refers to "rules or guidelines that are often not directly taught but assumed to be known" (Smith Myles, et al., 2004, p.5), such as idioms, metaphors, and body language. Mainstream schools are often focused on academic content rather than on the development of social skills, including the explicit explanation of the "hidden curriculum", or "unwritten rules" that people follow in social interactions (Smith Myles, et al., 2004). *The Hidden Curriculum on the Go* apps (one for children, and one for adults) explain behaviours, rules and expectations in diverse social situations and environments.

Students with ID are often naive when it comes to social interactions, which leads to their increased vulnerability. They are commonly victims of neglect and abuse (Horner-Johnson & Drum, 2006), bullying (Reiter & Lapidot-Lefler, 2007), or become offenders themselves (Holland, Clare, & Mukhopadhyay, 2002). Therefore developing their understanding of often complex social situations and potential dangers is of utmost importance. *The Staying Safe and Safer Strangers Social Stories* app includes two community safety social stories. The safer strangers' story is focused on which strangers are safer and good to approach for help, while the second story deals with what to do when a student gets lost.

Self-Determination

According to Wehmeyer (1996, p.24), self-determination refers to "acting as the primary causal agent in one's life and making choices and decisions regarding one's quality of life free from undue influence or interference". One's ability to act in a self-determined way depends on a number of factors, including environmental (such as a person's school, and living environment) and individual ones (for example a level of support needs). Mobile technology can be used as an important tool, which has the potential to increase one's self-determination and minimize the impact of barriers to self-determined behaviour. Furthermore, it can provide "valuable ways to promote self-management and self-instruction" (Ayres, Mechling, & Sansosti, 2013, p.263), such as allowing a student with intellectual disabilities to complete their tasks in an appropriate sequence by using instructional videos or photos.

In order to support students' self-determination, teachers and parents need to provide space for students to choose the types of apps they want to use. Providing a choice between relevant apps to students with intellectual disabilities should be a common and best practice. Educators and parents must understand that iPad apps that are effective may not be interesting to the student. If the student is not interested in engaging with the app, they likely will not.

Strnadová, Cumming, & Marquez (2014) conducted a study examining how teachers and parents perceive iPad integration and its effects on the education of students with high support needs. The results indicated that both parents and teachers were satisfied with students' increased self-determination, which was described by one of the participating parents in the following way: *"She points to it and sometimes verbally says, 'iPad' and at other times needs prompting before verbally asking for it. (...) She will choose which apps she wants to use independently and she works out how to use new apps very quickly."* (Parent 3 in Strnadová et al., 2014)

Adult Education

One of the many things that adults with intellectual disabilities have in common with their typically developing peers, is that they are eager to learn new skills which are directly related to the knowledge they need for a specific reason (Bowman & Plourde, 2012). There are times in their adult life, when people with intellectual disabilities can benefit from using mobile technology. These include increasing skills for (semi) independent living, employment, learning and acquiring skills for successful parenting, and for recreational and leisure activities. The portability of mobile learning devices certainly allows for iPods/ iPads to be used with frequent access across different environments, which is crucial for individuals with intellectual disabilities in order to better acquire and master new skills.

Areas of functioning that specifically lend themselves to be assisted by mobile technology include the further development of social and communication skills. The *Conversation Builder Teen* is a useful app allowing teenagers and adults with intellectual disabilities to develop their conversational skills, proper use of pragmatics, and abstract language. The *Between the Lines Advanced* app allows not only for expanding the vocabulary, but also for interpreting body language, using problem solving and answering "why" questions. The *Personal Social Skills - Workplace* allows learner to practice skills specifically related to appropriate behaviour in the workplace. The *Social Success* app is focused on development of skills such as life skills, narrative skills, and problem solving (e.g., eating in a restaurant, dealing with relationships).

The importance of the development of self-determination skills over the life-span cannot be over-estimated. The *It's My Future!* app was developed to help adults with intellectual disabilities engage in meaningful participation in their annual planning meetings. It includes self-paced videos focused on topics such as decision-making, goal setting, community living, employment, and leisure activities.

Instructional videos on iPods and iPads are tools that can be used by adults with intellectual disabilities to learn more autonomous behaviour. There is an increasing body of research examining the usefulness of mobile technology for this purpose. For example, Davidson (2012) successfully used iPods to teach adults with intellectual disabilities some of the skills important for independent living (cooking, using a washing machine, managing a budget or using a stove).

The ability to manage one's time and personal scheduling is fundamental for independent living, employment, transportation, and recreation (Green, Hughes, & Ryan, 2011). Individuals with intellectual disabilities often struggle with time management skills, due to their "cognitive limitations in working memory or abstract concepts regarding time" (Green, Hughes, & Ryan, 2011, p.14). Therefore, *iCalendar* can be a useful tool for adults with intellectual disabilities to manage their time successfully. *iCalendar* allows users to manage their own calendar as well as invite others to meetings. The case manager of the adult with ID could set the calendar for them and they would receive notifications of appointments. This control of the calendar could gradually be released to the user.

The social inclusion of individuals with intellectual disabilities is also reflected by how many of them serve as researchers for technology studies as opposed to serving as the research participants. (Barnes, 2004; Bigby et al., 2014; Stevenson, 2010). In their inclusive research study about the well-being of aging women with intellectual disabilities, Strnadová et al. (2014) utilised mobile technology (specifically iPads) as an assistive technology. While there were a number of advantages of doing this, such as the increased self-determination of the researchers with intellectual disabilities, and an increased quality of relationships in their daily lives; there were also some downfalls of using iPads for this population of researchers. One of the researchers experienced tremors, which limited her use of the iPad, while two other researchers were limited by their fine motor skills, and thus needed to seek help to plug in their devices to charge them (Cumming et al., 2014).

Besides potential issues with motor skills, there are other barriers to using mobile technology for people with intellectual disabilities. The impact of this limited access to mobile technology was emphasized by Davidson (2012, p.22), who highlighted that individuals with intellectual disabilities "have faced issues with the new knowledge economy because much information previously available in paper is now exclusively available online" due to their low literacy skills. Amongst the reasons causing this exclusion are financial issues sometimes experienced by this population, given their commonly lower socioeconomic status, which is mainly due to the lack of post-secondary educational opportunities,, the lesser likelihood of participating in the labour force and the lower likelihood of being employed full-time (AIHW, 2008). Davidson's study (2012) highlighted the common financial problems of individuals with intellectual One of the participants with ID, who was using the iPod in order to develop skills for independent living, explained why she could not continue to watch the instructional videos at home, since she lived in a home without electricity, and therefore was not able to charge her iPod. Other potential barriers include physical factors associated with ageing, such as a possible lack of fine motor skills (Davidson, 2012; Cumming et al., 2014) and/or vision problems.

It is obvious that while mobile technology presents a powerful tool for increased inclusion of adults with intellectual disabilities in wider society, it is not a "miracle tool" with a potential to address each and every individual need in this population.

CONCLUSION

The needs of students with ID vary greatly. Research has indicated success in using mobile technology to support students with ID in learning a variety of skills (Friedlander & Besko-Maughan, 2012; Hager, 2010; Seeton, 2009; Ramdoss, et al., 2011; Ramdoss, Lang, et al., 2012; Ramdoss, Machalicek, et al., 2012; Ramdoss, Mulloy, et al. 2011).

Using Universal Design for Learning and understanding the important features of mobile application, educators can make informed decisions about which applications are going to be the most effective for their students. While educators are encouraged to implement these technologies with their students, they are equally encouraged to make these choices using the provided framework and information. This chapter detailed applications, which are available for students with ID in the areas of communication behaviour, academics, social skills, self-determination, and adult education. As the selection of mobile applications is ever-growing and changing, rather than providing a list of applications and where they can be found here, the authors encourage the reader to locate the apps they find interesting in the appropriate place for the platform they are using.

It should be noted however, that technology is never a panacea nor is it a replacement for traditional evidence-based teaching. This necessitates professional development for teachers in order to develop their skills in selecting appropriate applications to suit the needs of each student, and implementing the technology into classroom teaching and learning effectively. This form of technology holds much promise for the future. It is portable, inexpensive, and through the use of apps can grow with each individual student. With proper implementation and integration with effective teaching, mobile technology will be a non-stigmatizing, customizable efficacious educational support for students with intellectual disabilities.

REFERENCES

Alberto, P., & Troutman, A. (2009). *Applied behavior analysis for teachers* (8th ed.). Upper Saddle River, NJ: Prentice Hall.

American Psychiatric Association. (2013). *Diagnostic and statistical manual of mental disorders* (5th ed.). Arlington, VA: American Psychiatric Publishing.

Arthur-Kelly, M., Foreman, P., Bennett, D., & Pascoe, S. (2008). Interaction, inclusion and students with profound and multiple disabilities: Towards an agenda for research and practice. *Journal of Research in Special Educational Needs, 8*(3), 161–166. doi:10.1111/j.1471-3802.2008.00114.x

Aslan, S., & Reigeluth, C. M. (2011). A trip to the past and future of educational computing: Understanding its evolution. *Contemporary Educational Technology, 2*(1), 1–17.

Australian Institute of Health and Welfare (AIHW). (2008). *Disability in Australia: Intellectual disability*. Canberra: AIHW.

Ayres, K. M., Mechling, L., & Sansosti, F. J. (2013). The use of mobile technologies to assist with life skills/independence of students with moderate/severe intellectual disability and/or autism spectrum disorders: Considerations for the future of school psychology. *Psychology in the Schools, 50*(3), 259–271. doi:10.1002/pits.21673

Barnes, C. (2004). "Reflections on Doing Emancipatory Disability Research." In J. Swain, S. French, C. Barnes, C. Thomas (Eds.), Disabling Barriers--Enabling Environments (pp. 47-53). London: Sage Publications.

Beirne-Smith, M., Patton, J. R., & Kim, S. H. (2006). *Mental Retardation. An introduction to intellectual disabilities*. United States of America: Pearson Prentice Hall.

Bigby, C., Patsey, F., & Ramcharan, P. (2014). Conceptualising inclusive research with people with intellectual disability. *Journal of Applied Research in Intellectual Disabilities, 27*(1), 3–12. doi:10.1111/jar.12083 PMID:24390972

Bowman, S. L., & Plourde, L. A. (2012). Andragogy for teen and young adult learners with intellectual disabilities: Learning, independence, and best practices. *Education, 132*(4), 789–798.

Browder, D., Ahlgrim-Delzell, L., Spooner, F., Mims, P. J., & Baker, J. (2009). Using time delay to teach literacy to students with severe developmental disabilities. *Exceptional Children, 75*, 343–364.

Browder, D. M., Spooner, F., Ahlgrim-Delzell, L., Harris, A., & Wakeman, S. (2008). A meta-analysis on teaching mathematics to students with significant cognitive disabilities. *Exceptional Children, 74*(4), 407–432.

Brown, T., Prendergast, L., & Woodfin, L. (2011). Use of the iPad for students with significant intellectual disabilities. *Innovations and Perspectives.* http://www.ttacnews.vcu.edu/2011/09/use-of-the-ipad-for-students-with-significant-intellectual-disabilities/

Burke, R. V., Andersen, M. N., Bowen, S. L., Howard, M. R., & Allen, K. D. (2010). Evaluation of two instruction methods to increase employment options for young adults with autism spectrum disorders. *Research in Developmental Disabilities, 31*(6), 1223–1233. doi:10.1016/j.ridd.2010.07.023 PMID:20800988

CAST. (2011). *About UDL.* Retrieved from http://www.cast.org/udl/index.html

Cihak, D., Fahrenkrog, C., Ayres, K., & Smith, C. (2010). The use of video modeling via a video iPod and a system of least prompts to improve transitional behaviors for students with autism spectrum disorders in the general education classroom. *Journal of Positive Behavior Interventions, 12*(2), 103–115. doi:10.1177/1098300709332346

Cohen, L., & Spenciner, L. J. (2005). *Teaching students with mild and moderate disabilities:Research-based practices*. Upper Saddle River, NJ: Pearson Merrill Prentice Hall.

Courtade, G., Spooner, F., & Browder, D. M. (2007). Review of studies with students with significant cognitive disabilities which link to science standards. *Research and Practice for Persons with Severe Disabilities*, *32*(1), 43–49. doi:10.2511/rpsd.32.1.43

Courtade, G. R., Browder, D. M., Spooner, F., & DiBiase, W. (2010). Training teachers to use an inquiry-based task analysis to teach science to students with moderate and severe disabilities. *Education and Training in Autism and Developmental Disabilities*, *45*(3), 378–399.

Cumming, I., Strnadová, I., Knox, M., & Parmenter, T. (2014). Mobile technology in inclusive research: Tools of empowerment? *Disability & Society*, *29*(7), 11–14. doi:10.1080/09687599.2014.886556

Cumming, T. (2007). Virtual reality as assistive technology. *Journal of Special Education Technology*, *22*(2), 55–58.

Cumming, T. (2013). Mobile Learning as a tool for students with EBD: Combining evidence based practice with new technology. *Beyond Behavior*, *23*(1), 1–6.

Davidson, A.-L. (2012). Use of mobile technologies by young adults living with an intellectual disability: A collaborative action research study. *Journal on Developmental Disabilities*, *18*(3), 21–32.

Fitzgerald, G. E. (2005). Using technologies to meet the unique needs of students with emotional/behavioral disorders: Findings and directions. In D. Edyburn, K. Higgins & R. Boone (Eds.), Handbook of special education technology research and practice (pp. 335-354). Whitefish Bay, WI: Knowledge by Design, Inc.

Flores, M., Musgrove, K., Renner, S., Hinton, V., Strozier, S., Franklin, S., & Hil, D. (2012). A comparison of communication using the Apple iPad and a picture-based communication system. *Augmentative and Alternative Communication*, *28*(2), 74–84. doi:10.3109/07434618.2011.644579 PMID:22263895

Glidden, L. M. (2008). *International Review of Research in Mental Retardation*. San Diego: Elsevier.

Green, J. M., Hughes, E. M., & Ryan, J. B. (2011). The use of assistive technology to improve time management skills of a young adult with an intellectual disability. *Journal of Special Education Technology*, *26*(3), 13–20.

Gresham, F. M. (2002). Teaching social skills to high-risk children and youth: Preventive and remedial strategies. In M. R. Shinn, H. M. Walker & G. Stoner (Eds.), Interventions for academic and behavior problems II: Preventive and remedial approaches (pp. 403-432). Bethesda, MD: National Association of School Psychologists.

Hansen, D. L., & Morgan, R. L. (2008). Teaching grocery store purchasing skills to students with intellectual disabilities using a computer-based instruction program. *Education and Training in Developmental Disabilities*, *43*(4), 431–442.

Heward, W. L. (2013). *Exceptional Children: An Introduction to Special Education*. Upper Saddle River, NJ: Pearson.

Holland, T., Clare, I. C. H., & Mukhopadhyay, T. (2002). Prevalence of 'criminal offending' by men and women with intellectual disability and the characteristics of 'offenders': Implications for research and service development. *Journal of Intellectual Disability Research*, *46*(1), 6–20. doi:10.1046/j.1365-2788.2002.00001.x PMID:12061335

Horner-Johnson, W., & Drum, C. E. (2006). Prevalence of maltreatment of people with intellectual disabilities: A review of recently published research. *Mental Retardation and Developmental Disabilities Research Reviews, 12*(1), 57–69. doi:10.1002/mrdd.20097 PMID:16435331

Individuals With Disabilities Education Act (IDEA), 20 U.S.C. § 1400 (2004).

Jimenez, B. A., Browder, D. M., & Courtade, G. R. (2008). Teaching an algebraic equation to high school students with moderate developmental disabilities. *Education and Training in Developmental Disabilities, 43*(2), 266–274.

Lyons, G., & Cassebohm, M. (2012). The education of Australian school students with the most severe intellectual disabilities: Where have we been and where could we go? A discussion primer. *Australasian Journal of Special Education, 36*(1), 79–95. doi:10.1017/jse.2012.8

Neitzel, J., & Wolery, M. (2009). *Steps for implementation: Time delay.* Chapel Hill, NC: The National Professional Development Center on Autism Spectrum Disorders, Frank Porter Graham Child Development Institute, The University of North Carolina.

Ornelles, C. (2007). Providing classroom-based intervention to at-risk students to support their academic engagement and interactions with peers. *Preventing School Failure, 51*(4), 3–12. doi:10.3200/PSFL.51.4.3-12

Palmer, S. B., Wehmeyer, M. L., Davies, D. K., & Stock, S. E. (2012). Family members' reports of the technology use of family members with intellectual and developmental disabilities. *Journal of Intellectual Disability Research, 56*(4), 402–414. doi:10.1111/j.1365-2788.2011.01489.x PMID:21988242

Parmenter, T. (2011). What is intellectual disability? How is it assessed and classified? *International Journal of Disability Development and Education, 58*(3), 303–319. doi:10.1080/1034912X.2011.598675

Parsons, S., & Mitchell, P. (2002). The potential of virtual reality in social skills training for people with autism spectrum disorders. *Journal of Intellectual Disability Research, 46*(5), 430–443. doi:10.1046/j.1365-2788.2002.00425.x PMID:12031025

Reiter, S., & Lapidot-Lefler, N. (2007). Bullying among special education students with intellectual disabilities: Differences in social adjustment and social skills. *Intellectual and Developmental Disabilities, 45*(3), 174–181. doi:10.1352/1934-9556(2007)45[174:BASESW]2.0.CO;2 PMID:17472426

Schuchardt, K., Gebhardt, M., & Maehler, C. (2010). Working memory functions in children with different degress of intellectual disability. *Journal of Intellectual Disability Research, 54*(4), 346–353. doi:10.1111/j.1365-2788.2010.01265.x PMID:20433572

Simonsen, B., Fairbanks, S., Briesch, A., & Myers, D. (2008). Evidence-based practices in classroom management: Considerations for research to practice. *Education & Treatment of Children, 31*(3), 351–380. doi:10.1353/etc.0.0007

Smith Myles, B., Trautman, M. L., & Schelvan, R. L. (2004). *The Hidden Curriculum: Practical solutions for understanding unstated rules in social situations.* Autism Aspergers Publishing, Co.

Stevenson, M. (2010). Flexible and Responsive Research: Developing Rights-Based Emancipatory Disability Research Methodology in Collaboration with Young Adults with Down Syndrome. *Australian Social Work*, *63*(1), 35–50. doi:10.1080/03124070903471041

Strnadová, I., Cumming, T., & Marquez, E. (2014). Parents' and teachers' experiences with mobile learning for students with high support needs. *Special Education Perspectives.*, *23*(2), 43–55.

Tomlinson, C. A. (2008). The goals of differentiation. *Educational Leadership*, *66*(3), 26–30.

Wehmeyer, M. (1996) Self-determination as an educational outcome: Why is it important to children, youth and adults with disabilities? In D. Sands & M. Wehmeyer (Eds.), Self-Determination Across the Life Span: Independence and Choice for People with Disabilities (pp. 15-34). Baltimore, MD: Brookes.

Wehmeyer, M. L., Palmer, S., Smith, S. J., Davies, D., & Stock, S. (2008). The efficacy of technology use by people with intellectual disability: A single-subject design meta-analysis. *Journal of Special Education Technology*, *23*(3), 21–30.

Zirpoli, T. J., & Melloy, K. J. (2007). *Behavior management: Applications for teachers* (5th ed.). Upper Saddle River, NJ: Prentice-Hall.

ADDITIONAL READING

Braddock, D., Rizzolo, M., Thompson, M., & Bell, R. (2004). Emerging technologies and cognitive disability. *Journal of Special Education Technology*, *19*(4), 49–56.

Campigotto, R., McEwen, R., & Demmans Epp, C. (2013). Especially social: Exploring the use of an iOS application in special needs classrooms. *Computers & Education*, *60*(1), 74–86. doi:10.1016/j.compedu.2012.08.002

Cumming, T., Draper Rodriguez, C., & Strnadová, I. (2013). Aligning iPad applications with evidence-based practices in inclusive and special education. In S. Keengwe (Ed.), Pedagogical applications and social effects of mobile technology integration (55-78). Hershey, PA: IGI Global. doi:10.4018/978-1-4666-2985-1.ch004

Cumming, T., & Strnadová, I. (2012). The iPad as a pedagogical tool in special education: Promises and possibilities. *Special Education Perspectives*, *21*(1), 34–46.

Draper Rodríguez, C., Strnadová, I., & Cumming, T. (2014). Using iPads with students with disabilities: Lessons learned from students, teachers and parents. *Intervention in School and Clinic*, *49*(4), 244–250. doi:10.1177/1053451213509488

Fernández-López, A., Ródriguez-Fortíz, M., Rodríguez-Almendros, M. L., & Martínez-Segura, M. J. (2013). Mobile learning technology based on iOS devices to support students with special education needs. *Computers & Education*, *61*, 77–90. doi:10.1016/j.compedu.2012.09.014

Reid, G., Strnadová, I., & Cumming, T. (2013). Expanding horizons for students with dyslexia in the 21st century: Universal design and mobile technology. *Journal of Research in Special Educational Needs*, *13*(3), 175–181. doi:10.1111/1471-3802.12013

Strnadová, I., Cumming, T., & Draper Rodriguez, C. (2014). Incorporating mobile technology into evidence-based practices for students with autism. In N. Silton (Ed.), Innovative technologies to benefit students on the autism spectrum (35-52). Hershey, PA: IGI Global. DOI: doi:10.4018/978-1-4666-5792-2.ch003

Van der Meer, L. et al.. (2011). Teaching functional use of an iPod-based speech-generating device to individuals with developmental disabilities. *Journal of Special Education Technology*, *26*(3), 1–11.

Watts, L., Brennan, S., & Phelps, R. (2012). iPadiCan: Trialling iPads to support primary and secondary students with disabilities. *Australian Educational Computing*, *27*(2), 4–12.

KEY TERMS AND DEFINITIONS

Augementative and Alternative Communcation (AAC): forms of communication other than speech which allows students to communicate wants and needs.

Intellectual Disabilities: a disability which is displayed through adaptive behaviors and cognitive abilities that are measured 2 standard deviations below the mean.

Mobile Technology: various types of portable technology, including mobile smart phones, personal digital assistants (PDAs), and tablet devices such as the iPad.

Self-Determination: skills, which allow students to engage in goal-directed behaviour.

Students with High Support Needs: students with most severe intellectual disabilities. They have commonly communication, sensory and/or physical disabilities and need extensive support in all aspects of life.

Universal Design for Learning: an approach to teaching that aims to make materials, lessons, and assessments accessible through the means of representation, expression and engagement.

Chapter 3
Using iPads and Mobile Technology for Children with Developmental Disabilities:
Facilitating Language and Literacy Development

Lisa A. Proctor
Missouri State University, USA

Ye Wang
Teachers College, Columbia University, USA

ABSTRACT

With increasing access to iPads and mobile technology in both home and school settings, evidence regarding how best to use this technology to enhance language and literacy learning is lacking, particularly for children with developmental disabilities. As a comprehensive review, this chapter discusses the use of iPads and mobile technology in the language and literacy development of this population. It concludes that while iPads and mobile technology provide opportunities for language and literacy development, the inherent challenges and limitations of this technology warrant attention from parents, educators and speech-language pathologists. iPads and mobile technology may be a valuable accelerator for the language and literacy development of children with developmental disabilities if used properly; however, improper or careless usage can become a distraction that further delays the communication development of this population.

INTRODUCTION

Given that the first iPad was introduced only five short years ago, the impact on education for children both with and without disabilities is striking. Although there is frequent access to iPads, iPods, iPhones and other mobile technology devices using iOS, Android, and Windows operating systems in both home

DOI: 10.4018/978-1-4666-8395-2.ch003

and school environments, evidence regarding how best to use this technology to enhance language and literacy learning is lacking particularly for children with developmental disabilities. This chapter provides a comprehensive review of the role of iPads and mobile technology in the language and literacy development of children with developmental disabilities.

First, this chapter provides information on categorizing the primary function of various applications targeting language and literacy development in order for parents and professionals to better understand how this technology can be utilized to achieve educational goals. The types of applications discussed include communication applications that provide an Augmentative and Alternative Communication (AAC) system for children with complex communication needs. These applications are contrasted with applications that are specifically designed to provide stimuli for expanding receptive and expressive language. Furthermore, applications that specifically target components of written language (i.e., literacy) development are reviewed.

Within these three categories of applications targeting language and literacy development (i.e., apps for communication, apps to facilitate language, and apps to facilitate literacy), we first provide information on populations for whom the applications are appropriate, the theoretical basis for use of mobile technologies, and practical rationales for their use. Second, research on evidence-based practice associated with the use of different applications is discussed. Third, the chapter provides challenges and potential solutions associated with using iPads and mobile technology for language and literacy development. Each section ends with a summary as well as additional resources for comparing and contrasting available applications.

The goal of the chapter is to provide readers with a comprehensive overview on the potential of iPads and mobile technology to facilitate the language and literacy development of children with developmental disabilities. In addition, the chapter proffers guidance regarding the use of iPads and mobile technology to achieve best practices in facilitating the language and literacy skills of this population.

BACKGROUND

In the brief interval since its introduction, the iPad has had a major impact in many educational and therapeutic situations including communication options for persons with complex communication needs (CCN) (Light & McNaugton, 2012; McNaughton & Light, 2013; RERC on Communication Enhancement, 2011), facilitating language development (Fernandez, 2011a), and literacy instruction for children who are typically developing and for children with disabilities (Beschoner & Hutchinson, 2013). The iPad is of course one of many mobile technologies that provide apps for education and communication. In addition to iPads there are numerous tablets available on the Android operating platform (Higginbotham & Jacobs, 2011) as well as a number of different smartphones that can also be used with apps albeit with a smaller display. However, due to the popularity of the iPad, this chapter focuses on the use of the iPad tablet as well as the iPhone and iPod Touch that were used to introduce many of the apps now used on the iPad. This approach is justifiable since there was much development with Apple-based apps before the introduction of the iPad (Fernandes, 2011b) and the fact that much research examining the use of mobile technologies for AAC has involved the iPod Touch (Achmadi et al., 2012; Kagohara et al., 2013; Kagohara et al., 2010; Kagohara et al., 2012). Additionally, the ideas developed in this chapter are easily adapted to similar devices produced by other manufacturers.

The iPad's "multifunctional, engaging platform" provides a singular means for data collection, motivators, and therapy materials (Gosnell, 2011) and it was being used as a communication device for children with disabilities, being provided to classrooms, or made available through instructional technology departments (An & Alon, 2013). The iPad has had a "seismic" impact on the field of AAC (McNaughton & Light, 2013; RERC on Communication Enhancement, 2011), revolutionized speech-language therapy (Fernandes, 2011a), and created the potential for anytime and anywhere literacy learning opportunities (Hutchinson, Beshorner, & Schmidt-Crawford, 2012).

Within one year of the introduction of the iPad (March, 2011), an informal electronic survey revealed that among the respondents who had iDevices, over half used the iPad in therapy (Fernandes, 2011a). Bruno-Dowling (2012) reported on a survey conducted by the Pennsylvania Speech-Language-Hearing Association revealing that 62.2% of the respondents, primarily SLPs, used the iPad for work. The uses of the iPad varied and included AAC intervention, data collection, therapy materials, training, and emails. Scuito (2013) surveyed individuals working with children who are deaf and hard of hearing regarding their use of the iPad. Many of the respondents used the iPad to increase speech and language skills with some applications for literacy use noted. Benefits of use of the iPad included motivation it provided to students as well as the convenience it provided in terms of availability of therapy materials. Many of the professionals using the iDevices had purchased them with their own funds (Fernandes, 2011a; Scuito, 2013).

In addition to its seeming ability to motivate and provide easy access to a plethora of therapy and educational materials, another appealing aspect of the iPad is its versatility (King, Thomeczek, Voreis, & Scott, 2014). The iPad can be used for mainstream computer functions such as checking email, note-taking, browsing the Internet, and storing photographs, videos, and music. In educational contexts, the iPad can provide an additional method of instruction and would be considered part of instructional technology. In other instances, it provides adaptive services for persons with disabilities as an assistive technology. Built in features such as the calendar app and video feedback and recording, may be used by speech-language pathologists (Fernandez, 2011a) Additionally, there are apps designed to assess and treat articulation, provide a communication device and facilitate language development (Fernandes, 2011a). In addition to being versatile, the iPad is considered "cool", sophisticated, and reasonably priced (Sailers, 2010) as well as socially acceptable (Alliano, Herriger, Koutsoftas, & Bartlotta, 2012).

Despite all of these positive qualities of the iPad and similar mobile technologies, there is concern regarding its implementation and use (King et al., 2013; RERC on Communication Enhancement, 2011). As with any technology, there needs to be functional guidance in the use of technology (Parette, Hourcade, Blum, Watts, Stoner, Wojcik & Chrismore, 2013). This chapter reviews the use of the iPad as a communication option for persons with complex communication needs and as a tool in language and literacy interventions.

AUGMENTATIVE AND ALTERNATIVE COMMUNICATION

AAC provides important communication options for individuals with complex communication needs. These options may include unaided modalities such as gestures and sign language, low-tech communication boards and picture exchange systems, and speech-generating devices (Beukelman & Mirenda, 2013). A speech-generating device in simple terms is a portable computer with a touch screen interface that provides voice output when an individual selects a symbol or set of symbols. Although there are similarities across many of the devices that are currently available, they may vary in a number of features including size, symbols used to activate messages, access methods, and additional features (Beukelman & Mirenda, 2013). These different modalities as well as variations in speech-generating devices are necessary because AAC supports the communication of a variety of individuals including those with intellectual disabilities, autism spectrum disorders (ASD), and severe speech and physical impairments (Beukelman & Mirenda, 2013). An important aspect of AAC clinical intervention has been finding the communication system or device best matched to each specific individual (Beukelman & Mirenda, 2013; Light & McNaughton, 2012; McBride, 2011; RERC on Communication Enhancement, 2011), providing intervention to facilitate functional use of the device or system (Beukelman & Mirenda, 2013; Kagohara et al., 2012; Kagohara et al., 2013; Light & McNaughton, 2012), and provision of technical support (RERC on Communication Enhancement, 2011).

The Use of Mobile Technologies in AAC

From the use of desktop computers to alternative access technologies, AAC has evolved along with the changes in computer technologies (Lanyon, 2012; Shane, Blackstone, Vanderheiden, Williams, & De-Ruyter, 2012). The most recent and significant change has been the use of smart phone and tablet mobile technologies as speech-generating devices. Since the iPhone version of Proloquo2go was introduced, mobile devices have been used as speech-generating devices (Sennott, 2011). However, the introduction of the iPad in particular has dramatically changed AAC (Sennott, 2011). This is in part because the larger screen on the iPad provided more options regarding AAC versus the iPhone or iPod Touch (Bradshaw, 2013). In the field of AAC, mobile technologies have provided a new option for individuals with complex communication needs. There are now available communication apps that when used on a tablet, "mimic" dedicated devices including symbol based communication systems, text to speech communication system, and a combination of the two (Alliano et al., 2012). These apps are being utilized with individuals across a range of ages and disabilities. Most iDevices are used as individuals' only high tech systems, but some are used in conjunction with another device (Niemeijer, Donnellan, & Robledo, 2012; Rummell-Hudson, 2011). The mobile technologies are similar to traditional AAC devices in that they provide touch screens, processing power, and speech output (Hershberger, 2011). In fact,

"The user interfaces of these AAC tools largely are iterations of the previous software, and the hardware features may have added some unique features in multi-touch capabilities, but for the most part they are relatively similar to what has been offered previously... What has changed dramatically is the pricing, availability, and exposure of these AAC tools" (Sennott, 2011, p. 4)

Through the use of a mobile device and a "communication app", there are now available cheaper and more portable options to traditional speech-generating devices that also provide access to the numerous additional activities/apps provided by these devices (McNaughton & Light, 2013). Just one year after the introduction of the iPad, there was estimated to be over 100 communication apps available (RERC on Communication Enhancement, 2011). The mainstream nature of these systems has generated a consumer driven model and empowered families to seek out communication options for their children (Hershberger, 2011; RERC on Communication Enhancement, 2011; Rummell-Hudson, 2011). In some instances, iPads and communication apps are being purchased by families independent of speech-language pathologists and educators (Costello, Shane, & Caron, 2012; Meder, 2012). Family members of individuals with ASD as well as professionals working with this population have, in particular, embraced the use of mobile technologies as speech-generating devices (Rummell-Hudson, 2011). iPads are now being used with individuals who had previously used dedicated AAC systems as well as for individuals who previously did not have access to speech-generating devices (Niemeijer et al., 2012). The popular media, the fields of special education and speech-language pathology, and related fields have provided anecdotal reports of the use of the iPad and other mobile technologies for communication of children with disabilities (Lanyon, 2012). This can only be characterized as a major change in the field of AAC (RERC on Communication Enhancement, 2011). Despite the enthusiasm, it is important to step back and examine the evidence supporting the use of these systems, understand the challenges, and consider factors associated with their success (McNaughton & Light, 2013; RERC on Communication Enhancement, 2011).

Using iPads as Communication Devices: Evidenced-Based Practice

Although the clinical application of these devices has far surpassed evidence regarding their use, there is observational, exploratory and single subject design research to support the use of communication systems (Flores et al., 2012; Kagohara et al., 2013; King et al., 2013). King and colleagues (2013) observed the iPad use of six children with ASD who were nonverbal. On average the children's use of the iPad involved AAC apps 36% of the time. Although this was a descriptive study and did not provide specific information on use of the communication apps, it did provide evidence that mobile technologies with communication apps are being used as speech-generating devices for children with developmental disabilities. In another exploratory study by An and Alon (2013), the authors examined how school settings were using iPads. One pattern observed was the individual use of iPads for children with developmental disabilities for communication.

Kagohara and colleagues (2013) provided a systematic review of the use of iPad/iPod/iPhone with individuals with developmental disabilities and eight of the studies reviewed dealt with communication. Overall, the systematic review found that mobile technologies (e.g., iPhone, iPod, and iPad) held promise as communication systems for persons with developmental disabilities. One of the limitations of the evidence provided by the review was that the studies primarily provided information on the use of the iPad for the communicative function of requesting. Kagohara, et al. (2012), however, specifically examined the use of iPods and subsequently iPads both with the Proloquo2Go communication application to teach two children with developmental disabilities to name objects. In the initial study, the students were taught to use the iPod Touch to answer open-ended and closed-ended questions. Time-delay, least-to-most prompting hierarchy and discriminative reinforcement were used to elicit correct responses to closed-ended questions. Both participants were successful at learning to name 12 pictures when provided with a response group of four. In a follow-up intervention, Kagohara et al. (2012) increased the number of targeted items to 18 and increased the number of items on the display including distracter items. The switch from the iPod Touch to the larger iPad allowed for the increased number of line drawings displayed. Both participants were successful in responding to closed-ended questions to learn to name pictures via the speech-generating device. Overall the authors concluded that the iPad could be used for the communicative function of naming in addition to requesting.

Another concern related to existing evidence on the use of the iDevices as a communication system for persons with developmental disabilities is the level of independence with use of these devices (Achmadi et al., 2012). Achmadi and colleagues (2012) investigated the ability of children with developmental disabilities who had previously been taught to make requests using an iPod Touch and Proloquo2go to learn to navigate and make multiple step requests using the same device and software. Using systematic instructional strategies, the two students were successfully taught to turn on the device, "swipe" the slide bar in order to unlock the device, select a desired category and then make a selection. Compared to traditional AAC devices, the iPad does require different motor patterns, such as swiping, tapping, expanding, and squeezing, which are unique to mobile technologies (Shane et al., 2012). Kagohara et al. (2010) used behavioral intervention strategies to teach a young man how to access icons on the iPod Touch. Initially, it was thought that problems with fine motor skills interfered with the use of the mobile technology. However, upon further analysis, the issue seemed to be the sensitive nature of the touch screen and responses to the student's unsuccessful attempts at activating the device. Through errorless training, the young man was able to make a selection and activate a speak display icon. This case study illustrated that appropriate instruction may be needed for the successful use of mobile technologies for communication.

Mobile technologies have been successful in helping children to make simple requests and name pictures. In addition, children with disabilities have been taught to navigate software associated with communication apps and have learned to use the sensitive touch screens provided by these technologies. When considering the research associated with the use of iPads as speech-generating devices, it is also important to note that the iPad and corresponding apps work in much the same way as dedicated AAC devices (Sennott, 2011). Consequently, research supporting speech-generating devices may also support the use of the iPad, especially if the vocabulary representation, screen display and voice output are similar. However, the numerous and differing apps now available for the iPad do provide challenges related to documenting the effectiveness of the iPads for communication (Lanyon, 2012).

One question often faced in selecting AAC systems is whether to use low-tech options, unaided options or speech-generating devices. The lower cost of mobile technologies with communication apps has increased consideration of speech-generating devices versus low-tech options. Speech generating devices may provide a motivation for communication (van der Meer, Didden et al., 2012).

Flores and colleagues (2012) compared the use of pictures on the iPad with low-tech use of pictures for children with developmental disabilities. Although the results were mixed, two of the children in the study were anecdotally reported to prefer the iPad as the mode of communication compared to low-tech pictures and communication with the iPad was better or equivalent to communication with picture cards. In addition, the adults working with the children seemed to prefer the iPad due to factors related to ease of use and preparation of materials. Van der Meer, Kagohara et al., (2012) compared the use of the iPod Touch with Proloquo2Go to sign language with four children with developmental disabilities. Three of the children showed a preference for the speech-generating device (iPod Touch) and one child showed a preference for the sign language modality. Van der Meer, Didden et al. (2012) conducted a similar study that compared the iPod Touch to Picture Exchange and signs. All four of the children who participated learned to use the iPod Touch to make simple requests and three of the four children showed a preference for the speech-generating device. Choice making was used to examine communication mode preference in the early stages of intervention and the mode chosen by a child was subsequently used more efficiently. Although it is important to consider when selecting an AAC system, speech-generating devices provided through mobile technologies, are a viable and often preferred communication mode for children with developmental disabilities (Flores et al., 2012; van der Meer, Didden et al., 2012; van der Meer, Kagohara et al., 2012).

Since the iPad represents an evolution of aspects of AAC technology that has been around for decades, future research should concentrate on differences in functionality in iPads and dedicated AAC devices. As with all speech-generating devices assessment, individualization, instructional strategies and communication partner training must be considered (Light & McNaughton, 2012). Much of the research presented used behavioral strategies and wasn't compared to other instructional options. As with these dedicated devices, more information is needed regarding the best language systems and displays. More information is also needed regarding long term and functional use of the systems. iPads obviously provided the AAC field with a new method of communication for individuals with complex communication needs and have been a major change in the field of AAC (McNaughton & Light, 2013; RERC on Communication Enhancement, 2011). However, despite the benefits and "game changing" (McLeod, 2011) nature of the iPad, its use as a speech-generating device is not without challenges (Gosnell, Costello, & Shane, 2011a; McNaughton & Light, 2013; RERC on Communication Enhancement, 2011).

Challenges Regarding Use of iPads as Speech-Generating Devices

Assessment

One major concern has been that the popularity and ease of acquiring these systems might result in a lack of appropriate assessment and "feature matching" prior to device acquisition (Gosnell et al., 2011a; Gosnell, Costello, & Shane, 2011b; McBride, 2011). Families appear to be purchasing iPads and communication apps independently of professional input (Costello et al., 2013; RERC on Communication Enhancement, 2011); however, families report needing more information on how to use the technology with their children (Meder, 2012). Professionals and families are not only faced with making the decision between communication modality (speech-generating device, low tech pictures, and unaided systems including sign), they must also decide on whether to select between either a dedicated AAC device or a mobile technology with an app, or a combination of the two. When deciding on whether to use a dedicated AAC device or a mobile technology with a communication app, some factors discussed include: appropriate research and development used in developing apps (RERC on Communication Enhancement, 2012), new models of assessment to correspond to the use of mobile technologies and AAC (Gosnell et al., 2011b; McNaughton & Light, 2013), focus on communication including a range of communicative functions (McNaughton & Light, 2013), appropriate intervention (McNaughton & Light, 2013), different methods of access (Chappell, 2011; McNaughton & Light, 2013), and continued research (McNaughton and Light, 2013; RERC on Communication Enhancement, 2011). In addition, despite the low cost of mobile technologies, new funding options (RERC on Communication Enhancement, 2011) and access to device trials (Costello et al., 2013) need to be explored. These decisions become more complicated as manufacturers develop devices from tablet computers, apps become available on manufacturer's devices and publically available, and the variety of apps increases.

Gosnell and colleagues (2011b) emphasize the importance of using stable frameworks for looking at each individual using AAC to determine needs and not relying on "... guesswork, media coverage, public testimonials, or recommendations from well-meaning friends and family" (p. 88). They provide the following guidance: decide whether an iDevice is most appropriate, compare the apps and their features, match person's needs to a particular app and provide clinical trials of the apps. Comparing apps may be challenging given the number of apps and the rate at which AAC apps are developed and updated (Lanyon, 2012). Gosnell and colleagues (2011b) also provide a matrix to examine various apps including purpose of use, output, representation, the display, feedback features, rate enhancement, access of the device, motor competencies, and support. The features and matrix are provided on a chart through Boston Children's Hospital Augmentative Communication Program (Boston Children's Hospital, n.d.). The chart can be used to determine the most appropriate app by finding the one that has the needed features. The authors stressed that in addition to the information provided by the matrix, it is important to include client input in the decision making process. It may be helpful to narrow down the apps reviewed based on reliable resources. Alliano and colleagues (2012) used the matrix developed by Gosnell and colleagues (2011b) to review 21 AAC apps. First, they divided the apps into three categories – symbols only, symbols and text, and text to speech. They narrowed down the apps for review by examining app ratings from Spectronics, a web site that provides ratings, as well as reviewer ratings from the iTunes stores. From a group of 150 apps, they were able to narrow down their comparison to 21 apps with several in each of the specific categories.

Numerous websites provide descriptions of available apps (Lanyon, 2012). For instance, the AAC TechConnect website (AAC TechConnect, n.d.) provides free information on the communication apps that are currently available. Also for a monthly fee the website will provide an app assistant that helps in the selection of the communication app. The website and blog PrAACtical AAC also provides resources to assist in app selection. In order to have hands-on experiences with the apps, families and professionals should also be aware of free and trial access to apps. For example, Tobii Dynavox provides a free download of a professional version of their application to speech language pathologists who are members of the American Speech-Language-Hearing Association (ASHA).

Accessibility

Although there are a number of factors discussed regarding selecting between dedicated AAC devices and apps, one of the most frequently discussed is access. "The wonderful new touch technology found in the latest computing platforms is not so wonderful if you cannot touch it" (Sennott, 2011, p. 5). AAC began as a way to provide communication to individuals with physical disabilities and a large part of the evolution of the field has been the development of access methods for persons with severe physical disabilities (Shane et al., 2012). Although this now includes eye tracking, head tracking, and scanning, much of the mobile technology targeting children requires adequate physical movement (Fager, Bardach, Russell, & Higginbotham, 2012). Accessing the touch screen on an iPad may be different than dedicated devices, and mobile devices may not have the same ability to provide access to individuals with severe physical disabilities (Chappell, 2011). Families and professionals must be aware of access options provided by the iPad in order to determine if it is the right communication system for a child with physical access needs. One important step is familiarity with the accessibility features provided by the devices (Fager et al., 2012; Fernandes, 2011a) as well as keeping current with the changes in adaptations/development that help to make iPads more accessible. For example, switch activation is now facilitated by the BlueTooth Technology provided by these devices (Dolic, Pibernik, & Bota, 2012). Although switch activation began to emerge in 2012, as of 2012 there was still limited use for eye gaze and head control (Fager et al., 2012). Companies such as Enabling Devices, RJ Cooper and Associates, Inc., and Ablenet provide accessories and access technologies to assist children with physical and cognitive disabilities in accessing these systems. For example, Enabling Technologies has developed a mounting system specific for the iPad (Alliano et al., 2012).

Development and Support

The use of communication apps with mobile technologies is continuing to evolve. However, developers of apps continue to utilize software designs and vocabulary displays similar to those of traditional AAC despite the need for innovation in AAC (Light & McNaughton, 2012; McNaughton & Light, 2013). It is important that the development of new apps and solutions include not only the input of software developers, but individuals with expertise in communication. Historically, development has been done by the AAC manufacturers and has been part of the cost of the dedicated AAC system (Hershberger, 2011; RERC on Communication Enhancement, 2011). With the addition of mobile technologies and the emphasis on software versus hardware, AAC developers and manufactures are facing a new industry paradigm and their response to this change will have a major impact on the development of AAC software (Hershberger, 2011). At the time of this writing many companies had developed apps for the iPad as well as changed their hardware to utilize already existing tablet platforms. Finally individuals with complex communication disorders need to be included in app development (RERC on Communication Enhancement, 2011; Steele & Woronoff, 2011).

Another hidden cost associated with dedicated AAC devices has been the support provided to consumers by consultants (Hershberger, 2011). It is still unclear how this support will be provided since the apps are not purchased through the device manufacturers, but rather are purchased through the Apple iTunes store. Since the familiarity level with the iPad technologies varies among families, the need for support may also vary. Niemeijer and colleagues (2012) found from both professionals and families that the professionals working with individuals using AAC including those using iPads, iPhones, iPod Touches lack knowledge regarding AAC. It appears that despite devices being purchased prior to assessment, parents wanted support prior to acquiring the device as well as after the device was acquired. This may include support on how to help the child learn to use the device (Meder, 2012) as well as technical support (RERC on Communication Enhancement, 2011).

SUMMARY

iPads and communication apps provide an inexpensive and familiar communication mode for many persons wiht complex communication needs. Families and professionals need, as always, to match the individual to the most appropriate communication system. The plethora of apps and the ever-changing technology provide challenges in this process. Regardless, mobile technologies have been a watershed development in the field of AAC. Research is needed and all stakeholders need to consider access, support, funding, and ongoing development.

Summary of the use of iPads and mobile technology for AAC:

1. iPads and other mobile technologies provide an affordable option for speech-generating devices for persons with complex communication needs.
2. Professionals and families should become familiar with mobile technologies and the advantages of this technology over laptop and desktop computers. This may include a better understanding of the advantages of the solid-state drive provided by tablet computers (Lanyon, 2012).

3. Speech-language pathologists and educators need to learn about the differences between dedicated AAC devices and mobile devices with communication apps and how to select which is best for an individual client. These differences may include cost, funding availability, selection and access options, vocabulary representation, availability, organization of the software applications, and technical and implementation support. However, it is also important to remember that this is a constantly evolving area of development.

4. Families and professionals need access to and information about the numerous apps available. Although it isn't possible to list all communication apps currently available, examples of specific apps include *Proloquo2go (*Assistiveware), *TouchChat HD- AAC* (Silver Kite), *Avaz Pro- AAC app for Autism* (Avaz Together), *LAMP Words for Life* (Prentke Romich Company), *GoTalk Now* (Attainment Company), *Scene Speaks* (Good Karma Applications, Inc.), and *SPEAKall* (SPEAK MODalities LLC). There are internet resources to provide feature comparisons and decision-making guidance as well as methods for obtaining free, trials, and/or reduced priced options for downloading apps.

5. iPads are multifunctional and thus allow access to other computer functions. Niemiejer and colleagues (2012) found that individuals using the iPad for primary purposes of communication used it for entertainment and learning as well. It is also important to consider how the iPad will be used and/or integrated with other technologies including dedicated AAC systems. In some instances, it may be appropriate to use Guided Access to limit the apps available to an individual.

6. Using the iPad for communication is much like using dedicated AAC devices. Existing evidence on AAC should be used in implementation of the iPad. This would include having the appropriate vocabulary, page organization and display (Light & McNaughton, 2012) as well as providing appropriate instructional strategies and partner training (Meder, 2012).

7. Professionals need to find ways to keep current on the changes that are continually occurring. As an initial step, this can include information from trusted blogs and websites (Gosnell et al., 2011b) and information provided by ASHA. For example, ASHA has available Live and On Demand Webinars.

8. As with all new technology, privacy and security issues must keep pace with the technology (RERC on Communication Enhancement 2011). AAC devices by their nature contain personally identifiable information and protection of this information needs to be a consideration.

LANGUAGE INTERVENTION

Language intervention involves speech-language pathologists in collaboration with parents and teachers, including teachers of the deaf and hard of hearing and teachers of special education, to advance the communication abilities of children with language difficulties. Intervention involves facilitating communication including receptive and expressive language for infants/toddlers and preschoolers with language delays, school age children with language disorders, children with intellectual and physical disabilities, children with ASD, and children with hearing impairments. Language intervention approaches and strategies can range from behavioral approaches that discuss the stimuli and prompts used to elicit responses and are considered more structured to social-interaction approaches that involve providing less structured activities with adult interaction styles designed to facilitate language (Kaderavek, 2011). In addition to specific approaches or styles of interactions, speech-language pathologists and educators have historically used a variety of materials and activities to target language goals including storybook reading, play activities, and pictures and word stimulation. The goal in selecting activities and materials is to maximize children's communication skill (DeCurtis & Ferrer, 2011). The specific materials and activities are selected by the age and communication skills of the children, the intervention approaches utilized by the speech-language pathologists or educators, and evidenced-based practice guidelines.

Mobile Technologies and Facilitating Language

Since the early 1980's personal computers have been used as an intervention tool for preschool-aged children with speech and language disorders that was found to have benefits (Cochran & Nelson, 1999). The use of technology became an option for facilitating the language of children with more significant disabilities (Schery & O'Connor, 1992, 1997). These computer-assisted interventions often involved adaptations and additional hardware such as expanded keyboards when targeting language goals via the computer along with targeted language structures presented through the computer software (Schery & O'Connor, 1992). Despite their common use, microcomputers presented challenges relative to access/portability of system (Schery & O'Connor, 1992), and required adaptations (e.g. touchscreens) in order for direct feedback from child input. The introduction of the iPhone and the subsequent introduction of the iPad with their ease of use and portability has resulted in technology becoming a common material used by speech-language pathologists for reinforcing/motivating participation as well as serving as a therapy tool (DeCurtis & Ferrer, 2011; Fernandes, 2011a). There are anecdotal reports explaining that iPads are motivating, versatile, time savers, and effective therapy tools if used appropriately (Mumy, 2012). Students are reported to enjoy the touch screens provided by tablets compared to the mouse often used with a personal computer (Sailers, 2010) and the iPad Touch screens allow children to hear, see, and feel during learning activities (Fernandes, 2011a). iPads are believed to aid children in the learning process (Sailers, 2010).

iPad applications used in speech and language therapy include those that provide stimuli for production of targeted speech sounds. In fact, the first app specifically designed for speech and language therapy was designed to allow speech-language pathologists the opportunity to select targeted sounds and to have all of their picture stimuli stored on their iPhones (Fernandes, 2011b). These first apps were designed to provide a presentation platform for speech sound stimuli, which clearly offered benefits to speech-language pathologists. These apps allowed them to use small iPhones, devices they already owned to provide therapy materials (e.g., picture cards) and to track data (Fernandes, 2011b). Quickly following these apps targeting articulation were apps that targeted language goals (Fernandes, 2011b). Dedicated apps (software designed for a specific purposes) are being used to target receptive and expressive language. In addition, there are creative uses of apps not specifically developed to facilitate language and versatile iPad features (e.g. photo and video capabilities) to facilitate language (Gosnell, 2011).

For at least the early stages of smart phones and tablets, the use of these apps and mobile technologies appeared to catch on more quickly within the field of speech-language pathology compared to other comparable fields such as occupational therapy and physical therapy. This may in part have been due to the play-based nature of speech-language pathology as well as possible limitations in traditional therapy materials (Fernandes, 2011b). In time, apps that targeted numerous communication and language intervention goals became available. When considering language and communication with iPads, there may, of course, be overlaps with apps on AAC when the child's communication mode is AAC and a child is learning language through that mode. The focus of this section of the chapter, however, is the use of apps and other iPad functions to facilitate language learning across modalities rather than the use of iPad apps that specifically serve as the child's communication modality.

There are now apps available that provide methods for targeting joint attention, vocal imitation, turn-taking, following directions, vocabulary building, elicitation of spontaneous utterances (DeCurtis & Ferrer, 2011) as well as improving length and complexity of utterances (DeCurtis & Ferrer, 2011; Gosnell, 2011; Rummell-Hudson, 2011). In fact there appears to be an "app" for almost all conceivable language intervention goals (Mumy, 2012).

In addition to the variation in the targeted language goals, the population of children with whom the iPad is used ranges from toddlers with language delays (Artemenko, 2014; DeCurtis & Ferrer, 2011; Snape & Mailo, 2013) to older children with ASD (Brady, 2012; Chadron, 2012; Lee et al., 2013) and children who are deaf and hard of hearing (Scuito, 2013). The rationale for the use of the iPad in language intervention is its ability to provide multisensory learning (Fernandes, 2011a). Furthermore, the engaging and motivating nature of the iPad can create opportunities for communication (Decurtis & Ferrer, 2011). The number of speech-language pathologists, educators, and parents reporting the use of iPads for learning is increasing and there are numerous blogs discussing the benefits of iPads for therapy (Fernandes, 2011b).

However, despite the overwhelming enthusiasm, there is concern that for language intervention, iPads will be used in almost all therapy sessions and other traditional materials will be abandoned (Mumy, 2012). Consequently, it is imperative to take a step back to determine if this is improving the intended language skills. In other words, how do speech-language pathologists, educators, and parents best use iPads to develop better expressive vocabularies, to produce longer and more complex utterances, and to engage more appropriately with individuals in their environments compared to children receiving services when this technology was not available or was used in a limited fashion?

Evidenced-Based Practice in Using iPads for Language Intervention

When observing children who are nonverbal using iPads in the classroom, King et al. (2014) noted that in addition to AAC apps, the children used apps that were designed to improve language skills. However, the authors noted that, frequently, the children were seen using the apps independently and did not consistently attend to the aspects of the apps that highlighted the targeted language structure. Although the observational nature of this study did not provide information on expressive language gains via the iPad apps geared to improve language, it did provide evidence that children with disabilities were using iPads and language apps in their classrooms. However, the use may have been independent and children may have not utilized the apps in the intended manner. Similar concerns regarding whether certain iPad apps promoted interaction and increased expressed language skills were raised by McNab (2013). McNab reported on the second phase of a three-phase study that involved providing families with iPads and corresponding story book apps. Some parents reported concerns that their children missed the opportunities for person-to-person interaction when reading stories on the iPad compared to engagement in storybook reading with hard copies. In addition, there were some concerns reported relative to "distracting" features of the apps in terms of shared reading for interactive language (Vaala & Takeuchi, 2012). It should be noted that the parents in this phase of McNab's study were not provided with instruction relative to dialogic storybook reading and the use of the iPad.

Lee et al. (2013) used the iPad in conjunction with discrete trial training to teach specific language skills. Two children participated in the study and the goal for the first child was to increase two word responses after looking at a picture, and for the second child the goal was to increase receptive language. In this alternative-treatment-design study, the stimuli were varied between low-tech strategies and the use of the iPad. The study also included choice opportunities for the children regarding instructional modality. Both participants indicated a preference for the iPad condition and providing the participants with a choice was associated with a reduction in challenging behaviors. The child working on receptive language increased skills and decreased challenging behaviors, but the expressive language of the other child did not vary regardless of the instructional modality. The authors concluded that the iPad held promise as a language-learning tool.

Lorah, Crouser, Gilroy, Tincani and Hantula (2014) used the iPad to teach children to discriminate between pictures. The iPad provided a method for changing the stimulus prompts, motivating the children, and assisting at least some of the children in learning to discriminate between pictures. Sandvik, Smordal, and Oserud (2012) investigated the use of an app with a behaviorist perspective "the apps provide a quick and immediate feedback of reinforcement" and an app with a constructionist perspective, "immersive experiences such as those provided by mobile investigation or games" (p. 209) on the language use of kindergarten-aged children. The children used the iPad in teacher facilitated interactions and peer groups. In addition, there were opportunities for the use of a large display to share the iPad display. Through analysis of children's conversations when using the iPad in these different contexts, the authors concluded that the iPad provides "useful and purposeful" (p. 216) language and literacy interaction.

Cardon (2012) examined the use of the iPad to increase language and language related skills for four young children with ASD by using the iPad to provide video modeling. Parents of children with ASD were taught to use video modeling to teach imitation skills with specific prompts and to praise their children. The parents in the study were able to use the iPad to create appropriate video models and to show these models to their children. All of the children increased their imitation skills and, to varying degrees, the children demonstrated increases in expressive language. Three of the four children demonstrated increases in receptive language. This study added to the literature on the successful use of video modeling to teach language skills to children with ASD and it highlighted the versatility and ease of using the iPad. These studies and anecdotal reports have provided some initial evidence for the use of the iPad for language learning and student preference for the iPad. More research is needed to understand the benefits of the multitude of iPad functions and apps across various populations and language goals.

Despite the enthusiasm for the iPad and the anecdotal reports on its benefits, data driven research on the use of the iPad has been limited (King et al., 2014). There is guidance regarding apps that target language skills supported by theory and research (Brady, 2012). However, it is important that adults provide support and guidance so children will use the apps for the intended purposes and receive the intended benefits. "Today, apps are available that will help children develop increased vocabulary for verbs in different tense levels, practice 'wh' questions skills, sort categories, and more. Many times it is not about what features the apps provide, but how SLPs use their skills with the app to promote language development. Creativity can make any app a useful tool for promoting language learning" (Fernandes, 2011a, p. 38). This means that when using iPads for language development, speech-language pathologists and teachers should still consider what are the appropriate apps, interactions styles, and additional support such as large displays to promote language learning.

Challenges Regarding Using iPads for Language Intervention

Matching the Language Goal to an Appropriate App or iPad Function

Determining whether the iPad is useful in language intervention is dependent on the language skills targeted, the manner in which the iPad is used and the instructional strategies that are used in conjunction with the iPad. For example, vocabulary development of school age children is developed through direct instruction, repeated exposure to target words, use of the words in a variety of contexts and visual organizers (Steele & Mills, 2011). Since iPads can provide multisensory and engaging introductions to vocabulary as well as easy access to graphic organizers such as *Inspiration Maps VPP* (Inspiration Software, Inc., n.d.), the iPad seems a good fit for targeting this goal albeit with the need to ensure use of the target vocabulary in other contexts.

In a different scenario, the goal may be expressive vocabulary during storybook reading with a toddler. A story may be on the iPad with interactive features (touching pictures that provide an action, highlighting words). Although these features may have benefits for the child in terms of overall literacy development, some children may wish to interact with the iPad independently rather than engaging in a shared reading experience (McNab, 2013). If the goals of the shared book reading are face-to-face interaction, for each child, the speech-language pathologist, educator, or parent may need to consider whether hard copy books or e-books best serve this purpose (Vaala & Takeuchi, 2012).

Another option may be to use the iPad as one aspect of the intervention and create other activities that correspond to the iPad application (Graham, 2011; Mumy, 2012). Graham (2011) discussed how she used a virtual lemonade stand, the *Lemonade Stand* app (Social Entertainment Technologies, LLC), to facilitate language in individual and group settings. Cochran and Nelson (1999) provided guidance on activities completed before and after activities on computers to illustrate how technology can be integrated into other components of language intervention and this guidance seems appropriate for iPad use. For example apps that provide animation and music for popular songs and fingers plays such as "The Wheels on the Bus" and the "Itsy Bitsy Spider" may be used to introduce the songs and corresponding motions. As the child becomes familiar with the sequences of the songs, routine-based intervention can be used to provide the child with communication opportunities. Blogs and websites provide resources on creative uses of iPads that are intended to provide interactions. The very multifunctional aspect of the iPad as well as the multitude of apps available that are designed for language interaction or can be creatively used for language intervention means that the iPad in conjunction with other language learning activities can be used to facilitate a wide variety of language skills. For expressive language in particular, this means consideration has to be given to the interaction that is occurring because of the iPad as well as when the child is using the iPad.

Ensuring Use of the iPad for Meaningful Communication and Interaction

Since the initial use of personal computers to increase language skills, it has been important "… to distinguish between effects that result from technology alone and effects that are improved by technology but derive from the interaction between individuals" (Collisson & Long, 1993, pp. 179-180). For language intervention, the iPad should serve as a tool to increase interaction between the adult and child or the child and peers. Many apps designed to facilitate language development were not designed for the child to use independently (Fernandes, 2011a) and it is the responsibility of speech-language pathologists and/or educators to help parents understand that the goal is to use the iPad to increase communication (Decurtis & Ferrer, 2011). Mumy (2012) stated, "The crux of the matter is, in addition to our digital reality, the other reality I see is that children still must learn to interact with people in addition to machines. There is still much to be said for the meeting of the eyes, for the exchange of words between humans, for appropriate physical contact, for the manipulation of objects in one's hands, and so forth, so we must not write-off valuable non-techie resources and materials that are still available to us" (p. 2). This may involve training parents not just how to operate the technology, but also about how to use the iPad to promote interaction. This may involve creating thematic activities that occur both before and after the use of the iPad app (Mumy, 2012).

Summary

The iPad has provided a useful resource for language intervention for children with communication difficulties. Like the incorporation of personal computers into therapy, speech-language pathologists must consider how to select appropriate software based on the learning goals as well as to determine how cognitive, visual and motor skills may impact access and make appropriate adaptations (Cochran & Nelson, 1999). Speech-language pathologists, educators, and families need to ensure that the iPad is used as one of many materials to accomplish goals and that meaningful interactions continue to be the focus of language intervention. Similar to learning about dedicated versus generic software for personal computers (Cochran & Nelson, 1999), professionals need to find appropriate resources for learning about apps, creative uses of apps, and integrating the app with other educational and intervention activities. Blogs and websites may provide important information that may not yet be available through traditional resources such as textbooks.

Summary of the use of iPads and mobile technology for language intervention:

1. iPads are increasingly used as "therapy materials" for speech-language pathologists and special education professionals, including language intervention for infants/toddlers and school-aged children with language delays including children with a variety of developmental disabilities.

2. Speech-language pathologists and educators need to become familiar with the functions/capabilities of the iPad. This could range from understanding the video features for video modeling, creating music on the iPad and knowing how they can be used to promote language. For example, a music teacher in New York used "music apps" on the iPad including *Thumb Jam* to help students with disabilities participate in a high school band (Westervelt, 2014). Although the intended purpose was to play music, the teacher reported increased verbalization and socialization for students because of the motivation and engagement that playing music on the iPad provided.

3. Speech language pathologists and educators need to become familiar with the apps available including those with specific purposes and those that can be adapted to target a variety of language goals. For infants and toddlers this may include interactive books (e.g., Five Little Monkeys Jumping on the Bed (Oceanhouse Media)), music and songs, (e.g., The Wheels on the Bus (Duck Duck Moose, Inc.)) and interactive games (e.g., Peekaboo Barn (Night and Days Studio), Toca Doctor (Toca Boca), My PlayHome (Playhome Software Ltd), iTouchiLearn Morning Routines (iTouchiLearn), and My Talking Tom (Outfit7)). Examples of apps specific to language learning for school-aged children include Story Builder, Rainbow Sentences, and Conversation Builder (Mobile Education Store) and Sentence Ninja and Syntax City (Smarty Ears Apps). In reviewing the apps, speech-

language pathologists and educators need to be aware of the goals targeted by the app, the types of intervention strategies supported by the app, and how apps can be adapted/utilized for language learning. In addition, it is important to be aware of the various functions and features of the various apps. For example, many of the apps targeting syntax (e.g., *Syntax City* and *Rainbow Sentences*) allow students to record their utterance productions as well as create sentences through picture and written stimuli. Finally, there are several apps to assist children with ASD in successfully participating in daily activities and could be considered apps to provide positive behavioral supports. These include, *the First Then Visual Schedule* app *(Good Karma Applications).* They may also be viewed as apps that assist in language learning since they provide additional input to the individual. A comprehensive list of currently available apps is beyond the scope of this chapter, however, multiple Internet resources provide lists and reviews. For example, Snape & Maiolo, 2013 provide a comprehensive resource related to apps and speech-language pathology. Another listing of language apps includes Spectronics (n.d.a). GeekSLP (n.d.) is another available resource in addition to blogs such as Sublime Speech (n.d.). Just 4-5 years ago there were only 1-2 blogs, now there are numerous blogs that provide information on apps (Fernandes, 2011b).

4. In order to evaluate the use of the iPad, it is imperative that, first, the therapy goals be clear and the iPad be considered a tool to target these goals.

5. For language goals, especially expressive language goals, it is important to realize that the iPad should be used as a tool to promote interaction and that children should be using the iPad with a communication partner. Sailers (2010) provides examples of using the iPad to increase engagement in group therapy by requiring children to show the iPad screen to the group as they are developing their sentences via the iPad.

6. Speech-language pathologists and educators also need to consider the unknowns regarding large amounts of exposure to technology on development especially for young children as well as understanding the features of technology that make it more or less beneficial. The field should be aware of the ongoing information on the role of technology with young children (Christakis, 2014).

7. In the absence of a literature base, clinicians need to use their clinical expertise when using an app. This includes the realization that many apps have great flexibility and can target goals for which they might not have been designed. There is also the realization that just because a developer of an app purports that the app increases a particular skill it doesn't necessarily mean it will. The clinician has to use his/her knowledge of evidenced-based practices and expertise as well as consideration of individual clients to determine the most appropriate use of the iPad app for language intervention.

8. Therapists and educators don't need to abandon more traditional therapy tools (Mumy, 2012) and communication methods (DeCurtis & Ferrer, 2011). One tool (e.g. the iPad) is not sufficient for all children in all contexts (Mumy, 2012). Therapists should consider how to use the iPad with other therapy materials.

9. Therapists should be systematic when incorporating iPads into therapy. For example, DeCurtis and Ferrer (2011) provided "The 7 Ps of Using Mobile Technology Therapy". These included developing a rationale for the use of the mobile technology, consider the age and developmental level of the children, how much time will be spent using the device, what is the intended purpose of the app, what is the best positioning when using the app (side by side versus face to face), how will the app facilitate the child's plan and shared enjoyment and how will the app facilitate "real-life" learning.

10. As part of the decision making process, it is important to remember that not all children respond in the same way to technology. Understanding why the iPad is more appealing to some children versus others still seems unclear (Lee et al., 2013).

LITERACY INTERVENTION

Literacy development and intervention is expansive in terms of the many skills to be addressed in order for a child to become literate. This includes the development of traditional print literacy that begins at the emergent literacy stage and continues to conventional literacy skills (Erickson, Hatch, & Clendon, 2010; Kaderavek, 2011). Emergent literacy skills develop prior to formal literacy instruction and include the development of oral language development, print awareness and book knowledge, phonological and phonemic awareness, and early writing (Kaderavek, 2011). Conventional reading instruction may include phonemic awareness if these skills are not fully developed, but specifically address a child's ability to decode as well as the development of reading fluency, comprehension, and vocabulary (National Reading Panel, 2000).

In today's new digital world, children are expected to develop skills related to New and Multiple Literacies associated with the use of computer technologies (Cubelic & Larwin, 2014; see the review of New and Multiple Literacies on Paul & Wang, 2012). Emergent literacy development also needs to be expanded to include familiarity with literacy through digital modalities (Beschorner & Hutchison, 2013). New and Multiple Literacies for children with developmental disabilities might also be considered as *functional literacy*, which is the ability to obtain information through multiple pathways from the environment and use it to make decisions and choices, modify the environment and acquire pleasure (Alberto, Fredrick, Hughes, McIntosh, & Cihak, 2007). The most important feature of functional literacy is multimodal, which encourages children with developmental disabilities not only to discern information conveyed in multiple forms but also to use various modes of expression, such as verbal language and AAC devices.

Literacy development and instruction is of course important for all children including children with disabilities. Despite a greater understanding of how best to help all children become literate, many children, including those with different disabilities, may not achieve their literacy potential. For example, individuals with developmental disabilities including physical disabilities are at risk in terms of literacy development (Machalicek, Sanford, Lang, Rispoli, Molfenter, & Mbesha, 2010). Kliewer, Biklen, Kasa-Hendrickson (2006) called for "a science of literacy for all" (p. 163) to provide every child with opportunities to develop as literate citizens, particularly the labeled children who are still legally segregated from "valued access to the citizenship tools of literacy" (p. 164).

With appropriate literacy instructional approaches and adequate literacy practices, most children and adolescents with developmental disabilities are capable of accessing and utilizing information from traditional reading and writing to various degrees. Meanwhile, everyone, including children and adolescents with moderate or severe developmental disabilities for whom the cognitive and/or physical demands of traditional reading and writing are too great, should have the choice of using New and Multiple Literacies as alternative literacy achievement standards (Paul & Wang, 2012). No one should be denied the opportunity to acquire and utilize information through multiple pathways.

Helping children to become "literate" is a collaborative process among teachers, learning disabilities specialists, speech-language pathologists and families. Classroom teachers, especially those working with young children (i.e., preschool and early elementary age), have a primary responsibility for helping children to learn to read. However, parent involvement is vital to this process particularly in the stage of emergent literacy (Kaderavek, 2011). In addition, ASHA has outlined the role of the speech-language pathologists in literacy assessment and intervention (ASHA, 2001), and ASHA clearly emphasizes the need for speech-language pathologists to become involved in literacy instruction, particularly for children with speech and language difficulties. Families and professionals must find optimal methods of literacy instruction for all children. The introduction of the iPad has provided both a new instructional technology to enhance the literacy instruction of children who are typically developing and children with language disorders as well as an important form of assistive technology for children with disabilities who require technologies to become literate.

Mobile Technologies and Literacy Instruction

The use of technology to improve literacy instruction is not novel. Desktop and laptop computers along with specialized software programs have been used in instruction to improve reading and writing skills. However, the role of mobile devices on literacy learning and technology in the new millennium was not envisioned (Masterson, Apel, & Wood, 2002). Mobile technologies provide a new and exciting opportunity for literacy learning. Since tablets are engaging and intuitive, they have the potential to impact "a widely diverse group of young learners" (Cubelic & Larwin, 2014, p. 58). In addition, tablets can provide "ubiquitous learning" that does not require children to be in front of a computer as well as affording easier transitions between home and school use (Hutchinson et al., 2012; Northup & Killeen, 2013). In addition to providing children with ways to learn about traditional print literacy, integration of these new technologies into classrooms promote understanding of New and Multiple Literacies, which the International Reading Association has stated is needed for young children (Northrop & Killeen, 2013). iPads and literacy apps are increasingly being used in schools as tools for promoting literacy instruction (Dobler, 2012; Manko 2013/2014) as well as collaboration and socialization among children (Dobler, 2012; Oladunjoye, 2013). The use of the iPad for literacy instruction may involve the goal of providing an iPad to each child (An & Alon, 2013; Manko, 2014), iPads provided to a classroom and shared amongst children (An & Alon, 2013; Dobler, 2012), or school iPads that may be checked out from the instructional technology department (An & Alon, 2013). Regardless of the model used for making iPads available for classroom use, it is important to understand how iPads influence literacy learning.

Evidenced Based Practice in using iPads for Literacy Intervention

"Although little research has been done on the use of iPads and smartphones as learning tools, past experiences with technology can help guide the use of tablets in the classroom" (Northup & Killeen, 2013, p. 532). Based on emerging evidence, computers and specialized software were used to assist with narrative development, writing skills, reading comprehension, and spelling skills (Wood & Masterson, 1999). The introduction of the iPad has resulted in a need to shift the research focus of literacy and technology to this new modality. There are anecdotal reports of the use of iPads to facilitate reading instruction and assessment helping to improve standardized tests scores (Manko, 2014) and the use of the iPad to provide individualized reading instruction (Dobler, 2012).

Oladunjoye (2013) utilized classroom observations and teacher interviews to better understand the role of iPads as a part of Information and Communication Technology in the literacy development of preschool age children. The children were observed to use iPads for writing, and to develop phonological awareness using the *School Style* app. Analysis of teacher interviews revealed that teachers perceived iPads as facilitating the literacy development of the children in their classrooms. Hutchinson et al. (2012) reported a case study of a fourth grade classroom that used the iPads in conjunction with the "TPACK" (technological pedagogical content knowledge) framework. The authors describe the purpose of the framework as understanding how teachers use these different areas of knowledge to integrate technology into classrooms. In this study, the iPads provided digital books which in turn offered digital support, word-by-word tracking, picture animation, and voice recordings. The iPad implementation started by reviewing the literacy curriculum and then integrated the technology into that curriculum. For example, in order to provide comprehension of stories, the authors utilized the app *Doodle Buddy*, which gave children a chance to draw pictures and used visualization to aid in the comprehension of stories. iBooks were used to support independent reading and the *Strip Designer* app was used for story retelling. The result of the study was an illustration of how the iPad can be a viable tool for addressing literacy goals in the classroom.

Beschorner and Hutchison (2013) also stressed the importance of guidelines when implementing technology. They provided iPads and apps that corresponded to emergent literacy to two preschool classrooms for a period of seven weeks. The apps selected allowed for problem solving, decision making, and interactivity and included the *Magnetic ABCs* app and the *Storykit* app. They also provided opportunities for reading, writing, listening, and speaking, the important roots of early literacy. "The results of this study suggest that the iPad and other similar tablets can be used in multiple ways as an instructional tool to support the teaching of emergent literacy in the early childhood classroom (p. 20)." Themes that developed in terms of literacy activities included digital environmental print, emergent writing using digital technology, functions of writing, connecting reading, writing, speaking, listening, and social learning. The authors concluded that the iPad helped the children to learn about digital technology and provided a means to learn important emergent literacy skills. In a multisite study, Simpson, Walsh, and Rowsell (2013) used observation as well as student and teacher reflections to understand the interactions of student pairs while reading with the iPad. Their analysis emphasized the importance of touch and collaboration in how children were learning to read via the iPad.

Cubelic and Larwin (2014) incorporated appropriate apps into teacher-created lessons targeting first sound fluency (e.g., *ABC Phonic, Build a Word*), phoneme segmentation fluency (e.g. *Skill Builder Spelling, Phonics Monster 1*), and nonsense word fluency (e.g., *Bee Sees, ABC Touch & Learn*). They found that at the end of the school year the children in the experimental group, the children provided with corresponding apps, did better with first letter segmentation and decoding. One interesting finding was the interaction between years of teaching and the impact of the iPad technology. For the control group, the children who did not have access to iPad apps, teachers' years of experience was positively linked with student learning. However, for the experimental group, students of teachers with fewer years of experience did best in developing these early literacy skills.

Qualitative investigation on the use of the iPad in classroom settings has also been conducted with children with disabilities. Flewitt, Kuchikova, and Messer (2014) observed iPad use in classroom with children with a range of disabilities. Their observations focused on the role of touch in the use of the iPads. They noted the role of the lightweight and flexible iPad in motivating students, creating independence, providing feedback, and allowing for adaptation. They asserted that the iPad provided touch engagement that allowed for the children's participation in literacy activities.

In addition, as to the use of apps specifically designed to improve literacy instruction, the iPad has been used to provide video modeling to improve the literacy abilities of individuals with ASD (Kagohara, Sigafoos, Achmadi, O'Reilly, & Lancioni, 2011). Kagohara and colleagues (2011) investigated the use of video modeling via the iPad to teach two children with ASD to use the spell check function of a word processing program. Both of the children in the study were able to learn to use the spell check function with the assistance of video modeling from the iPad.

Combined with information on the use of personal computers to support literacy instruction (Masterson et al., 2002; Wood & Masterson, 1999) and more recent information specific to iPads, there is growing evidence that technology can be useful in supporting literacy instruction.

Challenges Regarding Using iPads for Literacy Intervention

Ensuring that Technology is a Tool to Support the Curriculum

To support literacy development for all children, the iPad needs to support the literacy curriculum. In addition, curricula will need to be adapted to include important New and Multiple Literacies and the skills children need to learn relative to these new technologies. How the iPad is used to support the curriculum is an important consideration. Northrop and Killeen (2013) provide a framework for early literacy that involved a "Gradual Release Model". The important aspects of the model is matched to the child's level and ensuring that the child understands the literacy content of the apps. Within this model, the teacher models and provides guided instruction and then independence for the child. They stress that it isn't the technology alone that increases the child's performance, but matching the technology, which is motivational and fun to the child. Northup and Killeen provided examples of apps that focused on phonics apps (letter formation, letter sounds, and blending of simple words). They recommended teaching the concept without the app and then teacher "think-aloud" when teaching the child to use apps to ensure the child isn't clicking through the app without understanding the literacy content.

Providing Appropriate Adaptations for Children with Disabilities

One aspect of literacy instruction for individuals with disabilities is to consider the unique contributions of technology. For example, children with complex communication needs may not be able to use subvocal articulation in spelling novel words. Consequently, technology in the form of computerized "sounding out" of words was used to enhance the spelling abilities of a child using an AAC. In a single subject design, McCarthy, Beukelman, and Hogan (2011) used a computer with specialized software to produce individual sounds and blends of targeted words. This use of technology was successful in facilitating the child's spelling skills. Technology can provide children with significant intellectual disabilities with ways to engage in emergent literacy activities, learn to read words, and develop text comprehension. Assistive technology can also help to minimize the learning challenges faced by these children as well as the physical challenges of children with sensory and physical disabilities (Erickson et al., 2010). Technology may provide adapted writing (e.g., stamps, expanded keyboards), adapted books, books on computer, and talking word processors (Koppenhaver & Erickson, 2003).

Tablet technologies including the iPad are accessible and easily used by the vast majority of children. The role of "touch" in learning may provide a motivational method for literacy learning (Flewitt et al., 2014). Although children with physical disabilities may be able to adapt how they physically interact with the iPad or use it with support (Flewitt et al., 2014), as with use of iPads for AAC, consideration needs to be given to accessibility of the iPad for children with physical disabilities. More research is needed regarding the use of the iPad to facilitate the literacy development of children with disabilities (Oladjunjoye, 2013). However, its use with diverse learners seems promising. Flewitt and colleagues (2014) concluded after qualitative analysis of the iPad for literacy instruction with children with disabilities, "Together with the teachers, we therefore argue that engagement with iPads through touch offered this highly diverse group of students more accessible routes into literacy than traditional literacy resources" (p. 114).

SUMMARY

The iPad, like the personal computer, has become an important aspect of literacy instruction. This isn't just in terms of how they support traditional literacy learning, but also in terms of children learning to live in a digital world. Although the very recent introduction of the iPad prevents the existence of abundant research, research on personal computers and the research that is available on iPad support its use. It is important that iPads be incorporated into the literacy curriculum, appropriate instructional strategies be employed, and that the iPad's ability to bridge home and school be considered. In addition, specific use with children with disabilities should continue to be explored. Although it is exciting for educators and families alike, professionals are faced with the challenge of keeping current on the available apps and their functions.

Summary of the use of iPads and mobile technology for literacy intervention:

1. The use of computer technology for literacy instruction has transitioned from primarily personal computers to the inclusion of the iPad and other mobile technologies. These mobile technologies are providing literacy support to all stages of traditional literacy as well as exposure to New and Multiple literacies.

2. For most children, iPads and apps can provide instructional technology that supports the literacy curriculum. This requires educators to clearly define literacy skills and be aware of apps and iPad functions that target these skills.

3. In order for educators to fully utilize the iPad, it is important they become familiar with the apps that are available. Literacy apps may range from interactive books (e.g., to letter-sound correspondence and early phonics (e.g., *Starfall ABCs,* Starfall*),* drawing and early writing (e.g., *Doddle Buddy for iPads,* Pinger apps), early reading/decoding (e.g., *Starfall Learn to Read*, Starfall), and creating stories (e.g. *Picotello*, AssistiveWare)). As with communication and language apps, blogs and webpages such as "apps for early literacy" available through Spectronics (n.d.b) may provide helpful information.

4. There should be a systematic process and framework for introducing apps to children in order to support literacy learning. Models such as the "Gradual Release Model" (Northrop & Killeen, 2013) provide guidance related how to incorporate use of the iPad into teaching a specific skill.

5. Adaptations are needed to provide the most appropriate technology for children with disabilities. This includes becoming knowledgeable regarding accessibility features available on the iPad (Fernandes, 2011a).

6. Providing appropriate literacy instruction to children with disabilities should include the use of assistive technologies (Erickson et al., 2010). Therefore understanding the many ways that assistive technology including the iPad can provide children with disabilities with access to literacy learning is imperative.

7. Professionals should use existing information regarding the benefits of traditional computers when considering how iPads can promote literacy. For example Rankin-Erickson, Wood, Beukelman, and Beukelman (2003) used the word processing program Write:OutLoud on a desktop computer to assist first grade students in decoding selected words in stories. This type of activity could be easily adapted to a tablet computer such as the iPad.

8. The use of tablet computers can be used to bridge literacy learning between home and school environments, which needs to be an important aspect of iPad use. An important feature of the iPad is its portability as well as its ease of use.

9. Similar to the use of the iPad for language development, how best to integrate iPad technologies and traditional teaching materials should continue to be explored. For example, hard copy books may still be preferred for shared reading by some parents. E-books, however, may provide literacy support when parents are unable to read with the child (Vaala & Takeuchi, 2012)

10. Training and support needs to be provided. This should not just involve finding out about apps, but about how to systematically use the apps. This should include training related to understanding iPad operating systems and upgrades (Fernandes, 2011c). Although this may include working with teachers reluctant to use technology (Cubelic & Larwin, 2014), training may not be as difficult as anticipated due to the intuitive nature of the iPad (Manko, 2014).

11. Another important consideration is how the use of the iPad can be coordinated with other technologies such as Smart Boards. Projecting the images of the iPad onto a larger display may provide opportunities for student collaboration (Sandvik et al., 2012).

12. Consideration should be given to benefits beyond those of specific literacy skills. Oladunjoye (2013) discusses how the iPad provided an impetus for social interaction. The author described how both apps with a constructivist perspective (e.g., child creates a car) and a behaviorist perspective (e.g., child had to provide the correct response) created opportunities for social interactions between children.

13. There are several models of how iPads are used in classrooms (e.g., individual use, shared classroom iPads) (An & Alon, 2013) or by speech-language pathologists (Fernandes, 2011a). How best to provide access to the iPads and current apps should be a consideration.

CONCLUSION

Focused on three primary functions of applications targeting language and literacy development, this chapter introduces the use of iPads and mobile technology for AAC, language intervention and literacy intervention for children with developmental disabilities. It starts with comparison of iPads and mobile technology and dedicated AAC devices including information on cost, funding, support for families and professionals, and adaptations for specific populations such as those with limited physical access. AAC provides a mode of communication for individuals with a range of disabilities including those with intellectual disabilities, ASD, and severe speech and physical disabilities. Mobile technologies and iPads specifically have revolutionized the field of AAC by providing an alternative method for developing a speech-generating device (McNaughton & Light, 2013). Current research documenting the effectiveness of iPads and mobile technology as communication devices is provided. Additionally, resources for learning about and comparing the currently available iPad and mobile technology communication applications are discussed.

The use of iPad and mobile technology in facilitating language intervention for children with developmental disabilities is explored. While communication applications provide a mode of communication to assist individuals with limited functional communication, other applications simply provide a stimulus for facilitating receptive and expressive language. These applications have become a frequently used tool for speech-language pathologists and educators working with children with a range of developmental disabilities. How these applications differ from other educational formats including more traditional computer programs are discussed as well as the evidence supporting these programs is presented.

Similarly, there are numerous iPad and mobile technology applications that address the development of literacy skills. These include early storybook reading, phonological awareness, and early writing. They are being used for a host of populations including children who are typically developing, children with intellectual disabilities, children with ASD and children who are deaf or hard of hearing. The chapter categorizes the specific skills addressed by the applications and how they can be incorporated into a comprehensive literacy program.

iPads and mobile technology can be effective tools in facilitating language and literacy development for children with developmental disabilities. However, parents, educators and speech-language pathologists should be cautious due to the technology's inherent challenges and limitations. For example, the quality of different apps vary since not all developers necessarily have the adequate expertise and experience working with children, let alone children with developmental disabilities. Second, the numerous apps and ever-changing technology makes it challenging to match the individual to the most appropriate devices/apps. Substantial training for children, parents and professionals is needed to ensure the optimal use of the app or device function. Third, it is critical to match the language/literacy goals and curricula to an appropriate app or iPad function, which does not always occur in practice. Furthermore, parents and professionals should ensure that the use of the iPad and mobile technology enhances communication and interaction between the child and adults/peers rather than allowing the child to withdraw. It can be problematic when children, both with developmental disabilities and typically developing, become too dependent on technology – children who already have difficulties with social interactions may be encouraged to interact with technology instead of people. This may inadvertently reinforce their avoidance of social interactions and not promote their building relationships with people. Finally, parents and professionals need to provide appropriate adaptations for children with disabilities. For example, children with severe physical disabilities may need particular assistance in using iPads and mobile technology. Used properly, iPads and mobile technology may be a valuable accelerator of language and literacy development of children with developmental disabilities; whereas improper or careless use can cause the technology to be a distraction that further delays the communication development of this population.

ACKNOWLEDGMENT

The authors would like to thank Nicole Molumby for her assistance in locating resources for this chapter.

REFERENCES

AAC TechConnect. (n.d.). *AAC TechConnect*. Retrieved April 3, 2015 from http://www.aactechconnect.com

Ablenet. (n.d.). *Ablenet*. Retrieved April 3 from http://www.ablenetinc.com

Achmadi, D., Kagohara, D. M., van der Meer, L., O'Reilly, M., Lancioni, G. E., Sutherland, D., & Sigafoos, J. et al. (2012). Teaching Advance operation of an iPod-based speech-generating device to two students with autism spectrum disorders. *Research in Autism Spectrum Disorders*, 6(4), 1258–1264. doi:10.1016/j.rasd.2012.05.005

Alberto, P. A., Fredrick, L., Hughes, M., McIntosh, L., & Cihak, D. (2007). Components of visual literacy: Teaching logos. *Focus on Autism and Other Developmental Disabilities*, 22(4), 234–243. doi:1 0.1177/10883576070220040501

Alliano, A., Herriger, K., Koustsoftas, A. D., & Bartlotta, T. E. (2012). A review of 21 iPad applications for augmentative and alternative communication purposes. *SIG 12 Perspectives on Augmentative and Alternative Communication, 21*(2), 60-71. doi:10.1044/aac21.2.60

American Speech-Language-Hearing Association. (2001). *Roles and responsibilities of speech-language pathologi ts with respect to reading and writing in children and adolescents* [Guidelines]. Retrieved on April, 3, 2015 from http://www.asha.org/policy/GL2001-00062.htm#sthash.3521rREs.dpuf

An, H., & Alon, S. (2013). iPad implementation models in K-12 school environments: An exploratory study. In R. McBride & M. Searson (Eds.), *Proceedings of Society for Information Technology & Teacher Education International Conference 2013* (pp. 3005-3011). Chesapeake, VA: AACE.

Artemenko, S. (2014). App-titude: Apps that excite our youngest clients: These interactive apps feature visuals that make word-learning and talking fun for tots. *The ASHA Leader, 19*(2), 38–39. doi:10.1044/ leader.APP.19022014.38

Attainment Company. (n.d.). *Attainment Company.* Retrieved April 3, 2015 from http://www.attainment-company.com/assistive-technology

Avaz Together. (n.d.). *Avaz Together.* Retrieved April 3, 2015 from http://www.avazapp.com/features/

Beschorner, B., & Hutchinson, A. (2013). iPads as a literacy teaching tool in early childhood. *International Journal of Education in Mathematics, Science, and Technology, 1*(1), 16–24.

Beukelman, D. R., & Mirenda, P. (2013). *Augmentative and alternative communication: Supporting children and adults with complex communication needs* (4th ed.). Baltimore, MD: Paul H. Brookes Publishing.

Boston Children's Hospital. (n. d.). *Augmentative communication program handouts and resources.* Retrieved August 13, 2014 from http://www.childrenshospital.org/centers-and-services/programs/a-_-e/ augmentative-communication-program/downloads

Bradshaw, J. (2013). The use of augmentative and alternative communication apps for the iPAD, iPod and iPhone: An overview of recent developments. *Tizard Learning Disability Review, 18*(1), 31–37. doi:10.1108/13595471311295996

Brady, L. (2012). iPad Apps can support evidence-based practice. *Speech Therapy for Autism: Technology, Speech Therapy and Autism.* Retrieved June 25, 2014, from http://proactivespeech.wordpress.com/ author/proactivespeech/page/2/

Bruno-Dowling, S. (2012). *How many SLPs are really using iPads?* Retrieved June 26, 2014 http:// community.advanceweb.com/blogs/sp_1/archive/2012/03/13/how-many-slps-are-really-using-ipads.aspx

Cardon, T. (2012). Teaching caregivers to implement video modeling imitation training via iPad for their children with autism. *Research in Autism Spectrum Disorders, 6*(4), 1389–1400. doi:10.1016/j. rasd.2012.06.002

Chapple, D. (2011). The evolution of augmentative communication and the importance of alternative access. *SIG 12 Perspectives on Augmentative and Alternative Communication, 20*(1), 34-37. doi:10.1044/aac20.1.34

Christakis, D. A. (2014). Interactive media use at younger than the age of 2 years: Time to rethink the *American Academy of Pediatrics Guideline? JAMA Pediatrics, 168*(5), 399–400. doi:10.1001/jamapediatrics.2013.5081 PMID:24615347

Cochran, P. S., & Nelson, L. K. (1999). Technology applications in intervention for preschool-age children with language disorders. *Seminars in Speech and Language, 20*(3), 203–218. doi:10.1055/s-2008-1064018 PMID:10480492

Collisson, B. A., & Long, S. H. (1993). Computer-assisted language intervention: What difference does the clinician make? *Language, Speech, and Hearing Services in Schools, 24*(3), 179–180. doi:10.1044/0161-1461.2403.179

Cooper, R. J., & Associates. Inc. (n.d.). Apps, ipads accessories, software and hardware for persons with special needs. Retrieved April 3, 2014 from http://www.rjcooper.com

Costello, J. M., Shane, H. C., & Caron, J. (2013). *AAC, mobile devices and apps: Growing pains with evidenced based practice.* Boston Children's Hospital. Retrieved June 28, 2014 from http://www.vantatenhove.com/files/papers/AACandApps/CostelloShaneCaron-WhitePaper.pdf

Cubelic, C. C., & Larwin, K. H. (2014). The use of iPad technology in the kindergarten classroom: A quasi-experimental investigation of the impact on early literacy skills. *Comprehensive Journal of Educational Research, 2*(4), 47–59.

DeCurtis, L. L., & Ferrer, D. (2011, September 20). Toddlers and technology: Teaching the techniques, *The ASHA Leader*. Retrieved June 25, 2014, from http://www.asha.org/Publications/leader/2011/110920/Toddlers-and-Technology.htm#2

Dobler, E. (2012). Using iPads to promote literacy in the primary grades. *Reading Today, 29*(3), 18–19.

Dolic, J., Pibernik, J., & Bota, J. (2012). Evaluation of mainstream table devices for symbol based AAC communication. *KES-AMSTA'12 Proceedings of the 6th KES international conference on Agent and Multi-Agent Systems: Technologies and Applications* (pp. 251-260). Berlin: Springer-Verlag. doi:10.1007/978-3-642-30947-2_29

Duck Duck Moose. (n.d.). *Duck Duck Moose: Award winning education apps for children.* Retrieved April 3, 2015 from http://www.duckduckmoose.com

Enabling Devices. (n.d.) *Assistive technology – Products for people with disabilities.* Retrieved April 3 from https://enablingdevices.com/catalog

Erickson, K. A., Hatch, P., & Clendon, S. (2010). Literacy, assistive technology, and students with significant disabilities. *Focus on Exceptional Children, 42*(5), 1–16.

Fager, S., Bardach, L., Russell, S., & Higginbotham, J. (2012). Access to augmentative and alternative communication: New technologies and clinical decision making. *Journal of Pediatric Rehabilitation Medicine: An Interdisciplinary Approach, 5*(1), 63–51. doi:10.3233/PRM-2012-0196 PMID:22543893

Fernandez, B, (2011a). iTherapy: The revolution of mobile devices within the field of speech therapy. *SIG 16 Perspectives on School-Based Issues, 12*(2), 35-40. doi:10.1044/sbi12.2.35

Fernandez, B. (2011b). Is the iPad revolutionizing speech therapy? From an SLP & app developer. *ASHA Sphere*. Retrieved June 25, 2014, from http://blog.asha.org/2011/06/07/is-the-ipad-revolutionizing-speech-therapy-from-an-slp-app-developer/

Fernandez, B. (2011c). Calling all SLPs and teachers to update the iOS system on their iPads & IPods. *ASHA Sphere*. Retrieved June 25, 2014, from http://blog.asha.org/2011/04/26/calling-all-slps-and-teachers-to-update-the-ios-system-on-their-ipads-ipods/

Flewitt, R., Kucirkova, N., & Messer, D. (2014). Touch the virtual, touching the real: iPads and enabling literacy for students experiencing disability. *Australian Journal of Language and Literacy, 37*(2), 107–116.

Flores, M., Musgrove, K., Renner, S., Hinton, V., Strozier, S., Franklin, S., & Hill, D. (2012). A comparison of communication using the Apple iPAD and a picture based system. *Augmentative and Alternative Communication, 28*(2), 74–84. doi:10.3109/07434618.2011.644579 PMID:22263895

GeekSLP. (n.d.). *GeekSLP.com: Your source of educational apps and technology information.* Retrieved April 3, 2015 from http://www.geekslp.com

Good Karma Applications. (n.d.). *Good karma applications.* Retrieved April 3, 2015 from http://www.attainmentcompany.com/assistive-technology

Gosnell, J. (2011). Apps: An emerging tool for SLPs; A plethora of apps can be used to develop expressive, receptive, and other language skills. *The ASHA Leader.* Retrieved June 26, 2014 from http://www.asha.org/publications/leader/2011/111011/apps--an-emerging-tool-for-slps.htm

Gosnell, J., Costello, J., & Shane, H. (2011a). There isn't always an app for that! *SIG 12 Perspectives on Augmentative and Alternative Communication, 20(1),* 7-8. doi:10.1044/aac20.1.7

Gosnell, J., Costello, J., & Shane, H. (2011b). Using a clinical approach to answer "what communication apps should we use?" *SIG 12 Perspectives on Augmentative and Alternative Communication, 20(3),* 87-96. doi:10.1044/aac20.3.87

Graham, M. (2011). *Who wants lemonade?* Retrieved June 26, 2014 http://all4mychild.com/blog/?p=168

Hershberger, D. (2011). Mobile technology and AAC apps from an AAC developer's Perspective. *SIG 12 Perspectives on Augmentative and Alternative Communication, 20(1),* 28-33. doi:10.1044/aac20.1.28

Higginbotham, J. & Jacobs, S. (2011). The future of the android operating system for augmentative and alternative communication. *SIG 12 Perspectives on Augmentative and Alternative Communication, 20*(2), 52-56. doi:10.1044/aac20.2.52

Hutchinson, A., Beschorner, B., & Schmidt-Crawford, D. (2012). Exploring the use of the iPad for literacy learning. *The Reading Teacher, 66*(1), 15-23. doi: 10:1002/TRTR01090

Inspiration Software, Inc. (n.d.). *Inspiration Software, Inc.* Retrieved April 3, 2015 from http://www.inspiration.com

iTouchiLearn Apps. (n.d.). *iTouchiLearn apps: Mobile apps for early learners.* Retrieved April 3, 2015 from http://itouchilearnapps.com

Kaderavek, J. N. (2011). *Language disorders in children: Fundamental concepts in assessment and intervention.* Boston, MA: Allyn & Bacon Publishing.

Kagohara, D. M., Sigafoos, J., Achmadi, D., O'Reilly, M., & Lancioni, G. (2011). Teaching children with autism spectrum disorders to check the spelling of words. *Research in Autism Spectrum Disorders, 6*(1), 304–310. doi:10.1016/j.rasd.2011.05.012

Kagohara, D. M., van der Meer, L., Achmadi, D., Green, V., O'Reilly, M., Lancioni, G., & Sigafoos, J. et al. (2012). Teaching picture naming to two adolescents with autism spectrum disorders using systematic instruction and speech-generating devices. *Research in Autism Spectrum Disorders, 6*(1), 1224–1233. doi:10.1016/j.rasd.2012.04.001

Kagohara, D. M., van der Meer, L., Achmadi, D., Green, V., O'Reilly, M. F., Mulloy, A., & Sigafoos, J. et al. (2010). Behavioral intervention promotes successful use of an iPod-Based communication device by an adolescent with autism. *Clinical Case Studies, 9*(5), 328–338. doi:10.1177/1534650110379633

Kagohara, D. M., van der Meer, L., Ramdoss, S., O'Reilly, M. F., Lancioni, G. E., Davis, T. N., & Sigafoos, J. et al. (2013). Using iPods and iPads in teaching programs for individuals with developmental disabilities: A systematic review. *Research in Developmental Disabilities, 34*(1), 147–156. doi:10.1016/j.ridd.2012.07.027 PMID:22940168

King, A. M., Thomeczek, M., Voreis, G., & Scott, V. (2014). iPad use in children and young adults with Autism Spectrum Disorder: An observational study. *Child Language Teaching and Therapy, 30*(2), 159–173. doi:10.1177/0265659013510922

Kliewer, C., Biklen, D., & Kasa-Hendrickson, C. (2006). Who may be literate? Disability and resistance to the cultural denial of competence. *American Educational Research Journal, 43*(2), 163–192. doi:10.3102/00028312043002163

Koppenhaver, D. A., & Erickson, K. (2003). Natural emergent literacy supports for preschoolers with autism and severe communication impairments. *Topics in Language Disorders, 23*(4), 283–293. doi:10.1097/00011363-200310000-00004

Lanyon, H. (2012). *The iPad and augmentative and alternative communication. Unpublished Graduate Research Project.* Springfield, MO: Missouri State University.

Lee, A., Lang, R., Davenport, K., Moore, M., Rispoli, M., van der Meer, L., . . . Chung, C. (2013). Comparison of therapist implemented and iPad-assisted interventions for children with autism. *Developmental Neurorehabilitation.* Retrieved June 25, 2014, from http://informahealthcare.com/doi/abs/10.3109/17518423.2013.830231

Light, J., & McNaughton, D. (2012). Supporting the communication, language, and literacy development of children with complex communication needs: State of the Science and Future Research Priorities. *Assistive Technology, 24*(1), 34-44. doi: 10. 1080/10400435.2011.684717

Lorah, E. R., Crouser, J., Gilroy, S. P., Tincani, M., & Hantula, D. (2014). Within stimulus prompting to teach symbol discrimination using an iPad speech generating device. *Journal of Developmental and Physical Disabilities, 26*(3), 335–346. doi:10.1007/s10882-014-9369-1

Machalicek, W., Sanford, A., Lang, R., Rispoli, M., Molfenter, N., & Mbesha, M. K. (2010). Literacy interventions for students with physical and developmental disabilities who use aided AAC: A systematic review. *Journal of Developmental and Physical Disabilities, 22*(3), 219–240. doi:10.1007/s10882-009-9175-3

Manko, J. (2013/2014). Technology driven literacy instruction: Liberty Elementary's iPad initiative. *Reading Today, 31*(3), 35.

Masterson, J. J., Apel, K., & Wood, L. A. (2002). Technology and literacy: Decisions for the new millennium. In K. G. Butler & E. R. Silliman (Eds.), *Speaking, Reading, and Writing in Children with Language Learning Disabilities* (pp. 273–293). Mahwah, NJ: Lawrence Erlbaum Associates Publishers.

McBride, D. (2011). AAC evaluations and new mobile technologies: Asking and answering the right questions. *SIG 12 Perspectives on Augmentative and Alternative Communication, 20(1),* 9-16. doi:10.1044/aac20.1.9

McCarthy, J. H., Beukelman, D. R., & Hogan, T. P. (2011). Impact of computerized "sounding out" on spelling performance of a child who use AAC: A preliminary report. *SIG 12 Perspectives on Augmentative and Alternative Communication, 20(4),* 119-124. doi:10.1044/aac20.4.119

McLeod, L. (2011). Game Changer. *Perspectives on AAC, 20*(1), 17–18. doi:10.1044/aac20.1.17

McNab, K. (2013). *Bridging the digital divide with iPads: Effects on early literacy.* Paper presented at the conference of the International Society for Technology in Education, San Antonio, TX.

McNaughton, D., & Light, J. (2013). The iPad and Mobile Technology Revolution: Benefits and Challenges for Individuals who require Augmentative and Alternative Communication. *Augmentative and Alternative Communication, 29*(2), 107–116. doi:10.3109/07434618.2013.784930 PMID:23705813

Meder, A. (2012). *Mobile media devices and communication applications as a form of augmentative and alternative communication: An assessment of family wants, needs, and preferences.* Unpublished Master's Thesis, University of Kansas.

Mobile Education Store. (n.d.). *Mobile Education Store: Apps.* Retrieved April 3, 2015 from http://mobile-educationstore.com/category/apps

Mumy, A. P. (2012). One-dimensional speech-language therapy: Is the iPad Alone Enough. *ASHA Sphere.* Retrieved June 25, 2014, from http://blog.asha.org/2012/06/05/one-dimensional-speech-language-therapy-is-the-ipad-alone-enough/

National Reading Panel. (2000). Teaching children to read: An evidenced-based assessment of the scientific research literature on reading and its implications for reading instruction. Retrieved June 27, 2014 from http://nationalreadingpanel.org/Publications/summary.htm

Niemeijer, D., Donnellan, A. M., & Robledo, J. A. (2012). Taking the pulse of augmentative and alternative communication on iOS. *AssistiveWare*. Retrieved June 25, 2014, from http://www.assistiveware.com/taking-pulse-augmentative-and-alternative-communication-ios

Night and Day Studios. (n.d.). *Night and Day Studios.* Retrieved April 3, 2015 http://www.nightanddaystudios.com

Northup, L., & Killeen, E. (2013). A framework for using iPads to build early literacy skills. *The Reading Teacher, 66*(7), 531–537. doi:10.1002/TRTR.1155

Oceanhouse Media. (n.d.). *Oceanhouse Media.* Retrieved April 3, 2015 from http://www.oceanhousemedia.com

Oladunjoye, O. K. (2013). *iPad and computer devices in preschool: A tool for literacy development among teachers and children in preschool.* Unpublished Master's thesis, Stockholm University, Sweden. Retrieved June 27, 2014 from http://www.diva-portal.org/smash/get/diva2:640202/COVER01

Outfit7 (n.d.). *Outfit7.* Retrieved April 3, 2015 from http://outfit7.com/apps/talking-tom-cat-1/

Parette, H. P., Hourcade, J. J., Blum, C., Watts, E. J., Stoner, J. B., Wojcik, B. W., & Chrismore, S. B. (2013). Technology user groups and early childhood education: A preliminary study. *Early Childhood Education Journal, 41(3),* 171-179. Doi: 10:1007/s10643-012-0548-3.

Paul, P., & Wang, Y. (2012). *Literate thought -- Understanding comprehension and literacy.* Sudbury, MA: Jones & Bartlett.

Pinger apps (n.d.). *Pinger apps.* Retrieved April 3, 2015 from https://www.pinger.com/content/apps.html

Playhome Software, Ltd. (n.d.). *My playhome.* Retrieved April 3, 2015 from http://www.myplayhome-app.com

PrAACtical AAC. (n.d.) *PrAACtical AAC supports for language learning.* Retrieved April 3, 2015 from http://praacticalaac.org

Prentke Romich Company. (n.d.). *Lamp Words for Life.* Retrieved April 3, 2015 from https://aacapps.com

Rankin-Erickson, J. L., Wood, L. A., Beukelman, D. R., & Beukelman, H. M. (2003). Early computer literacy; first graders use the "talking" computer. *Reading Improvement, 40*(3), 132–144.

RERC on Communication Enhancement. (2011, March 14). *Mobile devices and communication apps: An AAC-RERC white paper.* Retrieve June 27, 2014, from http://aac-rerc.psu.edu/index.php/pages/show/id/46

Rummel-Hudson, R. (2011). A revolution at their fingertips. *SIG 12 Perspectives on Augmentative and Alternative Communication, 20*(1), 19-23. doi:10.1044/aac20.1.19

Sailers, E. (2010). *How I became the speech guy with an iPad.* Retrieved June 26, 2014 from http://blog.asha.org/2010/09/21/how-i-became-the-speech-guy-with-an-ipad/

Sandvik, M., Smordal, O., & Osterud, S. (2012). Exploring iPads in practitioners' repertoires for language learning and literacy practices in kindergarten. *Nordic Journal of Digital Literacy, 7*(3), 204–220.

Schery, T., & O'Connor, L. C. (1992). The effectiveness of school-based computer language intervention with severely handicapped children. *Language, Speech, and Hearing Services in Schools, 23*(1), 43–47. doi:10.1044/0161-1461.2301.43

Schery, T., & O'Connor, L. C. (1997). Language intervention: Computer training for young children with special needs. *British Journal of Educational Technology, 28*(4), 271–279. doi:10.1111/1467-8535.00034

Scuito, E. W. (2013). The iPad: Using new technology for teaching reading, language, and speech for children with hearing loss. *Independent Studies and Capstones: Paper 676.* Program in Audiology and Communication Sciences, Washington University school of Medicine. St. Louis, MO. Retrieved June 26, 2014 from http://digitalcommons.wustl.edu/pacs_capstones/676/

Sennott, S. (2011). An introduction to the special issue on new mobile AAC technologies. *SIG 12 Perspectives on Augmentative and Alternative Communication, 20*(1), 3-6. doi:10.1044/aac20.1.3

Shane, H. C., Blackstone, S., Vanderheiden, G., Williams, M., & DeRuyter, F. (2012). Using AAC technology to access the world. *Assistive Technology, 24*(1), 3–13. doi:10.1080/10400435.2011.64871 6 PMID:22590795

Silver Kite. (n.d.). *Silver Kite: The assistive technology solution center.* Retrieved April 3, 2015 from http://www.assistiveware.com

Simpson, A., Walsh, M., & Rowsell, J. (2013). The digital reading path: Research modes and multidirectionality with iPads. *Literacy, 47*(3), 123–130. doi:10.1111/lit.12009

Smarty Ears Apps. (n.d.). *Smarty Ears Apps.* Retrieved April 15, 2015 from http://smartyearsapps.com

Snape, J., & Maiolo, B. (2013). *Using iPads in Speech Pathology.* Independent Living Centre WA. Retrieved June 26, 2014 from http://ilc.com.au/wp-content/uploads/2013/08/ilc_tech_using_ipads_in_speech_pathology.pdf

Speak MODalities. (n.d.) *Speak MODalities.* Retrieved on April 3, 2015 from http://speakmod.com/products/speakall/

Spectronics. (n.d.a). *Top 10 apps for language development.* Retrieved April 3, 2015 from http://www.spectronicsinoz.com/online/resource/top-10-apps-for-language-development/

Spectronics. (n.d.b). *Apps for early literacy series.* Retrieved April 3, 2015 from http://www.spectronicsinoz.com/online/resource/apps-for-early-literacy-introduction/

Starfall. (n.d.). *Starfall.* Retrieved April 3, 2015 from http://www.starfall.com

Steele, R. & Moromoff, P. (2011). Design challenges of AAC apps, on wireless portable devices, for persons with Aphasia. *SIG 12 Perspectives on Augmentative and Alternative Communication, 20*(2), 41-51. doi:.10.1044/aac20.2.41

Steele, S. C., & Mills, M. T. (2011). Vocabulary intervention of school-age children with language impairment: A review of evidence and good practice. *Child Language Teaching and Therapy, 27*(3), 354–370. doi:10.1177/0265659011412247 PMID:25104872

Sublime Speech. (n.d.). *Sublime speech: Speech therapy with a twist.* Retrieved April 3, 2015 from http://sublimespeech.com/tag/aac

Tobii Dynavox. (n.d.). *AAC software.* Retrieved on April 3, 2015 from http://www.tobiidynavox.com/software/#freeresources

TOCA BOCA. (n.d.). *TOCA BOCA.* Retrieved April 3, 2015 from http://tocaboca.com

Vaala, S., & Takeuchi, L. (2012). *Parent co-reading survey: Co-reading with children on iPads: Parents' perceptions and practices.* New York, NY: The Joan Ganz Cooney Center. Retrieved June 27, 2014, from http://www.joanganzcooneycenter.org/wp-content/uploads/2012/11/jgcc_ereader_parentsurvey_quick-report.pd

van der Meer, L., Didden, R., Sutherland, D., O'Reilly, M. F., Lancioni, G. E., & Sigafoos, J. (2012). Comparing three augmentative and alternative communication modes for children with developmental disabilities. *Journal of Developmental and Physical Disabilities*, *24*(5), 451–468. doi:10.1007/s10882-012-9283-3

van der Meer, L., Kagohara, D., Achmadi, D., O'Reilly, M. F., Lancioni, G. E., Sutherland, D., & Sigafoos, J. (2012). Speech-generating devices versus manual signing for children with developmental disabilities. *Research in Developmental Disabilities*, *33*(5), 1658–1669. doi:10.1016/j.ridd.2012.04.004 PMID:22554812

Westervelt, E. (June 11, 2014). *iPads allow kids with challenges to play in high school's band.* Retrieved June 27, 2014, from http://www.wbur.org/npr/320882414/ipads-allow-kids-with-challenges-to-play-in-high-schools-band

Wood, L., & Masterson, J. J. (1999). The use of technology to facilitate language skills in school-age children. *Seminars in Speech and Language*, *20*(3), 219–232. doi:10.1055/s-2008-1064019 PMID:10480493

Write:OutLoud. (1993). Wauconda, IL: Don Johnston Developmental Equipment.

ADDITIONAL READING

Beukelman, D. R., Fager, S., Ball, L., & Dietz, A. (2007). AAC for adults with acquired neurological conditions: A review. *Augmentative and Alternative Communication*, *23*(3), 230–242. doi:10.1080/07434610701553668 PMID:17701742

Binger, C., Ball, L., Dietz, A., Kent-Walsh, J., Lasker, J., Lund, S., & Quach, W. et al. (2012). Personnel roles in the AAC assessment process. *Augmentative and Alternative Communication*, *28*(4), 278–288. doi:10.3109/07434618.2012.716079 PMID:23256859

Bopp, K. D., Brown, K. E., & Mirenda, P. (2004). Speech-language pathologists' roles in the delivery of positive behavior support for individuals with developmental disabilities. *American Journal of Speech-Language Pathology*, *13*(1), 5–19. doi:10.1044/1058-0360(2004/003) PMID:15101810

Branson, D., & Demchak, M. (2009). The use of augmentative and alternative communication methods with infants and toddlers with disabilities: A research review. *Augmentative and Alternative Communication*, *25*(4), 274–286. doi:10.3109/07434610903384529 PMID:19883287

Costigan, F. A., & Light, J. (2010). A review of preservice training in augmentative and alternative communication for speech-language pathologists, special education teachers, and occupational therapists. *Assistive Technology*, *22*(4), 200–212. doi:10.1080/10400435.2010.492774 PMID:21306066

Diamandis, P. H., & Kotler, S. (2012). *Abundance: The future is better than you think*. New York: Free Press.

Falloon, G. (2013, October). Young students using iPads: App design and content influence on their learning pathways. *Computers & Education*, *68*, 505–521. doi:10.1016/j.compedu.2013.06.006

Fried-Oken, M., Beukelman, D. R., & Hux, K. (2012). Current and future AAC research considerations for adults with acquired cognitive and communication impairments. *Assistive Technology*, *24*(1), 56–66. doi:10.1080/10400435.2011.648713 PMID:22590800

Ganz, J. B., Earles-Vollrath, T. L., Heath, A. K., Parker, R. I., Rispoli, M. J., & Duran, J. B. (2011). A meta-analysis of single case research studies on aided augmentative and alternative communication systems with individuals with autism spectrum disorders. *Journal of Autism and Developmental Disorders*, *42*(1), 60–74. doi:10.1007/s10803-011-1212-2 PMID:21380612

Goldin, C., & Katz, L. F. (2008). *The race between education and technology*. Cambridge, MA: Harvard University Press.

Heft, T. M., & Swaminathan, S. (2002). The effects of computers on the social behavior of preschoolers. *Journal of Research in Childhood Education*, *16*(2), 162–174. doi:10.1080/02568540209594982

Hutchison, A., & Reinking, D. (2011). Teachers' perceptions of integrating informatioini and communication technologies into literacy instruction: A national survey in the U.S. *Reading Research Quarterly*, *46*(4), 308–329.

Kucrikova, N., Messer, D., Sheehy, K., & Panadero, C. F. (2014, February). Children's engagement with educational iPad apps: Insights from a Spanish classroom. *Computers & Education*, *71*, 175–184. doi:10.1016/j.compedu.2013.10.003

Martin, F., & Ertzberger, J. (2013, October). Here and now mobile learning: An experimental study on the use of mobile technology. *Computers & Education*, *68*, 76–85. doi:10.1016/j.compedu.2013.04.021

Plowman, L., & Stephen, C. (2005). Children, play, and computers in preschool education. *British Journal of Educational Technology*, *36*(2), 145–158. doi:10.1111/j.1467-8535.2005.00449.x

Plowman, L., Stephen, C., & McPake, J. (2010). Supporting young children's learning with technology at home and in preschool. *Research Papers in Education*, *25*(1), 93–113. doi:10.1080/02671520802584061

Schlosser, R. W., & Sigafoos, J. (2009). Navigating evidence-based information sources in augmentative and alternative communication. *Augmentative and Alternative Communication*, *25*(4), 225–235. doi:10.3109/07434610903360649 PMID:19903133

Shane, H. C., Laubscher, E. H., Schlosser, R. W., Flynn, S., Sorce, J. F., & Abramson, J. (2012). Apply technology to visually support language and communication in individuals with autism spectrum disorders. *Journal of Autism and Developmental Disorders*, *42*(6), 1228–1235. doi:10.1007/s10803-011-1304-z PMID:21691867

Simeonsson, R. J., Bjorck-Akesson, E., & Lollar, D. J. (2012). Communication, disability, and ICF-CY. *Augmentative and Alternative Communication*, *28*(1), 3–10. doi:10.3109/07434618.2011.653829 PMID:22364533

Wang, X. C., & Ching, C. C. (2003). Social construction of computer experience in a first-grade classroom: Social processes and mediating artifacts. *Early Education and Development*, *14*(3), 335–361. doi:10.1207/s15566935eed1403_4

Wilkinson, K. M., Light, J., & Drager, K. (2012). Considerations for the composition of visual scene displays: Potential contributions of information from visual and cognitive sciences. *Augmentative and Alternative Communication*, *28*(3), 137–147. doi:10.3109/07434618.2012.704522 PMID:22946989

Williams, M. B., Krezman, C., & McNaughton, D. (2008). "Reach for the stars": Five principles for the next 25 years of AAC. *Augmentative and Alternative Communication*, *24*(3), 194–206. doi:10.1080/08990220802387851

KEY TERMS AND DEFINITIONS

Conventional Reading Skills: Conventional reading skills may include phonemic awareness if these skills are not fully developed, but specifically addresses a child's ability to decode as well as the development of reading fluency, comprehension, and vocabulary (NRP, 2000).

Emergent Literacy Skills: Emergent literacy skills develop prior to formal literacy instruction and include the development of oral language development, print awareness and book knowledge, phonological and phonemic awareness, and early writing.

Functional literacy: Functional literacy is the ability to obtain information through multiple pathways from the environment and use it to make decisions and choices, modify the environment and acquire pleasure.

Gradual Release Model: Northrop and Killeen (2013) propose a "gradual release model" as a framework for early literacy. The important aspects of the model is matching to the child's level and ensuring that the child understands the literacy content of the apps. Within this model, the teacher models and provides guided instruction and then independence for the child. They stress that it isn't the technology alone that increases the child's performance, but matching the technology which is motivational and fun to the child. Northup and Killen provided examples of apps that focused on phonics apps (letter formation, letter sounds, and blending of simple words). They recommended teaching the concept without the app and then teacher "think-aloud" when teaching the child to use the app to ensure the child isn't clicking through the app without understanding the literacy content.

Language Development and Intervention: Language development and intervention involves learning new concepts and vocabulary, developing expressive vocabulary, increasing length of utterance, learning new grammatical structures, and improving pragmatic skills.

Literacy Development and Intervention: Literacy development and intervention is expansive in terms of the many skills to be addressed in order for a child to become literate. This includes the development of traditional print literacy that begins at the emergent literacy stage and continues to conventional literacy skills.

Speech-generating Device: A speech-generating device is essentially a portable computer with a touch screen interface that provides voice output when an individual selects specific word or message.

Chapter 4
Early Literacy and AAC for Learners with Complex Communication Needs

Janis Doneski-Nicol
Northern Arizona University, USA

Jody Marie Bartz
Northern Arizona University, USA

ABSTRACT

Augmentative and Alternative Communication (AAC) systems are a common assistive technology (AT) intervention for learners with complex communication needs (CCN) – those learners who are unable to use speech and language as a primary mode of communication. AAC systems can be a powerful intervention; however, these systems must be integrated with strong, early and conventional literacy instructional opportunities. In this chapter, we provide parents, educators, researchers, academics, and other professionals with the most up to date and innovative information as well as practical resources regarding early literacy and AAC for learners with CCN. Emphasis will be on young children with CCN in preschool and early elementary school settings. Features of AAC systems and evidence-based literacy assessment and intervention, as well as the benefits and challenges, are presented to provide the reader with information on the current state of the field. The chapter concludes with directions for future research and provides a comprehensive list of resources and organizations.

INTRODUCTION

Learners with complex communication needs (CCN) face barriers to using speech and/or language as their primary communication mode. Learners with CCN are a heterogeneous population often with developmental disabilities, which may include autism, cerebral palsy, intellectual disability or other disabilities. Approximately 3.5 million persons in the United States do not have the speech skills to meet their communication needs on a daily basis (Beukelman & Miranda, 2005). Prevalence rates of 3-6% have been reported for school-aged learners (Matas, Mathy-Laikko, Beukelman & Legresley, 1985),

DOI: 10.4018/978-1-4666-8395-2.ch004

while Binger and Light (2006) report that for preschoolers receiving special education, the prevalence of CCN may be as high as 12%. Sign language skills may be introduced but may be potentially inadequate for independent and total communication. Without the ability to speak and, in a large percent of these learners, without the ability to use sign language as a meaningful mode of communication, these learners may have severely limited communication opportunities.

A common intervention for learners with CCN is the provision for augmentative and alternative communication (AAC) systems. Picture symbols representing words or phrases are selected by others and provided as a means to facilitate communication by pointing, directly or indirectly, to a desired symbol/ message. These symbols are presented in a variety of mediums from paper-based arrays to high tech computer based systems. Novel and independent communication requires literacy skills to compose and supplement messages that may not be available on AAC systems (Millar, Light, & McNaughton, 2004). Without literacy skills, learners who use AAC systems may encounter immediate and future long-term consequences which include: (a) decreased participation across settings, (b) decreased educational options, and (c) decreased options for independence and employment (Fallon, Light, McNaughton, Drager & Hammer, 2004; Millar, Light, McNaughton, 2004).

Gus Estrella, an individual with CCN, captured the power of literacy for persons with complex communication needs.

The words I was given were words that would produce pictures, not words that would make language. And they wanted me to master a language? I was also given piles of sentences and criticized for not using them. I don't know about you, but I don't think in terms of preformed sentences. Sometimes I even change my thought half way through the sentence, and I have also been known to throw in a very descriptive word, when the mood strikes me! I can think of few things more dehumanizing and even demeaning than selecting canned sentences from a list. And seeing that the subject matter you want to talk about is nowhere to be found! What gives communication joy is when you tell your partner something he or she doesn't already know, and perhaps you didn't know yourself what you were going to say until you were halfway through composing your sentences! (Estrella, 1997)

Learners with CCN who use AAC systems are often deprived of reading and writing skill instruction, which Estrella (1997) believes is necessary for "communication joy." Estrella was empowered with access to AAC systems and conventional literacy for full communication opportunities. Without these skills, learners have severe limitations throughout their lifespan (Koppenhaver, Hendrix, & Williams, 2007; Millar, Light & McNaughton, 2004).

It is well established in the literature that individuals with CCN can develop literacy skills (Koppenhaver, Hendrix, & Williams, 2007; Light, McNaughton, Weyer, & Karg, 2008; Lund & Light, 2006). Instruction can result in positive language, communication and literacy outcomes for children with CCN. A significant need exists to translate literacy research for learners with CCN into the literacy practices of homes, schools, and community programs (Light, McNaughton, Weyer, & Karg, 2008). Bringing the educational significance of literacy interventions to the forefront will afford ALL learners the opportunity to develop reading and literacy skills beyond the emergent level.

Since the 1970s, reading and writing instruction for learners with disabilities, has focused on functional skills such as sight words, which were necessary for survival (e.g., stop, women's, exit, etc.). These 'functional skills' do not provide ongoing support for literacy development. Indeed, they do not support literacy for independence (Browder, Spooner, & Bingham, 2004). This chapter challenges the reader to consider early and conventional literacy instruction as the most appropriate educational intervention for all learners, no matter how the learners may be labeled (e.g. developmental and intellectual disabilities). This chapter will provide direction across literacy assessment and instruction for educational teams, inclusive of families, teachers, related services personnel, and administrators, for learners with CCN who use AAC systems. This chapter considers the unique needs of learners with CCN and the power of literacy for these learners. This chapter will capture the early preschool and elementary stage when learners are acquiring early literacy skills and gradually transitioning to conventional literacy skills. Solid literacy foundations are necessary for children in this learning range to support ongoing success of reading and writing for learning in upper grades. Without solid literacy foundations, learning can stall.

Readers of this chapter will:

- Understand the significant impact of literacy skills for learners with CCN and significant support needs.
- Analyze opportunity and access literacy barriers and facilitators for learners with CCN.
- Understand current evidence-based assessment and instructional practices related to early literacy, AAC and learners with CCN.

BACKGROUND

Complex Communication Needs and Significant Support Needs

Learners with CCN require Assistive Technology (AT) tools and strategies to communicate across environments and with communication partners. Learners with CCN, considering the World Health Organization's International Classification of Functioning, Disability and Health model, often have health conditions, which significantly affect body functions and structures. These conditions are compounded by environmental factors as well as by personal factors, which directly impact participation across activities (Simeonsson, Bjorck-Akesson & Lollar, 2012). These heterogeneous learners may present with whole ranges of communication, language, intellectual, motor, visual, and hearing skills (Light & McNaughton, 2012b). Each learner has a unique profile, which may necessitate significant support needs. Individual learner needs must be considered in planning for communication and literacy learning.

Alternative and Augmentative Communication Systems

AAC systems must be established for learners with CCN as a means to participate in and benefit from literacy instruction. AAC systems are not a single communication device or a single letter board to augment communication. Rather, AAC systems consider the multiple modes of communication which may be used to support a learner with CCN, including gestures, sign language, picture symbol languages and letters to write messages (ASHA, 2004; Calculator, 2013).

Learners with CCN require opportunities to develop and practice communication and language skills beginning at an early age. "Postponing the consideration of AAC strategies when behaviors and physical conditions suggest high risk for delayed or impaired speech can be detrimental to a child's long-term speech and language development" (Cress & Marvin, 2003, p, 267). Early language, communication and literacy development services for children with CCN should be directly linked to AAC and should be provided early (Romski & Sevcik, 2005). While families and educational teams express concern that the provision of AAC systems will delay the development of speech, this myth has been dispelled across the research (ASHA, 2004; Blischak, Lombardino & Dyson, 2003; Millar, Light & Schlosser, 2006; Schlosser & Wendt, 2008). Early AAC interventions with infants and toddlers have increased intentional communication and aided the speech production abilities of these learners (Branson & Demchak, 2009; Romski, Sevcik, Adamson, Cheslock, Smith, Barker & Bakeman, 2010). Presentation of AAC early, provides opportunities for literacy activities as well as the development of conventional literacy skills.

Purposes of Communication and Communication Competencies

The provision of an AAC system is only the first step in developing meaningful communication. Learners with CCN must develop communication for the purpose of expressing wants and needs, information transfer, social closeness, and social etiquette (Light, 1998). An AAC system is only meaningful if educational teams facilitate ongoing opportunities for communication as well as development of communication competencies. Light (1998) identified four levels of communication competencies: (1) operational, (2) linguistic, (3) social and (4) strategic. Learners with CCN must develop operational skills specific to AAC systems including the skills of using symbols of the system(s) and the hardware of the system(s). Linguistic competence integrates both receptive and expressive language skills as well as AAC system symbol knowledge to create meaningful communication messages. Learners must also develop social competencies which include the rules involved in social interactions as well as the knowledge and judgment necessary to initiate, maintain, and terminate communication interactions. Finally, across communication competencies, learners with CCN must develop strategies that sustain communication and prevent and or overcome communication breakdowns through strategic competency skills (Light, 1998). Establishment of AAC systems and communication competencies should be integrated within literacy instruction.

Early Literacy

The term "literacy" is a broad term and a powerful skill for ALL learners. This chapter will focus on literacy from a traditional early literacy perspective, addressing the early skills necessary to read and write for a specific purpose and to support communication for learners with CCN. However, a necessary understanding, before moving forward in this chapter, is expressed by Hannon (2000): "We should be wary of promoting literacy as if it were self-evident as an end in itself. It is, rather, a means by which learners can reach goals which they may value for themselves" (p. 7).

Early literacy is a developmental stage, involving early experiences across reading, writing, and oral language. Early literacy skills are the reading and writing behaviors of young children which occur prior to conventional literacy skills, and are related to or predictive of conventional literacy skills (NELP, 2008; Sulzby, 1989). The National Early Learning Panel (NELP) (2008) identified the following early literacy skills as strong predictors of later conventional reading and writing skills: (1) alphabet knowledge, (2) phonological awareness, (3) rapid naming tasks, (4) writing or writing one's name and (5) phonological short-term memory. Weaker predictive evidence for oral language and concepts about print as well as perception skills was also identified. It should be noted that teaching sight words or symbol reading are not recommendations of the National Early Literacy Panel.

Conventional Literacy

The transition from early literacy to conventional literacy is a process of developing independence in reading and writing activities with the ultimate goal of independence to successfully read, comprehend, and compose desired materials (Kaderavek & Rabidoux, 2004). The National Reading Panel (2000) identified the instructional pieces of phonemic awareness, phonics, fluency, guided oral reading, teaching of vocabulary words and reading comprehension strategies as the pieces of a total reading instruction package to support attainment of independent and conventional literacy.

Power of Literacy for Learners with CCN

For learners without speech, literacy is one of the most powerful communication supports in society today. Literacy has a significant impact on quality of life across self-esteem, self-determination, independence, information gathering, organization, learning and entertainment for learners with CCN (Downing, 2005). The consequences for learners with CCN who fail to develop conventional literacy skills are more significant than simply not being able to read and write desired materials. While strong AAC language systems provide a first means for effective and efficient communication, literacy provides the power of supplementing these AAC language systems for full novel and independent communication (Light & McNaughton, 2009; Strum, Spadorcia, Cunningham, Cali, Staples, Erickson, Yoder & Koppenhaver, 2006). Without literacy skills, learners with CCN are dependent upon others to develop their communication message options (Beukelman & Mirenda, 2013). Literacy is a key to independence for learners with CCN. Christy Brown expresses this independence:

I drew it - the letter "A." There it was on the floor before me... I looked up. I saw my mother's face for a moment, tears on her cheeks...I had done it! It had started the thing that was to give my mind its chance of expressing itself...That one letter, scrawled on the floor with a broken bit of yellow chalk gripped between my toes, was my road to a new world, my key to mental freedom. (Brown, 1954, p. 17)

Early and conventional literacy opportunities for learners with CCN are significantly reduced or constrained by factors such as: attitudinal barriers, low expectations, limited opportunities, limited means of accessing literacy, limited time and age (Downing, 2005; Forts & Luckasson, 2011; Koppenhaver, Hendrix & Williams, 2007). Browder, Gibbs, Ahlgrim-Delzell, Courtade, Mraz, and Flowers (2008) further exposed these factors in their statement that "not everyone would agree that this population can or should be taught to read" (p.270). Most learners with CCN do not achieve conventional literacy skills, and those that do rarely attain skills beyond the second grade level (Sturm, Spadorcia, Cunningham, Cali, Staples, Erickson, Yoder & Koppenhaver, 2006). As the least powerful are the last to become literate, literacy is a source of conflict across history and can be viewed as a means of perpetuating discrimination (Hannon, 2000). In many cases learners with complex communication needs are considered to be "the least powerful." As stated by Koppenhaver (2000):

Unfortunately, our field has often treated emergent literacy as an end goal rather than a starting place. That is, practitioners have been quicker to accept emergent literacy and nonconventional performance than to consider how to move the student on to conventional reading and writing. (p. 273)

Literacy instruction can result in positive language, communication and literacy outcomes for learners with CCN. However, a history of limited literacy instruction for learners with CCN leaves deficits in the evidence-based practices from which learners may develop these powerful skills (Spooner, Rivera, Browder, Baker, & Salas, 2009). Results of research and evidence-based practices must be translated into daily practices of educational teams (Light, McNaughton, Weyer, & Karg, 2008).

No longer viewed as a set of particular skills, literacy refers to a status that accords people the opportunities and supports to communicate, given the skills and capacities they have and can develop. To be literate is to have status, respect, and accommodation from others, to have skills in communication (verbal, written, sign, gestural, or other language), and to have access to the information and technologies that make possible self-determined participation in the communication processes of one's communities and broader society (Ewing, 2000, p.1).

OPPORTUNITY BARRIERS AND FACILITATORS TO LITERACY

Barriers and facilitators to literacy can be framed through the constructs of opportunities and access (Beukelman & Mirenda, 1989). Opportunities are created by educational teams and situations that are out of the control of the learner whereas access is directly related to the learner and their educational team. Limited opportunities to literacy interactions, activities, and explicit instruction may be created by educational teams and situations which learners with CCN are unable to control, thus often creating immediate barriers across the lifespan (Beukelman & Mirenda, 1998). Opportunities to develop literacy skills require collaborative educational teams to provide access and recognize opportunities for literacy instruction above and beyond the emergent literacy level for learners with CCN, thus facilitating opportunity for independent communication (Erickson, Hatch & Clendon, 2010; Fallon, 2008; Koppenhaver, 2000). When opportunities are provided to ALL children, opportunity barriers are broken down and facilitators emerge. This chapter will present the reader with barriers and facilitators to literacy achievement for learners with CCN.

Policy

Educational teams must consider and implement two policies for learners with CCN including the Individuals with Disabilities Education Improvement Act (IDEIA) (2004) and No Child Left Behind (NCLB) (2001). IDEIA sets high achievement standards for all children with disabilities and guides special education services. Under IDEIA an Individual Education Plan (IEP) is developed for learners with disabilities by the educational team. The educational team must consider and document the AT needs of the individual learner necessary to meet IEP goals and objectives. NCLB (2001) enacted assessment, accountability, and Adequate Yearly Progress requirements for education agencies. Highly qualified teachers must provide instruction to all children. Literacy is a high NCLB priority and educational agencies are required to close achievement gaps and ensure that all children are reading at grade level by the end of third grade. These policies should facilitate educational teams' high expectations and literacy instruction for all learners.

Attitudes

Attitudes of educational teams can facilitate or directly create barriers to literacy instruction for learners with CCN. It is necessary to "embrace the 'zero reject' philosophy that has become widely accepted over the past 10 years and to remember that no one is "too anything" to benefit from either AAC instruction or the opportunity to develop in the area of literacy" (Mirenda, 2001, p. 1). Educational teams must assume the least dangerous assumption (Donnellan, 1984) that learners with CCN possess the competence and the ability to develop conventional literacy levels and must be provided with evidence-based explicit instruction and opportunities to develop language, communication and literacy. Denying these givens is a dangerous assumption which may lead to denying potential access to literacy.

Knowledge and Skill

Implementing successful assessment and intervention across literacy requires levels of knowledge and skills of reading, writing, and complex communication needs. The absence of this knowledge has been identified as a critical barrier to the development of literacy skills for learners with CCN (Sturm, et al., 2006). Educational teams must work collaboratively to (a) understand core literacy (reading and writing) instruction across grade levels, (b) maximize instructional time for all learners and (c) make knowledge-based curricular decisions that enable all students to access literacy (Sturm, et al., 2006).

Significant efforts to ensure that educators have these skill-sets across reading, writing, and communication prior to entry into the classroom, are necessary. Conner, Alberto, Compton, and O'Connor (2014) indicated, that combinations of professional development strategies including "coaching, linking student assessment data to instruction, using technology and participating in communities of practice, can support teacher's learning and implementation of research-based reading instruction" (p. xi). Pre-service preparation should include CCN and AAC instruction as well as comprehensive literacy skills and knowledge (Fallon, 2008, Pufpaff & Yssel, 2010). Continuing education opportunity offerings for educational teams should also be available to address effective literacy instruction for learners with CCN (Fallon, 2008).

Environment

Educational environments can serve as both facilitators and barriers to literacy success. Curriculum is shaped by educational environments and settings (Smith, 2000). Learners with complex communication needs are educated in a wide range of educational settings. These settings must be considered within the IEP process and the general education classroom should be the first setting considered and the initial starting point for all learners. This is the setting where all learners should be educated.

Learners with CCN in general education classrooms may be provided with educational and related services through a "push-in" model, which provides special education and related services in the general education classroom. While this service level may meet the needs of many learners and should be the initial attempted service model for literacy instruction, there may be intensive instruction needs that require consideration of a "pull-out" model of service, temporarily removing students from their general education classrooms and providing services in an alternative setting. The dynamics of classrooms often guide these decisions. However, educators must consider the lack of educational opportunities which may occur when learners are placed in alternative settings for educational instruction. Inclusive environments provide learners with CCN the benefit of interactions with peers who may provide rich modeling opportunities for natural communication, and direct instruction. Further, inclusive school environments provide rich literacy instruction across age-appropriate activities (Ruppar, 2013). One might consider the incredible richness of a kindergarten classroom.

Instructional Time

Learners in grades 1-3 engage in "extensive and repeated opportunities to build a range of reading skills" (Sturm, et al., 2006, p. 32). Engagement (Allington, 1977) and instruction time directly increase literacy skills for all learners (Sonnenschein, Stapleton, & Benson, 2010). Learners should receive 90-120 minutes of literacy instruction daily (Gunning, 2005). For struggling readers, the difference between 30 minutes and 60 minutes of instruction is significant (Harn, Linan-Thompson, & Roberts, 2008), and some students may require 60-90 minutes of additional daily instruction to make adequate literacy progress (Torgesen, Houston, Rissman, & Kosanovich, 2007). Instructional time must be reserved to facilitate literacy opportunities.

Competing Priorities

Educational teams face barriers to providing daily literacy instruction time in classrooms. These barriers may include personal care, therapies, and medical needs (Browder, Mims, Spooner, Ahlgrim-Delzell & Lee, 2008). Additionally, implementation of AT tools and strategies, which can support access to communication and learning, are often time-consuming (Copley & Ziviani, 2004). Educational teams must identify dedicated and integrated literacy instruction across all activities with appropriate AT supports, including opportunities during personal care, therapies, and medical procedures. Collaborative education teams should employ regular meetings and develop supports and accountability systems to facilitate success for learners with CCN (Hunt, Soto, Maier, Müller, & Goetz, 2002).

ACCESS BARRIERS AND FACILITATORS TO LITERACY

Access barriers are directly related to the individual strengths and needs of the learner with CCN and their educational team's ability to address these (Beukelman & Mirenda, 1998). Two conceptual models for AT decision making, the *Human, Activity, Assistive Technology (HAAT)* and the *Student, Environment, Tasks, and Tools (SETT)* provide models for identifying a learner's strengths and needs matched to the features of AT, applying best practice and potential predictive models for considering AT (Cook & Polgar, 2008; Giesbrecht, 2013). The core concepts of these two models provide for the construction of meaningful interactions between the learner, their desired activities and environments and the AT necessary to support activities. These models provide an opportunity for educational teams and learners to identify specific access barriers to successful literacy instruction and to systematically and consistently identify the AT tools necessary for success. Coupled with the Wisconsin Assistive Technology Initiative (WATI) *AT Checklist,* a form that provides categorical lists of AT tools, consideration of AT tools and strategies for all learners including AT for communication, reading, the motor aspects of writing, composition of writing and overall access to materials and instructional tools, can begin (Gierach, 2009).

Language and Communication

Many learners with CCN encounter challenges across expressive and receptive language and communication skills. From birth, children begin to develop both spoken and written language skills. These skills are interrelated and develop concurrently (Foley, 2003). However, learners with CCN may struggle to attain competence in both receptive and expressive language. This is further compounded by reduced expressive language opportunities, which further reduce language skills (Light, 1997). Educational teams must understand the language and communication profile of each individual learner with CCN. No learner profile will be the same across this heterogeneous group of learners and no assumptions should be made regarding language and communication of these learners as a group. Rather educational teams must facilitate the understanding of current profiles of learners and identify next steps in supporting ongoing development of language and communication that should occur concurrently, with both early and conventional literacy instruction.

Intellectual

The educational team must also understand the intellectual strengths and needs of learners with CCN. Each learner will have a unique profile. When considering the intellectual needs of learners with CCN, it is important to recognize the barriers that many standardized tests place on learners with CCN, including speech, motor, and experience barriers. "Standardized testing procedures may result in low levels of performance that conceal underlying competencies and lead to misjudgments about abilities (Olswang, Feuerstein, Pinder & Dowden, 2013, p. 4)." Educational teams should consider dynamic assessment as a means to determine levels of intellectual skills and needs for specific intervention (Olswang, Feuerstein, Pinder & Dowden, 2013). Dynamic assessment, applied by Vygotsky, integrates teaching into the process of assessment. This combined method allows educational teams to determine how a learner may respond to immediate instruction and modifications during assessment tasks which appear difficult for the learner. This process includes the use of qualitative indicators and cognitive strategies. (Gindes, 1995). Dynamic assessment provides understanding of the present power, capacity and attitude of the learner.

Physical Access

Learners with CCN present with diverse physical needs. These learners may have developmental disabilities that may include physical access limitations and barriers to accessing AAC systems and literacy materials. Prior to considering specific techniques for accessing AAC systems and literacy materials, educational teams should consider the seating and positioning needs of learners with CCN who have complex physical needs. Costigan and Light (2011) recommend the following guidelines for consideration: "(a) providing appropriate equipment for functional weight bearing, (b) positioning the pelvis for stability and mobility and (c) pursuing proper body alignment" (Costigan & Light, 2011, p. 233). These considerations may increase access to AAC, literacy activities, and participation.

With the seating and positioning needs of a learner addressed, educational teams must then identify the AT tools and strategies which provide access to AAC and literacy. Multiple access techniques and/or strategies should be considered and identified as learners with CCN may have varied positions, medication levels, tone, and fatigue, throughout the day. Access techniques may include eye tracking, head tracking, and scanning as well as modified pointers and keyguards to facilitate access (Fager, Bardach,

Russell, & Higginbotham, 2012). Educational teams can facilitate access to all activities and environments through collaborative teaming and consideration of the individual needs of the learner and the environments and tasks the learner desires to engage in.

Sensory/Perceptual

Learners with CCN may encounter additional challenges specific to hearing and vision deficits. Learners with CCN and sensory and/or perceptual impairments require educational teams who actively involve vision and hearing specialists to determine the most appropriate modes to deliver literacy instruction. The scope of this chapter does not provide for children with significant vision or hearing loss. Educational teams who work with children with significant sensory and/or perceptual needs should consider the Deaf-Blind Model Classroom Resources of the Center for Literacy and Disability Studies (http://www.med. unc.edu/ahs/clds/resources/deaf-blind-model-classroom-resources) as a supplement to this discussion.

AAC Systems

Learners with CCN present with many strengths and challenges across various modes of communication. The availability of appropriate AAC systems with features to support language and literacy matched to the individual needs of the learner must be available. Learner profiles impact the selection of communication systems provided to the learner. To support literacy development, learners with CCN require AAC systems which support language development and provide access to reading instruction, including opportunities to communicate sounds, sound chunks, syllables, words, phrases, and sentences (Sturm, et al., 2006).

When selecting language and vocabulary messages for learners, it is important to include syntactic, semantic and pragmatic functions of language on AAC systems (Banajee, Dicarlo, Buras Stricklin, 2003). High frequency core vocabulary lists, which represent approximately 80% of the words which the general population uses in communication across ages and activities, should be considered for learners with CCN (Banajee, Dicarlo, & Buras Stricklin, 2003; Marvin, Beukelman, & Bilyeu, 1994; Balandin & Iacono, 1999; Stuart, Beukelman, & King, 1997; Fried-Oken & More, 1992). Core vocabulary words may include: *I, me, that, go, more, finished, some, help*, etc. (A number of core vocabulary lists may be accessed at http://www.minspeak.com/CoreVocabulary.php#.U_JKq6DfK6k). Introduction and the teaching of core vocabulary for learners with CCN provide access to language and literacy instruction in the classroom (Van Tatenhove, 2009).

It is necessary to provide AAC systems early and offer many opportunities to use them across activities, environments, and communication partners. While AAC systems initiate support, communication partner skills must also be developed and in place to support learning (Van Tatenhove, 2009). The Improving Partner Applications of Augmentative Communication Techniques (ImPAACT) Program holds promise in providing instruction for families and educational teams to use AAC systems to increase the production of multisymbol AAC messages in literacy activities. This program employs the sequence of "(1) Pretest and commitment to instructional program, (2) Strategy description, (3) Strategy demonstration, (4) Verbal practice of strategy steps, (5) Controlled practice and feedback, (6) Advanced practice and feedback, (7) Posttest and commitment to long-term strategy use and (8) Generalization of strategy use (Kent-Walsh, Binger, & Malani, 2010, p. 157)." Planning for AAC system selection, vocabulary selection and partner training can facilitate access to literacy.

Literacy

The individual strengths and needs of learners with CCN impact their access to literacy instruction, as does inappropriate and severely limited literacy instruction. Repeated opportunities and a broad range of authentic literacy activities must be available to learners with CCN including explicit instruction. Instruction must go beyond access to storybook reading and include oral and written literacy activities. These activities must be adapted to provide appropriate access to support the individual needs of each learner with CCN (Sturm, et al., 2006). Facilitating literacy through assessment and instruction addresses the barriers which learners with CCN encounter and facilitates access to independent communication and literacy engagement.

EARLY LITERACY ASSESSMENT AND INSTRUCTION

Many opportunity and access barriers to literacy instruction and achievement for learners with CCN have been identified and must be systematically addressed to allow successful literacy instruction through evidence-based practices and AT tools and strategies. Educational teams must recognize barriers, which prevent literacy opportunities for learners with CCN and understand that "impairment can become especially disabling when a society fails to provide the necessary accommodations for performing competence" (Savarese & Savarese, 2012, p. 103). Teaching both early literacy skills and then conventional literacy skills requires that educational teams provide time for assessment, instruction, use appropriate and effective techniques, identify and implement the most appropriate adaptations to facilitate participation, support high levels of motivation and plan for ongoing progress monitoring (McNaughton & Light, 2010).

Assessment

Educational teams should assess the early literacy skills of ALL learners including the skills of phonemic awareness, letter-naming fluency, concepts about print, word reading, oral language and vocabulary (Connor, Alberto, Compton, & O'Connor, 2014). Connor, Alberto, Compton, and O'Connor (2014) also recommend the use of dynamic assessment to allow intervention strategies to be tested within assessment sessions. The following assessment/screening practices align with the Institute of Educational Sciences recommendations and modifications which are necessary for learners with CCN and are guided by current literature. Many of the assessment modifications can also be used within instruction. When selecting assessment and instruction modifications for learners with CCN, attention must be given to how modifications are made and if modifications maintain assessment of what was intended to be assessed. Further, understanding if modifications place additional cognitive and motor demands on the learner and how this may alter assessment results, is necessary.

Phonemic Awareness

Phonemic awareness is the ability to notice, think about, and work with individual sounds within words. Between kindergarten and early second grade, learners master phonemic awareness skills of phoneme matching, phoneme isolation, phoneme blending, phoneme segmentation and phoneme manipulation. Learners with CCN are limited in their ability to use speech as a means to work with individual sounds and words. The use of symbols as a means to assess and develop phonemic awareness skills is effective. However, considerations of symbol understanding as well as physical access to selection of a symbol response must be considered (Light, McNaughton, Werg, & Karg, 2008; Dahlgren Sandberg, Smith, & Larsson, 2010).

Phonemic Matching

Phonemic matching requires learners to identify words which begin with the same sound. Assessment for learners with CCN can be conducted through the use of a stimulus picture and four response picture options. The learner is asked, after hearing the stimulus word, which response picture has the same first sound (Peeters, Verhoeven, Moor, Balkom & van Leeuwe, 2009). Another approach is indicating if a sound occurred at the beginning of a word after it was stated by an evaluator (Dahlgren Sandberg, Smith, & Larsson, 2010).

Phoneme Isolation

Phoneme isolation skills involve identifying individual sounds in initial, medial and final positions in words. For an alternative response method, learners with CCN can indicate if pairs of words, spoken by an evaluator, share phonemes in a specific word position (Dahlgren Sandberg, Smith, & Larsson, 2010).

Phoneme Blending

Phoneme blending asks that learners use individual sounds (/c/, /a/, /t/), provided by an evaluator, and combine these sounds to form a word (*cat*). Oral responses are typically required. Learners with CCN can be provided with symbol sets to select the formed word (Light, McNaughton, Werg, & Karg, 2008; Dahlgren Sandberg, Smith, & Larsson, 2010).

Phoneme Segmentation

Phoneme segmentation requires that learners indicate the sounds heard in a word, again requiring an oral response. Presentation of an individual sound and asking a learner with CCN to select a symbol, which begins with, ends with or contains the sound in the middle, can replace the oral response (Light, McNaughton, Werg, & Karg, 2008).

Phoneme Manipulation

Learners who have mastered phoneme manipulation skills are able to demonstrate the ability to say or identify words, which have an initial or final sound, removed or replaced with alternative sounds. During phoneme manipulation activities, learners with CCN can select a symbol, which corresponds with the new word (Dahlgren Sandberg, Smith, & Larsson, 2010).

Letter-Naming Fluency

The ability to name letters accurately and fluently is referred to as letter-naming fluency. Letter identification activities can be modified for learners with CCN through the presentation of six print letter response choices and the oral presentation of the letter to identify (Hander & Erickson, 2007).

Concepts about Print

Learners typically master concepts about print in kindergarten, understanding that (a) print has meaning and can be used for different purposes, (b) there is a relationship between print and speech, (c) there are differences between letters and words, (d) words are separated by spaces, (e) there are differences between words and sentences and (f) punctuation marks the end of a sentence. Understanding the parts of a book as well as the beginning, middle, and end of a story and that text is read from the left to the right and from the top to the bottom of a page of print, are also developed concepts of print. Assessment of learners with CCN should include assessment of behaviors and responsiveness during book reading and understanding the purpose and function of storybooks (Bellon-Harn & Harn, 2008; Browder, Mims, Spooner, Ahlgrim-Delzell, & Lee, 2009; Skoto, Koppenhaver, & Erickson, 2004). Concepts about Print (Clay, 1993) can be modified with multiple choice and yes/no questions (Hanser & Erickson, 2007).

Word Reading Skills

Learners develop both sight word and word decoding skills which extend beyond sight word knowledge. Letter sound correspondence skills should be assessed to determine early skills in word decoding. Providing a letter sound orally and asking the learner to locate the letter, from an array, which pairs with the sound provides a modification to oral requirements. This may be facilitated on a computer keyboard, letter board or AAC system (Light, McNaughton, Werg, & Karg, 2008).

Assessment of word reading skills can be conducted using a number of modifications to replace oral responses. Word reading can be assessed by asking learners with CCN, who are given a set of symbols, to read a word and match the word to a symbol (Light, McNaughton, Werg, and Karg, 2008; Dahlgren Sandberg, Smith, & Larsson, 2010). Dahlgren Sandberg, Smith, and Larsson (2010) also asked learners to participate in a series of word reading assessments including: indicating if a written word is a real word, selecting a correct print pseudoword presented orally by an evaluator, having learners identify the boundaries of three words from a letter chain sequence (e.g., helpwenthot) and reading a sentence and matching sentence content to a picture from an array of seven options. Clearly, many options are available to assess word-reading skills.

Oral Language Skills

Learner's oral language, including phonological, semantic, syntactic and pragmatic language skills, influence their access to and their understanding of reading and writing. Learners use both expressive and receptive oral language knowledge to produce and comprehend spoken and written language. Assessment of oral language skills includes the complex measures of grammar, defining words, and listening comprehension, which are significant factors in predicting conventional literacy skills (Lonigan, Allan, & Lerner, 2011; NELP, 2008). Learners with CCN will benefit from assessment across these areas as well as access to modified assessments and instruction with integrated use of AAC systems.

Vocabulary Knowledge

Learners must use the words they hear to begin to make sense of the words they encounter in print. Vocabulary knowledge interacts across all literacy skills. The Peabody Picture Vocabulary Test (PPVT) can provide information on vocabulary skills of learners with CCN, using picture stimulus plates to allow for responses through pointing or modified pointing (head or mouth pointer, toe pointing, or eye gaze) (Erickson, Hanser, Hatch, & Sanders, 2009; Ferreira, Rönnberg, Gastafson, & Wengelin, 2007). Dynamic assessment of vocabulary knowledge, before, during and after literacy activities, is also valuable in the assessment process.

Comprehensive assessment tools that have been used to gauge literacy skills of learners with CCN include the Preschool and Primary Inventory of Phonological Awareness (PIPA) and the Sheffield Early Literacy Development Profile (Mathisen, Arthur-Kelly, Kidd & Nissen, 2009). The Literacy Rubric (Staugler, 2007) also provides an informal tool to monitor progress in describing literacy behaviors of learners and can be useful in creating a visual profile of emergent and early literacy skills.

Early Writing Skills

Many of the early literacy skills highlighted earlier contribute to the assessment of early writing skills for learners. Assessment of early writing skills requires that learners with CCN have access to writing opportunities and tools. Assessment should include understanding of the learner's use of drawing and scribbling letters or letter like forms, salient beginning sounds and beginning, middle, and ending sounds (Cabell, Tortorelli, & Gerde, 2013).

Early writing requires that learners have exposure and access to both symbols and letters, preferably integrated within their AAC systems (Johnston, Davenport, Kanarowski, Rhodehouse & McDonnell, 2009). Often letters are removed from AAC systems or are not provided since educational teams identify them as unnecessary. Consider this story of a young man with an AAC system that utilized a symbol-based language system, paired with a computer keyboard option, to produce text to speech messages. This young man had early understanding of the function of print and letters. When notes were sent to and from home/school, this young man would use his AAC device keyboard to type and then listen to the words of the notes through the voice output of the AAC system. This process of literacy development for him was significant. The presence of a keyboard provided for independent literacy skill development.

MEANINGFUL LITERACY EXPERIENCES

Meaningful literacy experiences for ALL learners support continued lifelong literacy skill development. Motivation to read and write may be facilitated through a variety of teaching strategies, routines, praise and reinforcement, building of excitement, cooperative learning and use of manipulatives (letter stamps, toys and materials to write about, etc.). Educational teams should approach literacy instruction planning through considerations of meaningful literacy experiences which may include learner-focused literacy activities, social media opportunities and literacy applications.

Learners Focused Literacy Activities

All learners benefit from reading and writing experiences which are motivating. One means to motivate learners is to make literacy activities personal, related to the learner and his/her life (Deci, 1992; Guthrie, McRae, & Klauda, 2007; Hulleman, Godes, Hendricks, & Harackiewicz, 2010). A number of strategies can be employed to make literacy personal, including:

- Reading books about valued topics for learners,
- Participating in self-selected reading and writing,
- Writing books with and about learners, and
- Publishing books for other learners to read.

Social Media

Social media provides unique opportunities for self-expression, interaction and social inclusion for learners with CCN. Social media can be facilitated through texting, chats, instant messaging, email and a plethora of social networking sites. Social media tools offer an opportunity for self-representation without the potential barriers present during face-to-face communication situations (Light & McNaughton, 2012a; Hynan, Murray, & Goldbart, 2014). Further, social media, such as blogging, provides an opportunity for learners to develop as writers (McGrail & Davis, 2011). Selection of letters, words, or AAC system symbols can be used as a means to input text into a social media tool, and collaborative peer activities can provide supports for early communicators and literacy learners. Learners using many higher technology AAC systems, based on computer or mobile platforms, have immediate means to input text from communication devices into social media tools.

Literacy Applications

A large set of literacy applications for both mobile devices and computers is available to support early literacy engagement and learning. Unfortunately, only a limited emerging evidence base is available to identify outcomes of these tools for learners with disabilities. Multimodal e-books and literacy applications may serve as beneficial and enjoyable instructional tools to help children persist in learning through the use of sound, illustration, animation and video. Educational teams must select the most appropriate modes of instruction for learners and consider the potential distractions of applications. Further, the need for scaffolding from teachers or parents is strongly recommended across current studies (Kazakoff-Lane, 2010; Korat, Shamir, & Arbiv, 2011; Kucirkova, Messer, Critten, & Harwood, 2014; Neumann & Neumann, 2014; Morgan, 2013; Macaruso & Rodman, 2011; Salmon, 2013; Spooner, Ahlgrim-Delzell, Kemp-Inman, & Wood, 2014; Wild, 2009).

EARLY READING INSTRUCTION METHODS AND STRATEGIES

Literacy instruction methods and strategy recommendations are available across the evidence-based literature specific to learners with CCN. The instructional evidence-based practices across storybook reading, alphabet knowledge and phonemic awareness, word reading and decoding and writing will be discussed followed by a discussion of integrated literacy and AAC instruction.

Storybook Reading with Learners

Storybook reading is a prevalent theme across the literature for learners with CCN. Storybook reading provides a rich interactive context to support language development (Kent-Walsh, Binger, Hashman, 2010). Reading with learners develops motivation for reading and supports world knowledge, language concepts and sentence structures. Further, reading exposes learners to written genres and opportunities to develop comprehension and inference skills (Beukelman & Mirenda, 2013; Strum & Clendon, 2004). Storybook interactions are critical in the development of early foundations of literacy skills and in the later development of conventional literacy skills (DaFonte, Pufpaff, & Taber-Doughty, 2010). Learners develop concepts of turning the pages, pointing to pictures, naming pictures and discussing content. Developing engaging and enjoyable book reading routines is only a starting point and should lead to introducing instructional activities within storybook reading (Stephenson, 2010).

Interactive storybook reading experiences are key to literacy development, however, research indicates that learners with CCN experience less joint book reading activities and are typically passive participants in these experiences, which results in decreased preparation for reading instruction (Iacono, 2004). The integration of AAC systems in storybook reading activities and instruction are critical for participation and learning, however, the use of AAC systems during storybook reading activities is low for learners with CCN (Peeters, Verhoeven, Moor, Balkom & van Leeuwe, 2009).

Providing effective scaffolding during storybook reading activities is a key to opportunity and access for learners with CCN. Evidence-based scaffolding strategies that go beyond pointing to text and illustrations include:

- Embedded AT and augmentative communication supports,
- Positioning AT, AAC, and storybook materials to facilitate physical access for learners and communication partners,
- Engaging learners through labeling, commenting, relating storybooks to learners, providing natural responses and providing modeling and expansion of utterances,
- Using wh- open ended questions including prediction or inference questions,
- Completing repeating story lines,
- Facilitating opportunities for responses through wait time,
- Utilizing a prompting hierarchy to encourage initiation of a response and
- Integration of story-related manipulatives

(Bellon-Harn & Harn, 2008; Skoto, Kopenhaver, & Erickson, 2004; Rosa-Lugo & Kent-Walsh, 2008; Binger, Kent-Walsh, Ewing, & Taylor, 2010; Kent-Walsh, Binger, & Hasham, 2010; Stephenson, 2010; Soto & Dukhovny, 2008; Browder, Mims, Spooner, Ahlgrim-Delzell, & Lee, 2008). Training is necessary to support educational teams and communication partners in employing these scaffolding methods (Skoto, Kopenhaver, & Erickson, 2004; Rosa-Lugo & Kent-Walsh, 2008; Binger, Kent-Walsh, Ewing, & Taylor, 2010; Kent-Walsh, Binger, & Hasham, 2010).

The use of AAC systems during storybook reading activities can be supported through both visual scene displays and symbol grid displays (Wood Jackson, Wahlquist, & Marquis, 2011). Symbol introduction within storybook routines increase learner use of line drawings and pointing to book illustrations within these routines (Stephenson, 2010). AAC system vocabulary and symbol learning can be facilitated during storybook reading including use of multi-word utterances. Setting appropriate vocabulary targets, expecting learner participation, providing multiple opportunities to use the vocabulary, ensuring time for responses and providing corrective feedback and praise are key interventions (Soto & Dukhovny, 2008).

Providing access to storybook reading for learners with CCN requires planning. It is essential to help learners access books across environments. Learners with CCN could benefit from adapted books, book routines and e-book activities (Erickson, Kopenhaver, Yoder, & Nance, 1997; Light & Kelford Smith, 1993; Stephenson, 2010). While books may be abundant in environments, it is important to ensure that children with CCN and others with significant need can physically navigate to these books or request these books.

Modifications to books can increase physical access for learners with CCN and significant support needs. Modifications may include:

- Increasing space between pages for ease of page-turning (page fluffers or popsicle stick page extenders).
- Creating alternative durable/turnable pages (hard picture album pages, book pages in plastic bags, and laminated pages) (Fenlon, McNabb, Pidlypchak, 2010).

Books must also be physically positioned during reading activities to facilitate access to both learners with CCN and their communication partners (Skoto, Kopenhaver, & Erickson, 2004). Without appropriate positioning of books, visual and physical barriers prevent full engagement in literacy activities. Commercial and homemade book holders (PVC pipe book holders, binder clips to position and hold books open, etc.) can support positioning and access.

Storybook adaptations to increase engagement of learners include 1) using the student's name as the main character, 2) adding a repeated story line for the main idea of the book, 3) presenting a surprise element and 4) providing sensory materials and objects to supplement the reading activity (Browder, Mims, Spooner, Ahlgrim-Delzell, & Lee, 2008). Individualized or adapted books can also be created for or with learners with CCN through authentic publishing opportunities, including rewriting the original text of books, using old calendar or magazine picture pages to write about, or writing novel stories about events, supplemented by personal photographs. Opportunities and access are facilitated through reading and writing.

Multimedia applications provide platforms for the presentation of instructional materials to support learners (Coleman, 2009; Spooner, Ahlgrim-Delzell, Kemp-Inman, & Wood, 2014). Scaffolding can be provided to learners who have a difficult time accessing books physically or decoding and comprehending the text of a book, using multimedia and electronic text tools. Multimedia presentation tools such as PowerPoint and other multimedia computer and mobile device applications, provide options for creating books and materials with recorded voice, music, video, pictures, and more. The use of multimedia tools provides multiple options to meet the individual needs of learners (Rivera, 2013). Multimedia tools may also support early literacy instruction through the creation of motivating and individualized pages with interactive and auditory components for sound blending, phoneme segmentation, letter-sound correspondence and sight word recognition. Other multimedia resources include *Tar Heel Reader* (TarHeelReader. org), which provides a large set of multimedia accessible books for learners and the electronic book resources of *Bookshare* (Bookshare.org). For learners with CCN and significant motor support needs, access can be facilitated to books created in multimedia and electronic formats. The right click of the mouse to change a slide in PowerPoint can be facilitated through a commercial computer or mobile device "switch interface" or home-made "Mouse House" (http://www.lburkhart.com/mhouse.htm). To provide comprehensive access to multimedia and electronic text, additional AT tools for access should be considered by educational teams.

Alphabet Knowledge and Phonemic Awareness

Alphabet knowledge and phonemic awareness skills are achievable by learners with CCN (Card & Dodd, 2006; Dahlgren Sandberg, 2006). Explicit instruction of phoneme-grapheme correspondence, segmentation, phonemic manipulation and encoding of CVC word skills can result in literacy success for learners with CCN (Blischak, Shah, Lombardino, & Chiarella, 2004).

Evidence-based strategies include:

- Use of letter tiles for letter sound-correspondence activities, accompanied by praise and a prompting hierarchy to teach correct responses (Blischak, Shah, Lombardino, & Chiarella, 2004).
- Using a prompting hierarchy to teach letter-sound correspondence and spelling of CVC combinations through 1) a prompt to touch the letter that says __ or spell ___ followed by modeling of the correct response, 2) following two or more sessions of 80% or higher performance adding a five second delay before modeling, 3) if an incorrect response occurs repeat directions with a model, 4) when a correct response occurs, the learners are allowed to participate in a brief but engaging activity with the teacher (Johnston et al., 2009).
- Teaching letter/sound correspondence and phoneme awareness within story reading contexts (Truxler & O'Keefe, 2007).
- Providing instruction on sound blending and segmentation within a structured sound awareness and analysis context, with a direct focus on print to sound translation (Truxler & O'Keefe, 2007).

Light and McNaughton (2009) provide additional suggestions for selection of the letter sound correspondence to teach, including: lower-case letters first, letters and sounds that occur more frequently in children's books, separation of letters which are visually or auditorily similar, short vowels first (since there are fewer code rules associated with short vowels) and single letter instruction before consonant clusters. Further, it is recommended that letter sounds be taught before letter names to decrease competing information which can create confusion for learners.

Teaching alphabet knowledge and phonological awareness does not often involve high technology AT tools. Rather they utilize AAC systems with no-technology adaptations, which all educational teams can employ. Educational teams must implement these instructional techniques, consider the most appropriate amounts and intensity of instruction and, through ongoing assessment, identify barriers to successful instruction (Blischak, Shah, Lombardino & Chiarella, 2004).

Word Reading and Decoding

Learners are ready for instruction in word decoding skills when they are able to do some sound blending and know some letter-sound correspondences. Learners with CCN do not need to master all the letter names; rather just a few letter sounds are necessary to progress in literacy instruction. These are the only identified prerequisites to begin to decode words and move forward as a reader and writer. Decoding skills are beyond the level of presenting the same word continuously and developing a sight word inventory. Decoding skills provide the foundation to understand how to read any presented word.

Pairing picture symbols with text has been used as an intervention to teach reading to many learners with CCN. Unfortunately, this practice may actually limit progress in reading. Picture symbols, which have multiple meanings or are abstract in their meaning, may increase reading confusion (Erickson, Hatch & Clendon, 2010). It has been documented that learning to read words, paired with pictures, is more difficult than learning an individual word (Fossett & Mirenda, 2006; Pufpaff, Blischak, & Lloyd, 2000; Singh & Solman, 1990; Solman & Wu, 1995). There is, however, a benefit to using picture symbols in the process of teaching word reading through an active matching of the word to the picture (Fossett & Mirenda, 2006).

Evidence-based word reading and decoding instructional methods for learners with CCN include:

- Decoding and sight word instruction during share storybook reading using a process of read, pause, and providing time for the learner to fill in the blank (NRP, 2000),
- Integrated phonological awareness, decoding and sight word instruction (Browder, Gibbs, Ahlgrim-Delzell, Courtade, Mraz & Flowers, 2008),
- Direct instruction techniques including: 1) providing explanations of the correct responses, 2) leading students to make a correct response, and 3) providing opportunities for independent responses (Fallon, Light, McNaughton, Drager, & Hammer, 2004),
- Use of highly motivating words for the individual learner (e.g., Mind Craft) (Hanser and Erickson, 2007),
- Begin with letter combinations and word families which occur frequently (Hanser & Erickson, 2007),
- Direct explicit instruction on single word reading, with a focus on matching single sounds to the initial sounds of words, telescoping sounds into words and reading single VC (verb-consonant) and CVC (consonant-vowel-consonant) words (Fallon, Light, McNaughton, Drager, & Hammer, 2004),
- Providing sound blending instruction: saying the word slowly, extending each phoneme, then asking the learner to blend the word silently, and finally having the learner say or indicate the word from an array of symbols (Light & McNaughton, 2009), and
- Providing phoneme segmentation instruction through selecting a letter that is the first sound in a word or a symbol that begins with the same sound (Fallon, Light, McNaughton, Drager, & Hammer, 2004; Light & McNaughton, 2009).

EARLY WRITING INSTRUCTION METHODS AND STRATEGIES

Early writing has been well documented in the literature as a foundation for reading development skills (Jones, Reutzel, & Fargo, 2010). Writing requires physical access to activities and the complex integrated skills of reading, writing, speaking and listening. "Development of conventional writing skills will be enhanced when children, who use AAC, have rich background knowledge, access to a broad range of vocabulary to express that knowledge, and the communication competence to convey their background knowledge using a range of AAC systems" (Strum, 2003, p. 9). Many writing opportunities are necessary for learners with CCN (Erickson & Koppenhaver, 1995; Foley and Wolter, 2010; Millar, Light, & McNaughton, 2004; NRP, 2000). Developmentally appropriate practices for early writing require daily writing activities, supporting development from stages of scribbles to letter/word writing. Explicit modeling, scaffolding, connections between reading and writing, encouragement of inventive spelling, availability of writing materials, meaningful writing, words in the environment, group writing and writing activities provide for the development of early literacy skills (Gerde, Bingham, & Wasik, 2012; Strum, 2003).

Learners with CCN and significant support needs may require extra support to access the physical writing process, including a variety of writing utensils, adapted utensils, writing templates, prewritten words or phrases, word processing, computer accessibility features, alternative keyboards, word prediction and voice recognition software (Foley & Staples, 2006). AAC systems can also provide significant support for the motor and composition aspects of the writing process, assuming that the available language is valuable within the writing process (Foley & Staples, 2006). Computer and mobile device-based AAC systems transfer text-based messages, composed with AAC system picture symbols, to word processing type software and applications. This process uses writing with symbols, a process which should be an integrated beginning to writing but never an end.

The composition of written materials may be supported through highly motivating picture supports to write about, word supports (pictures with words, word walls, word banks, dictionaries, etc.), fill in the blank activities, repeated line writing activities, writing templates, adult or peer-shared writing activities, word processing software, talking word processors, multimedia software, outlining tools and visual webbing/planning software (Hanser & Erickson, 2007; Lane, 2008; Light, McNaughton, Weyer & Karg, 2008; Lorenz, Green, Brown, 2009). Tools that educational teams may consider include: Tar Heel Reader's "Write a Book" option (Fenlon, McNabb, Pidlypchak, 2010), graphic organizers (Inspiration™, Kidpiration™, Popplet™, Bubbl™, SpiderScribe™, etc.), and outlining tools such as Draftbuilder™. Opportunities to write, which are meaningful and authentic-beyond copying-(National Reading Panel, 2000) are most important in offering opportunities to write. Ongoing assessment and high expectations will also facilitate this process.

Integrated Literacy and AAC Instruction

It is necessary to conclude this early literacy discussion with a consideration of comprehensive AAC core based language systems as a means to integrate literacy, language and communication development. Core vocabulary, available on a select number of AAC systems, provides access to literacy learning. Hanser and Erickson (2007) and Mathisen, Arthur-Kelly, Kidd and Nissen (2009) used the Minspeak™ Unity™, core-based, language system to integrate language and literacy instruction. The Unity language system provides a unique core and fringe vocabulary, which is developmental and supports communication, language and literacy learning. Utilizing the unique features of Unity, these studies demonstrated how access to a developmental core based language system and teaching of this language system in conjunction with literacy instruction can provide opportunities for communication, language, and literacy skill development and result in effective literacy outcomes for students. Educational teams should consider core based AAC language systems such as, *Unity,* for all learners. Key elements to consider in this process include:

- Weekly planning,
- Explicit, structured, and systematic instruction,
- Targeting of specific vocabulary within books and activities,
- Word identification and spelling instruction,
- Homework for school and home, and
- Visual supports to aid in finding vocabulary on a Unity based AAC system (Hanser & Erickson, 2007; Mathisen, Arthur-Kelly, Kidd & Nissens, 2009)

CONVENTIONAL LITERACY SKILLS

Five core areas discussed by the National Reading Panel are important to literacy instruction for all children: phonemic awareness, phonics, vocabulary, fluency, and comprehension. While the primary focus of this chapter has been on early literacy, the ultimate goal for all learners is to promote strong conventional literacy skills. The following briefly discusses key conventional literacy skills.

Phonemic Awareness

Children who have developed phonological skills and phonemic awareness are able to match, blend, segment and manipulate the sounds of speech. These skills are significant in the development of reading skills and should be incorporated into early literacy programs (Ehri, Nunes, Stahl, & Willows 2001).

Phonics

Phonics instruction teaches children relationships between letters and the individual sounds of spoken language. Maclean (1988) discusses phonics as "a path breaker for beginners" (p. 514). Phonics instruction teaches children to use these relationships to read and write words (NICHD, 2001).

Vocabulary

Phonological awareness, phonemic awareness, and phonics provide a foundation for developing the skills of vocabulary, fluency and comprehension in reading. Vocabulary instruction is important in the process of learning to read since vocabulary knowledge aids in the decoding of words and comprehension of reading materials (NICHD, 2001; Blachowicz, Fisher, Ogle, & Watts-Taffe, 2006). Reading, hearing, using, and speaking with vocabulary can provide a rich environment for vocabulary learning across the curriculum (Blanchowicz, et al., 2006). The key for learners with CCN is to access vocabularies and vocabulary learning, integrated with strong language access across AAC systems.

Fluency

Fluency instruction provides children with the skills to read text accurately and quickly (NICHD, 2001). "Fluency is manifested in accurate, rapid, expressive oral reading and is applied during, and makes possible, silent reading comprehension." (Pikulski & Chard, 2005, p. 510). Learners with CCN require opportunities to develop fluency with strong AAC language systems supported by text to speech. Further, silent reading comprehension must be explicitly taught, reinforced and assessed (Erickson, Koppenhaver, Yoder, & Nance, 2007). Building of fluency skills can be supported through repeated reading, read-alongs and paired readings with fluent readers (Foley & Wolter, 2010).

Comprehension

Each of the reading skills discussed above contributes to the goal of reading instruction. Comprehension instruction teaches children to read purposefully, to gather information or to enjoy the pleasure of reading while at the same time reading actively using their knowledge and experience to understand and enjoy text (NICHD, 2001). Learners with CCN benefit from instructional techniques including comprehension monitoring, summarization, graphic and semantic organizers, response opportunities, generating questions and learning to recognize text structures (NRP, 2000).

FUTURE RESEARCH DIRECTIONS

Two key studies should be considered in identifying future research directions across literacy and learners with CCN. Pufpaff (2008) and Light, McNaughton, Weyer, and Karg (2008) studied the implementation of comprehensive literacy programs for two learners with CCN. PufPaff's research is engaged in the Building Blocks reading program, based on the Four Blocks literacy framework, while Light et al. researchers employed intensive evidence-based literacy instruction components. Pufpaff (2008) identified significant barriers to the literacy curriculum using the constructs of opportunity barriers and access barriers for a student with significant support needs in an inclusive kindergarten classroom. Opportunity barriers included minimal planning, no delineation of education team member roles and limited support and training for the general education teacher. Access barriers for the student included challenging behaviors, fine motor impairment and a lack of functional speech. The student was not provided with an appropriate AAC system, effective instructional practices were not employed and peers were not prepared or provided with training. These opportunity and access barriers require additional attention in future research.

Light et al. (2008) demonstrated the effects of the researcher-provided intervention in a self-contained environment with 55 hours of intervention provided over 16 months to a learner with CCN and significant support needs. Instruction included letter-sound correspondences, sight-word recognition, sight-word decoding, application of skills in shared reading, reading and understanding of simple sentences, keyboarding skills and typing simple personalized stories. During phase one, the student acquired nine letter-sound correspondences. She was able to read 30 words with greater than 90% accuracy, and she applied single-word reading skills in shared reading activities with greater than 90% accuracy. During phase two, she acquired eleven new letter-sound correspondences, learned about 30 additional new words and applied reading skills in shared reading activities with greater than 90% accuracy. She located letter-sounds on the keyboard with greater than 80% accuracy and typed short sentences with some oral scaffolding support. The outcomes of this research require additional attention in generalized settings, when implemented by educational teams.

We need to successfully translate these research results into daily practices in schools, homes, and community programs so that individuals who require AAC have the opportunities and effective instruction needed to ensure that they develop the literacy skills that they require to attain their full potential. (Light, McNaughton, Weyer, and Karg, 2008, p. 130)

Assessment

Understanding the literacy profiles of learners with CCN is complex. Three significant areas require investigation (1) Which formal and informal assessments should be used to develop a literacy profile for a learner with CCN? (2) What modifications to formal and informal assessments are appropriate for learners and do not increase cognitive or physical demands during the assessment process? and (3) How can the literacy profiles of learners with CCN inform instruction?

Intervention

Literacy intervention research needs to shift to educational and home settings in order to enhance evidence-based understanding and instruction in generalizable environments for learners with CCN. Much of the current research exists within a researcher provided context; a transition to natural environments is necessary.

Teacher Education

Educational teams must have knowledge and skills across literacy and learners with CCN. How to achieve this level of knowledge and to support educational teams in the classroom is a necessary next step in research. Further, understanding how the family, as a member of this team, can develop both knowledge and skill to supplement literacy instruction in the home must be well understood to support learners.

FUTURE THEMES

When successfully implemented and when aligned with evidenced-based practices, AT tools and strategies are powerful. AAC systems provide opportunities for the establishment and development of communication. However, AAC systems provide only a partial solution for learners with CCN. Learners with CCN, also require significant opportunity and instruction in literacy to support novel and independent communication as well as ongoing opportunities in today's society. This chapter has challenged the reader to consider the role of literacy for learners using AAC systems and how AAC systems and AT tools and strategies can support literacy learning across home, schools, and the community.

CONCLUSION

Opportunity and access to early and conventional literacy instruction should be provided to ALL children. Educational teams must assess current skills across language, literacy, and communication and develop comprehensive instructional plans across home, school, and community to enhance the literacy instruction opportunities and access for learners with CCN. AAC systems, supplemented by the most appropriate AT tools and strategies, must be in place across environments to support literacy development. Literacy skill development is NOT symbol recognition and functional environmental sign instruction. Literacy instruction should align to current evidence-based instructional practices recognized for all children as the foundation for conventional literacy skills. This should allow all children the basic human rights of communication and literacy and will thus support the ultimate human right, communication.

REFERENCES

Allington, R. L. (1977). If they don't read much, how they ever gonna get good? *Journal of Reading, 21*, 57–61.

American Speech-Language-Hearing Association. (2004). *Roles and responsibilities of speech-language pathologists with respect to augmentative and alternative communication: technical report* [Technical Report]. Available from www.asha.org/policy

Balandin, S., & Iacono, T. (1999). Crews, wusses, and whoppas: Core and fringe vocabularies of Australian meal-break conversations in the workplace. *Augmentative and Alternative Communication, 15*(2), 95–109. doi:10.1080/07434619912331278605

Banajee, M., Dicarlo, C., & Burass Stricklin, S. (2003). Core vocabulary determination for toddlers. *Augmentative and Alternative Communication, 19*(2), 67–73. doi:10.1080/0743461031000112034

Bellon-Harn, M. L., & Harn, W. E. (2008). Scaffolding strategies during repeated storybook reading an extension using a voice output communication aid. *Focus on Autism and Other Developmental Disabilities, 23*(2), 112–124. doi:10.1177/1088357608316606

Beukelman, D., & Mirenda, P. (1989). *Augmentative and Alternative Communication: Management of Severe Communication Impairments*. Baltimore: Brookes Publishing.

Beukelman, D., & Mirenda, P. (2005). *Augmentative and Alternative Communication: Management of Severe Communication Impairments*. Baltimore: Brookes Publishing.

Beukelman, D., & Mirenda, P. (2013). *Augmentative and Alternative Communication: Management of Severe Communication Impairments*. Baltimore: Brookes Publishing.

Binger, C., Kent-Walsh, J., Ewing, C., & Taylor, S. (2010). Teaching educational assistants to facilitate the multisymbol message productions of young students who require augmentative and alternative communication. *American Journal of Speech-Language Pathology, 19*(2), 108–120. doi:10.1044/1058-0360(2009/09-0015) PMID:19948759

Binger, C., & Light, J. (2006). Demographics of preschoolers who require AAC. *Language, Speech, and Hearing Services in Schools, 37*(3), 200–208. doi:10.1044/0161-1461(2006/022) PMID:16837443

Blachowicz, C. L., Fisher, P. J., Ogle, D., & Watts-Taffe, S. (2006). Vocabulary: Questions from the classroom. *Reading Research Quarterly, 41*(4), 524–539. doi:10.1598/RRQ.41.4.5

Blischak, D. M., Lombardino, L. J., & Dyson, A. T. (2003). Use of speech-generating devices: In support of natural speech. *Augmentative and Alternative Communication, 19*(1), 29–35. doi:10.1080/0743461032000056478

Blischak, D. M., Shah, S. D., Lombardino, L. J., & Chiarella, K. (2004). Effects of phonemic awareness instruction on the encoding skills of children with severe speech impairment. *Disability and Rehabilitation, 26*(21-22), 1295–1304. doi:10.1080/09638280412331280325 PMID:15513729

Branson, D., & Demchak, M. (2009). The use of augmentative and alternative communication methods with infants and toddlers with disabilities: A research review. *Augmentative and Alternative Communication, 25*(4), 274–286. doi:10.3109/07434610903384529 PMID:19883287

Browder, D., Gibbs, S., Ahlgrim-Delzell, L., Courtade, G. R., Mraz, M., & Flowers, C. (2008). Literacy for students with severe developmental disabilities: What should we teach and what should we hope to achieve? *Remedial and Special Education, 30*(5), 269–282. doi:10.1177/0741932508315054

Browder, D. M., Mims, P. J., Spooner, F., Ahlgrim-Delzell, L., & Lee, A. (2008). Teaching elementary students with multiple disabilities to participate in shared stories. *Research and Practice for Persons with Severe Disabilities, 33*(1-2), 3–12. doi:10.2511/rpsd.33.1-2.3

Browder, D. M., Spooner, F., & Bingham, M. A. (2004). Current practices in alternate assessment and access to the general curriculum for students with severe disabilities in the United States of America. *Australasian Journal of Special Education, 28*(2), 17–29. doi:10.1080/1030011040280203

Brown, C. (1954). *My left foot*. London: Secker & Warburg.

Cabell, S. Q., Tortorelli, L. S., & Gerde, H. K. (2013). How do I write…? Scaffolding preschoolers' early writing skills. *The Reading Teacher, 66*(8), 650–659. doi:10.1002/trtr.1173

Calculator, S. N. (2013). Use and acceptance of AAC systems by children with Angelman Syndrome. *Journal of Applied Research in Intellectual Disabilities, 26*(6), 557–567. PMID:23606637

Card, R., & Dodd, B. (2006). The phonological awareness abilities of children with cerebral palsy who do not speak. *Augmentative and Alternative Communication, 22*(3), 149–159. doi:10.1080/07434610500431694 PMID:17114160

Clay, M. (1993). *An observation survey of early literacy achievement*. Portsmouth, NH: Heinemann.

Coleman, M. B. (2009). PowerPoint" Is Not Just for Business Presentations and College Lectures: Using" PowerPoint" to Enhance Instruction for Students with Disabilities. *Teaching Exceptional Children Plus, 6*(1), 1–13.

Connor, C. M., Alberto, P. A., Compton, D. L., & O'Connor, R. E. (2014). *Improving Reading Outcomes for Students with or at Risk for Reading Disabilities: A Synthesis of the Contributions from the Institute of Education Sciences Research Centers (NCSER 2014-3000)*. Washington, DC: National Center for Special Education Research, Institute of Education Sciences, U.S. Department of Education. This report is available on the IES website at; http://ies.ed.gov/

Cook, A. M., & Polgar, J. M. (2008). *Introduction and Framework. Cook & Hussey's Assistive Technologies: Principles and Practice*. St. Louis, MO: Mosby.

Copley, J., & Ziviani, J. (2004). Barriers to the use of assistive technology for children with multiple disabilities. *Occupational Therapy International, 11*(4), 229–243. doi:10.1002/oti.213 PMID:15771212

Costigan, F. A., & Light, J. (2011). Functional seating for school-age children with cerebral palsy: An evidence-based tutorial. *Language, Speech, and Hearing Services in Schools, 42*(2), 223–236. doi:10.1044/0161-1461(2010/10-0001) PMID:20844273

Cress, C. J., & Marvin, C. A. (2003). Common questions about AAC services in early intervention. *Augmentative and Alternative Communication, 19*(4), 254–272. doi:10.1080/0743461031000598242

Da Fonte, M. A., Pufpaff, L. A., & Taber-Doughty, T. (2010). Vocabulary use during storybook reading: Implications for children with augmentative and alternative communication needs. *Psychology in the Schools, 47*(5), 514–524.

Dahlgren Sandberg, A. (2006). Reading and spelling abilities in children with severe speech impairments and cerebral palsy at 6, 9, and 12 years of age in relation to cognitive development: A longitudinal study. *Developmental Medicine and Child Neurology, 48*(08), 629–634. doi:10.1017/S0012162206001344 PMID:16836773

Dahlgren Sandberg, A., Smith, M., & Larsson, M. (2010). An analysis of reading and spelling abilities of children using AAC: Understanding a continuum of competence. *Augmentative and Alternative Communication, 26*(3), 191–202. doi:10.3109/07434618.2010.505607 PMID:20874081

Deci, E. L. (1992). *The relation of interest to the motivation of behavior: A self-determination theory perspective.* Hillsdale, NJ, England: Lawrence Erlbaum Associates, Inc.

Donnellan, A. M. (1984). The criterion of the least dangerous assumption. *Behavioral Disorders, 9*(2), 141–150.

Downing, J. E. (Ed.). (2005). *Teaching literacy to students with significant disabilities: Strategies for the K-12 inclusive classroom.* Thousand Oaks, CA: Sage. doi:10.4135/9781483328973

Ehri, L. C., Nunes, S. R., Stahl, S. A., & Willows, D. M. (2001). Systematic phonics instruction helps students learn to read: Evidence from the National Reading Panel's meta-analysis. *Review of Educational Research, 71*(3), 393–447. doi:10.3102/00346543071003393

Erickson, K., Hanser, G., Hatch, P., & Sanders, E. (2009). *Research-based practices for creating access to the general curriculum in reading and literacy for students with significant intellectual disabilities. Monograph prepared for the Council for Chief State School Officers (CCSSO) Assessing Special Education Students (ASES) State Collaborative on Assessment and Student Standards (SCASS).* Retrieved From: http://idahotc.com/Portals/15/Docs/IAA/10-11%20Docs/Research_Based_Practices_Reading_2009.pdf

Erickson, K., & Koppenhaver, D. (1995). Developing a literacy program for children with severe disabilities. *The Reading Teacher, 48,* 676–684.

Erickson, K. A., Hatch, P., & Clendon, S. (2010). Literacy, assistive technology, and students with significant disabilities. *Focus on Exceptional Children, 42*(5), 1–16.

Erickson, K. A., Koppenhaver, D. A., Yoder, D. E., & Nance, J. (1997). Integrated communication and literacy instruction for a child with multiple disabilities. *Focus on Autism and Other Developmental Disabilities, 12*(3), 142–150. doi:10.1177/108835769701200302

Estrella, G. (1997). *1997 Edwin and Esther Prentke AAC Distinguished Lecturer.* Retrieved from: http://www.aacinstitute.org/Resources/PrentkeLecture/1997/GusEstrella.html

Ewing, G. (2000). Update from the executive director. *Incoming, 2*(7), 1. Retrieved January 12, 2005, from hp://www.mtml.ca/newslet/ july00/page1.htm

Fager, S., Bardach, L., Russell, S., & Higginbotham, J. (2012). Access to augmentative and alternative communication: New technologies and clinical decision-making. *Journal of Pediatric Rehabilitation Medicine, 5*(1), 53–61. PMID:22543893

Fallon, K. A., & Katz, L. (2008). Augmentative and alternative communication and literacy teams: Facing the challenges, forging ahead. *Seminars in Speech and Language, 29*(2), 112–119. doi:10.1055/s-2008-1079125 PMID:18645913

Fallon, K. A., Light, J., McNaughton, D., Drager, K., & Hammer, C. (2004). The effects of direct instruction on the single-word reading skills of children who require augmentative and alternative communication. *Journal of Speech, Language, and Hearing Research: JSLHR, 47*(6), 1424–1439. doi:10.1044/1092-4388(2004/106) PMID:15842020

Fenlon, A. G., McNabb, J., & Pidlypchak, H. (2010). So Much Potential in Reading!" Developing Meaningful Literacy Routines for Students With Multiple Disabilities. *Teaching Exceptional Children, 43*(1), 42–48.

Ferreira, J., Rönnberg, J., Gustafson, S., & Wengelin, Å. (2007). Reading, why not? Literacy skills in children with motor and speech impairments. *Communication Disorders Quarterly, 28*(4), 236–251. doi:10.1177/1525740107311814

Foley, B., & Staples, A. (2006). Assistive technology supports for literacy instruction. *SIG 12 Perspectives on Augmentative and Alternative Communication, 15*(2), 15-21.

Foley, B., & Wolter, J. A. (2010). Literacy intervention for transition-aged youth: What is and what could be. In D. McNaughton & D. Beukelman (Eds.), *Language, Literacy, and AAC Issues for Transition- Age Youth* (pp. 35–68). Baltimore, MD: Brookes.

Foley, B. E. (2003). Language, literacy, and AAC: Translating theory into practice. *SIG 12 Perspectives on Augmentative and Alternative Communication, 12*(1), 5-8.

Forts, A. M., & Luckasson, R. (2011). Reading, writing, and friendship: Adult implications of effective literacy instruction for students with intellectual disability. *Research and Practice for Persons with Severe Disabilities, 36*(3-4), 121–125. doi:10.2511/027494811800824417

Fossett, B., & Mirenda, P. (2006). Sight word reading in children with developmental disabilities: A comparison of paired associate and picture-to-text matching instruction. *Research in Developmental Disabilities, 27*(4), 411–429. doi:10.1016/j.ridd.2005.05.006 PMID:16112841

Fried-Oken, M., & More, L. (1992). An initial vocabulary for nonspeaking preschool children based on developmental and environmental language sources. *Augmentative and Alternative Communication, 8*(1), 41–56. doi:10.1080/07434619212331276033

Gerde, H. K., Bingham, G. E., & Wasik, B. A. (2012). Writing in early childhood classrooms: Guidance for best practices. *Early Childhood Education Journal, 40*(6), 351–359. doi:10.1007/s10643-012-0531-z

Gierach, J. (2009). Assessing Students' Needs for Assistive Technology (ASNAT): A resource manual for school district teams, 5th Eds. Milton, WI: Wisconsin Assistive Technology Initiative. (nod). Retrieved From www.wati.org

Giesbrecht, E. (2013). Application of the human activity assistive technology model for occupational therapy research. *Australian Occupational Therapy Journal, 60*(4), 230–240. doi:10.1111/1440-1630.12054 PMID:23888973

Gindis, B. (1995). The social/cultural implications of disability: Vygotsky's paradigm for special education. *Educational Psychologist, 30*(2), 77–81. doi:10.1207/s15326985ep3002_4

Gunning, T. G. (2005). Creating literacy instruction for all students. Boston, MA: Pearson Higher Ed.

Guthrie, J. T., McRae, A., & Klauda, S. L. (2007). Contributions of concept-oriented reading instruction to knowledge about interventions for motivations in reading. *Educational Psychology, 42*(4), 237–250. doi:10.1080/00461520701621087

Hannon, P. (2000). *Reflecting on literacy in education*. New York, NY: Routledge Falmer.

Hanser, G. A., & Erickson, K. A. (2007). Integrated word identification and communication instruction for students with complex communication needs preliminary results. *Focus on Autism and Other Developmental Disabilities, 22*(4), 268–278. doi:10.1177/10883576070220040901

Harn, B. A., Linan-Thompson, S., & Roberts, G. (2008). Intensifying instruction does additional instructional time make a difference for the most at-risk first graders? *Journal of Learning Disabilities, 41*(2), 115–125. doi:10.1177/0022219407313586 PMID:18354932

Hulleman, C. S., Godes, O., Hendricks, B. L., & Harackiewicz, J. M. (2010). Enhancing interest and performance with a utility value intervention. *Journal of Educational Psychology, 102*(4), 880–895. doi:10.1037/a0019506

Hunt, P., Soto, G., Maier, J., Müller, E., & Goetz, L. (2002). Collaborative teaming to support students with augmentative and alternative communication needs in general education classrooms. *Augmentative and Alternative Communication, 18*(1), 20–35. doi:10.1080/aac.18.1.20.35

Hynan, A., Murray, J., & Goldbart, J. (2014). 'Happy and excited': Perceptions of using digital technology and social media by young people who use augmentative and alternative communication. *Child Language Teaching and Therapy, 30*(2), 175–186. doi:10.1177/0265659013519258

Iacono, T. A. (2004). Accessible reading intervention: A work in progress. *Augmentative and Alternative Communication, 20*(3), 179–190. doi:10.1080/07434610410001699744

Individuals With Disabilities Education Improvement Act, 20 U.S.C. (2004). Retrieved from: http://idea.ed.gov/download/statute.html

Johnston, S. S., Davenport, L., Kanarowski, B., Rhodehouse, S., & McDonnell, A. P. (2009). Teaching sound letter correspondence and consonant-vowel-consonant combinations to young children who use augmentative and alternative communication. *Augmentative and Alternative Communication, 25*(2), 123–135. doi:10.1080/07434610902921409 PMID:19444683

Jones, C., Reutzel, D. R., & Fargo, J. D. (2010). Comparing two methods of writing instruction: Effects on kindergarten students' reading skills. *The Journal of Educational Research, 103*(5), 327–341. doi:10.1080/00220670903383119

Kaderavek, J. N., & Rabidoux, P. (2004). Interactive to independent literacy: A model for designing literacy goals for children with atypical communication. *Reading & Writing Quarterly, 20*(3), 237–260. doi:10.1080/10573560490429050

Kazakoff-Lane, C. (2010). Anything, anywhere, anytime: The promise of the animated tutorial sharing project for online and mobile information literacy. *Journal of Library Administration*, *50*(7/8), 747–766. doi:10.1080/01930826.2010.488961

Kent-Walsh, J., Binger, C., & Hasham, Z. (2010). Effects of parent instruction on the symbolic communication of children using augmentative and alternative communication during storybook reading. *American Journal of Speech-Language Pathology*, *19*(2), 97–107. doi:10.1044/1058-0360(2010/09-0014) PMID:20181850

Kent-Walsh, J., Binger, C., & Malani, M. (2010). Teaching partners to support the communication skills of young children who use AAC: Lessons from the ImPAACT Program. *Early Childhood Services (San Diego, Calif.)*, *4*(3), 155–170.

Koppenhaver, D. (2000). Literacy in AAC: What should be written on the envelope we push? *Augmentative and Alternative Communication*, *16*(4), 270–279. doi:10.1080/07434610012331279124

Koppenhaver, D. A., Hendrix, M. P., & Williams, A. R. (2007). Toward evidence-based literacy interventions for children with severe and multiple disabilities. *Seminars in Speech and Language*, *28*(1), 79–89. doi:10.1055/s-2007-967932 PMID:17340385

Korat, O., Shamir, A., & Arbiv, L. (2011). E-books as support for emergent writing with and without adult assistance. *Education and Information Technologies*, *16*(3), 301–318. doi:10.1007/s10639-010-9127-7

Kucirkova, N., Messer, D., Critten, V., & Harwood, J. (2014). Story-Making on the iPad When Children Have Complex Needs Two Case Studies. *Communication Disorders Quarterly*, 1525740114525226.

Lane, K., Harris, K. R., Graham, S., Weisenbach, J. L., Brindle, M., & Morphy, P. (2008). The effects of self-regulated strategy development on the writing performance of second-grade students with behavioral and writing difficulties. *The Journal of Special Education*, *41*(4), 234–253. doi:10.1177/0022466907310370

Light, J. (1997). "Let's go star fishing": Reflections on the contexts of language learning for children who use aided AAC. *Augmentative and Alternative Communication*, *13*(3), 158–171. doi:10.1080/07434619712331277978

Light, J. (1998). Toward a definition of communication competence for individuals using augmentative and alternative communication systems. *Augmentative and Alternative Communication*, *5*(2), 137–144. doi:10.1080/07434618912331275126

Light, J., & Kelford Smith, A. (1993). Home literacy experiences of preschoolers who use AAC systems and of their nondisabled peers. *Augmentative and Alternative Communication*, *9*(1), 10–25. doi:10.1080/07434619312331276371

Light, J., & McNaughton, D. (2009). *Accessible Literacy Learning: Evidence-based reading instruction for individuals with autism, cerebral palsy, Down syndrome, and other disabilities*. San Diego, CA: Mayer-Johnson.

Light, J., & McNaughton, D. (2012a). Supporting the communication, language, and literacy development of children with complex communication needs: State of the science and future research priorities. *Assistive Technology*, *24*(1), 34–44. doi:10.1080/10400435.2011.648717 PMID:22590798

Light, J., & McNaughton, D. (2012b). The changing face of augmentative and alternative communication: Past, present, and future challenges. *Augmentative and Alternative Communication, 28*(4), 197–204. do i:10.3109/07434618.2012.737024 PMID:23256853

Light, J., McNaughton, D., Weyer, M., & Karg, L. (2008). Evidence-based literacy instruction for individuals who require augmentative and alternative communication: A case study of a student with multiple disabilities. *Seminars in Speech and Language, 29*(2), 120–132. doi:10.1055/s-2008-1079126 PMID:18645914

Lonigan, C. J., Allan, N. P., & Lerner, M. D. (2011). Assessment of preschool early literacy skills: Linking children's educational needs with empirically supported instructional activities. *Psychology in the Schools, 48*(5), 488–501. doi:10.1002/pits.20569 PMID:22180666

Lorenz, B., Green, T., & Brown, A. (2009). Using Multimedia Graphic Organizer Software in the Prewriting Activities of Primary School Students: What Are the Benefits? *Computers in the Schools, 26*(2), 115–129. doi:10.1080/07380560902906054

Lund, S. K., & Light, J. (2006). Long-term outcomes for individuals who use augmentative and alternative communication: Part I-what is a "good" outcome? *Augmentative and Alternative Communication, 22*(4), 284–299. doi:10.1080/07434610600718693 PMID:17127616

Macaruso, P., & Rodman, A. (2011). Efficacy of computer-assisted instruction for the development of early literacy skills in young children. *Reading Psychology, 32*(2), 172–196. doi:10.1080/02702711003608071

Maclean, R. (1988). Two paradoxes of phonics. *The Reading Teacher, 41*(6), 514–517.

Marvin, C., Beukelman, D., & Bilyeu, D. (1994). Vocabulary-use patterns in preschool children: Effects of context and time sampling. *Augmentative and Alternative Communication, 10*(4), 224–236. doi:10.1080/07434619412331276930

Matas, J., Mathy-Laikko, P., Beukelman, D., & Legresley, K. (1985). Identifying the nonspeaking population: A demographic study. *Augmentative and Alternative Communication, 1*(1), 17–31. doi:10.1080/07434618512331273491

Mathisen, B., Arthur-Kelly, M., Kidd, J., & Nissen, C. (2009). Using MINSPEAK: A case study of a preschool child with complex communication needs. *Disability and Rehabilitation. Assistive Technology, 4*(5), 376–383. doi:10.1080/17483100902807112 PMID:19484639

McGrail, E., & Davis, A. (2011). The influence of classroom blogging on elementary student writing. *Journal of Research in Childhood Education, 25*(4), 415–437. doi:10.1080/02568543.2011.605205

McNaughton, D., & Light, J. (January, 2010). *Evidence-based literacy intervention for individuals with complex communication needs*. Assistive Technology Industry Association, Orlando, FL. Retrieved from: http://aac-rerc.psu.edu/_userfiles/file/ATIA%202010%20%20literacy%20HO%202%20page.pdf

Millar, D. C., Light, J. C., & McNaughton, D. B. (2004). The effect of direct instruction and writer's workshop on the early writing skills of children who use augmentative and alternative communication. *AAC: Augmentative & Alternative Communication, 20*(3), 164–178. Retrieved from http://search.ebscohost.com/login.aspx?direct=true&db=rzh&AN=2005025249&site=ehost-live&scope=site

Millar, D. C., Light, J. C., & Schlosser, R. W. (2006). The impact of augmentative and alternative communication intervention on the speech production of individuals with developmental disabilities: A research review. *Journal of Speech, Language, and Hearing Research: JSLHR, 49*(2), 248–264. doi:10.1044/1092-4388(2006/021) PMID:16671842

Mirenda, P. (2001). Beneath the surface. *Augmentative and Alternative Communication, 17*(1), 1–1. doi:10.1080/aac.17.1.1.1

Morgan, H. (2013). Multimodal children's e-books help young learners in reading. *Early Childhood Education Journal, 41*(6), 477–483. doi:10.1007/s10643-013-0575-8

National Early Literacy Panel. (2008). *Developing early literacy: Report of the National Early Literacy Panel.* Washington, DC: National Institute for Literacy.

National Institute of Child Health and Human Development (NICHD). NIH, DHHS. (2001). Put Reading First: The Research Building Blocks for Teaching Children to Read (N/A). Washington, DC: U.S. Government Printing Office.

National Reading Panel. (2000). *Teaching children to read: An evidence-based assessment of the scientific research literature on reading and its implications for reading instruction* [on-line]. Retrieved From: http://www.nichd.nih.gov/publications/nrp/report.cfm

Neumann, M. M., & Neumann, D. L. (2014). Touch screen tablets and emergent literacy. *Early Childhood Education Journal, 42*(4), 231–239. doi:10.1007/s10643-013-0608-3

No Child Left Behind Act of 2001, Pub. L. No. 107-110, 115 Stat. 1425 (2002). Retrieved June 26, 2014, from http://www.ed.gov/policy/elsec/leg/esea02/107-110.pdf

Olswang, L. B., Feuerstein, J. L., Pinder, G. L., & Dowden, P. (2013). Validating dynamic assessment of triadic gaze for young children with severe disabilities. *American Journal of Speech-Language Pathology, 22*(3), 449–462. doi:10.1044/1058-0360(2012/12-0013) PMID:23813200

Peeters, M., Verhoeven, L., de Moor, J., van Balkom, H., & van Leeuwe, J. (2009). Home literacy predictors of early reading development in children with cerebral palsy. *Research in Developmental Disabilities, 30*(3), 445–461. doi:10.1016/j.ridd.2008.04.005 PMID:18541405

Pikulski, J. J., & Chard, D. J. (2005). Fluency: Bridge between decoding and comprehension. *The Reading Teacher, 58*(6), 510–519. doi:10.1598/RT.58.6.2

Pufpaff, L. A. (2008). Barriers to participation in kindergarten literacy instruction for a student with augmentative and alternative communication needs. *Psychology in the Schools, 45*(7), 582–599. doi:10.1002/pits.20311

Pufpaff, L. A., Blischak, D. M., & Lloyd, L. L. (2000). Effects of modified orthography on the identification of printed words. *American Journal of Mental Retardation, 105*(1), 14–24. doi:10.1352/0895-8017(2000)105<0014:EOMOOT>2.0.CO;2 PMID:10683705

Pufpaff, L. A., & Yssel, N. (2010). Effects of a 6-week, co-taught literacy unit on preservice special educators' literacy-education knowledge. *Psychology in the Schools, 47*(5), 493–500.

Rivera, C. J. (2013). Multimedia shared stories: Teaching literacy skills to diverse learners. *Teaching Exceptional Children, 45*(6), 38–45.

Romski, M., & Sevcik, R. A. (2005). Augmentative communication and early intervention: Myths and realities. *Infants and Young Children, 18*(3), 174–185. doi:10.1097/00001163-200507000-00002

Romski, M., Sevcik, R. A., Adamson, L. B., Cheslock, M., Smith, A., Barker, R. M., & Bakeman, R. (2010). Randomized comparison of augmented and nonaugmented language interventions for toddlers with developmental delays and their parents. *Journal of Speech, Language, and Hearing Research: JSLHR, 53*(2), 350–364. doi:10.1044/1092-4388(2009/08-0156) PMID:20360461

Rosa-Lugo, L. I., & Kent-Walsh, J. (2008). Effects of parent instruction on communicative turns of Latino children using augmentative and alternative communication during storybook reading. *Communication Disorders Quarterly, 30*(1), 49–61. doi:10.1177/1525740108320353

Ruppar, A. L. (2013). Authentic literacy instruction in inclusive environments for students with severe disabilities. *Teaching Exceptional Children, 46*, 44–50.

Salmon, L. G. (2014). Factors that affect emergent literacy development when engaging with electronic books. *Early Childhood Education Journal, 42*(2), 85–92. doi:10.1007/s10643-013-0589-2

Savarese, E. T., & Savarese, R. J. (2012). Literate lungs: One autist's journey as a reader. *Research and Practice for Persons with Severe Disabilities, 37*(2), 100–110. doi:10.2511/027494812802573594

Schlosser, R. W., & Wendt, O. (2008). Effects of augmentative and alternative communication intervention on speech production in children with autism: A systematic review. *American Journal of Speech-Language Pathology, 17*(3), 212–230. doi:10.1044/1058-0360(2008/021) PMID:18663107

Simeonsson, R. J., Bjorck-Akesson, E., & Lollar, D. J. (2012). Communication, disabilities, and the ICF-CY. *Augmentative and Alternative Communication, 28*(1), 3–10. doi:10.3109/07434618.2011.65 3829 PMID:22364533

Singh, N. N., & Solman, R. T. (1990). A stimulus control analysis of the picture-word problem in children who are mentally retarded: The blocking effect. *Journal of Applied Behavior Analysis, 23*(4), 525–532. doi:10.1901/jaba.1990.23-525 PMID:2074241

Skoto, B. G., Koppenhaver, D. A., & Erickson, K. A. (2004). Parent reading behaviors and communication outcomes in girls with Rett Syndrome. *Exceptional Children, 70*(2), 145–166. doi:10.1177/001440290407000202

Smith, M. K. (1996, 2000). Curriculum theory and practice. In *The encyclopaedia of informal education.* Retrieved from www.infed.org/biblio/b-curric.htm

Solman, R. T., & Wu, H. M. (1995). Pictures as feedback in single word learning. *Educational Psychology, 15*(3), 227–244. doi:10.1080/0144341950150301

Sonnenschein, S., Stapleton, L. M., & Benson, A. (2010). The relation between the type and amount of instruction and growth in children's reading competencies. *American Educational Research Journal, 47*(2), 358–389. doi:10.3102/0002831209349215

Soto, G., & Dukhovny, E. (2008). The effect of shared book reading on the acquisition of expressive vocabulary of a 7 year old who uses AAC. *Seminars in Speech and Language*, *29*(2), 133–145. doi:10.1055/s-2008-1079127 PMID:18645915

Spooner, F., Ahlgrim-Delzell, L., Kemp-Inman, A., & Wood, L. A. (2014). Using an iPad2® with systematic instruction to teach shared stories for elementary-aged students with autism. *Research and Practice for Persons with Severe Disabilities*, *39*(1), 30–46. doi:10.1177/1540796914534631

Spooner, F., Rivera, C. J., Browder, D. M., Baker, J. N., & Salas, S. (2009). Teaching emergent literacy skills using cultural contextual story-based lessons. *Research and Practice for Persons with Severe Disabilities*, *34*(3-4), 102–112. doi:10.2511/rpsd.34.3-4.102

Staugler, K. (2007). Literacy Rubric: Informal Literacy Assessment Tool. https://wvde.state.wv.us/osp/ supporting- literacy/documents/Literacy%20Rubric.pdf

Stephenson, J. (2010). Book Reading as an Intervention Context for Children Beginning to Use Graphic Symbols for Communication. *Journal of Developmental and Physical Disabilities*, *22*(3), 257–271. doi:10.1007/s10882-009-9164-6

Stuart, S., Beukelman, D., & King, J. (1997). Vocabulary use during extended conversations by two cohorts of older adults. *Augmentative and Alternative Communication*, *13*(1), 40–47. doi:10.1080/074 34619712331277828

Sturm, J. (2003). Writing in AAC. *The ASHA Leader*, *8*(16), 4–5.

Sturm, J. M., & Clendon, S. A. (2004). Augmentative and alternative communication, language, and literacy: Fostering the relationship. *Topics in Language Disorders*, *24*(1), 76–91. doi:10.1097/00011363-200401000-00008

Sturm, J. M., Spadorcia, S. A., Cunningham, J. W., Cali, K. S., Staples, A., Erickson, K., & Koppenhaver, D. A. (2006). What happens to reading between first and third grade? Implications for students who use AAC. *Augmentative and Alternative Communication*, *22*(1), 21–36. doi:10.1080/07434610500243826 PMID:17114156

Sulzby, E. (1989). Assessment of emergent writing and children's language while writing. In L. Morrow & J. Smith (Eds.), The role of assessment in early literacy instruction. Englewood Cliffs, NJ: Prentice-Hall.

Torgesen, J., Houston, D., Rissman, L., & Kosanovich, M. (2007). Teaching All Students to Read in Elementary School: A Guide for Principals. *Center on Instruction*. Retrieved From: http://www.fcrr.org/ Interventions/pdf/Principals%20Guide-Elementary.pdf

Truxler, J. E., & O'Keefe, B. M. (2007). The effects of phonological awareness instruction on beginning word recognition and spelling. *Augmentative and Alternative Communication*, *23*(2), 164–176. doi:10.1080/07434610601151803 PMID:17487629

Van Tatenhove, G. M. (2009). Building language competence with students using AAC devices: Six challenges. *SIG 12 Perspectives on Augmentative and Alternative Communication*, *18*(2), 38-47.

Wild, M. (2009). Using computer-aided instruction to support the systematic practice of phonological skills in beginning readers. *Journal of Research in Reading*, *32*(4), 413–432. doi:10.1111/j.1467-9817.2009.01405.x

Wood Jackson, C., Wahlquist, J., & Marquis, C. (2011). Visual supports for shared reading with young children: The effect of static overlay design. *Augmentative and Alternative Communication*, *27*(2), 91–102. doi:10.3109/07434618.2011.576700 PMID:21592004

ADDITIONAL READING

Binger, C., & Kent-Walsh, J. (2012). Selecting skills to teach communication partners: Where do I start? *SIG 12 Perspectives on Augmentative and Alternative Communication*, 21(4), 127-135.

Connor, C. M., Alberto, P. A., Compton, D. L., & O'Connor, R. E. (2014). *Improving Reading Outcomes for Students with or at Risk for Reading Disabilities: A Synthesis of the Contributions from the Institute of Education Sciences Research Centers (NCSER 2014-3000)*. Washington, DC: National Center for Special Education Research, Institute of Education Sciences, U.S. Department of Education. This report is available on the IES website at; http://ies.ed.gov/

Erickson, K., Hanser, G., Hatch, P., & Sanders, E. (2009). *Research-based practices for creating access to the general curriculum in reading and literacy for students with significant intellectual disabilities.* Monograph prepared for the Council for Chief State School Officers (CCSSO) Assessing Special Education Students (ASES) State Collaborative on Assessment and Student Standards (SCASS). Retrieved From: http://idahotc.com/Portals/15/Docs/IAA/10-11%20Docs/Research_Based_Practices_Reading_2009.pdf

Florida Department of Education. (2003). *Cool tools informal reading assessments.* Retrieved from: http://www.paec.org/itrk3/files/pdfs/readingpdfs/cooltoolsall.pdf

Gierach, J. (2009). *Assessing Students' Needs for Assistive Technology (ASNAT): A resource manual for school district teams, 5th Eds.* Milton, WI: Wisconsin Assistive Technology Initiative. (n.d.). Retrieved From www.wati.org

Keefe, E. B., & Copeland, S. R. (2011). What is literacy? The power of a definition. *Research and Practice for Persons with Severe Disabilities*, *36*(3), 92–99. doi:10.2511/027494811800824507

Koppenhaver, D., & Williams, A. (2010). A conceptual review of writing research in augmentative and alternative communication. *Augmentative and Alternative Communication*, *26*(3), 158–176. doi:10.3109/07434618.2010.505608 PMID:20874079

Light, J., & McNaughton, D. (2012). Supporting the communication, language, and literacy development of children with complex communication needs: State of the science and future research priorities. *Assistive Technology*, *24*(1), 34–44. doi:10.1080/10400435.2011.648717 PMID:22590798

Light, J. L., McNaughton, D., Weyer, M., & Karg, L. (2008). Evidence-based literacy instruction for individuals who require augmentative and alternative communication: A case study of a student with multiple disabilities. *Seminars in Speech and Language*, *29*(2), 120–132. doi:10.1055/s-2008-1079126 PMID:18645914

Michael Barker, R., Saunders, K. J., & Brady, N. C. (2012). Reading instruction for children who use AAC: Considerations in the pursuit of generalizable results. *Augmentative and Alternative Communication*, *28*(3), 160–170. doi:10.3109/07434618.2012.704523 PMID:22946991

National Early Literacy Panel. (2008). *Developing early literacy: Report of the National Early Literacy Panel*. Washington, DC: National Institute for Literacy.

National Reading Panel. (2000). *Teaching children to read: An evidence-based assessment of the scientific research literature on reading and its implications for reading instruction* [on-line]. Retrieved From: http://www.nichd.nih.gov/publications/nrp/report.cfm

Pufpaff, L. A. (2008). Barriers to participation in kindergarten literacy instruction for a student with augmentative and alternative communication needs. *Psychology in the Schools*, *45*(7), 582–599. doi:10.1002/pits.20311

Ruppar, A. L. (2013). Authentic literacy and communication in inclusive settings for students with significant disabilities. *Teaching Exceptional Children*, *46*(2), 44–50.

KEY TERMS AND DEFINITIONS

Augmentative and Alternative Communication (AAC): AAC is a broad term used to describe methods to support persons who are unable to use speech and/or language as a primary mode of communication. AAC systems include many modes of communication including sign language, use of symbols to communicate, written communication, and a wide range of dedicated communication devices.

Complex Communication Needs: Learners with complex communication are a heterogeneous population who require AAC system supports for successful expressive and receptive communication.

Conventional literacy: Conventional literacy skills are those skills which support a learner in reading a wide variety of text genres and comprehending these materials and writing for a large set of audiences with strong composition.

Dynamic assessment: Dynamic assessment, a Vygotsky concept, integrates teaching into the process of assessment. This combined method allows educational teams to determine how a learner may respond to immediate instruction during specific assessment tasks, which may appear difficult for the learner.

Early literacy: Early literacy skills are oral, reading, and writing skills which emerge between birth and early elementary school through exposure to language and literacy activities as well as direct instruction. Early literacy skills include print awareness, letter knowledge, vocabulary, phonological awareness, and narrative skills.

Least Dangerous Assumption: Least Dangerous Assumption is a concept coined by Donnellan (1984). If a child is at an appropriate age, similar to the age of their peers, and is not communicating, reading, or writing the least dangerous assumption is to simply provide the instruction that one would provide to all children. The least dangerous effect of this decision would be that the child might not learn to communicate, read, or write. The most dangerous decision is to not provide instruction and thus the child is surely never to attain these skills. In the absence of proof that a child cannot learn, assume the least dangerous solution.

Chapter 5
The Use of Mobile Technologies for Students At-Risk or Identified with Behavioral Disorders within School-Based Contexts

Frank J. Sansosti
Kent State University, USA

Peña L. Bedesem
Kent State University, USA

ABSTRACT

Students at-risk or identified with behavioral disorders often present complex challenges to educators. The purpose of this chapter is to: (a) highlight the benefits and challenges of using mobile technologies within school-based contexts; (b) provide a brief overview of the contemporary research regarding the use of mobile devices for improving the outcomes of students with behavioral disorders within schools; and (c) offer essential techniques, methods, and ideas for improving instruction and management for students with behavioral difficulties via mobile technologies. Taken together, the intent is to call attention to the evidence that supports the use of mobile technologies for students who are at-risk or identified with behavioral disorders in schools, raise awareness of those strategies that appear to be the most effective for such students and assist service providers in providing accountable education.

BACKGROUND AND SIGNIFICANCE

Students who exhibit behavioral and learning problems present complex challenges for schools (Cook, Landrum, Tankersley, & Kauffman, 2003). Typically, students with behavioral problems are those who have been identified, or who are at risk of being identified as having a disability, and who exhibit one or more of the following behaviors: (a) attention problems; (b) hyperactivity; (c) aggressive behavior(s);

DOI: 10.4018/978-1-4666-8395-2.ch005

(d) withdrawn behavior(s); (e) bizarre behavior(s); (f) poor academic performance; (g) difficulties with memory; and/or (h) poor language abilities (Vaughn & Bos, 2012). While any student can demonstrate behavioral problems, most often, individuals who qualify for special education and related services under the *Individuals with Disabilities Education Improvement Act* (IDEIA, 2004) categories of Emotional Disturbance, Specific Learning Disabilities, and Other Health Impaired (which encompasses many children diagnosed with Attention Deficit Hyperactivity Disorder; ADHD) constitute the majority of focus within school-based settings. Historically, such students have been described as the toughest to teach, the most often segregated, and the most likely to fail (Cook et al., 2003). Hypothesized reasons for such detrimental outcomes rest upon the notion that students who exhibit behavioral problems often are judged by others to be disruptive, disobedient, and engaging in behaviors that impede learning (Alisauskas & Simkiene, 2013). According to Berger (1995) and Swaggart (1998) students with behavioral problems often: (a) waste time during academic assignments, (b) engage in academic content less frequently, (c) demonstrate increased inattentiveness and impulsivity, (c) exhibit poor social skills, and (d) require increased instructional attention and effort from teachers. Taken together, such areas of deficit likely result in incomplete schoolwork, lack of instructional gains, and frustrated educators.

As a group, students with behavioral problems represent a large portion of those students receiving special education instruction in schools. As part of the IDEIA, each state's Department of Education (DOE) and the U.S. Department of Education (USDOE) are required to record specific childhood disabilities for each school year. In 2012, the total number of students between the ages of six and 21 receiving special education and related services for Emotional Disturbance (ED), Specific Learning Disabilities (SLD), and Other Health Impaired (OHI) combined was close to three and a half million (IDEA Data Center, 2014). It is possible that the number of children receiving special education under these categories is a gross underestimate of the actual frequency of services necessary to support the education of those who are at-risk or have been identified as having behavioral problems. This is due to the fact that some children may not be included in IDEIA counts because they attend private schools, are home schooled, or do not meet eligibility criteria for special education but require some level of supportive services. Moreover, aside from the exact number of students served, placement in general education settings has become a dominant service delivery issue for students with behavioral difficulties. Data from the Office of Special Education Programs (IDEA Data Center, 2014) suggest that students with behavioral difficulties increasingly are served in inclusive settings. Specifically, 43% of students with Emotional Disturbance received their special educational instruction in the general education curriculum. Similarly, 62% of students identified as Other Health Impaired and 64% of those identified as having a Specific Learning Disability were educated within general education classrooms.

Given the percentages of students receiving services within inclusive contexts, combined with the fact that these statistics likely are underestimates of the true number of students who need support, educators likely face challenges instructing and managing students with behavioral problems. As such, school professionals not only need to be prepared to support children with behavioral problems, but also be aware of the evidence-based practices that are available. Moreover, as technology begins to permeate educational programming, educators need to identify the most promising and helpful tools that can be deployed readily within classroom contexts to assist in supporting the education of students with behavioral difficulties. The awareness and understanding of the use of mobile technologies for individuals with disabilities who demonstrate behavioral problems has particular relevance to the field of education, as practitioners increasingly have been called upon to support the educational needs of such students. Moreover, it is highly likely that parents and advocates frequently request the use of mobile technologies within school-based settings due to the proliferation of inexpensive devices (e.g., iPads) and dedicated applications geared to a variety of behaviors such as attention, emotional regulation, and social skills, to name a few.

The use of mobile technologies for enhancing the outcomes of students who exhibit behavioral disorders is a relatively new area of research, but one that has demonstrated great potential. Researchers have identified that the use of mobile technologies can result in increased task completion of students with moderate intellectual disabilities (e.g., Mechling, Gast, & Fields, 2008; Mechling, Gast, & Seid, 2010); increased self-monitoring for students with emotional and behavioral disorders (e.g., Bedesem, 2012; Blood et al., 2011; Gulchak, 2008); and improved on-task performance (e.g., Cihak, Wright, & Ayres, 2010; Davies, Stock, & Wehmeyer, 2002; Spriggs, Gast, & Ayres, 2007). Such positive outcomes likely result from an increased interest level among students, leading to a greater likelihood of intervention adherence and follow through (Taber-Dougty, 2005).

USE OF MOBILE TECHNOLOGIES FOR EDUCATIONAL PROGRAMMING

The understanding and use of mobile technologies within the realm of education is not new. In fact, the broad term *Assistive Technology Device* was first codified under the *Technology-Related Assistance for Individuals with Disabilities Act*, of 1988, and was defined as "any item, piece of equipment, or product system, whether acquired commercially off the shelf, modified, or customized, that is used to increase, maintain, or improve functional capabilities of individuals with disabilities." This definition was modified further by the IDEIA of 2004 to exclude any surgically implanted medical devices. Although this definition captures just about any technological device, the majority of assistive technology in schools is typically packaged technology programs such as text-to-speech programs, word-prediction programs, and screen magnifiers (Edyburn, 2004). However, with the widespread and continually emerging use of technology-based instruction and intervention, we provide more precision to the definition. Included in this definition is the notion that ubiquitous technologies, such as mobile technology, can be repurposed as assistive technology (Bouck, Shurr, Tom, Jasper, Bassette, Miller, & Flanagan, 2012). Today, mobile technologies represent any electronic device that accepts, processes, stores, and/or outputs data at high speeds. These may include mobile devices like smartphones (e.g., Android, iPhone) and tablets (e.g., iPad, Kindle Fire). A generally accepted definition within education defines the use of mobile technologies in the classroom as mobile learning. Specifically, mobile learning is a method of teaching and learning centered on the use of small, maneuverable devices, such as smartphones, iPads/tablets, iPods, and all other handheld devices which offer some form of wireless connectivity (Keegan, 2005). Taken together, mobile technologies and mobile learning refer, generally, to those portable technological instruments that can be used in a variety of locations (flexibility, adaptability) and permit access to specific programs and/or apps designed to encourage the active use of information that enables the acquisition and development and/or application of skills. In a similar way, Brazuelo and Gallego (2011) defined mobile learning as "the educational system that facilitates the construction of knowledge, the resolution of learning problems, and the development of a variety of skills and abilities in an autonomous way, anywhere, thanks to portable mobile devices (p.17)."

Benefits and Challenges of Using Mobile Technologies in School-Based Contexts

There are several benefits of using mobile technology in school-based contexts. Probably one of the most obvious benefits is the prevalence and functionality of such technology. Mobile devices such as smart phones (e.g., iPhones, Androids), iPods, and tablet computers (e.g., iPad, Kindle, Galaxy) are owned and used by school-age children and adults on a daily basis. Mobile devices can be used for communication (e.g., phone, text messaging, email, video conference), organization (e.g., calendar, planner, notebook), research (e.g., Internet browser), and entertainment (e.g., camera, books, music, videos, games), and, can be purchased for a relatively low price. The ability to purchase high quality digital devices at prices significantly lower than the cost of desktop and laptop computers also may assist in closing the gap between students who have access to technology and those who do not have access to technology. For example, many Title 1 schools are making a significant effort to level the playing field for their students by providing mobile devices for use at school and at home. According to the most recent Speak Up survey (2014), over 25% of high school students in Title 1 schools said that they have a school provided tablet to use for schoolwork, compared to only 13% of high school students in non-Title 1 schools. The same trend is seen in Title 1 elementary and middle schools where students in grades 3-5 (22%) and grades 6-8 (24%) are assigned a school tablet.

Researchers have posited that another benefit of using mobile technologies is "increased engagement, motivation, achievement, enthusiasm for learning, and enhanced student understanding (Lin, Fulford, Ho, Iyoda, & Ackerman, 2012, p. 132)." With respect to technology-supported learning environments, however, research focusing on students' motivation is limited. As technology becomes more prevalent in school-based contexts, it is imperative that we understand how technology-supported learning activities effects motivation. Consequently, Ciampa (2014) applied Malone and Lepper's (1987) motivation theory as a theoretical framework for how the use of mobile devices for classroom instruction relates to a student's motivation to learn. Ciampa's study focused on what elementary students and an elementary teacher reported as motivational elements for the use of mobile technology in the classroom. Ciampa found that six categories emerged as elements of mobile technology that stimulate intrinsic motivation (challenge, sensory and cognitive curiosity, control) and extrinsic motivation (competition, cooperation, recognition), all of which coincide with Malone and Lepper's six elements that motivate students to learn. As such, it is possible that the use of mobile technologies for students with behavioral problems is highly motivating, since it allows and encourages students to utilize their technical knowledge and experiences and permits them to engage in self-directed learning activities (West, 2012).

Another benefit of using mobile technologies that is specific to students with disabilities is that mobile technologies can be used as assistive technology. As mentioned previously, although the language used to define assistive technology under the *Technology-Related Assistance for Individuals with Disabilities Act* is broad, schools typically use packaged programs to assist students with disabilities. However, these packaged programs are costly (Bouck, Shurr, Tom, Jasper, Bassette, Miller, & Flanagan, 2012). The functionality of mobile devices makes them potentially more cost effective than many assistive technology packages. Additionally, mobile devices have touch screens that are user friendly and some mobile devices even include built-in accessibility options that are customizable. For example, they can provide text-to-speech, zoom, and mono audio to meet individual needs, and apps can be selected based on personal preference (Douglas, Wojcik, & Thompson, 2012). For these reasons, researchers have begun to explore the use of mobile technologies to assist students with moderate to severe disabilities (e.g., Achmadi et al., 2012; Kagohara et al., 2013; Mintz, Branch, March, & Lerman, 2012; Neely, Rispoli, Camargo, Davis, & Boles, 2013)

Although there are several benefits to the use of mobile technology in school-based contexts, there are challenges that also should be considered. For instance, the literature provides little guidance as to the best practices for incorporating mobile technologies into school environments (Campigotto, McEwin, & Epp, 2013). Application developers and the media support the use of mobile technologies by showing images of what this technology is capable of doing for education but often leave out *how* educators can actually use mobile technology to teach on a daily basis. How to use mobile technology might be even more challenging for educators of students with behavior problems. Educators need to take into consideration the emotional/behavioral and academic needs of a student before using mobile technologies in the classroom. Without guidance on how to identify and use appropriate mobile technologies and applications for students with behavior problems, educators are often left to randomly choose what might benefit these students. This "trial and error" approach may waste valuable instruction time and result in minimal positive outcomes.

CONTEMPORARY UTILIZATION OF MOBILE TECHNOLOGIES IN SCHOOLS

Educators typically use mobile technologies in school-based contexts to increase behavior and academic outcomes for students with behavioral problems. Behavior outcomes can include attention to task, emotion regulation, social skills, and organization. Academic outcomes can include performance accuracy, self-regulated learning, and functional skills. Although research in these areas is considered to be in its infancy, researchers have begun to demonstrate the benefits of using mobile technologies for students with behavioral problems.

Examples of Mobile Technologies for Increasing Behavior Outcomes

Researchers have looked to mobile technology to increase positive behavior in classroom contexts by exploring its use as a way for students with behavior problems to monitor their own behavior. Teaching students self-monitoring skills not only places the responsibility of behavior back on the student, but also allows the educator to focus on content instruction. Gulchak (2008) used a digital mobile device as a self-monitoring system for an 8-year old student with an emotional and behavioral disorder (EBD). Alarms on the daily calendar of the personal digital assistant (PDA) cued the student to determine if he was on-task or off-task and recorded the answer using a drop-down menu on the mobile device. Results of the study supported the use of a handheld computer as an all-inclusive self-monitoring device. Self-monitoring increased student's on-task behavior from 64% to 98%. Gulchak also reported that, at the start of the study, the student expressed excitement about using the PDA. Blood, Johnson, Ridenour, Simmons, and Crouch (2011) employed an even more commonly used digital mobile device for their study. Blood and colleagues taught a 10-year old student with EBD to use an iPod Touch to provide video modeling and as a self-monitoring cueing device. The student increased his time on task from 44% during baseline to 99% during the intervention phase. In 2012, Bedesem examined the use of mobile phones to change and support behavior in educational settings. Bedesem taught middle school students with mild to moderate disabilities (e.g., ADHD, SLD) how to self-monitor their on-task behavior in an inclusive general education classroom. The total mean for both participants increased from 45% in the baseline phase to 71% during the intervention phase. The results of these studies demonstrate the potential of mobile technologies to support positive classroom behavior among students with behavioral difficulties.

Examples of Mobile Technologies for Increasing Academic Outcomes

The research examining strategies for increasing academic outcomes for students with behavioral problems is not as robust as those examining strategies for increasing behavioral outcomes. While authors suggest a multitude of ways in which educators can use mobile technologies to increase the academic performance of students (e.g., Aronin & Floyd, 2013; Parette, & Blum, 2014), few studies supporting the use of mobile technologies specifically for students with behavioral problems have been conducted. McClanahan, Williams, Kennedy, and Tate (2012) used a series of apps on an iPad to teach a fifth-grade struggling reader with ADHD. Results of this case study demonstrated that the device not only helped the student focus attention, it facilitated his becoming more fluent in reading. Comparisons of pre- and post assessments not only showed that the student had gained one year's growth in reading within a six week time period, but also gained confidence and a sense of being in control of his learning. In a comparative study of worksheets and iPads, Haydon et al. (2013) demonstrated the differential effects of worksheets and iPads on the percentage of correct responses on various math problems (i.e., coin, fractions, patterns, operations). Specifically, three students diagnosed with emotional disturbance solved more math problems correctly in less time and demonstrated higher levels of active student engagement when using iPads.

Despite a limited number of research studies specifically examining the use of mobile technologies for promoting academic skills in students with behavioral disorders, it is possible to extrapolate the findings of research investigating the use of mobile technologies with other student populations. For example, Van Laarhoven, Johnson, Van Laarhoven-Myers, and Grider (2009) used a video-prompting procedure on an iPod to help instruct a young man with developmental disabilities to complete vocational tasks in a competitive work setting. Mechling, Gast and Seid (2009) adapted this approach with a personal digital assistant (PDA) to teach cooking skills to a group of individuals with autism spectrum disorder and to a group of students with moderate intellectual disability (Mechling, Gast, & Seid, 2010) when using both video and photographic prompts. Similarly, Mechling and Seid (2011) used video and photographic prompts on a PDA to assist pedestrian travel by students with moderate intellectual disability. More recently, Walser, Ayres, and Foote (2012) used an iPhone and a video-modeling procedure to instruct a group of high school students with moderate intellectual disability to prepare food. Such examples are applicable to individuals with or at-risk for behavioral disorders and should be used as a guide for developing and implementing a variety of intervention strategies. Aside from the outcomes indicated in each of these studies, authors cited engagement, portability and accessibility of the devices, as well as how using everyday technology in the classroom connects students who have behavior problems with their peers, as reasons to support the use of mobile technologies to improve academic outcomes for students.

Application of Mobile Technologies in Classroom Environments

Given the rapid proliferation of mobile devices within schools, we believe that educators have an excellent opportunity to embrace and use this technology to enhance the educational experiences of students with behavioral disorders. However, we argue that the implementation of mobile technology in classrooms needs to be performed in a careful and deliberate manner to ensure learning and the development of students. To ensure that students are working at an independent instructional level, and accessing and working with the desired content, educators should follow a four-step process that we illuminate below:

Step 1: *Teach the Content without Technology*. It is important first to teach the content explicitly before using any device/app. Technology can be used routinely for practicing skills, but it is no substitute for direct instruction. Directly teaching students provides the foundation for building successive applied skills to master particular content. While students find the use of technology engaging, such engagement can be fleeting or, at times, addictively distracting. Moreover, the long-term outcomes of using technology as a formal education have not been proven. As such, we posit that educators are the primary agents of good, formal education. Mobile technologies are a method for amplifying pedagogical capacity by creating a portable interactive, adaptive, and student-centered learning environment.

Step 2: *Explain and Model with Technology*. During this step, educators should introduce the device and/or app as a way for students to practice what they have learned through direct instruction. To ensure that students are successful, explain and model how to use the device/app with students.

Step 3: *Provide Guided Practice*. After students appear to have grasped the information and the use of technology to enhance their learning, it is essential to allow time for guided practice. During guided practice, the objective is to ensure that students understand both how to use a device/app and understand the content a device/app is using. At this stage, it may be helpful to create a list of guiding questions that can be used to help students learn and provide a quick check to ensure that students are able to integrate and apply the information correctly.

Step 4: *Allow Time of Independent Practice*. At this stage, students have a solid understanding of the content and how to use a mobile device to enhance their learning. As such, students are ready to use the device for independent practice to hone their skill development. Within educational contexts, devices can be made available during center time and/or independent seat time. To extend learning, have students use the concepts in a variety of activities. Now that students have demonstrated their ability to engage independently with the content, it is possible to collaborate with parents to continue learning at home (carryover of lessons/interventions across multiple settings).

By applying the above steps in practice, educators gradually shift from teacher-centered to student-centered instruction. This permits teachers to scaffold and guide students' understanding of material. Additionally, such a process allows teachers to make adjustments and provide feedback as necessary.

CONSIDERATIONS FOR SCHOOL-BASED PRACTICE

The Necessity of Data Collection and Evaluation

Data collection is the one step that is most often ignored or performed irregularly in the assessment of and intervention for academic, behavioral, and social difficulties in students at-risk or identified as having a behavioral disorder (Sansosti, Powell-Smith, & Cowan, 2010). However, there are several undeniable reasons for frequently collecting data as a critical part of demonstrating student improvement when using computer-based technologies. First, through data collection, it is possible to determine if the effects of particular computer-based approaches/strategies are favorable. Without data, educators may not be able to notice a student's improvements from his or her initial performance to his/her current behavior. Second, systematic data collection allows for formative evaluation. That is, data collected while a strategy or an intervention is being implemented, allows educators to identify problems early on in the process and make changes during the course of the intervention rather than waiting to see if it was successful after several weeks or months (Alberto & Troutman, 2013). Third, collecting data is the ultimate tool for accountability! As a result of educational reform efforts, beginning with the No Child Left Behind Act (NCLB; 2001) and extended by the IDEIA (2004), educators are required to select appropriate instruction strategies that are evidence-based. Therefore, it is essential that data be gathered for *all* aspects of instruction. In this era of evidence-based accountability, educators are responsible for results and educational planning. This is particularly true when implementing mobile technologies for students with behavioral disorders, which, relatively speaking is still 'new' and constantly emerging. Therefore, it is vital to have reliable and valid data demonstrating that the use of a particular device or app is effective at creating change in student academic, behavioral, and/or social performance. Quality data not only permits educators and educational teams to make appropriate programming decisions for students who are at-risk for or identified as having a behavioral disorder but also delivers legally defensible practices. Readers interested in understanding the methods and procedures for collecting and graphing data should refer to the Alberto and Troutman (2013) text, which includes sample instruments and strategies that can be used readily within a variety of educational settings.

Collection of data for the mere sake of collecting data is a fruitless activity unless the data are evaluated. For the most part, visual inspection of a graph will indicate whether or not the desired treatment effects were obtained. As part of a visual inspection of graphs, educators will want to provide information regarding changes in the mean data that occur from baseline to intervention. More recently, Parker and Hagan-Burke (2007) and Parker, Vannest, and Brown (2009) suggest using the improvement rate difference (IRD) to supplement visual inspection of graphs and for calculating effect size. IRD has been used for decades in the medical field (referred to "*risk reduction*" or "*risk difference*") to describe the absolute change in risk that is attributable to an experimental intervention. This metric is valued within the medical community due to its ease of interpretation as well as the fact that it does not require specific data assumptions for confidence intervals to be calculated (Altman, 1999). IRD represents the difference between two proportions (baseline and intervention). More specifically, it is the difference in improvement rates between baseline and intervention phases (Higgins & Green, 2009; Parker et al., 2009). By knowing the absolute difference in improvement, practitioners can determine the effect of an intervention and if the change in behavior is worth repeating. To calculate IRD, a minimum number of data points are removed from either baseline or intervention phases to eliminate all overlap. Data points removed from the baseline phase are considered "improved," meaning they overlap with the intervention. Data points removed from the intervention phase are considered "not improved," meaning they overlap with the baseline. The proportion of data points "improved" in baseline is then subtracted from the proportion of data points "improved" in the intervention phase ($IR_I - IR_B = IRD$). The maximum IRD score is 1.00 or 100% (all intervention data exceed baseline). An IRD of .70 to 1.0 indicates a large effect size, .50 to .70 a moderate effect size, and less than .50 a small or questionable effect size (Parker et al., 2009). An IRD of .50 indicates that half of the scores between the baseline and treatment phases were overlapping so there is only chance-level improvement. One distinct advantage of IRD is that it affords the ability to calculate confidence intervals. Practitioners can interpret the width of a confidence interval as the precision of the approach (large intervals indicate that the IRD is not trustworthy, whereas narrow intervals indicate more precision).

Professional Development Needs

Pre-Service Training of Educational Staff

University trainers should provide more guidance and direct instruction to develop teacher competence in mobile technology use in the classroom, in general, as well as the more specific application for students at-risk for or identified with behavioral disorders. However, such training should be embedded within coursework pertaining to curriculum, instruction, and intervention rather than within technology specific courses. Technology specific courses may be insufficient to train future educators how to best use technology to support learning because, in these courses, technology may become an abstraction without specific regard to the practices or context of instructing students. Instead, trainers should model and explain a traditional instructional approach and/or intervention and then demonstrate and incorporate technology-based examples of that same instruction/intervention. In so doing, trainees stand a better chance of understanding the relationship and value of the technological application and, in turn, are better equipped to implement the use of mobile technologies within the classroom.

In addition to instruction, trainers should require specialized, "hands-on" learning projects during student teaching, practicum, and/or internships that require students to utilize various didactic mobile technologies with students in the classroom. Such projects should focus on the development, implementation, data collection, and evaluation of the use of mobile technologies. This application not only has the benefit of teaching students the logistics of intervention development and implementation; it also has the added benefit of demonstrating to those in the field how the research conducted at the university level can be applied effectively within a classroom context.

Ongoing Professional Development Needs for Educational Staff

Given the increased use of mobile technologies in classrooms, combined with requests by parents and advocates for educators to use a variety of technological supports for students with or at-risk for behavioral disorders, there exists a need for current practitioners to engage in a host of ongoing professional development activities. As such, educational staff must continually seek to strengthen and broaden their skill-set to remain relevant and effective. Perhaps the quickest way to gain immediate information about emerging technologies is through attendance at professional conferences. Although conference sessions typically excel at providing attendees breadth, they often fall short in delivering in-depth information and practice with technological tools. Given this limitation, technology-specific conferences likely will offer workshops and trainings allowing attendees an opportunity to explore the available technologies and observe applications of such within a variety of contexts. However, there is a danger in the technology becoming an abstraction where the focus is more on the technology than on how it relates to practice.

Another, less structured, strategy is to allot time over the year to explore software demonstrations that often are available free of charge online or in device-specific "app stores." This clearly places the onus on the educator to seek out different mobile technology applications (not to mention that the practitioner needs to possess basic skills to operate a mobile device, etc.). Finding potential interventions is not likely the greatest challenge. Instead, the challenge rests in separating those that are likely to work from those that are unlikely to benefit a student.

Finally, efforts should be made to create collaborative projects that benefit both researchers and educators. That is, researchers/consultants who have familiarity with mobile technologies should work with educators/schools to develop a supportive infrastructure. Both the educational staff and researcher/consultant can work together to identify the needs of buildings (or the larger district) and align those technologies that best meet the needs of students. Once the needs are identified, the researcher/consultant can provide ongoing training/coaching with educational staff and other student support services personnel. Once this small team of individuals has the foundation, they can provide a trainer-of-trainers approach to others within their building(s). While the building (district) teams are implementing mobile technologies with students, the researcher/consultant can provide ongoing, supportive technical assistance (e.g., troubleshooting difficulties, modeling application of strategies, observing the schools progression). In so doing, it is likely that schools can increase their capacity to use mobile technologies to support the education of students at-risk for or with behavioral disorders, as well as provide the much-needed applied research.

FUTURE RESEARCH DIRECTIONS

Our review of the literature demonstrates that there is much work to be done to ensure the potential benefits of mobile technologies are truly realized for children with or at risk for behavioral problems. While the extant research has demonstrated that the use of mobile technologies can be leveraged to support classroom behavior, there is limited research on how mobile technologies can be used to increase long-term academic outcomes. Although there exists a wide range of educational applications designed to increase academic performance, including applications for test preparation, productivity, complex calculations, and applications for demonstrating knowledge and practicing skills in the basic content areas (i.e., math, reading, science, social studies) there is little to no empirical evidence for the effectiveness of such educational applications. That being the case, there are several areas where additional research is warranted. First, researchers should focus on *how* teachers should use technology to support evidence-based practices. Proponents of the use of mobile technology in classrooms often instruct teachers to simply integrate mobile technology into their instruction and behavior management plans without providing explicit instructions on how to do so. Without explicit instruction, teachers are left to randomly choose how they integrate mobile technology and which applications they use, which may or may not benefit students with behavioral problems. Therefore, more research is needed on 'best practices' for integrating mobile technology in the classroom and how to choose appropriate applications to support evidence-based practices. This not only will provide a starting point for teachers, but also will provide a baseline for further research on the use of mobile technology for students with or at risk for behavioral difficulties. Second, future research should focus on *if* and *to what degree* the use of mobile technologies can increase the academic performance of students with behavioral problems when these devices are paired with evidence-based practices. This area of research also could include examining moderating variables that may influence the effectiveness of mobile technology and applications such as gender, age/grade, setting, and disability. This knowledge would add to the literature base and provide evidence to support the use of mobile technologies and applications in the classroom-based contexts for students at risk for and with behavioral problems. Third, future research should attempt to isolate those factors that determine effectiveness. Scant information is available to assist educators in identifying which factors alone lead to successful implementation. For example, studies should be designed and conducted to examine *who* is most likely to benefit from the use of technology-based strategies, as well as *what* environmental variables must be present for long-term educational outcomes to be produced.

SUMMARY

Reaching the needs of students at risk for or identified with behavioral disorders can be a daunting task, even for the most seasoned of educators. However, the use of mobile technologies like smartphones and tablets affords educators the ability to improve student interest and engagement, thereby increasing the potential for promoting positive student outcomes. To date, mobile technologies have been used successfully to increase behavior and academic outcomes for students with behavioral problems across a variety of educational contexts. As such, we posit an effort to increase the use of mobile technologies as a supplemental tool for teaching students with behavioral problems. In so doing, educators may be able to provide higher quality instruction that has a greater likelihood of long-term success.

REFERENCES

Achmadi, D., Kagohara, D. M., van der Meer, L., O'Reilly, M. F., Lancioni, G. E., Sutherland, D., & Sigafoos, J. et al. (2012). Teaching advanced operation of an iPod-based speech-generating device to two students with autism spectrum disorders. *Research in Autism Spectrum Disorders*, 6(4), 1258–1264. doi:10.1016/j.rasd.2012.05.005

Alberto, P. A., & Troutman, A. C. (2013). *Applied behavior analysis for teachers* (9th ed.). Pearson.

Alisauskas, A., & Simkiene, G. (2013). Teachers' experiences in educating pupils having behavioural and/or emotional problems. *Specialusis Ugdymas*, 28, 62–72.

Altman, D. G. (1999). *Practical statistics for medical research*. Bristol, UK: Chapman & Hall.

Aronin, S., & Floyd, K. K. (2013). Using an iPad in inclusive preschool classrooms to introduce STEM concepts. *Teaching Exceptional Children*, 45(4), 34–39.

Bedesem, P. L. (2012). Using cell phone technology for self-monitoring procedures in inclusive settings. *Journal of Special Education Technology*, 27(4), 33–46.

Berger, J. (1995). Self-instruction: Lessons from Charlotte. *LD Forum, 20*, 20-22.

Blood, E., Johnson, J. W., Ridenour, L., Simmons, K., & Crouch, S. (2011). Using iPod Touch to teach social and self-management skills to an elementary student with emotional/behavioral disorders. *Education & Treatment of Children*, 34(3), 299–322. doi:10.1353/etc.2011.0019

Bouck, E. C., Shurr, J. C., Tom, K., Jasper, A. D., Bassette, L., Miller, B., & Flanagan, S. M. (2012). Fix it with TAPE: Repurposing technology to be assistive technology for students with high-incidence disabilities. *Preventing School Failure*, 56(2), 121–128. doi:10.1080/1045988X.2011.603396

Campigotto, R., McEwin, R., & Epp, C. D. (2013). Especially social: Exploring the use of an iOS application in special needs classrooms. *Computers & Education*, 60(1), 74–86. doi:10.1016/j.compedu.2012.08.002

Ciampa, K. (2014). Learning in the mobile age: An investigation of student motivation. *Journal of Computer Assisted Learning, 30*(1), 82–96. doi:10.1111/jcal.12036

Cihak, D. F., Wright, R., & Ayres, K. M. (2010). Use of self-modeling static-picture prompts via a handheld computer to facilitate self-monitory in the general education classroom. *Education and Training in Autism and Developmental Disabilities, 45,* 136–149.

Cook, B. G., Landrum, T. J., Tankersley, M., & Kauffman, J. M. (2003). Bringing research to bear on practice: Effective evidence-based instruction for students with emotional or behavioral disorders. *Education & Treatment of Children, 26,* 345–361.

Davies, D. K., Stock, S. E., & Wehmeyer, M. L. (2002). Enhancing independent task performance for individuals with mental retardation through use of a handheld self-directed visual and audio prompting system. *Education and Training in Mental Retardation and Developmental Disabilities, 37,* 209–218.

Douglas, K. H., Wojcik, B. W., & Thompson, J. R. (2012). Is there an app for that? *Journal of Special Education Technology, 27*(2), 59–70.

Edyburn, D. L. (2004). Rethinking assistive technology. *Special Education Technology Practice, 5*(4), 16–23.

Edyburn, D. L. (2013). Critical issues in advancing the special education technology evidence base. *Exceptional Children, 80*(1), 7–24.

Gulchak, D. J.Daniel J. Gulchak. (2008). Using a mobile handheld computer to teach a student with an emotional and behavioral disorder to self-monitor attention. *Education & Treatment of Children, 31*(4), 567–581. doi:10.1353/etc.0.0028

Haydon, T., Hawkins, R., Denune, H., Kimener, L., McCoy, D., & Basham, J. (2012). A comparison of iPads and worksheets on math skills of high school students with emotional disturbance. *Behavioral Disorders, 4,* 232–243.

Higgins, J. P. T., & Green, S. (2009). *Cochrane Handbook for Systematic Reviews of Interventions.* The Cochrane Collaboration. Available from www.cochrane-handbook.org

IDEA Data Center. (2014). *2012 IDEA Part B Child Count and Educational Environments.* Retrieved from https://explore.data.gov/Education/2012-IDEA-Part-B-Child-Count-and-Educational-Envir/5t72-4535

Individuals with Disabilities Education Improvement Act of 2004, 20 U.S.C.§ 614 *et seq.*

Kagohara, D. M., van der Meer, L., Ramdoss, S., O'Reilly, M. F., Lancioni, G. E., Davis, T. N., & Sigafoos, J. et al. (2013). Using iPods and iPads in teaching programs for individuals with developmental disabilities: A systematic review. *Research in Developmental Disabilities, 34*(1), 147–156. doi:10.1016/j.ridd.2012.07.027 PMID:22940168

Keegan, D. (2005). *The incorporation of mobile learning into mainstream education and training.* Retrieved from http://www.mlearn.org.za/CD/papers/keegan1.pdf

Lin, M., Fulford, C. P., Ho, C. P., Iyoda, R., & Ackerman, L. K. (2012). *Possibilities and challenges in mobile learning for k-12 teachers: A pilot retrospective survey study.* Proceedings from IEEE Seventh International Conference on Wireless, Mobile, and Ubiquitous Technology in Education (pp. 132-136). Retrieved from http://doi.ieeecomputersociety.org/10.1109/WMUTE.2012.31

Malone, T. W., & Lepper, M. R. (1987). Making learning fun: A taxonomy of intrinsic motivations for learning. *Aptitude. Learning and Instruction, 3*, 223–253.

McClanahan, B., Williams, K., Kennedy, E., & Tate, S. (2012). A breakthrough for Josh: How use of an iPad facilitated reading improvement. *TechTrends: Linking Research and Practice to Improve Learning, 56*(3), 20–28. doi:10.1007/s11528-012-0572-6

Mechling, L., Gast, D. L., & Fields, E. A. (2008). Evaluation of a portable DVD player and system of least prompts to self-prompt cooking task completion by young adults with moderate intellectual disabilities. *The Journal of Special Education, 42*(3), 179–190. doi:10.1177/0022466907313348

Mechling, L. C., Gast, D. L., & Seid, N. H. (2009). Using a personal digital assistant to increase independent task completion by students with autism spectrum disorder. *Journal of Autism and Developmental Disorders, 39*(10), 1420–1434. doi:10.1007/s10803-009-0761-0 PMID:19466534

Mechling, L. C., Gast, D. L., & Seid, N. H. (2010). Evaluation of a personal digital assistant as a self-prompting device for increasing multi-step task completion by students with moderate intellectual disabilities. *Education and Training in Autism and Developmental Disabilities, 45*, 422–439.

Mechling, L. C., & Seid, N. H. (2011). Use of a hand-held personal digital assistant (PDA) to self-prompt pedestrian travel by young adults with moderate intellectual disabilities. *Education and Training in Autism and Developmental Disabilities, 46*, 220–237.

Mintz, J., Branch, C., March, C., & Lerman, S. (2012). Key factors mediating the use of a mobile technology tool designed to develop social and life skills in children with autistic spectrum disorders. *Computers & Education, 58*(1), 53–62. doi:10.1016/j.compedu.2011.07.013

Neely, L., Rispoli, M., Camargo, S., Davis, H., & Boles, M. (2013). The effect of instructional use of an iPad on challenging behavior and academic engagement for two students with autism. *Research in Autism Spectrum Disorders, 7*(4), 509–516. doi:10.1016/j.rasd.2012.12.004

No Child Left Behind Act of 2001, 20 U.S.C. § 6301 *et seq.*

Parette, P. H., & Blum, C. (2014). Using flexible participation in technology-supported, universally designed preschool activities. *Teaching Exceptional Children, 46*(3), 60–67.

Parker, R. I., & Hagan-Burke, S. (2007). Median-based overlap analysis for single case data: A second study. *Behavior Modification, 31*(6), 919–936. doi:10.1177/0145445507303452 PMID:17932244

Parker, R. I., Vannest, K. J., & Brown, L. (2009). The improvement rate difference for single case research. *Exceptional Children, 75*, 135–150.

Sansosti, F. J., Powell-Smith, K. A., & Cowan, R. J. (2010). *High functioning autism/Asperger syndrome in schools: Assessment and Intervention.* New York, NY: Guilford Press.

Spriggs, A. D., Gast, D. L., & Ayres, K. M. (2007). Using picture activity schedule books to increase on-schedule and on-task behaviors. *Education and Training in Developmental Disabilities, 42,* 209–223.

Swaggart, B. L. (1998). Implementing a cognitive behavior management program. *Intervention in School and Clinic, 33*(4), 235–238. doi:10.1177/105345129803300406

Taber-Doughty, T. (2005). Considering student choice when selecting instructional strategies: A comparison of three prompting systems. *Research in Developmental Disabilities, 26*(5), 411–432. doi:10.1016/j.ridd.2004.07.006 PMID:16168881

Van Laarhoven, T., Johnson, J. W., Van Laarhoven-Myers, T., Grider, K. L., & Grider, K. M. (2009). The effectiveness of using a video iPod as a prompting device in employment settings. *Journal of Behavioral Education, 18*(2), 119–141. doi:10.1007/s10864-009-9077-6

Vaughn, S., & Bos, C. S. (2012). *Strategies for teaching students with learning and behavior problems.* Upper Saddle River, NJ: Pearson.

Walser, K., Ayres, K. M., & Foote, E. (2012). Effects of a video model to teach students with moderate intellectual disabilities to use key features of an iPhone. *Education and Training in Autism and Developmental Disabilities, 47,* 319–331.

West, D. M. (2012). *Digital schools: How technology can transform education.* Washington, D.C.: Brookings Institution Press.

KEY TERMS AND DEFINITIONS

Assistive Technology: Any type of equipment that can be used to increase, maintain, or improve functional capabilities of student with disabilities.

Educational Technology: Effective use of technological tools to support and enhance teaching and learning.

Individuals with Disabilities Education Improvement Act: (IDEIA; 2004): IDEIA is the Federal law that entitles students with disabilities to a free appropriate public education that is individualized to meet specific educational needs.

Mobile Application: A computer program designed to run on smartphones, tablets, and other mobile devices.

Mobile Technology: Any portable electronic device that accepts, processes, and stores data at high speeds (e.g., smart phone, tablet computer).

Students with Behavioral Disorders: Children who exhibit inappropriate behavior and/or feelings over an extended period of time that adversely affects their education.

Students with Disabilities: Students with disabilities are students who have been identified, assessed, and determined to be eligible for special education services under the Individuals with Disabilities Education Act.

Chapter 6
Recent Advances in Augmentative and Alternative Communication:
The Advantages and Challenges of Technology Applications for Communicative Purposes

Toby B. Mehl-Schneider
City University of New York, USA

ABSTRACT

With the increased development of mobile technologies, such as smartphones and tablets (i.e. iPhone, iPad), the field of augmentative and alternative communication (AAC) has changed rapidly over the last few years. Recent advances in technology have introduced applications (apps) for AAC purposes. These novel technologies could provide numerous benefits to individuals with complex communication needs. Nevertheless, introducing mobile technology apps is not without risk. Since these apps can be purchased and retrieved with relative ease, AAC assessments and collaborative evaluations have been circumvented in favor of the "quick fix"-simply ordering a random app for a potential user, without fully assessing the individual's needs and abilities. There is a paucity of research pertaining to mobile technology use in AAC. Therapists, parents and developers of AAC applications must work collaboratively to expand the research pertaining to the assessment and treatment of children who utilize AAC mobile technologies for communication purposes.

INTRODUCTION

Augmentative and Alternative Communication (AAC) is a general term for all means of communication, other than verbal speech output, that are used for expressing "thoughts, needs, wants and ideas" (American Speech-Language-Hearing Association, 2014). The terminology of 'AAC' includes a vast

DOI: 10.4018/978-1-4666-8395-2.ch006

range of techniques and systems that is utilized to enhance existing communication abilities and to enable effective communication, where it is lacking, in order to improve one's communicative ability and, therefore, his/her quality of life.

This chapter will broadly discuss various types of AAC systems as well as the diversity of children with developmental disorders who use the AAC systems to communicate or to assist in their communicative interaction. Individuals who utilize AAC on a daily basis use the system to communicate and increase social and communicative interaction in a number of settings and situations. Each particular user has his or her specific complex communication needs (CCN), requiring different AAC means to assist in communicating with family and friends, as well as to increase language and literacy skills (Light & McNaughton, 2012). Additionally, this chapter will address various ways to access AAC systems and equipment for the purpose of effective communicative output, based on the specific AAC user's abilities and limitations.

Recent advances in AAC will be highlighted. The rapid evolution of technology in recent decades has brought with it significant changes to the field of AAC. With the development of mobile high technology devices, such as smartphones and tablets (i.e. iPhone, iPad), communication applications (apps) have become more easily accessible to children with various developmental and communication needs. Numerous advantages of these devices have been noted as devices have become more acceptable and more mainstream (Bradshaw, 2013). This chapter will include some examples of recent, popular AAC apps and will highlight other resources (i.e. articles, websites) which enumerate and describe potential apps for communicative purposes. However, the chapter will also delineate some notable concerns to consider when using these technological apps as the AAC user's principal communicative system. The paper will conclude with some functional limitations in the current AAC research in this area, as well as discuss some important research and work in the field which has yet to be accomplished. Some recommendations and suggestions will be proposed in the conclusion as well.

AUGMENTATIVE AND ALTERNATIVE COMMUNICATION: AN OVERVIEW

Augmentative and alternative communication (AAC) refers to any and all assisting communicative functions which 'augment' or serve as 'alternatives' for verbal vocalizations. In addition to verbal speech, these can include any vocalizations, gestures, facial expressions or AAC devices. Furthermore, AAC systems can include light tech tools, such as an alphabet board or communication book (McBride, 2011).

AAC systems are utilized by individuals who require adaptive support for expressive communication, such as reading and writing. People from all age groups, socioeconomic groups, races and religions use AAC as a means to communicate expressively. Children and adults alike who require assistance with expressive communication due to both congenital and acquired language impairments will use AAC systems to communicate with their family and peers. Individuals with congenital impairments such as cerebral palsy, autism, mental retardation and developmental apraxia of speech, use AAC systems as a form of expressive communication which allows them to partake in daily social interactions. These children may require use of AAC devices due to significant communicative needs in their social, family, educational and community environments (Light & McNaughton, 2012). Individuals with acquired impairments which result in profound communication difficulties, such as amyotrophic lateral sclerosis (ALS), stroke, traumatic brain injury, multiple sclerosis (MS) and spinal cord injury, often require some form of AAC for expressive output purposes (Beukelman & Mirenda, 1998).

Professional Collaboration during Assessment and Treatment

There are a myriad of professionals who are part of a collaborative team to assess, evaluate and provide therapy to children and adults with AAC needs. As each member of the team is a professional with a specific specialty, it is crucial that the various specialists collaborate with one another during the assessment process, in order to enable the individual with AAC needs to receive the most appropriate AAC system. Professionals that are important collaborators for an AAC team include the speech-language pathologist, occupational therapist, physical therapist, psychologist, guidance counselor and social worker. Teachers and vocational counselors can contribute important information about using a system to meet educational objectives while computer technologists/engineers can assist in choosing and modifying software programs for the AAC user as needed. Once the most beneficial system is chosen, the various team members must collaborate on the most effective course of treatment for the purpose of continually increasing and improving the individual's communicative skills via the AAC system.

There are numerous ways that professionals can join together as a collaborative team. Multidisciplinary teams, interdisciplinary teams and transdisciplinary teams have been formed to assess and evaluate the needs of the AAC user in order to make individual-specific decisions about proper AAC systems and therapeutic treatment. On a multidisciplinary team, the individual specialist independently assesses and provides a course of treatment, while on an interdisciplinary team, each team member evaluates the AAC user individually, but collaborates together to provide the most beneficial therapeutic intervention. On a transdisciplinary team, both the assessment and treatment of the AAC user is a collaborative and mutual team effort, requiring the specialists to have knowledge of the other disciplines involved and a responsibility for the AAC user as a complete individual (Beukelman & Mirenda, 1998).

However, whether a multidisciplinary, interdisciplinary or transdisciplinary team is formed by the professionals and specialists treating the individual with AAC needs, the ultimate goal is effective communication among all team members. In the evaluation process, there is a multitude of knowledgeable specialists in the field of AAC, who are charged with the responsibility of locating the best AAC system for the particular AAC user at the particular stage in his or her communicative development. An AAC assessment and evaluation process cannot be completed within a vacuum; the most beneficial intervention plans can only be determined following a collaborative process. Furthermore, the team members must contribute to shared objectives and goals for treatment purposes in order to consistently assist the individual AAC user in communicating effectively.

The objective of each collaborative evaluation is to identify the present skills and difficulties of the individual. By assessing his or her daily communication abilities and impairments as well as his or her specific communication needs and desires, the clinical team can match the most appropriate device to the specific AAC user (McBride, 2011).

Augmentative and Alternative Communication Devices

The results and recommendations of the collaborative team of therapists and specialists in conjunction with the AAC user and his or her family will determine the traditional AAC device requested and ordered for communicative purposes. The available devices differ greatly from one another in terms of their communicative capabilities, complexities, sophistication, and price ranges.

Access

During an assessment for the proper AAC system, the treating therapists and specialists evaluate the individual user's ability to access the AAC system, thus determining what mode of access is best for that particular AAC system user. Users of AAC systems can access and select vocabulary items via direct selection or scanning techniques. Direct selection refers to directly choosing a particular icon from a selection set of vocabulary words and messages for the purpose of expressive communication. Use of direct selection on AAC systems includes finger-powered light pointers, optical pointers or head-sticks to directly select a particular desired vocabulary item.

Scanning techniques, on the other hand, refer to a technique in which the many items on the AAC display are scanned prior to the AAC user's vocabulary selection. In this technique, the AAC user is not directly selecting a particular item, usually due to the fact that he or she does not exhibit the motor control necessary to select the particular item directly. During this type of item selection, the vocabulary items are displayed and scanned by an electronic device or facilitator, either in a visual or auditory linear way, circular scanning, row-column scanning or group-item scanning. In each of these types of scanning techniques, the individual AAC user must scan through numerous undesired items until he or she can express the desired item (Beukelman & Mirenda, 1998).

In visual linear scanning, each particular item is highlighted, one by one, row by row, until the target is highlighted and the AAC user selects his/her desired communicative item. Similarly, in auditory linear scanning, each item is announced aloud, one by one, by either a synthetic voice, recorded human voice or human facilitator until the AAC user selects the particular desired item. Circular scanning refers to items displayed in circular formation, identified one at a time until the desired item is selected. The items are usually scanned by an arrow, one by one, similar to a hand on a clock moving in a circular fashion around the clock's numbers. Row-column and group item scanning refer to the identification of a group of items by the AAC user, whether in a row, column or specified group of items, and removing the options until he/she comes to his/her desired selection. The purpose of this kind of scanning is to increase scanning efficiency (Beukelman & Mirenda, 1998).

Additionally, there are various selection control techniques that can be used to select the desired item in the scanning process, namely directed (inverse), automatic (regular) and step scanning. Each of these selection control techniques is personalized for the particular AAC user based on his or her physical abilities--both gross and fine motor skills-- as well as to the user's visual and cognitive skills.

Vocabulary

Augmentative and alternative communication systems must include the necessary vocabulary for expressive communication purposes. The specific AAC system employed by an individual must include both a core vocabulary of frequently spoken words and messages that are utilized effectively by many other AAC users or by non-AAC users in similar environments and contexts. In addition, the system must also include a fringe vocabulary, referring to words and messages that are specialized and specific in nature for the particular AAC user. Having these words at his or her disposal is crucial for the AAC user since the AAC system is personalized and creates the language output needs for the individual user (Beukelman & Mirenda, 1998). Currently, there are many representative symbols for the vocabulary needs of the AAC user, ranging from Google images and digital pictures to specialized vocabulary, such as the popular Mayer Johnson Picture Communication Symbols (PCS), DynaSyms and SymbolStix to name a few (Light & McNaughton, 2012). Close family, caregivers and friends should have input in choosing the vocabulary words in order to further the expressive output capabilities of the AAC user. However, the most significant informer of necessary terminology is the individual, who will ultimately utilize the AAC system. Some AAC users may or may not be able to provide this crucial information depending on the individual's age and cognitive abilities (Beukelman & Mirenda, 1998).

Research in the field of AAC has determined that augmentative and alternative means of communication assist the individual user with his or her communication output without obstructing or hindering speech output in any way. In fact, AAC devices have enhanced and expanded children's speech production (Schlosser & Wendt, 2008). Millar, Light and Schlosser (2006) investigated the outcome of AAC treatment on speech production of individuals--both children and adults--with developmental disorders. Of the twenty-three studies reviewed by the authors, six studies, consisting of twenty-seven cases, provided the most beneficial evidential analysis for determination of study results. Following this literature review, Millar et al. (2006) determined that 89% of the 27 cases demonstrated increased speech production, although the gains were modest at best. The remaining 11% of cases did not demonstrate any increase in speech production, but did not demonstrate any decrease either. Therefore, AAC has been found to be a beneficial means of immediate communication by providing a mechanism for language output as needed. Additionally, AAC has proven to be useful for prompting and priming an individual child to speak aloud.

MOBILE TECHNOLOGY TOOLS FOR AAC: BENEFITS OF AAC APPS

Recent advances in mobile technology have provided the general public with numerous choices of applications (apps) for augmentative and alternative communication (AAC) purposes. These applications are broad and varied, ranging from simple, single-word communicative applications to applications with vocabularies of tens of thousands of words. Furthermore, there is a wide price range for these apps, from 'free' to hundreds of dollars. The only consistency about the applications is that they are all new, aiming to appeal to each individual AAC user as well as to therapists, families and friends.

Alliano, Herringer, Koutsoftas and Bartolotta (2012) reviewed numerous iPad applications which provide augmentative and alternative means of communication to those in need. The authors provide a comprehensive list of twenty-one iPad applications that includes AAC apps which use symbols only, those that use text-to-speech only, and those that use both symbols and text-to-speech (Alliano et al., 2012). These apps are a beneficial resource for speech-language pathologists in their quest for current augmentative and alternative communication tools for individuals with communication needs. Many recent articles, including an article by Alliano et al. (2012), have described the many benefits of AAC applications; these strengthened and supported their appeal to the AAC user and his or her family. Portability, cost effectiveness, social acceptability and ease of purchase are just some of the rationales for choosing mobile technology applications as a means of communication.

The ease of portability coupled with the significant power of mobile technology devices have made them extremely popular means of technology. Mobile technology devices, such as smartphones and tablets, are both smaller and lighter than many Speech-Generated Devices (SGDs) for AAC, making them more portable and versatile. These devices are easily accessible to the public and purchasing the necessary applications for AAC use is fairly simple for the individual user and his/her family.

Overall, mobile technology is also significantly cheaper than many popular SGDs for AAC users. With the reduced cost of these devices and the necessary applications, parents of children with AAC needs have the option of purchasing various apps to try out their functionality with little risk involved. Furthermore, many individuals have mobile technology devices like smartphones or tablets, thus obviating the need to purchase an additional device for AAC purposes. This limits the additional cost required to purchase AAC apps.

The ease of acquiring applications for the AAC user is another advantageous rationale for using mobile technology applications as a child's AAC means of communication. McBride (2013) discusses the significant allure and appeal of an easily attained and cheap AAC solution. AAC assessments can, at times, be lengthy ordeals, with numerous therapists from speech-language pathologists, occupational therapists, physical therapists and so forth, assessing the child, speaking to parents and teachers and writing up evaluations prior to ordering necessary communicative equipment. Even in the best case scenarios, an expedited assessment process is significantly longer than the time it would take a parent of a child with AAC needs to download an application. However, the ease of acquisition should *never* take the place of a formal assessment. This is a precarious and potentially dangerous decision and will be discussed later in the chapter.

Parents can enjoy an affordable option in purchasing many existing apps, thereby enabling their child to utilize a communication app with minimal expense risk. In case an application does not fulfill the needs of the child, the expense to the parent can be negligible; the parent may simply choose another application option for communication.

Applications and mobile technology can also be very beneficial for younger children. Apps on mobile technology devices will allow children to "have access to improved capacitive touch screens that are very sensitive to touch and can be activated reliably by infants and toddlers with CCN (complex communication needs)" (Light & McNaughton, 2012, p. 40).

Numerous AAC articles discuss the benefits of using mobile technology applications to help an individual with expressive communication. Many of these research articles discuss the applications in the context of "social acceptability," in which AAC users and clinicians alike deem forms of mobile technology as a more socially comfortable option for the AAC device user (McNaughton & Light, 2013; Alliano et al., 2012; Flores et al., 2012). The social acceptability of these devices for a myriad of functions may prompt and encourage the AAC user to utilize the device in more diverse settings. Since virtually one third of United States Internet users owned a mobile technology tablet in 2012 (Furman, 2012), the AAC user will feel more comfortable utilizing it as well, albeit for a personal communicative purpose. As these mobile technological devices are so universally acceptable, perhaps individual children may demonstrate a preference for using these devices over other SGDs, thus increasing their communicative performance.

As these mobile technology devices, such as the iPad, are used daily by the general public as a mainstream technology, the option of using an application on one of these devices for expressive output has become a more readily acceptable choice for individuals who require AAC. As McNaughton & Light (2013, p. 108) so aptly state, "Rather than being restricted to the use of specialized dedicated speech-generating devices (SGDs), many individuals who require AAC are now able to use mainstream technologies to meet their communication needs".

Traditional speech-generating AAC devices are not always readily used by individuals who need AAC tools to communicate, or are used only in specific contexts in which the AAC user is personally comfortable utilizing the device. The AAC user may refuse to utilize his or her traditional AAC device based on his or her personal feelings of uneasiness in a particular setting, such as with unfamiliar communication partners. In other instances, an AAC device may prove to be too bulky or cumbersome for the AAC user, prompting the AAC user to forgo bringing it or utilizing it in various daily situations (Alliano et al., 2012). In these cases, the use of an AAC app, used on a mobile device such as an iPad or iPhone, which can facilitate many AAC needs for communicative purposes, can come in handy.

AAC apps were created to fill the important gap between existing AAC devices in the current market and the novel technological availability of mobile technology. One such example,

Verbal Victor ™, is an app which was created by students at the Wake Forest University Computer Science Department to assist AAC users with promising, emerging cognitive skills, who have difficulty with device access due to fine motor control difficulties (Pauca & Guy, 2012). The students aimed to create an application which could be provided at a reasonable price, as opposed to high-tech AAC devices, which can cost thousands of dollars. With this goal in mind, they created Verbal Victor ™, an application for mobile technology systems for a specified population of AAC users. This particular app was released to the public in January 2011 and was downloaded from the Apple app store over 2,500 times by October 2011. This was a social entrepreneurship activity on behalf of the students who created and modified this application for AAC systems (Pauca & Guy, 2012). See Table 1 below for more information on Verbal Victor ™.

Table 1. Examples of popular AAC applications currently available (App Store, Apple, 2014)

Application	Manufacturer, Updated	Feature Descriptions	Price
Proloquo2Go™	(AssistiveWare, 2013)	• 14,000 SymbolStix™ symbols available for customization; import own photos/images • Communicate by direct selection of words/phrases • Customize grid size & buttons • Customize color, font, voice • Natural voice output with numerous genuine voice choices • Share messages on email and other social media apps • Proloquo2Go can be used on iPhone, iPod touch, iPad/iPad mini without internet connection	$219.00
Sono Flex™	(Tobii Technology, 2013)	• Core vocabulary & topic based vocabulary (pre-made) • 11,000 SymbolStix™ symbols available for customization; import own photos/images • Natural voice output with a variety of voices to choose from • Flexibility in vocabulary creation and customization • Sono Flex can be used on iPhone, iPod, iPad, regular PCs and on speech devices utilizing Tobii Communicator	$99.99
Speak It! Text to Speech™	(Future Apps Inc., 2013)	• Text-to-speech application • Simple; enter written/copied text and press "Speak it!" button • Natural sounding voice choices • Adjust volume, rate of speech, font size • Can be utilized on phone call • Visually highlights words when produced • Speak It! Text to Speech can be used on iPhone, iPod Touch and iPad	$1.99
TouchChat AAC™	(Silver Kite, 2014)	• Over 10,000 SymbolStix™ symbols available for customization; import own photos/images; can import/export vocabulary files • Adjustable button dwell time, release time; customized to meet needs of AAC user • Numerous voice choices • Customized grids, pages, messages and symbols • Message expansion enables communication in noisy environment • TouchChat-AAC for use on iPad, iPod or iPhone	$149.99
Verbal Victor™ 2.0	(Apps for the Greater Good LLC, 2013)	• For children with developmental delays, assisting with emerging language needs • Uses built in camera/microphone to create buttons/sounds • Enables category creation; simplifies navigation • Verbal Victor 2.0 can be used on iPhone, iPad, iPod touch; best on iPhone 5	$11.99

Similarly, Hewlett Packard recognized the need for professionals and families of children with AAC needs to have a forum from which they could present proposals and suggestions for AAC applications, thus allowing application programmers to develop these inspirational ideas into a reality (Alliano et al., 2012). On this website, http://www.hackingautism.org/, volunteer programmers attempt to use technology to "help those on the autism spectrum maximize their potential," as the website states.

Although there are numerous applications currently available, five popular applications are listed and described in Table 1 as examples of presently existing apps for AAC needs. The five applications listed below offer a small illustration of the numerous applications available for helping people meet their AAC needs. These applications were selected solely based upon their reviews in other research articles and are not determined to be more or less beneficial than the multitude of other applications not mentioned herein.

As the use of mobile technology applications in the field of AAC is relatively new, there is not a great deal of clinical research in this area. However, researchers have recently begun to investigate the use of apps for AAC as compared to using communication devices (i.e. DynaVox) for the purpose of overall communication competence. For instance, van der Meer, Sutherland, O'Reilly, Lancioni & Sigafoos (2012) conducted a study assessing both the acquisition of a certain means of communication as well as a preference for one means of communication over another. In this study they compared a SGD using an iPod Touch or an iPad versus manual signing and picture exchange communication.

The participants of this research study were four children with autism spectrum disorders. All four participants requested items using one or more of learned AAC communication modes. Of the four children, three children initially demonstrated a preference for using the SGD to communicate as compared to manual signing and picture exchange communication; the fourth child selected each of the AAC systems equally for communicative purposes. While three out of four study participants attained the study's noted criterion of requesting preferred items, only two of these three participants demonstrated a preference for the SGD during the maintenance stage. Consequently, van der Meer et al. (2012) surmised that a child's initial preferences for a mode of communication interaction should be reassessed following intervention to determine if the child continues to display the same feeling about the communication system, since the child's preferences may adjust and shift over time and affect his or her communication performance.

Achmadi, Kagohara, van der Meer, O'Reilly, Lancioni, Sutherland, Lang, Marschik, Green & Sigafoos (2012) evaluated how two adolescents with ASD learned to use an iPod Touch® for the purpose of requesting preferred items. This research study aimed to address the limitations of a previous study by van der Meer et al. (2011). In van der Meer's study, the system had always been on and turned to the appropriate page which did not provide the study participant with practice in turning on the device and navigating to the appropriate icon. Furthermore, in the previous study by van der Meer et al. (2011), only single responses were required, as opposed to multi-step response sequencing (i.e. first requesting 'snack' and then specifying the desired snack as a "cookie"). Hence, the study by Achmadi et al. (2012) focused on including multi-step response sequencing, a beneficial communication skill for effective communicative interaction. In the study by Achmadi et al. (2012), the adolescents successfully learned to turn on and unlock the iPod Touch® as well as to request preferred items in a multi-step requesting sequence, thereby increasing their communicative skill and communicative independence.

Flores et al. (2012) compared the frequency of communication using an iPad versus the frequency of communication using a non-electronic picture-based system. Initial findings demonstrated that five elementary school students with autism spectrum disorders (ASD) and developmental disabilities, who had previously communicated via a picture card system, communicated the same amount or an increased amount when provided with the iPad. Some of the children also demonstrated a preference for the iPad over the picture cards.

MOBILE TECHNOLOGY TOOLS FOR AAC: CHALLENGES OF AAC APPS

There is a significant problem with mobile technology AAC applications. As mobile technology apps have become commonplace over the last few years, the use of these apps for AAC needs has grown exponentially. However, many people are buying apps for their children without the assistance of professionals trained to assist children in their speech/language communication needs. In order to receive the proper device from a wealth of available AAC resources, a team of specially trained professionals, including speech-language pathologists, occupational therapists, physical therapists and others, should routinely evaluate and assess the needs and abilities of the child requiring some form of AAC, culminating in a collaborative request for the appropriate AAC device for the child's current abilities. The team should determine the appropriate size of the vocabulary by delineating the specific core and fringe vocabulary words necessary for the individual. Furthermore, the team should assess the individual for the most appropriate form of access necessary for optimal communication interaction.

Since these apps are readily available to the general public—in contrast to traditional AAC devices—parents are purchasing and providing communication apps for their children, oftentimes without the input of any trained therapists or specialists. Although these actions are undertaken with the best of intentions, the particular app or apps may not be appropriate for the particular child for a variety of reasons, further complicating the process of communication for this AAC user. For example, in the case of choosing an AAC app with an inappropriate vocabulary size, the individual user may become frustrated during his or her communication interaction, while a lack of familiar and child-specific words may result in confusion or circumlocution. Moreover, a parent or caregiver would need to make the determination for appropriate access alone, without the assistance of a trained professional, further mitigating the possibility of frustration on the part of the AAC user.

The appropriate means of communication is crucial for an individual child who requires AAC and a proper evaluation is essential for communicative success. The relative ease with which these AAC apps are acquired can mistakenly prompt a parent or caregiver of an AAC user, or potential user, to forgo the necessary evaluative process. Ease of availability does not determine that the app is a better form of AAC than a standard communication device, and does not substitute for a proper evaluation procedure.

In their research study of elementary school children, Flores et al. (2012) determined that students demonstrated errors in iPad activation; at times they did not touch the iPad correctly to select the particular icon. Similarly, Sennot and Bowker (2010) reported some difficulties with iPad activation, stating that the iPhone/iPod mobile technologies touch platform does not provide the appropriate access for an individual with a significant motor impairment. In their review of Proloquo2Go, an AAC app, Sennot and Bowker (2010, p. 143) state that the iPhone/iPod's "operating system does not allow adjustments to the screen sensitivity, activation-on-release, averaged activation, or any adjustments to the touch input," leading the authors to compare this app's operating system to other communication devices. They describe how these features are quite standard on "other communication devices, to adjust for tremors or to minimize accidental activations" (Sennot & Bowker, 2010, p. 143). Therefore, in some cases, apps may not constitute the best form of communication for certain individuals with motor disabilities.

Furthermore, Light & McNaughton (2012) explain how the available apps and technologies for AAC are not an effect or result of evidence-based practice. Mobile apps and technologies are unveiled quickly and are available almost immediately after production. Light & McNaughton (2102, p.36) state, "Essentially we are running apps reflecting designs from the 1980s/1990s on cutting edge 21st century hardware. This perpetuation of the status quo is both disappointing and problematic." The lack of research in this area, however, is not simply an aesthetics issue. The design and layout needs are important for the language, literacy and communicative needs of the individual child's AAC output, and the apps and technologies need to be redesigned to reflect the individual's needs.

There are numerous apps currently available to meet augmentative and alternative communication needs. Partial lists can be found in articles by Alliano et al. (2012) and Atticks (2012) which review a variety of apps for mobile technology that are used to augment and assist children and adults with a variety of communication needs in communicating effectively. Furthermore, the websites, AppsForAAC.net and speechbubble.org.uk are just two examples of websites which currently list and describe the existing applications for augmentative and alternative communication users, depicting their many features for assisting individuals with AAC needs.

LIMITATIONS AND FUTURE RESEARCH

Since the introduction of applications on mobile technology is such a new technology in the augmentative and alternative communication field, there is a dearth of research studies in the area of mobile technology use in AAC. While the existence of longitudinal research in this area is obviously lacking, there is also a lack of research about AAC applications which result in therapeutic evidence-based practice for treatment purposes. Recent studies are beginning to evaluate AAC apps that are utilized via mobile technology systems. In the past few years, studies have assessed some applications on these systems used by children with ASD (van der Meer et al., 2012), children with ASD or a developmental disability (Flores et al., 2012) as well as adolescents with ASD (Achmadi et al., 2012). As apps for AAC users become more prevalent, more research will be conducted in this area, both comparing static and dynamic communication devices with AAC apps, and evaluating the benefits and challenges of particular applications and the communicative effectiveness of the individual AAC user when using it as a communicative tool.

Attempting to bridge the gap between the clinical realities of the AAC user and the novel application technology for AAC users, Gosnell, Costello and Shane (2011) published an oft-quoted article titled *Using a clinical approach to answer 'what communication apps should we use?'* In this article, Gosnell et al. (2011) provide a significant initial framework for clinicians to utilize in selecting the proper and most appropriate augmentative and alternative communication application for their particular patient. Most importantly, Gosnell et al. (2011) noted that the most appropriate clinical approach in choosing a potential AAC app for a prospective user is to assess the needs of the particular individual, evaluating the personal communicative needs of that specific person. This is the identical AAC assessment approach used when evaluating a child or adult for a standard communication device. Alliano et al. (2012) then used the particular framework by Gosnell et al. (2011) to review twenty-one iPad applications, providing a supportive reference list for speech-language pathologists to assist them in choosing the correct application for the specific patient with AAC needs.

A crucial aspect of this future research is that augmentative and alternative communication assessments and evaluations must continue to be administered freely in order to effectively assess each potential AAC user on a case-by-case basis. McBride (2011, p. 15) explained that professionals in the field of AAC working with a child with AAC needs must "ensure that the AAC evaluation principles and procedures are being applied whenever AAC solutions are being considered". Although parents and caregivers merely aim to assist their child with AAC needs by purchasing an app or two for communicative purposes, they must be informed that simply buying an AAC application and providing for a child with complex communication needs may cause further harm than good. A collaborative team of trained professionals must personally evaluate the individual and reach specific conclusions regarding his or her communicative needs and requirements.

Furthermore, it behooves the professionals trained in the AAC field to work together as a collaborative team to determine which current applications are promising. An individual speech-language pathologist servicing an individual child using a specific application should keep detailed notes about the advantages and challenges of the particular app, in order to later collaborate with other speech-language pathologists in the AAC field as well as occupational therapists, physical therapists and teachers. The collaboration of therapists about the positive and negative aspects of an application can then be collected and provided to the app system creator/regulator, with the purpose of continually improving and enhancing the application.

Finally, much research is needed in this area of mobile technology applications for augmentative and alternative communication purposes. As in all areas of technological advancement, its expansion, growth and development is continually changing, transforming day by day, aiming to constantly progress and improve. In AAC research, however, the technological advancements must be reviewed and studied, determining the best current apps for children of various developmental disabilities and communication needs. Researchers in the field of AAC must be vigilant in using an appropriate framework for AAC evaluations, incorporating both communication devices and technological applications, as necessary. The American Speech Language Hearing Association (ASHA) could assist in this particular area to create a clear and comprehensive framework for the current assessment and selection of potential apps for communicative purposes. Furthermore, therapy for these children must be based on evidence-based practice, which can only result from consistent research in this area of study. With continued collaboration among parents, professionals and app developers as well as further research in this particular area of study, the use of mobile technology apps for AAC users may, one day, become a consistent and indispensable system for augmentative and alternative communication users.

REFERENCES

Achmadi, D., Kagohara, D. M., van der Meer, L., O'Reilly, M. F., Lancioni, G. E., Sutherland, D., & Sigafoos, J. et al. (2012). Teaching advanced operation of an iPod-based speech-generating device to two students with autism spectrum disorders. *Research in Autism Spectrum Disorders, 6*(4), 1258–1264. doi:10.1016/j.rasd.2012.05.005

Alliano, A., Herringer, K., Koutsoftas, A. D., & Bartolotta, T. E. (2012). A review of 21 iPad applications for augmentative and alternative communication purposes. *Perspectives on Augmentative and Alternative Communication, 21*(2), 60–71. doi:10.1044/aac21.2.60

Announcing the AAC-RERC white paper on mobile devices and communication apps. (2001). *Augmentative and Alternative Communication, 27*(2), 131-132.

Atticks, A. H. (2012). Therapy Session 2.0: From static to dynamic with the iPad. *SIG 15 Perspectives on Gerontology, 17*(3), 84-93.

Beukelman, D. R., & Mirenda, P. (1998). Augmentative and alternative communication: management of severe communication disorders in children and adults (2nd ed.). Paul H. Brooks Publishing Co., Inc.

Bradshaw, J. (2013). The use of augmentative and alternative communication apps for the iPad, iPod and iPhone: An overview of recent developments. *Tizard Learning Center Disability Review, 18*(1), 31–37. doi:10.1108/13595471311295996

Farrall, J. (2013). AAC Apps and ASD: Giving Voice to Good Practice. *SIG 12 Perspectives on Augmentative and Alternative Communication, 22*(3), 157-163.

Flores, M., Musgrove, K., Renner, S., Hinton, V., Strozier, S., Franklin, S., & Hil, D. (2012). A comparison of communication using the Apple iPad and a picture - based system. *Augmentative and Alternative Communication, 28*(2), 74–84. doi:10.3109/07434618.2011.644579 PMID:22263895

Furman, P. (2012, June 19). Tablets' popularity is through the roof, nearly one-third of U.S. Internet users have one: survey. *New York Daily News.*

Hewlett-Packard. (n.d.). Retrieved from http://www.hackingautism.org/

Light, J., & McNaughton, D. (2012). Supporting the communication, language, and literacy development of children with complex communication needs: State of the science and future research priorities. *Assistive Technology, 24*(1), 34–44. doi:10.1080/10400435.2011.648717 PMID:22590798

McBride, D. (2011). AAC evaluations and new mobile technologies: Asking and answering the right questions. *SIG 12 Perspectives on Augmentative and Alternative Communication, 20*(1), 9-16.

McNaughton, D., & Light, J. (2013). The iPad and mobile technology revolution: Benefits and challenges for individuals who require augmentative and alternative communication. *Augmentative and Alternative Communication, 29*(2), 107–116. doi:10.3109/07434618.2013.784930 PMID:23705813

Millar, D. C., Light, J. C., & Schlosser, R. W. (2006). The impact of augmentative and alternative communication intervention on the speech production of individuals with developmental disabilities: A research review. *Journal of Speech, Language, and Hearing Research: JSLHR, 49*(2), 248–264. doi:10.1044/1092-4388(2006/021) PMID:16671842

Pauca, V. P., & Guy, R. T. (2012, February). Mobile apps for the greater good: a socially relevant approach to software engineering. In *Proceedings of the 43rd ACM technical symposium on Computer Science Education* (pp. 535-540). ACM. doi:10.1145/2157136.2157291

Schlosser, R. W., & Wendt, O. (2008). Effects of augmentative and alternative communication intervention on speech production in children with autism: A systematic review. *American Journal of Speech-Language Pathology, 17*(3), 212–230. doi:10.1044/1058-0360(2008/021) PMID:18663107

Sennott, S., & Bowker, A. (2009). Autism, AAC, and Proloquo2Go. *SIG 12 Perspectives on Augmentative and Alternative Communication, 18*(4), 137-145.

Trembath, D., Balandin, S., Togher, L., & Stancliffe, R. J. (2009). Peer - mediated teaching and augmentative and alternative communication for preschool - aged children with autism. *Journal of Intellectual & Developmental Disability, 34*(2), 173–186. doi:10.1080/13668250902845210 PMID:19404838

van der Meer, L., Kagohara, D., Achmadi, D., Green, V. A., Herrington, C., Sigafoos, J., & Rispoli, M. et al. (2011). Teaching functional use of an iPod-based speech-generating device to individuals with developmental disabilities. *Journal of Special Education Technology, 26*(3), 1–11.

van der Meer, L., Sutherland, D., O'Reilly, M. F., Lancioni, G. E., & Sigafoos, J. (2012). A further comparison of manual signing, picture exchange, and speech-generating devices as communication modes for children with autism spectrum disorders. *Research in Autism Spectrum Disorders*, *6*(4), 1247–1257. doi:10.1016/j.rasd.2012.04.005

ADDITIONAL READING

Alliano, A., Herringer, K., Koutsoftas, A. D., & Bartolotta, T. E. (2012). A review of 21 iPad applications for augmentative and alternative communication purposes. *Perspectives on Augmentative and Alternative Communication*, *21*(2), 60–71. doi:10.1044/aac21.2.60

Beukelman, D. R., & Mirenda, P. (2013). Augmentative and alternative communication: supporting children and adults with complex communication needs: Fourth edition. Paul H. Brookes Publishing Co., Inc., Baltimore, Maryland, USA.

KEY TERMS AND DEFINITIONS

Application (App): A specialized program designed to fulfill a particular purpose as downloaded by a user to a mobile device.

Augmentative and alternative communication (AAC): An umbrella term used to describe a variety of different methods of communication that can assist people who have difficulty using verbal speech to communicate. AAC includes any aids, symbols, strategies and techniques that are used to increase communicative effectiveness.

Complex communication needs (CCN): An individual who has difficulty communicating using only verbal speech. This can result from speech/language or cognitive impairments.

Chapter 7
Selecting Computer–Mediated Interventions to Support the Social and Emotional Development of Individuals with Autism Spectrum Disorder

Kristen Gillespie-Lynch
City University of New York, USA

Patricia J. Brooks
City University of New York, USA

Christina Shane-Simpson
City University of New York, USA

Naomi Love Gaggi
City University of New York, USA

Deborah Sturm
City University of New York, USA

Bertram O. Ploog
City University of New York, USA

ABSTRACT

This chapter is designed to provide parents, professionals, and individuals with Autism Spectrum Disorder (ASD) with tools to help them evaluate the effectiveness of computer-mediated interventions to support the social and emotional development of individuals with ASD. Starting with guidelines for selecting computer-mediated interventions, we highlight the importance of identifying target skills for intervention that match an individual's needs and interests. We describe how readers can assess the degree to which an intervention is evidence-based, and include an overview of different types of experiments and statistical methods. We examine a variety of computer-mediated interventions and the evidence base for each: computer-delivered instruction (including games), iPad-type apps, virtual environments, and robots. We describe websites that provide additional resources for finding educational games and apps. We conclude by emphasizing the uniqueness of each individual with ASD and the importance of selecting interventions that are well-matched to the specific needs of each individual.

DOI: 10.4018/978-1-4666-8395-2.ch007

SELECTING COMPUTER-MEDIATED INTERVENTIONS TO SUPPORT THE SOCIAL AND EMOTIONAL DEVELOPMENT OF INDIVIDUALS WITH AUTISM SPECTRUM DISORDER

An increasing number of computer-mediated applications are becoming available to support the development of individuals with Autism Spectrum Disorder or ASD (Ploog, Scharf, Nelson, & Brooks, 2013). These applications are often believed to be highly effective and thus are widely used (Fletcher-Watson, 2014; Joshi, 2011), but currently there is limited scientific evidence that they are beneficial to the user. Limitations due to the lack of scientific evidence for the effectiveness of computer-mediated applications (which is not to say that they are *not* effective) may be attributable to the fact that the rate at which computer-mediated interventions for ASD are being developed far exceeds the rate at which research is being conducted to evaluate their effectiveness. Unfortunately, it can be daunting to sift through the proliferation of applications, to evaluate the (often limited) evidence supporting the effectiveness of a given application, and to determine if that application is likely to be useful for an individual with ASD.

The purpose of this chapter is to provide guidelines that help parents, professionals, and people with ASD evaluate and select computer-mediated applications to support the social and emotional development of individuals with ASD. We will provide readers with suggestions for how to select a computer-mediated application for a given individual by presenting evidence for the effectiveness of applications on a variety of platforms, including personal computers, handheld devices, and robots. Throughout this chapter, we will use the terms "computer-mediated" and "computer-based" to refer to all software-controlled interactions, regardless of platform. We will conclude with a synopsis of key points and recommendations for how to locate further information.

CORE DIFFICULTIES ASSOCIATED WITH ASD

ASD is defined by social difficulties and "restricted, repetitive patterns of behavior, interests, or activities" (American Psychiatric Association, 2013). Individuals with ASD often experience difficulties communicating with others and developing relationships. They may attend to people in different ways than typically developing individuals do (Ploog, 2010); for example, they may look less at eyes and faces while interacting (Speer, Cook, McMahon, & Clark, 2007). People with ASD may struggle with recognizing faces, understanding their own and others' more complex emotions (such as pride or jealousy), and regulating their own emotions (Chamak, Bonniau, Jaunay, & Cohen, 2008). Some difficulties in responding to others' faces and emotions may arise from unusual perceptual experiences associated with ASD, such as enhanced or atypical attention to details (Behrmann et al., 2006; Ploog, 2010). People with ASD are often interested in connecting with others but do not always know how to do so, which can lead to feelings of loneliness and depression (Jones et al., 2003).

Our focus in this chapter is computer-mediated applications that address the social-emotional challenges that people with ASD often encounter. However, to select effective computer-mediated applications, it is also essential to consider non-social characteristics associated with ASD that might contribute to social challenges and/or alter how an individual with ASD interacts with computerized interfaces. People with ASD often report atypical sensory experiences (APA, 2013; Bogdashina, 2003): These may include less responsiveness to a given sensory modality (e.g., not turning in response to a loud noise), more responsiveness to a given sensory modality (e.g., shielding one's eyes as if blinded by a light that others find less intense), variability in responsiveness to a given sensory modality (e.g., yelling in response to a scraping noise but not responding at all to a banging noise), or challenges integrating information across sensory modalities (e.g., difficulty using a person's tone of voice to help interpret his or her facial expression). Many people with ASD also experience motor difficulties including difficulty initiating movements, fine motor impairments (e.g., difficulty coordinating precise movements of the fingers which could affect the use of a computer mouse), and gross motor challenges (e.g., an unusual manner of walking; Provost, Lopez, & Heimerl, 2007).

These differences in the sensory-motor experiences of individuals with ASD may contribute to the challenges they face in understanding and responding to the relatively unpredictable world of social interactions (Ploog, 2010). However, individuals with ASD are often skilled at recognizing patterns in more predictable systems (such as calendars, train schedules, or computer programs) and at noticing details (Baron-Cohen et al., 2009). They often have focused special interests, which can provide opportunities for them to develop expertise and to connect with others with similar interests. Interactive technologies may aid people with ASD in exploring their interests and in overcoming some of the challenges they experience in face-to-face interactions (Benford, 2008; Jordan & Caldwell-Harris, 2012).

ARE INTERACTIVE TECHNOLOGIES HELPFUL FOR PEOPLE WITH ASD?

Computer-mediated intervention may help people with ASD interact with others by giving them opportunities to seek out people who share their interests, time to consider others' responses and edit their own, and practice interacting from the safety of a familiar place (Bagatell, 2010; Benford & Standen, 2009; Burke et al., 2010; Gillespie-Lynch, Kapp, Shane-Simpson, Smith, & Hutman, in press). Computers may appeal to individuals with ASD by building on their strengths and helping them cope with some of the difficulties that can make social interactions challenging, such as difficulties interpreting others' nonverbal behaviors (Müller, Schuler, & Yates, 2008).

People with ASD often find computer-based instruction enjoyable and motivating (Moore & Calvert, 2000), perhaps because computer-based information is organized according to predictable rules that may be well-matched to the literal and rule-based processing styles of many individuals with ASD (Murray, 1997; Swettenham, 1996). Indeed, Temple Grandin, an ASD expert who has ASD, views her own mind as operating much like an internet search engine (Grandin, 2009), which may be representative of some individuals with ASD. However, computer-based instruction may not be equally appealing and/or accessible to all individuals with ASD (Fletcher-Watson, 2014).

Computer-mediated applications can provide individualized one-on-one attention, immediate reinforcement, and consistency of treatment (e.g. by allowing users to engage with the same application at home and at school). In the following section, we will highlight steps that can be taken to select a computer-mediated application for a given individual (see Table 1 for an overview of potential steps to take when selecting an application). The following suggestions and guidelines were developed by the authors of this chapter based on scientific research including an informative article about how to evaluate computer-based interventions for ASD (Fletcher-Watson, 2014).

Table 1. Steps in Selecting Computer-Mediated Applications for Individuals with ASD

1) Select treatment goals: What skills does the person need/want help developing?
2) Select applications designed to achieve these goals
3) Examine others' ratings of the applications
4) Try out each application if possible: Is it customizable and user-friendly? Is it well-matched to the individual with ASD? Does he or she enjoy using it?
5) Search for research evidence of application efficacy: Consult scholar.google.com to see if scholar-reviewed research has been conducted to evaluate the application. Note that most applications will not yet have published research about them.
6) Evaluate research evidence of application efficacy: A) How many participants were there? Were they similar to the person the application is being evaluated for? B) How was the effectiveness of the intervention measured? Were observed benefits of the intervention related to your treatment goals? Did benefits of the intervention generalize to face-to-face interactions? C) What type of research design was used? **If an RCT was used:** Were participants randomly assigned to a control group? Were the results statistically significant?   **If a small-n design was used:** Was the baseline at least five sessions long? Was a graph provided to demonstrate changes from baseline following the intervention?
7) After selecting an application, determine how you will assess if it works
8) If you find no evidence that it works, repeat this process ☺

SELECTING A COMPUTER-MEDIATED APPLICATION FOR A SPECIFIC INDIVIDUAL WITH ASD

Is the Application Designed to Address Core Difficulties for the Individual?

A first step in evaluating the potential of an application is to determine what types of skills would maximize the individual's quality of life by helping him or her attain meaningful goals. In order to identify potential improvements in skills that could benefit an individual (or meet their treatment goals), one must not only identify what types of skills the individual needs help developing, but also what skills he or she does not need help with. For example, many people with ASD struggle to interpret emotions, while others do not (Harms et al., 2010). It is important to focus on treatment goals that do indeed represent difficulties for a given individual. Treatments goals may be ascertained through conversations with the individual with ASD and family members about their needs and interests, as well as by observations of the individual's social difficulties in a variety of situations.

Is the Application Designed to Achieve Treatment Goals?

It is essential to consider how social information is portrayed in a given application. For example, multimedia content (such as appealing graphics and music) may be particularly effective in capturing attention (Fletcher-Watson, 2014). Many people with ASD may not differ from people without ASD in their attention to *pictures* of faces, but may look differently at dynamic *videos or movies* of faces (Speer et al., 2007). Thus, applications that use videos of faces may be more effective in improving how people with ASD attend to faces than applications that rely solely on static images.

Does the Application Fit with Ongoing Treatment?

It is important to consider how the application will fit with possible ongoing, especially in-person, interventions. By planning overlap between computer-based and other interventions, one can maximize consistency and increase the likelihood that practiced skills will generalize to in-person interactions. It is also important to ensure that opportunities to engage with computer-mediated applications do not distract from in-person interactions. Despite the potential benefits of computers for supporting the development of social and emotional skills, people with ASD may spend less time engaged in social Internet activities (e.g. e-mail), and more time in relatively non-social computer-based activities, such as electronic games, relative to their peers without ASD (Mazurek & Wenstrup, 2013). Thus, one should evaluate the degree to which computer-based interventions (e.g., games that promote emotion recognition) support in-person social interactions as opposed to becoming undesirable replacements. An example of this undesirable use would involve playing a game to enhance face processing *instead* of interacting with live peers.

How Will Progress Be Evaluated?

After identifying applications that could address an individual's treatment goals, it is important to plan how one will evaluate progress. Ideally, evaluation of an intervention should consider progress both in terms of the specific computer-mediated application (e.g., moving up levels within a game designed to improve eye contact) as well as the generalization of skills to face-to-face interactions (e.g., looking more at peers during play). Current research evaluating the effectiveness of computer-mediated interventions to support the social and emotional development of individuals with ASD suggests that individuals with ASD may sometimes show improvements in social skills, as assessed within the application, while failing to generalize these skills when engaging with others in-person (Golan & Baron-Cohen, 2006). Consequently, computer-mediated applications may be most effective at supporting social development when used in conjunction with in-person interventions (Fletcher-Watson, 2014).

Is the Application Customizable?

Applications that can be personalized or customized to match the needs and goals of a given individual may be particularly beneficial because each individual with ASD is unique (Fletcher-Watson, 2014). Therefore, one should critically evaluate the match between an application and an individual's developmental level, learning goals, interests, sensory preferences, and motor capabilities. For example, using a mouse or a small touch-screen may be prohibitively challenging for an individual with fine-motor difficulties, whereas understanding written instructions may be challenging for an individual with reading difficulties. A key-evaluation criterion may be whether or not the application provides choices in terms of the types and intensities of sensory modalities in which instructions are delivered, the motor behaviors that are required to respond to the application, the learning goals, and the complexity of the task itself.

Is the Application User-Friendly?

For an application to be appealing it needs to strike a balance between being challenging and being manageable to use; this point of balance is specific to each individual. Although it may be possible to make a decision about whether a game is suitable based on a description, it is better to test a demo version of the game or borrow one from a friend. How much effort is required to get the game started is another factor to consider, and it is generally of value to have a game that is easy to set up for play with relatively little supervision. Indeed, the less time one has to spend on managing play, the more time will be available for other directly beneficial activities.

What Is the Educational and Entertainment Value of the Application?

Applications differ in the degree to which they encourage desirable social behaviors, are educational in other ways, and/or are entertaining. It is generally a good idea to try to balance these aspects, which, of course, do not need to be mutually exclusive. There may be applications that are very entertaining *and* rank high on encouraging behaviors that are desirable and address an individual's needs. (An example, not specifically designed for players with ASD is Sims®, a strategic life simulation game that is fun and challenging at a wide range of difficulty levels, but also allows the player to "build" families, communities, and entire cities with complex social fabric). For children uninterested in educational and/or social games, one might give the child permission to play a fun but less educational game only if the child first agrees to play a more educational, less fun game for a while. In this way, the child has been given an incentive to play a game of low interest, in order to play the game of high interest. This behavior-analytic approach is based on the scientifically validated, so-called Premack principle (e.g., Premack, 1962). In brief, it states that being allowed to engage in a preferred activity (such as playing a favorite computer game) can serve as a powerful reward or motivation to tackle a less preferred activity (such as playing a rather boring computer game). Parents have used this principle intuitively for a very long time and with great success when they tell their children something like "*First* do your homework, *then* you can play," with permission to play being the reward for successful homework completion.

Is There Evidence that the Application Is Effective?

After identifying potential applications that are well-matched to the treatment goals and characteristics of the individual with ASD, if available, one should evaluate the research basis for the effectiveness of the applications. One can often find published research in academic journals (meaning that the research has been reviewed by a community of scholars) by searching for the name of the application or its creators in Google Scholar (scholar.google.com). Even if a specific program has not been evaluated, one can look for applications with similar key features that have been evaluated. However, it might often be difficult to determine which aspects of a given intervention were or were not effective in promoting change, so one must be cautious when drawing conclusions. The next section will provide guidelines for evaluating the quality of research findings.

HOW TO EVALUATE RESEARCH ABOUT APPLICATIONS FOR INDIVIDUALS WITH ASD

As commercial applications are often not regulated by professional or scientific standards, it is important for consumers to be able to differentiate between good (i.e., therapeutically sound) applications, those that have not been tested sufficiently but may perhaps prove to be helpful, and others that are outright useless and ineffective, may cost a lot, and may even be harmful. As the rate of development of new applications is staggering, we have sketched out these general guidelines to assist parents in evaluating future products that are not yet on the market. The specific applications that will be discussed in this chapter may serve as examples for how to use these criteria when making a decision about obtaining a given application.

A Few Words about Scientific Evaluation

Some critics warn of science's rigorous data-driven approach that may appear excessively restrictive, and thus does not seem to adequately address consumers' urgent needs. Science does in fact have its shortcomings; for example, scientists are often reluctant to make potentially helpful, but still experimental treatments available to the public too quickly. This protects the consumer from potentially dangerous side effects. Science also protects against fraud and false claims as well as against well-intended but harmful products. Understandably, parents who are under a lot of emotional pressure because of their child's disability may be willing to try anything with the remote chance that it *might* be helpful. Risks may be underestimated when a decision is made based on an emotional reaction. Science tries to help people to make rational and sound decisions given the available knowledge; it offers people the best chance to actually identify products that might ultimately help and not harm the user.

Science attempts to evaluate treatments in such a way that the evaluation process itself is transparent to other researchers and to the public. When one estimates the correctness of evaluations, it is never entirely clear whether "App X is helpful" or "App Y is useless." As a result, scientists report estimated probabilities (between 0% and 100%), and accept that there is a certain chance of committing errors in their research. Indeed, statistics is how researchers assess the risks of claiming something is effective when it is not (false positives) and thinking something is not effective when in fact it is (false negatives). The specific ways of doing such assessments are beyond the scope of this chapter. For this chapter's purposes, it suffices to know that researchers typically accept at a maximum 5% chance of a false positive, that is, incorrectly concluding that an intervention is effective when in fact it is not. The chance of a false positive is reported as a significance level or p value less than .05. To assess the chance of a false negative is not as straightforward and depends on several factors (including the degree of effectiveness of the treatment itself). For practical purposes, false negatives are generally less critical than false positives because false negatives result, in the worst case, in simply not using a given treatment for which the degree of benefit was probably small to begin with.

How Many People Have Benefitted from this Application?

People generally agree that if you can show an *effect* on a lot of people (or a statistically significant finding), then it is more convincing and deemed more accurate than if you can show an effect on only a few people or only on one person. For example, anecdotal evidence that Child A was helped by a computer game is not as convincing as knowing that this game has benefited many children.

While the number of children who participated in a scientific evaluation study is one criterion for evaluating evidence that it works, most studies that evaluate applications do not involve many children. This is especially true in the early phases of product development when one just has a hunch that something might work. It is costly for researchers to involve many children in a study from the beginning. An additional factor pertains to interest in research participation: If parents have a choice between having their child join an exploratory study with little hope for personal benefits resulting from participation versus signing up their child for more hours of a proven, effective intervention, their choice for the proven intervention is understandable. Thus, conducting a scientifically sound evaluation study of a brand new product is often hindered just because it is difficult to recruit participants. This is why researchers very much appreciate if parents of children with ASD generously agree to let their children participate, even if there may not be any immediate and personal benefit for the participating children.

Fortunately, science has developed evaluation procedures that do not depend on very large numbers of participants for obtaining scientifically sound results (Shadish, 2014). In fact, it is possible to conduct a scientifically sound study with only one participant. Studies with one or a few participants often employ research designs that are commonly referred to as small-n designs (n refers to number of participants). In small-n designs, an individual's behavior is measured repeatedly while the environment in which the individual is tested is changed in a predictable way (i.e. by testing before the intervention, during the intervention, and after the intervention). If the individual's behavior changes in the same way every time he or she is in the same environment, this is considered evidence that that particular environment contributed to the behavior change. Small-n studies can be contrasted with studies wherein multiple participants are randomly assigned to different groups (i.e. a computer generates a number that decides for the researchers if the individual will receive an intervention or not). This procedure is known as random assignment and is used to control for random differences between individuals (i.e., individual differences are equally likely to show up in either of the two groups). This type of study is known as a randomized controlled trial (RCT). In RCT studies, individuals are either assigned to a group that receives the target intervention or to a control group that does not receive the target intervention. Differences between the group that receives the intervention and the control group are taken as evidence that the intervention is or is not effective.

Although RCT studies are considered by some the gold standard for testing the efficacy of an intervention (Lord et al., 2005), they are often conducted at a very slow pace relative to the rate at which technologies are developed. Small-n designs can be conducted more quickly and can thus provide important information about new applications. Although small-n designs appear to lack a control group and do not involve large numbers of participants, each participant in fact serves as his or her own control (as in comparing performance during intervention and baseline for a single individual). This method is often more effective than RCTs for highlighting differences between individuals in response to an intervention, but is less effective than RCTs for understanding the degree to which an intervention is generally effective for a diverse group of people.

In summary, if an application has been tested with more, rather than fewer children, it is generally preferable, as long as both studies were equally well-controlled. However, results of studies with very few participants can still be meaningful, if the research employs an appropriate design. In a peer-reviewed journal, the description of a study's research design is often described in the *Methods/Procedures* section of the scientific report.

Efficacy: Does the Application Really Work?

Efficacy is the capacity to produce an effect. In our context, it means: Does the application help children to improve in whatever area it claims to be helpful? For example, if an application is advertised to improve social skills in teenagers with ASD, is it really holding up to its promise? Efficacy is evaluated after researchers have evaluated the feasibility of an intervention, or the possibility that it is designed well enough that it could work. There are at least four aspects to consider when evaluating efficacy: (1) statistical significance, (2) clinical significance, (3) relative effectiveness, and (4) social validation.

Statistical Significance

The first refers to the question of whether an effect can be attributed to the actual workings of the application itself rather than to chance. This requires appreciation of the scientific method, including statistics as was outlined above. As also discussed above, the results of a research study are often backed-up by statistics that let a scientist estimate whether the obtained data were purely a chance outcome or, whether there is a reasonable hope (usually a 5% chance or p value of less than .05) that the promising results are due to the application and likely to occur again in the future for other children using it. (For an adamant critique of this view, however, see Branch, 2014.)

It is also important to keep in mind that statistical significance, when comparing groups of people, can obscure differences in responses to a treatment between *specific* individuals. Knowing that an intervention was effective for *other* individuals does not ensure that it will be effective for a *specific* individual. After selecting a promising application, it is essential to collect data on whether the application is actually helping the individual, while keeping in mind that change may begin gradually.

Another important statistical concept, effect size, refers to the degree of improvement. Over the past few years, it is increasingly expected that effect size should be reported for any scientific study (Shadish, 2014). Effect size is largely independent of statistical significance. For example, there could be a statistically significant (different from chance), yet negligible improvement (in effect size) in social skills, in a study involving hundreds of children. Such a negligible effect is so small that it is unlikely to actually help children, even though the improvement appears to be real and not due to chance.

Clinical Significance

Even if results are statistically significant and the effect is large, it does not necessarily mean that the results are very helpful for a particular individual. For example, it could be a reliable and truthful outcome that social behavior has improved by 100%, which seems very impressive. But if the level of social behavior has increased from, say, asking one spontaneous question during a day to asking two questions a day (a 100% increase!), it is not clear whether this reliable and superficially impressive 100% increase is going to make a real difference in the individual's life. So, when evaluating an application that significantly improves social skills (it produced a statistically significant result), one still must ask whether this improvement will make a meaningful difference.

Relative Effectiveness

This refers to the question of whether the application is doing a better job than another approach. For example, a game might present social situations to the player in the hopes that this will train socially relevant skills that are applicable for real-life situations. This may be true, but traditional approaches (e.g., role-playing with a parent) might be more effective and without a hefty price tag. Still, just because an application does not outperform a traditional approach, one may not want to dismiss it entirely, especially if the child is unwilling to engage in the more traditional educational activity. Generally, children like to play computer games, and if the application is engaging enough, the child may play it voluntarily and benefit from it. So when faced with a choice between a mildly effective application that the individual enjoys playing for a long time versus a highly effective, low-interest treatment which the individual avoids, one should consider using the application while continuing to look for applications that are both high-interest and effective.

One way to evaluate an application's relative effectiveness is to look for control groups in the research paper. A control group could be a group of participants who were exposed to a traditional approach and then compared to a group of children who played the game/app (as in a RCT; see Figure 1). Alternatively, a so-called *baseline* could provide an appropriate comparison. A baseline refers to data (e.g., level of social skills) that were taken before the child started playing the game (i.e. typically with the baseline measured over multiple observation sessions so one can assess any trend in the data); the baseline is then compared to data collected as the child uses the application over multiple sessions (as is common in a small-n design; see Figure 2). This design can also be viewed as a "before-after" design, with the baseline representing the "before treatment" condition. Either way, a proper comparison is critical. Otherwise, one has no way of knowing if a child's behavior really improved due to playing the application, or if it would have improved, perhaps even more, with an alternative method or no intervention.

Social Validation

Social Validation is related to the previous points, but adds a more pragmatic aspect to evaluation. Consider, for example, that a child has been using an application that has been shown to produce statistically and clinically significant results, with large effect sizes. But then one asks the child (if s/he can respond to such a question), parents, teachers, or friends and relatives, whether they actually perceive an improvement in, say, social skills, and the answer is "Not really!" This would be an example where social validation failed. Ideally, in order to know that an application is worth the money or time invested in it, one would want to know whether it has produced improvements that are noticeable to the child, parents, and the people around him or her. In many studies, social validation measures are published (for a landmark study about social validation, behavior treatment, and autism, see Schreibman, Koegel, Mills, & Burke, 1981) and these provide very solid, common-sense criteria for a parent to use to make a decision as to whether to obtain an application or not, without getting too bogged down with statistical and scientific detail.

Figure 1. Example figure from randomized controlled trial (RCT) design.

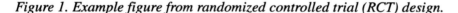
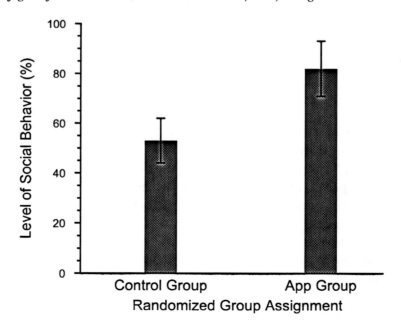

Figure 2. Example figure from small-n design.

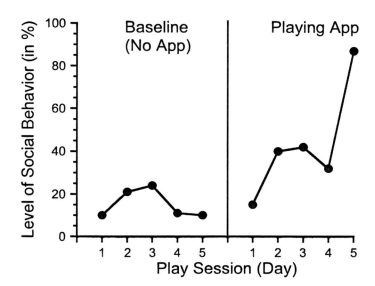

The next sections allow readers to apply the principles we have introduced in this section to evaluate the current state of the evidence for the effectiveness (or efficacy) of a range of different computer-mediated applications to support the social and emotional development of people with ASD.

SOCIAL-EMOTIONAL COMPUTER GAMES FOR INDIVIDUALS WITH ASD

To date, there have been only few scientifically rigorous tests concerning the efficacy of computerized games for improving social and emotional skills in individuals with ASD. As previously described, in a randomized controlled trial (RCT) researchers compare performance of an experimental group receiving a target intervention (e.g., playing a specific game aimed at improving face recognition) with a control group receiving either a different intervention or no intervention (see Figure 1). A commonly used control group is the wait-list control wherein the control group receives the intervention after the study has been completed. In this section, we report findings of several RCT studies (Tanaka et al., 2010; Hopkins et al., 2011; Golan & Baron-Cohen, 2006) testing the efficacy of interactive games in improving social and emotional skills for individuals with ASD.

Mind Reading

Golan and Baron-Cohen (2006) tested the effectiveness of *Mind Reading,* an interactive software resource designed to teach adults with high-functioning autism (HFA) or Asperger Syndrome the meanings of facial expressions and emotional tone of voice. *Mind Reading* (jkp.com/mindreading/) includes a library of audio and video clips representing 412 emotions and mental states, each performed by multiple actors (male and female of varying ethnicities and ages) to promote "generalization"—i.e., the participant's ability to apply learned skills to a variety of novel situations. *Mind Reading* defines each emotion with words and provides six silent films of faces, six voice recordings, and six written examples of situations that evoke that emotion. Users may browse the emotion library, use a learning center that provides lessons to teach about the different emotions, or enter the game zone to play any of five educational games.

To test the efficacy of *Mind Reading* in teaching adults with high-functioning autism (HFA; defined by an IQ in the normal range) to recognize complex emotions, Golan and Baron-Cohen (2006) conducted two RCT studies. In both studies, the experimental group was instructed to play *Mind Reading* games independently at home for two hours per week, for a total of twenty hours of training. In the first study, an experimental group consisting of 19 adults with HFA was compared to a control group of 22 individuals with HFA who did not receive any intervention. In the second study, an experimental group consisting of 13 adults with HFA used the software and attended weekly group sessions with a tutor who engaged them in role-play activities and discussions of emotions. This experimental group was compared with a control group consisting of 13 participants (also with HFA) who instead attended 10 sessions of social skills training. In both studies, the experimental group showed greater improvements from pre-test to post-test, relative to the control group, in recognizing complex emotions and mental states when presented with variations of the specific stimuli used during the *Mind Reading* training. However, even with the additional support of an in-person tutor in the second study, the experimental group failed to perform any better than controls on generalization tasks where they had to recognize emotions in pictures, audio recordings, and films that they had not seen during training. Thus, while *Mind Reading* software was effective in helping adults with HFA recognize emotions in the stimuli with which they were taught, it was not effective at helping them evaluate emotions in new stimuli. Additionally, around 25% of the participants in the *Mind Reading* training groups dropped out of the study, which suggests that the game may not have been particularly interesting or engaging for them.

The Transporters

More recently, Golan and colleagues (2009) used images from the *Mind Reading* software to build an animated television series *The Transporters* to improve emotion recognition in children with ASD. Although this intervention is not computer-mediated, we include it in this chapter because it applies the principles developed in the *Mind Reading* game to develop a video-based intervention for children. Evidence discussed below suggests that the *Transporters* may be more effective than the *Mind Reading* game. Although this improved effectiveness could be due to differences in the design of the two interventions, it could also be due to the fact that children are often more skilled at learning new social skills than adults because their brains are still developing rapidly. When considering the appropriateness of an application for a specific individual, it is always important to consider if the benefits reported with other users are likely to apply given the age and developmental level of the individual one hopes to assist.

This animated television series is available for purchase at thetransporters.com. *The Transporters* series is based around characters that are vehicles on which the faces of actors from the *Mind Reading* software have been grafted. Each 5-minute episode of *The Transporters* focuses on one of 15 emotions and mental states, including a number of complex emotions, for example, jealous and joking. *The Transporters* DVD contains quizzes for each episode that encourage children to match faces to each other, match faces to emotions, and match faces to situations; thus, the DVD includes interactive materials as well as videos for children to watch.

To evaluate the efficacy of *The Transporters* in teaching about emotions, Golan and colleagues conducted an RCT with 4- to 8-year-old children with HFA. Twenty children in the experimental group received *The Transporters* DVD and were compared to 19 children who did not participate in any intervention until after the study was over. Parents of children in the experimental group were instructed to have their child watch at least three episodes of *The Transporters* per day for a period of four weeks and to use the DVD guide to help their child to learn. The DVD guide encouraged parents to let their children watch the episodes repeatedly and to encourage them to look at the faces of the characters for emotional information. The guide also provided advice on how to engage children in discussions about the emotional themes of the episodes, including, for example, why people might respond to situations in different ways.

As pre- and post-intervention assessments of emotion recognition, children in the experimental and control groups were asked to (1) define emotion and mental state vocabulary words, (2) match situations taken from *The Transporters* episodes with characters' facial expressions, (3) match novel situations with facial expressions of *The Transporters* characters, and (4) match novel situations with facial expressions of unfamiliar actors (also taken from the *Mind Reading* software). Across all assessments, the experimental group showed significant gains whereas the control group did not. Importantly, their learning was not limited to tests involving images of *The Transporters* characters, but extended to faces of unfamiliar actors and included tests of their ability to describe emotions and mental states in words. Thus, the benefits from this approach generalized to novel situations.

Although the experimental group was required to watch only three episodes per day, many children watched the videos at much higher rates—indicating that the antics of the toy vehicles in *The Transporters* appealed to the children with ASD. Presumably by capitalizing on the children's intrinsic interests in vehicles and mechanical motion, *The Transporters* was effective in relating information about the characters' emotions and mental states successfully. Future studies are needed, however, to determine whether the observed gains extend to social functioning in real-life. Furthermore, it is unclear to what extent the observed benefits were linked to parental supports of children's learning (e.g., discussions of emotional concepts) and/or use of the interactive quizzes, and to what extent children would learn simply from watching the television programs on their own. Nevertheless, the results are very promising in suggesting that an animated television show might be a useful tool to foster interest in emotions and mental states in children with ASD. Finally, the knowledge gained from this DVD approach could easily be implemented in a more interactive application. For example, a game-like application might allow for player input with regard to how the characters in *The Transporters* act and react.

Junior Detective Training Program

The Junior Detective Training Program (sstinstitute.net/au/professionals/research) includes a computer game, small group activities, and parent trainings to support the social development of children with ASD. The main character in the computer game, the junior detective, specializes in decoding suspects' feelings from facial expressions, body postures and tone of voice. Through game play, children are encouraged to recognize complex emotions (such as guilt) in others and themselves using nonverbal and contextual cues. This knowledge is then applied in "virtual reality missions" focused on topics such as dealing with bullying or trying new things. In the social skills groups, children practice skills learned in the game and are provided with guidelines for social interaction. Parents are trained to encourage children to practice recognizing emotions in themselves and others at home.

In an efficacy study for the Junior Detective Training Program, 26 children with HFA were assigned to the training program and 23 were assigned to a wait-list control group (Beaumont & Sofronoff, 2008). Social skills questionnaires that parents filled out about their children at the beginning and end of the intervention revealed that children who participated in the training program may have improved more in their social skills than the control group. Participants in the training program also showed greater improvement in knowledge of emotion management techniques than participants in the control group. Assessments conducted five months after the intervention ended, suggested that these benefits were maintained (still apparent after the intervention was over).

Let's Face It!

Tanaka and colleagues (2010) tested the efficacy of *Let's Face It!* as a tool to enhance face recognition in children, adolescents, and young adults with ASD. *Let's Face It!* comprises a battery of interactive computer games that are available to download free of charge (web.uvic.ca/~letsface/letsfaceit). Tanaka et al. (2010) used a wait-list control design to test the effectiveness of seven *Let's Face It!* games at enhancing face-processing strategies. One of the games called 'ZapIt' required children to match faces across changes in facial expression, viewing angle, and clothing; another game called 'Splash' required children to splash faces that matched the identity of a target face. Throughout the intervention, parents were instructed to have their child play *Let's Face It!* games for a minimum of 100 minutes per week and to document through weekly logs their child's game play. The experimental group (42 participants with ASD, average age 10.5 years) played *Let's Face It!* for an average of 20 hours over an average period of 19 weeks while the control group (37 participants with ASD, average age 11.4 years) underwent whatever treatment they normally received.

To evaluate the efficacy of the intervention, the experimental and control groups were administered five tests measuring aspects of face recognition before and after the intervention. The experimental group showed larger gains relative to the control group on only one of the five tests of face recognition. While they improved in their ability to use a feature of the face (e.g., the eyes) to distinguish between faces that were otherwise identical, they did not improve relative to the control group in their ability to identify faces across changes in facial expression or orientation, nor in their ability to remember faces after a delay. Thus, the results provided limited evidence of benefits from short-term usage of a computer game involving face matching in improving aspects of face processing in children with ASD.

The research team that developed *Let's Face It!* has launched a new set of computerized games called *FaceStation*. Video demonstrations of new interactive games to support face processing in people with ASD are available online (centerforautismresearch.com/trial_interventions/computerized_gaming) and an efficacy study is in progress.

FaceSay

Hopkins et al. (2011) conducted an RCT to test the efficacy of *FaceSay* in enhancing emotion recognition and social interaction in children with ASD of varying cognitive levels. *FaceSay* is a virtual reality game available for purchase at facesay.com/social-skills-and-autism.html. Virtual reality environments use computer-technology to provide 3D experiences to mimic those experienced in real life. *FaceSay* uses realistic avatars and includes three games targeting different social skills: responding to joint attention (or looking where others are looking), recognizing facial expressions, and recognizing faces. In each game, a computer-animated avatar initiates interaction and asks the child to perform tasks requiring attention to faces or parts of faces. For example, in the "Amazing Gaze" game, the child is asked to follow the avatar's eyes to determine what the avatar is looking at. Hopkins et al. (2011) recruited 6- to 15-year-old children with low-functioning autism (LFA) and cognitive delays, and children with HFA without cognitive impairments. They randomly assigned them to experimental and control groups. The experimental group (11 participants with LFA, 13 participants with HFA) received bi-weekly 10- to 25-minute training sessions with *FaceSay* for a period of six weeks while the control group (14 participants with LFA, 11 participants with HFA) instead used *Tux Paint* open-source drawing software for children (tuxpaint.org). Children completed tests of emotion and face recognition and were observed interacting with their peers during recess both before and after intervention. In addition, parents completed a questionnaire about their children's social skills before and after intervention to assess a range of skills including cooperation, assertion, responsibility, and self-control.

Both LFA and HFA participants who viewed *FaceSay* showed larger gains in recognizing facial expressions from photographs in comparison to the control group. Only children with HFA showed improvement in recognizing the identities of individual faces following *FaceSay*. Importantly, both children with LFA and HFA showed improvements in interacting with their peers following *FaceSay* training. As discussed earlier, people with ASD often struggle with generalizing social skills they have learned from computer-mediated interventions to social interactions in the real world. *FaceSay* was effective at helping children with ASD, both those who were and were not cognitively delayed, generalize social skills learned on computers to real-life interactions. It is possible that virtual reality applications are more effective at supporting the development of real-life social skills relative to less realistic computer games because they are more likely to engage players to take on the roles of the characters.

Parents of children with LFA reported improvements in their children's social skills after *FaceSay* training (an example of social validation mentioned above). Similar trends reported by parents of children with HFA did not reach statistical significance, indicating a lack of social validation for children with HFA, as judged by statistical methods. Nevertheless, the *convergence of different types of evidence* (or similar improvements observed with tests, social interactions, and parent ratings) following *FaceSay* training suggests that realistic avatars might be effective in supporting the social and emotional development of children with ASD of varying cognitive levels. In the following section, we will discuss virtual-reality applications that are not specifically games to support individuals with ASD.

VIRTUAL-REALITY ENVIRONMENTS TO PROMOTE SOCIAL-EMOTIONAL DEVELOPMENT

Virtual-reality environments may be helpful for supporting the social development of people with ASD because they combine the benefits of computer-based instruction with stimuli that are more similar to real-life interactions, and thus are more likely to promote skills that generalize to in-person interactions. Virtual environments may be particularly beneficial for people with ASD because they provide opportunities to learn from mistakes without real-world consequences; guidance can be conveyed through experience rather than simply through words; and virtual realities can be flexibly altered to provide structured opportunities to explore (Standen & Brown, 2005).

In a preliminary study, Cheng, Chiang, Ye, and Cheng (2010) used a multiple-baseline design (similar in part to Figure 2) for three boys with HFA to evaluate the potential of virtual-reality to support empathy development. Their program uses 3D animation to create a virtual restaurant environment, and presents scripted situations that could elicit empathy, such as a passerby slipping and falling, as well as situations to elicit other emotions. Players select a realistic avatar and interact with other avatars, including a virtual teacher who poses questions about the situations (e.g., "How do you feel when..."). They use buttons to select expressions to convey emotions, and have the option of communicating with the teacher either with text or speech, which allows individuals with ASD with poor reading skills to use the system. Participants' responses to a computerized empathy rating scale administered during approximately 15 sessions suggested that they improved in empathy over the course of the training. However, empathy during real-life interactions or using stimuli that were not presented during training were not assessed. Indeed, one of the participants expressed boredom with being asked the same questions over and over. This study demonstrates feasibility (that an intervention designed in a user-friendly way may have the desired effects) but provides limited evidence of efficacy (that it did indeed improve empathy skills).

Collaborative virtual activities can be designed to support awareness of others among children with LFA (Holt & Yuill, 2014). Multi-user environments may provide unique and customizable supports to encourage not only social understanding (a common target of computer-mediated interventions) but also social interaction. In the study by Holt and Yuill (2014), four children with LFA were introduced to a computer-based game in which they sorted pictures from their favorite cartoons while seated next to a partner on his own computer. The game ran in two versions: 1) Using a collaborative interface, each computer depicted representations of the child's own and their partner's activity on the task, and they could only complete certain stages of the task by pressing a green "we agree" button and, 2) using a non-collaborative interface, each child worked on the same task on separate computers, but their own screen depicted only their own progress, and they did not have to attend to what their partner was doing or agree with him in order to move on. Participants showed more evidence of attending to the other child and higher engagement with the task (moving toward it or laughing) when using the collaborative interface. While preliminary, this study is exciting as it suggests that virtual environments can be designed to help cognitively delayed people with ASD enjoy working together.

Addressing the shortage of evidence-based interventions for young adults with ASD, a virtual reality Social Cognition Training was designed to improve the social skills, social cognition, and social functioning of young adults with ASD (Kandalaft, Dedehbani, Krawczyk, Allen, & Chapman, 2013). Eight young adults with ASD participated in this training study for five weeks. Participants used avatars (designed to resemble the participant) while interacting on a virtual Second Life island that included sites such as an office building, pool hall, and campground. An avatar of a coach directed participants to specific situations wherein they interacted with the avatar of a clinician. Ten social scenarios were presented including interacting with friends, meeting people, and job interviews. Each social scenario had related learning objectives such as reading others' emotions and interests, displaying one's own emotions, using appropriate language, and producing novel as opposed to rote responses. Participants were asked structured questions after the interactions to help them gain insight into their performance, and were then given opportunities to incorporate the feedback they had received in new situations (e.g., after discussing one job interview, they went on another). Social cognition was measured before and after the intervention by asking participants to identify emotions in pictures and voices. Recognition of pictures of emotions and emotion expressed through tone of voice improved across the course of the intervention. Importantly, emotion recognition improved with stimuli that had not been directly trained (in contrast to Golan & Baron-Cohen, 2006), suggesting good generalization. Participants reported that they had gained a lot of social experience from the intervention, which had improved their confidence in social situations. A limitation of the study design is that it lacked a control group; therefore, it remains unclear whether the observed improvements were due to the training or other changes that happened in participants' lives.

Stichter, Laffey, Galyen, and Herzog (2014) designed iSocial, a Virtual Learning Environment, to help adolescents with ASD learn skills such as emotion recognition in themselves and others, conversational skills, and problem solving. An educator situated at a distant college used the virtual environment to deliver lessons adapted from an in-person curriculum to three small cohorts of teens with ASD (11 total) at rural schools. Initial studies assessing the feasibility of the virtual curriculum provided feedback that helped researchers make the virtual environment socially engaging for the students. Virtual games (such as recognizing a character's facial expression to gain entrance to a castle) and collaborative activities (such as building a virtual restaurant) were used. Parents and teachers completed standardized questionnaires assessing participants' social symptoms and goal-orientation skills before and after the intervention. Student responses to assessments used in past studies to assess understanding of others' emotions did not provide evidence that their social skills had improved. However, some behavioral measures of cognitive flexibility improved. Parents indicated significant reductions in social symptoms and improvements in executive functioning (skills used to achieve goals such as planning), although teacher reports did not. The lack of a control group or observations of students' interactions with their peers make clear that additional evaluation is needed to establish efficacy.

The efficacy of job-interview training via virtual reality was assessed using a RCT with 16 adults with ASD in a virtual-reality group and 10 adults with ASD in a control group who received their usual treatment (Smith et al., 2014). The virtual training, available for purchase at jobinterviewtraining.net/meetmolly.aspx, consists of simulated job interviews and teaching of job interview skills, such as building a resumé, finding out about positions, and preparing questions to ask. Importantly, the behavior of the job interviewer varies based on the responses of the interviewee: The virtual reality system provides in-the-moment nonverbal feedback, offered by an onscreen job coach, and gives interviewees the option to receive verbal feedback by clicking the help button. It also offers scores on key aspects of performance and an opportunity to review audio and written transcripts of interviews that are coded for the quality of responses. Participants move from easy to hard interviews (where the interviewer is brusque and may ask illegal questions) based on their performance.

In-person role-plays of job interviews before and after the intervention revealed that participants who received the virtual reality training exhibited greater improvement during live interviews than their counterparts, which constitutes successful generalization of treatment effects (i.e., use of learned skills in untrained contexts). They reported that the system was easy to use, enjoyable, and that it prepared them for interviews, which constitutes successful social validation. These studies provide promising evidence that well-designed virtual reality environments are effective in supporting a range of social skills in individuals with ASD.

TABLET-BASED APPLICATIONS TO PROMOTE SOCIAL-EMOTIONAL DEVELOPMENT

While iPad®-type apps are one of the most popular computer-based applications for people with ASD, there are currently no published RCT studies evaluating their efficacy, although some are ongoing (Stephenson & Limbrick, 2013). However, small-n designs have yielded promising evidence that tablet-based instruction may be effective for people with ASD.

Murdock, Ganz, and Crittendon (2013) used an iPad® play story, depicting toy figures engaged in scripted dialogue about firefighters, to increase the play dialogue of four preschoolers of varying cognitive levels with ASD. A multiple-baseline design was used where each child's behavior was observed at least three times before training occurred (baseline). Then each child was exposed to the application at a different point in time in order to see if exposure to it yielded changes in the target behavior (i.e., adult-initiated dialogue about firefighters) that coincided with when the app was introduced. All participants showed an increase in play dialogue during at least some of the sessions after exposure to the application, compared to the baseline. Much of the dialogue was not scripted, which indicates that they generalized beyond the trained dialogues. However, one child began to refuse to participate during the intervention phase, so his play dialogue did not improve overall during intervention relative to baseline. This suggests that the play story may not have been equally engaging for all participants.

Video modeling (or simply demonstrating desired behaviors using video) may be more effective than live modeling for teaching skills to children with ASD (Charlop-Christy, Le, & Freeman, 2000). Cardon (2012) evaluated the effectiveness of a Video Modeling Imitation Training delivered via iPad®. Caregivers selected behaviors they wanted their children to learn and received training and a manual to help them create videos of themselves or siblings demonstrating desired skills using an iPad® to display them to their children with ASD. Parents provided in-person prompts and reinforcement to encourage their children to imitate the video models. The children showed more imitation after viewing the video models than they had during baseline, as well as improvements in their use of language. Furthermore, improved imitation was still apparent a week after the intervention stopped. However, the effectiveness of the iPad® intervention was not compared to an in-person intervention so this study does not provide information about the relative effectiveness of the iPad® intervention. These studies suggest that iPad® apps (and video modeling more generally) may be effective at supporting the social-emotional skills of people with ASD.

NEW APPLICATIONS TO PROMOTE SOCIAL-EMOTIONAL DEVELOPMENT

In the previous sections, we reviewed applications that have been tested, with more or less scientific rigor, to evaluate whether they can improve social and emotional skills. This section considers games currently under development. Although the efficacy of these applications has not yet been rigorously tested, we discuss their feasibility.

Robots

The first use of a robot as a remedial tool for children was in 1976 with a 7-year-old boy with autism (Weir & Emanuel, 1976, as cited in Duquette, Michaud, & Mercier, 2008). However, most research examining potential benefits of interactive robots in supporting the social development of people with

ASD is exploratory, and focused on demonstrating the feasibility as opposed to the efficacy of robots in intervention (Diehl, Schmitt, Villano, & Crowell, 2012). While many individuals with ASD may be more attentive to robots than to other toys or humans, this is not universal and more attention may not translate to more learning. For example, two children with ASD showed *more interest* in a robot but *less imitation* of the words it said than two children with ASD who interacted with a human (Duquette et al., 2008). However, note that the robot in this study was not designed to be interactive. In another study, six children with ASD and six typically developing children attended more to a robot than to a human, but required more prompts to look where the robot looked than to look where the human looked (Bekele, Crittendon, Swanson, Sarkar, & Warren, 2013).

Similar evidence that robots may elicit heightened interest, but that this interest may not necessarily translate into enhanced learning, is apparent in a recent report assessing the potential of the humanoid robot KASPAR for eliciting collaborative play among children with ASD (Wainer, Dautenhahn, Robins, & Amirabdollahian, 2014). Six children with ASD played a video game first with a robot and then with a human partner. The robot was designed to interact with people through simple gestures, speech, basic facial expressions, gaze following, and pointing. Although the children appeared more interested in and entertained by the robot, they exhibited more collaborative play and cooperation with the human partner. The researchers noted that these differences could be due to the fact that the children always played with the robot before they played with the human, but concluded that the robot should be altered in the future as children had struggled with the need to press buttons to communicate with the robot as the robot did not have the capacity to understand speech.

In the largest study to date of the interactions of children with ASD and robots, 24 children with autism were paired with a robot (a small dinosaur designed to express emotions and attention using body movements and vocalizations), a computer game, or an adult human (Kim et al., 2013) while another adult was present. Interactions involving the robot or the human were designed to be playful and similar in all obvious respects. Although the interviewer used a script to guide the interactions, the degree to which the interviewer stuck to the script (reflective of treatment fidelity) was not assessed. The computer game was not designed to elicit interaction. The children spoke more often when interacting with the robot than when interacting with the human or the computer game. These findings suggest that robots are intriguing to children with ASD and may elicit spontaneous speech; however, more research is needed to establish their effectiveness as an intervention tool.

LIFEisGAME

LIFEisGAME uses avatars to teach children to interpret facial expressions (Abirachel et al., 2011, Fernandes et al., 2011, Jain et al., 2012). In one mode, "Build a Face," the player is presented with three panels. The first contains a photo of a person with a well-defined emotion (e.g., happy, angry). The user selects an avatar to place in the second panel. This avatar can be a photo-realistic image or a cartoon image with exaggerated features (with a third class of avatars containing alien images). The third panel has an outline of the original face with overlaid "handles" controlling the eyebrows, eye shape, and mouth. The player directly manipulates these handles using a mouse. The goal of this game is to build the emotion on the avatar to match the original emotion. A touch-screen version of the game allows players to sketch directly on the avatar using strokes. In another mode of LIFEisGAME, a camera captures real-time images of the player that are mapped onto a dynamic avatar and animated as the user moves. This sophisticated technology allows players to receive feedback regarding their own facial expressions.

In several feasibility studies, researchers reported on user experiences with the game. They considered whether players enjoyed playing the game and which avatars the players selected, i.e., animals or people, 2D or 3D, cartoon or realistic images. In one study, 60% of the children imitated the facial expressions, but disliked the slow feedback of the real-time emotion change. Some players seemed to focus more on sketching than on matching the emotions. For more information, see portointeractivecenter.org/lifeisgame.

WEBSITES FOR iPAD®, iPHONE®, AND ANDROID®-BASED APPLICATIONS

Thus far, we have explored how researchers evaluate the effectiveness of computer-mediated applications in remediating difficulties associated with ASD; we have summarized several experiments utilizing interactive technologies to improve social skills and as part of that emotion and face recognition. We also provided details about some of the emerging games and applications under development that aim to support the social and emotional development of individuals with ASD. While these resources are meant to assist in the selection of technology to support people on the spectrum, our list is not exhaustive and the specific needs and interests of each individual with ASD should be considered. The following section describes websites that provide additional resources for finding applications for people with ASD.

Autism Speaks

The Autism Speaks website (autismspeaks.org) provides a plethora of resources for individuals with ASD, friends, family members, educators, and researchers. With the emergence of computer and tablet-based applications specifically designed for individuals with ASD and the general population, this site has recently expanded to provide a searchable database of applications (autismspeaks.org/autism-apps). Visitors to the site can browse applications or search them by keyword, skills targeted, supporting device, age group, and a star rating out of 5 stars. Presumably star ratings represent average ratings by users but specifics about how ratings are calculated including user comments are not evident. The applications range from *Developmental Reading,* an application designed for children aged 3-6 years to learn reading skills through their auditory and visual senses, to *Everyday Skills (Pocket Edition),* a functional skills application designed to help individuals develop independent living skills. As a significant strength of this site, each application has been given a supporting research rating that ranges from "Anecdotal" (no scientific studies available for the application), to "Research" (some related scientific studies but with no direct research support), to "Evidence" (authors of the site have determined that there is strong scientific evidence that supports the application's efficacy). Caution is warranted in interpreting these research ratings as specific criteria for evaluating research are not revealed. Nevertheless, links to relevant studies are often available next to each application.

Touch Autism

The Touch Autism site (Touchautism.com) provides a significantly shorter list of applications for both iPad® and iPhone®, designed specifically for children with ASD. Touch Autism was founded by a developer and a clinician who collaboratively build applications specifically for children with ASD. Their site currently lists a total of 26 applications (25 available for the iPad®, 25 for the iPhone®), ranging from *Conversation Social Stories,* an application that illustrates effective tools for communication (e.g., greetings, how to ask someone to play), to *Buzz Back* which was designed for individuals with auditory and visual impairments to illustrate cause-and-effect relationships through reinforcing vibrations on the iPhone®. A significant disadvantage of this site is that it does not provide visitors with a list of evidence-based research about any of the applications.

iAutism

The iAutism site (iautism.info) lists applications specifically created for individuals with ASD, available for iPad®, iPhone®, and Android® devices. Visitors can browse the entire list of applications or search for applications by device or category (i.e. Oral and Written Language, Token Reinforcement, or Games). Upon selecting an application, users are given a concise summary of the application and its cost to download; for a subset of applications, the site also provides a review of the application. Notably, iAutism also provides information about applications available in Spanish and other languages besides English. Although this site only provides anecdotal evidence on the efficacy of applications, it is interactive in nature, allowing visitors to post questions, comments, and provide feedback with other visitors about specific applications.

Apps for Autism

At the Apps-for-Autism site, available through appymall.com, users can browse a wide variety of applications, and they can search for applications that address their child's specific needs. Many of the applications on this site were not specifically designed for children with ASD, but the applications address skillsets appropriate for these children. Visitors can search the site by application category (i.e. Art, Language, and/or Music), grade, and/or skill coverage. Applications range from *Phonics Fun: Ending Sounds*, an application designed to assist children learning to read, to *Axel's Chain Reaction*, which blends fiction and non-fiction to help children develop comprehension skills. A strength is that the Apps-for-Autism site provides user-generated and site-generated reviews on most of the applications, but unfortunately it does not include research evidence on their efficacy.

Technology in Special Education

Even though the site was not designed specifically for individuals with ASD, Technology in Special Education (techinspecialed.com) lists over 800 education-based applications, grouped into subcategories ranging from Comprehension to Social Skills Development. The site claims that site experts have reviewed most of the applications listed, and most are free for children, parents, and educators to download. Visitors to the site can search for applications by the Goals/Skills they intend to develop in the user; applications range from those addressing social and emotional needs to applications that assist with breathing exercises. However, similar to many of the aforementioned sites, Technology in Special Education does not provide users with links to research to evaluate the efficacy of each application.

Bridging Apps

The Bridging Apps site (Bridgingapps.org) hosted by Easter Seals Disability Services, and not specifically focusing on ASD, allows visitors to browse over 1,300 applications available for a variety of devices. Visitors can search for applications by keyword, skill level, mobile device, and traits, with applications ranging from those addressing anxiety management to those designed to enhance general life skills. Upon selection, a brief summary is provided for each application with user feedback ratings and comments. This site also provides reviews by a special education teacher and certified therapist in the organization associated with Easter Seals. Although it provides anecdotal reviews from professionals, it does not provide empirical evidence of efficacy.

Apps for Children with Special Needs

This is one of the many sites developed specifically for children with special needs (a4cwsn.com). Visitors can browse through over 500 applications or search for specific applications based on keywords. A father of a child with ASD and a child with epilepsy provides reviews for each application, and recommends all those listed on the site. Applications range from *Avaz for Autism*, an iPad® application designed to help users develop their language skills, to *Time Timer*, a timer application for the iPad® that was designed to assist users with their time management skills. Research-based evaluations of applications are not easily accessible on this site.

CONCLUSION

Research is beginning to support the feasibility and efficacy of a range of different types of computer-based applications to support the social-emotional development of people with ASD, with virtual reality interventions emerging as particularly promising intervention tools. The increasing availability and diversity of computer- and tablet-based technologies provide parents, professionals, and people on the spectrum with many opportunities to tailor interventions to specific individual needs. With a great number of opportunities, the selection process has become more and more complex. In this chapter, we tried to guide the consumer through this selection process. As much as possible, people with ASD themselves should be involved in selecting, modifying, and (when applicable) designing applications to support their own development and the development of others with ASD.

One should also not feel limited to choosing applications that were designed specifically for people with ASD. Many of the applications that have been developed for the general public, as mentioned above, can also be effective for people with ASD when applied in a way that fits users' needs. Often-times technology-based interventions do not (and should not) function in isolation, but instead work best in conjunction with in-person interventions. By setting clear goals for what one hopes to gain from a given application, including how progress will be assessed, and by carefully evaluating evidence for its effectiveness, one can decide whether a given application is worth its cost in terms of time or money.

REFERENCES

Abirached, B., Zhang, Y., Aggarwal, J. K., Tamersoy, B., Fernandes, T., Miranda, J. C., & Orvalho, V. (2011, November). Improving communication skills of children with ASDs through interaction with virtual characters. In *Serious Games and Applications for Health (SeGAH), 2011 IEEE 1st International Conference on* (pp. 1-4). IEEE. doi:10.1109/SeGAH.2011.6165464

American Psychiatric Association. (2013). DSM 5. American Psychiatric Association.

Bagatell, N. (2010). From cure to community: Transforming notions of autism. *Ethos (Berkeley, Calif.)*, *38*(1), 33–55. doi:10.1111/j.1548-1352.2009.01080.x

Baron-Cohen, S., Ashwin, E., Ashwin, C., Tavassoli, T., & Chakrabarti, B. (2009). Talent in autism: Hyper-systemizing, hyper-attention to detail and sensory hypersensitivity. *Philosophical Transactions of the Royal Society of London. Series B, Biological Sciences*, *364*(1522), 1377–1383. doi:10.1098/rstb.2008.0337 PMID:19528020

Beaumont, R., & Sofronoff, K. (2008). A multi-component social skills intervention for children with Asperger syndrome: The Junior Detective Training Program. *Journal of Child Psychology and Psychiatry, and Allied Disciplines*, *49*(7), 743–753. doi:10.1111/j.1469-7610.2008.01920.x PMID:18503531

Behrmann, M., Thomas, C., & Humphreys, K. (2006). Seeing it differently: Visual processing in autism. *Trends in Cognitive Sciences*, *10*(6), 258–264. doi:10.1016/j.tics.2006.05.001 PMID:16713326

Bekele, E., Crittendon, J. A., Swanson, A., Sarkar, N., & Warren, Z. E. (2013). Pilot clinical application of an adaptive robotic system for young children with autism. *Autism*, *18*(5), 598–608. doi:10.1177/1362361313479454 PMID:24104517

Benford, P. (2008). *The use of Internet-based communication by people with autism*. Doctoral dissertation, University of Nottingham.

Bogdashina, O. (2003). *Sensory perceptual issues in autism and Asperger Syndrome: Different sensory experiences, different perceptual worlds*. London, UK: Jessica Kingsley Publishers.

Branch, M. (2014). Malignant side effects of nullhypothesis significance testing. *Theory & Psychology*, *24*(2), 256–277. doi:10.1177/0959354314525282

Burke, M., Kraut, R., & Williams, D. (2010). *Social use of computer-mediated communication by adults on the autism spectrum*. Paper presented at the 2010 ACM Conference on Computer Supported Cooperative Work, New York, NY.

Cardon, T. A. (2012). Teaching caregivers to implement video modeling imitation training via iPad for their children with autism. *Research in Autism Spectrum Disorders*, *6*(4), 1389–1400. doi:10.1016/j.rasd.2012.06.002

Chamak, B., Bonniau, B., Jaunay, E., & Cohen, D. (2008). What can we learn about autism from autistic persons? *Psychotherapy and Psychosomatics*, *77*(5), 271–279. doi:10.1159/000140086 PMID:18560252

Charlop-Christy, M. H., Le, L., & Freeman, K. A. (2000). A comparison of video modeling with in vivo modeling for teaching children with autism. *Journal of Autism and Developmental Disorders*, *30*(6), 537–552. doi:10.1023/A:1005635326276 PMID:11261466

Cheng, Y., Chiang, H., Ye, J., & Cheng, L. (2010). Enhancing instruction using a collaborative virtual learning environment for children with autistic spectrum conditions. *Computers & Education*, *55*(4), 1449–1458. doi:10.1016/j.compedu.2010.06.008

Diehl, J. J., Schmitt, L. M., Villano, M., & Crowell, C. R. (2012). The clinical use of robots for individuals with autism spectrum disorders: A critical review. *Research in Autism Spectrum Disorders*, *6*(1), 249–262. doi:10.1016/j.rasd.2011.05.006 PMID:22125579

Duquette, A., Michaud, F., & Mercier, H. (2008). Exploring the use of a mobile robot as an imitation agent with children with low-functioning autism. *Autonomous Robots*, *24*(2), 147–157. doi:10.1007/s10514-007-9056-5

Fernandes, T., Alves, S., Miranda, J., Queirós, C., & Orvalho, V. (2011). LIFEisGAME: A Facial Character Animation System to Help Recognize Facial Expressions. In *ENTERprise Information Systems* (pp. 423–432). Berlin, Germany: Springer. doi:10.1007/978-3-642-24352-3_44

Fletcher-Watson, S. (2014). A targeted review of computer-assisted learning for people with autism spectrum disorder: Towards a consistent methodology. *Review Journal of Autism and Developmental Disorders*, *1*(2), 87–100. doi:10.1007/s40489-013-0003-4

Gillespie-Lynch, K., Kapp, S. K., Shane-Simpson, C., Smith, D. S., & Hutman, T. (2014). Intersections Between the Autism Spectrum and the Internet: Perceived Benefits and Preferred Functions of Computer-Mediated Communication. *Intellectual and Developmental Disabilities*, *52*(6), 456–469. doi:10.1352/1934-9556-52.6.456 PMID:25409132

Golan, O., Ashwin, E., Granader, Y., McClintock, S., Day, K., Leggett, V., & Baron-Cohen, S. (2009). Enhancing emotion recognition in children with autism spectrum conditions: An intervention using animated vehicles with real emotional faces. *Journal of Autism and Developmental Disorders*, *40*(3), 269–279. doi:10.1007/s10803-009-0862-9 PMID:19763807

Golan, O., & Baron-Cohen, S. (2006). Systemizing empathy: Teaching adults with Asperger syndrome or high-functioning autism to recognize complex emotions using interactive multimedia. *Development and Psychopathology*, *18*(2), 591–617. doi:10.1017/S0954579406060305 PMID:16600069

Grandin, T. (2009). How does visual thinking work in the mind of a person with autism? A personal account. *Philosophical Transactions of the Royal Society of London. Series B, Biological Sciences*, *364*(1522), 1437–1442. doi:10.1098/rstb.2008.0297 PMID:19528028

Harms, M. B., Martin, A., & Wallace, G. L. (2010). Facial emotion recognition in autism spectrum disorders: A review of behavioral and neuroimaging studies. *Neuropsychology Review*, *20*(3), 290–322. doi:10.1007/s11065-010-9138-6 PMID:20809200

Holt, S., & Yuill, N. (2014). Facilitating other-awareness in low-functioning children with autism and typically-developing preschoolers using dual-control technology. *Journal of Autism and Developmental Disorders*, *44*(1), 236–248. doi:10.1007/s10803-013-1868-x PMID:23756935

Hopkins, I. M., Gower, M. W., Perez, T. A., Smith, D. S., Amthor, F. R., Wimsatt, C. F., & Biasini, F. J. (2011). Avatar assistant: Improving social skills in students with an ASD through a computer-based intervention. *Journal of Autism and Developmental Disorders*, *41*(11), 1543–1555. doi:10.1007/s10803-011-1179-z PMID:21287255

Jain, S., Tamersoy, B., Zhang, Y., Aggarwal, J. K., & Orvalho, V. (2012, May). An interactive game for teaching facial expressions to children with autism spectrum disorders. In *Communications Control and Signal Processing (ISCCSP), 2012 5th International Symposium* (pp. 1-4). IEEE. doi:10.1109/ISCCSP.2012.6217849

Jones, R., Quigney, C., & Huws, J. (2003). First-hand accounts of sensory perceptual experiences in autism: A qualitative analysis. *Journal of Intellectual & Developmental Disability*, *28*(2), 112–121. doi:10.1080/1366825031000147058

Jordan, C. J., & Caldwell-Harris, C. L. (2012). Understanding differences in neurotypical and autism spectrum special interests through internet forums. *Intellectual and Developmental Disabilities*, *50*(5), 391–402. doi:10.1352/1934-9556-50.5.391 PMID:23025641

Joshi, P. (2011, November 29). Finding good apps for children with autism. *Gadgetwise: The New York Times Blog*. Available at http://gadgetwise.blogs.nytimes.com/2011/11/29/finding-good-apps-for-children-with-autism

Kandalaft, M. R., Didehbani, N., Krawczyk, D. C., Allen, T. T., & Chapman, S. B. (2013). Virtual reality social cognition training for young adults with high-functioning autism. *Journal of Autism and Developmental Disorders*, *43*(1), 34–44. doi:10.1007/s10803-012-1544-6 PMID:22570145

Kim, E. S., Berkovits, L. D., Bernier, E. P., Leyzberg, D., Shic, F., Paul, R., & Scassellati, B. (2013). Social robots as embedded reinforcers of social behavior in children with autism. *Journal of Autism and Developmental Disorders*, *43*(5), 1038–1049. doi:10.1007/s10803-012-1645-2 PMID:23111617

Mazurek, M. O., & Wenstrup, C. (2013). Television, video game and social media use among children with ASD and typically developing siblings. *Journal of Autism and Developmental Disorders*, *43*(6), 1258–1271. doi:10.1007/s10803-012-1659-9 PMID:23001767

Moore, M., & Calvert, S. (2000). Brief report: Vocabulary acquisition for children with autism: Teacher or computer instruction. *Journal of Autism and Developmental Disorders*, *30*(4), 359–362. doi:10.1023/A:1005535602064 PMID:11039862

Mower, E., Black, M. P., Flores, E., Williams, M., & Narayanan, S. (2011). RACHEL: Design of an emotionally targeted interactive agent for children with autism. In *Multimedia and Expo (ICME), 2011 IEEE International Conference on* (pp. 1-6). IEEE.

Müller, E., Schuler, A., & Yates, G. B. (2008). Social challenges and supports from the perspective of individuals with Asperger syndrome and other autism spectrum disabilities. *Autism*, *12*(2), 173–190. doi:10.1177/1362361307086664 PMID:18308766

Murdock, L. C., Ganz, J., & Crittendon, J. (2013). Use of an iPad Play Story to Increase Play Dialogue of Preschoolers with Autism Spectrum Disorders. *Journal of Autism and Developmental Disorders*, *43*(9), 2174–2189. doi:10.1007/s10803-013-1770-6 PMID:23371509

Murray, D. K. C. (1997). Autism and information technology: therapy with computers. In S. Powell & R. Jordan (Eds.), *Autism and learning: a guide to good practice* (pp. 100–117). London, UK: David Fulton Publishers.

Ploog, B. O. (2010). Stimulus overselectivity four decades later: A review of the literature and its implications for current research in autism spectrum disorder. *Journal of Autism and Developmental Disorders*, *40*(11), 1332–1349. doi:10.1007/s10803-010-0990-2 PMID:20238154

Ploog, B. O., Scharf, A., Nelson, D., & Brooks, P. J. (2013). Use of computer-assisted technologies (CAT) to enhance social, communicative, and language development in children with autism spectrum disorders. *Journal of Autism and Developmental Disorders, 43*(2), 301–322. doi:10.1007/s10803-012-1571-3 PMID:22706582

Premack, D. (1962). Reversibility of the reinforcement relation. *Science, 136*(3512), 255–257. doi:10.1126/science.136.3512.255 PMID:14488597

Provost, B., Lopez, B. R., & Heimerl, S. (2007). A comparison of motor delays in young children: Autism spectrum disorder, developmental delay, and developmental concerns. *Journal of Autism and Developmental Disorders, 37*(2), 321–328. doi:10.1007/s10803-006-0170-6 PMID:16868847

Shadish, W. R. (2014). Statistical analyses of single-case designs: The shape of things to come. *Current Directions in Psychological Science, 23*(2), 139–146. doi:10.1177/0963721414524773

Smith, M. J., Ginger, E. J., Wright, K., Wright, M. A., Taylor, J. L., Humm, L. B., & Fleming, M. F. et al. (2014). Virtual reality job interview training in adults with autism spectrum disorder. *Journal of Autism and Developmental Disorders, 44*(10), 2450–2463. doi:10.1007/s10803-014-2113-y PMID:24803366

Speer, L. L., Cook, A. E., McMahon, W. M., & Clark, E. (2007). Face processing in children with autism effects of stimulus contents and type. *Autism, 11*(3), 265–277. doi:10.1177/1362361307076925 PMID:17478579

Standen, P. J., & Brown, D. J. (2005). Virtual reality in the rehabilitation of people with intellectual disabilities [review]. *Cyberpsychology & Behavior, 8*(3), 272–282. doi:10.1089/cpb.2005.8.272 PMID:15971976

Stephenson, J., & Limbrick, L. (2013). A review of the use of touch-screen mobile devices by people with developmental disabilities. *Journal of Autism and Developmental Disorders.* doi:10.1007/s10803-013-1878-8 PMID:23888356

Stichter, J. P., Laffey, J., Galyen, K., & Herzog, M. (2014). iSocial: Delivering the social competence intervention for adolescents (SCI-A) in a 3D virtual learning environment for youth with high functioning autism. *Journal of Autism and Developmental Disorders, 44*(2), 417–430. doi:10.1007/s10803-013-1881-0 PMID:23812663

Swettenham, J. (1996). Can children with autism be taught to understand false belief using computers? *Journal of Child Psychology and Psychiatry, and Allied Disciplines, 37*(2), 157–165. doi:10.1111/j.1469-7610.1996.tb01387.x PMID:8682895

Tanaka, J. W., Wolf, J. M., Klaiman, C., Koenig, K., Cockburn, J., Herlihy, L., & Schultz, R. T. et al. (2010). Using computerized games to teach face recognition skills to children with autism spectrum disorder: The Let's Face It! program. *Journal of Child Psychology and Psychiatry, and Allied Disciplines, 51*(8), 944–952. doi:10.1111/j.1469-7610.2010.02258.x PMID:20646129

Wainer, J., Dautenhahn, K., Robins, B., & Amirabdollahian, F. (2014). A pilot study with a novel setup for collaborative play of the humanoid robot KASPAR with children with autism. *International Journal of Social Robotics, 6*(1), 45–65. doi:10.1007/s12369-013-0195-x

KEY TERMS AND DEFINITIONS

Autism Spectrum Disorder (ASD): is a neurodevelopmental condition defined by social difficulties and restricted, repetitive behaviors and/or interests.

Computer-Mediated Interventions: are software-controlled forms of instruction such as iPad-type apps, virtual environments, and robots.

Evidence-Based Interventions: are instructional strategies that have been systematically evaluated and are believed to be effective according to current scientific knowledge.

Randomized Controlled Trial (RCT) Studies: assess interventions by assigning individuals to a group that receives an intervention or to a control group that does not receive the intervention.

Small-N Designs: are studies with one or a few participants where an individual's behavior is measured repeatedly while the environment in which the individual is tested is changed in a predictable way.

Social-Emotional Skills: allow one to form and maintain reciprocal relationships by recognizing and expressing one's own emotions and responding to others' perspectives.

Statistical Significance: indicates whether the obtained data are probably a chance outcome or, whether there is a reasonable hope (usually a 5% chance or p value of less than .05) that promising results are due to an intervention.

Chapter 8

Avatars, Humanoids, and the Changing Landscape of Assessment and Intervention for Individuals with Disabilities across the Lifespan

Emily Hotez
City University of New York – Hunter College, USA

ABSTRACT

In recent years, there has been a burgeoning field of research on the applications of virtual reality and robots for children, adolescents, and adults with a wide range of developmental disabilities. The influx of multidisciplinary collaborations among developmental psychologists and computer scientists, as well as the increasing accessibility of interactive technologies, has created a need to equip potential users with the information they need to make informed decisions about using virtual reality and robots. This chapter aims to 1) provide parents, professionals, and individuals with developmental disabilities with an overview of the literature on virtual reality and robot interventions in childhood, adolescence, and adulthood; and to 2) address overarching questions pertaining to utilizing virtual reality and robots. This chapter will shed light on the far-reaching potential for interactive technologies to transform therapeutic, educational, and assessment contexts, while also highlighting limitations and suggesting directions for future research.

BACKGROUND

In recent years, there has been an increasing body of research on the application of virtual reality and robots to children, adolescents, and adults with a wide range of developmental disabilities, including Attention Deficit Hyperactivity Disorder (ADHD); Autism Spectrum Disorders (ASD); Cerebral Palsy (CP) with and without Hemiplegia; Learning Disabilities (LD); Intellectual Disabilities (ID); and Down

DOI: 10.4018/978-1-4666-8395-2.ch008

Syndrome (DS). Moreover, a wide range of applications extends to individuals with deafness, visual impairments, diverse physical and motor disabilities, and multiple disabilities. These innovative technologies demonstrate the potential to transform the therapeutic, educational, and assessment contexts for individuals with disabilities and are of increasing interest to parents, professionals, and individuals with disabilities.

This chapter will address two particular innovative technologies that are representative of the changing landscape of assessment and intervention for individuals with disabilities across the lifespan: virtual reality and robots. *Virtual reality,* or a *virtual environment,* is a three-dimensional computer-based world, in which users can interact with objects or "avatars" (i.e., figures that resemble humans). These environments can be modified to resemble a wide range of settings, including classrooms, offices, and cafes. Virtual reality affords users the opportunity to repeatedly practice relevant skills in a safe environment. The extent to which the user is embedded in the scene is also highly variable, since some users may be able to watch themselves interacting in the scene, whereas other users may be represented by an avatar within a scene. Moreover, depending on the particular configuration within a virtual environment, users may also be able to receive direct feedback on their performance or interact with real people also using the program. Virtual reality can be accessed through a wide range of mediums, including videogames, head-mounted displays, or desktop computers (Parsons & Mitchell, 2002). Entirely distinct from virtual reality technology are *Robots,* technologies that "can interact with humans and show aspects of human-style social intelligence". Robots can also assume a wide range of forms, from "humanoids" (i.e., robots that resemble humans), to animal-resembling figures (Dautenhahn & Werry, 2004, p. 2). *Robotic systems* are robots that do not resemble an interactive agent like a human or animal; rather they are interactive configurations that may consist of gripper systems, switches, and buttons with which a user can engage (Prazak, Kronreif, Hochgatterer, & Furst, 2004).

RATIONALE

The driving force behind coordinating the goals of individuals with disabilities with interactive technology is the unique capability of technology to attract and maintain the interests of the users. Researchers have demonstrated the potential for virtual reality to promote children's participation in education, communication, and play settings (Chantry & Dunford, 2010). For example, Reid (2002) employed a virtual reality, play-based intervention (Mandala® GestureXtreme™) in which three school children with CP engaged in applications such as virtual drums, paint, and volleyball. Following the intervention, children showed greater self-efficacy, motivation, and engagement in play. In another study, Kim et al. (2013) investigated the potential for Pleo™, a social dinosaur robot to improve social interaction among children with ASD. The authors ascribed the robot's greater efficacy in eliciting children's social behaviors from the excitement and interest children spontaneously expressed towards it. The enjoyment that children experience from engaging with interactive technologies has also been demonstrated in older individuals, even if the intended outcome of the interactive technology was not achieved (e.g., ASD symptoms; Austin, Abbott, & Cabris, 2008). These findings underscore the potential for virtual reality and robots to serve as a highly motivating context for assessment, education, and therapy for individuals with disabilities across the lifespan.

The merging of virtual reality and robots with the fields of intervention and assessment affords developmental psychology researchers and clinicians unique advantages that are not always present in traditional intervention or assessment contexts. For example, while working with any population, researchers and clinicians often aim to enhance ecological validity (i.e., the extent to which the intervention or assessment context applies to the real world). Increasing the ecological validity of a particular intervention or assessment context is often accompanied by several limitations that impinge on the ability for professionals to draw firm conclusions about the success of a particular treatment (e.g., lack of control over surroundings). Virtual reality affords researchers the capacity to maximize ecological validity (i.e., simulating the real world), and control and manipulate the environment to meet individualized needs (Parsons, Rizzo, Rogers, & York, 2007). Alternatively, robots offer the unique advantage of engaging all of the users' physical senses (as opposed to virtual reality environments on computer screens). Robots have unique tactile properties that can engage users, without being as prohibitively expensive as animal therapeutic aids (Kim, Shic, & Scassellati, 2012). Psychologists often understand the efficacy of using robots as an intervention approach in the context of the developmental principle of "embodied interaction," which argues that human development occurs in the interaction between our bodies and the environment (Dautenhehn & Werry, 2004, p. 23).

VIRTUAL REALITY AND ROBOTS TODAY

In the past, several distinct barriers hindered the application of virtual reality and robots technology to the needs of individuals with disabilities. First, advanced technology was generally not designed to meet the needs of individuals with disabilities (Braddock, Rizzolo, Thompson, & Bell, 2004). Interactive technology researchers worked in isolation from psychological researchers, thus creating technology that did not necessarily stem from, or adapt to, the actual needs of the population (Kim, Paul, Shic, & Scassellati, 2012). Second, virtual reality and robots research had largely been published in and discussed in computer science journals, thus limiting dissemination of this emerging research to clinicians and researchers. Finally, the financial cost and highly technical expertise necessary for this technology had inhibited researchers, clinicians, and other stakeholders from demonstrating the success of such technologies empirically (Goldsmith & LeBlanc, 2004).

While these barriers have not yet been completely overcome, current and emerging collaborations between developmental psychologists, neuroscience researchers, computer science researchers, and engineers have created an influx of research on the potential for virtual reality and robots research to enhance the therapeutic, educational, and assessment contexts of individuals with disabilities. For example, the University of Southern California Institute for Creative Technologies is a collaborative research center comprised of a wide range of computer science researchers and social scientists who work towards utilizing immersive technologies such as virtual reality to solve problems and answer questions to improve the lives of individuals with disabilities. Another promising example of collaboration is Interactive Robotic Social Mediators as Companions (IROMEC), an interdisciplinary initiative that combines the field of robots with other disciplines such as cognitive science and developmental psychology.

In addition to the contribution of multidisciplinary collaborations, there is burgeoning research on making virtual reality and robots more accessible to individuals with disabilities. Accessibility can be readily observed in the availability of low-cost virtual reality interventions administered through at-home systems like Nintendo® Wii™ as well as through desktop virtual environments (i.e., virtual environments available through a desktop computer or laptop). Accessibility can also be observed in the extent to which researchers are tailoring technologies to better meet the needs of individuals with disabilities. This "evolution," is continuous, as researchers continuously refine and modify virtual environments to more effectively reflect the needs of the population and maximize the efficacy of the interventions (Strickland, McAllister, Coles, & Osborne, 2007). For example, researchers working with individuals with disabilities have surpassed many previous limitations of virtual reality technology (including the restrictions on mobility that arise from head-mounted displays) to create virtual environments in which the individual can move about freely and experience a greater level of immersion and engagement. In addition, researchers are investigating the potential to maximize the efficacy of robotic interventions with individuals with disabilities by using their input in designing robots. For example, researchers have asked for children's input about how particular robots should look (Robins, Dautenhehn, & Dubowski, 2006).

As multidisciplinary collaborations continue to create innovative technologies and interactive technologies begin to become more accessible to individuals with disabilities, there is a rising need to equip parents and individuals with disabilities with the information they need to make informed decisions regarding interactive technologies that can facilitate achievement of their specific goals. Virtual reality and robots have demonstrated a wide range of uses for individuals with disabilities across childhood, adolescence, and adulthood. While important developments are currently underway, there is presently a lack of research synthesis on the changing use of technology across the lifespan and how technology can meet the continuously changing goals for individuals with disabilities. More importantly, there is a dearth of information specifically directed towards helping parents and individuals with disabilities navigate decisions and considerations related to using innovative technologies.

CHAPTER OVERVIEW

This chapter aims to provide parents, professionals, and individuals with developmental disabilities with an overview of the state of the literature on virtual reality and robot interventions for children, adolescents, and adults that reflects the research that has emerged since the turn of the century. Specifically, this chapter will address common goals for virtual reality and robots among children, adolescents, and adults, that have been tailored to meet the evolving needs of individuals with disabilities (e.g., assessment, improving social skills, and enhancing physical and motor activity), as well as applications of virtual reality and robots specific to particular age groups (e.g., promoting play skills in children and independent living skills in adulthood). The current chapter is not meant to be an exhaustive review; rather, this chapter highlights important studies to show the progress and limitations of the field of virtual reality and robots for individuals with disabilities. To that end, each section will address relevant research findings the limitations of these findings, and proposed next steps. Finally, in addition to reviewing the existing research, this chapter also seeks to address select concerns and questions that many parents and individuals with disabilities may have in regard to utilizing virtual reality and robots. To accomplish this goal, this chapter will conclude by addressing four key questions: 1) if improved performance with virtual reality and robots generalizes to other contexts 2) if virtual reality and robots technologies are more effective than existing traditional therapeutic procedures 3) if virtual reality and robots are strong intervention approaches and 4) how individuals with disabilities can access virtual reality and robot technologies.

VIRTUAL REALITY AND ROBOTS IN CHILDREN

The scope of the use of virtual reality and robots in children has been far-reaching and continues to expand in addressing the needs of individuals with disabilities and their families with the consistent advent of innovations in technology. This section will focus on the use of virtual reality and robots in children in the following five domains: 1) assessment 2) social skills interventions 3) efforts to improve children's physical and motor abilities 4) enhancing play and 5) strengthening cognitive processes.

Assessment

Researchers have found virtual reality to effectively differentiate children with disabilities from typically developing children in several domains, rendering virtual reality a feasible assessment tool. This is particularly true for the Virtual Classroom which, as research demonstrates, has the potential to serve as an assessment tool for children with ADHD (Rizzo et al., 2000), and the Meal Maker, which has proven effective in differentiating children's functional abilities among children with Cerebral Palsy (CP) (Kirshner, Weiss, & Tirosh, 2011).

The Virtual Classroom

The virtual classroom simulates a classroom environment as well as auditory and visual distracters frequently experienced in a classroom environment, through sounds and images on a head-mounted display (Rizzo et al., 2006). For example, while the child sits in the classroom, there are typical classroom distracters present such as ambient classroom noise and activity occurring outside of the window. The child sits at a virtual desk within the classroom and is assessed in terms of his/her reaction time on a variety of attention tasks delivered visually, using the virtual blackboard, or auditorily, using the teacher's voice. Researchers and clinicians can change the settings of the virtual classroom context to investigate children with varying degrees of distractive stimuli (e.g., an auditory task with non-distractive stimuli or a visual task with distractive stimuli) (Gutiérrez-Maldonado, Letosa-Porta, Rus-Calafell, & Peñaloza-Salazar, 2009).

The Meal Maker

The Meal Maker is a game-like virtual kitchen environment that has served as a platform for the evaluation and treatment of specific aspects of functional performance for children with CP (Kirshner, Weiss, & Tirosh, 2011). In the Meal Maker, the user sits or stands in front of a green screen that permits the actual background to be subtracted and replaced by a virtual one. Participants see themselves in a mirror image on an LCD screen and are asked to wear a special glove that allows them to interact with objects in the virtual kitchen. The Meal-Maker includes two interactive options: the meal selection menu and the meal preparation menu. The meal selection menu option presents six recipes that differ in the number of ingredients, increasing from three to seven ingredients per meal. Selection of a specific recipe is made after the child's gloved hand hovers over one of the recipe icons on the meal selection menu. Once the child selects a recipe, he/she is transferred to the meal preparation menu, where he/she selects all ingredients associated with that recipe until the meal is completed.

Findings

There are two main conclusions that can be derived from this research. First, children find assessment more enjoyable in the context of virtual reality paradigms (Kirshner, Weiss, & Tirosh, 2011; Pollak, Shomaly, Weiss, Rizzo, & Gross-Tsur, 2010). This finding may be particularly useful in that children may engage more with the assessment if they are more highly motivated to do so. Second, virtual reality serves as a viable assessment context, given that both the Virtual Classroom and the Meal Maker were able to distinguish children with disabilities versus children without disabilities based on their performance. For example, just as in a standard classroom, children with ADHD are more affected by distractions and show a greater amount of difficulty performing tasks than those without ADHD in the virtual classroom (Adams, Finn, Moes, Flannery, & Rizzo, 2009; Parsons, Bowerly, Buckwalter, & Rizzo, 2007). Children with CP perform the Meal Maker tasks significantly more slowly, make significantly more errors, and select significantly more distracters than typically developing children when preparing a meal (Kirshner, Weiss, & Tirosh, 2011). Moreover, the ability to embed specific settings within each virtual environment affords researchers and clinicians the ability to distinguish particular impairments at a greater level of detail. While virtual reality clearly offers enormous potential in assessing children, findings must be interpreted with caution, given the sample restrictions in the aforementioned studies. For example, while ADHD indeed has a higher prevalence rate in males, research is needed to ascertain as to whether the Virtual Classroom can identify girls with ADHD, whose symptoms may present differently. Future research steps may include investigating the potential to utilize these particular virtual environments in an intervention context.

Social Skills

Virtual reality and robot researchers have extensively focused on utilizing interactive technology to improve children's social skills. Due to the nature of social interaction impairments in children with ASD, virtual reality and robot interventions for children's social skills have largely targeted children with ASD. Virtual reality interventions that improve social skills among children with ASD have used the Second Life® virtual programs (Ke & Im, 2013), as well as other collaborative virtual environment systems (Moore, Cheng, McGrath, & Powell, 2005). Similarly, since children with ASD appear to respond positively to robots like Pleo™, robots for children with ASD have been utilized as an intervention tool to address a wide range of social outcomes, like imitation (Boccanfuso & O'Kane, 2011).

Second Life®

Second Life® is a three-dimensional virtual world software available to the public (Second Life, 2015). One virtual reality-based social interaction program involves three social interaction tasks: (a) recognizing body gestures and facial expressions of a virtual communication partner (b) responding and maintaining interactions at a school cafeteria and (c) initiating and maintaining interactions at a birthday party (Ke & Im, 2013). An example of a school scenario is as follows: A target child, when spending his/her first day at the virtual school, meets with a peer in the school lobby. In order to befriend this peer, the child requests to identify what this peer likes or dislikes (e.g., animals, hobbies, academic subjects) based on the peer's facial expressions and body gestures.

Collaborative Virtual Environments

Two forms of virtual environments can be distinguished: a single user virtual environment (SVE) and a multiuser, collaborative virtual environment (CVE). In the SVE, the user is restricted to interacting with pre-programmed responses from the virtual environment. In a CVE, there can be more than one user and users can communicate with each other via personalized avatars. Researchers have tested the feasibility of utilizing a CVE among children with ASD (Moore, Cheng, McGrath, & Powell, 2005). The authors identified emotion recognition to be a key prerequisite for the success of a CVE. In effect, the authors tested an SVE system that incorporated avatar representations of four emotions (happy, sad, angry, and frightened) to see if children with ASD can meet the prerequisites required for participation in a CVE. In this study, the CVE had three stages through which the user had to progress. In stage 1, users were asked to match labels of emotions with avatars' depictions of those emotions. Stage 2 required users to predict the likely emotions caused by certain events. In Stage 3 of the system, the user is given an avatar representation of one of the emotions and is asked to select which of a number of given events he/she thinks may have caused this emotion. In a later study, the actual CVE was implemented with three children with ASD to test the feasibility of using a CVE to improve children's empathy (Cheng, Chiang, Ye, & Cheng, 2010).

Mobile Robots

Several robots have been developed to increase social skills among children with ASD. Tito the mobile robot is used to facilitate reciprocal interaction among children with low-functioning ASD (Duquette, Michaud, & Mercer, 2008). Children can interact with Tito, although Tito cannot imitate or interact with children in response. In contrast, the robot CHARLIE (Child-centered Adaptive Robot for Learning in an Interactive Environment) is a low-cost and highly interactive robot, which measures and adapts to a child's actions during interactive games (Boccanfuso & O'Kane, 2011). CHARLIE is equipped with a head and two arms, each with two degrees of freedom, and a camera and plays interactive imitation games using hand and face tracking. CHARLIE comes equipped with two autonomous interactive games: single- player ("Imitate Me, Imitate You") and two-player ("Pass the Pose"). In "Imitate Me, Imitate You", the robot has both passive and active game modes. In the passive mode, the robot waits for the child to initiate an interaction by raising one or both hands. In the second game mode, the robot initiates interactions. The "Pass the Pose" game engages two children in cooperative play by enlisting the robot as a mediator between two children, alternately initiating and imitating poses. These games are designed to increase attention, promote turn-taking skills and encourage child-led verbal and non-verbal communication through simple imitative play. It is also possible for CHARLIE to be operated by remote control (Boccanfuso & O'Kane, 2011, p. 342-343).

Findings

Results demonstrate the feasibility and efficacy for virtual reality to serve as a social skills intervention for children with ASD. In the Second Life® virtual world, children demonstrated increased performance in responding, initiating, greeting, and ending conversations in a positive manner during the intervention and showed improved social competence following the intervention (Ke & Im, 2013). Children with ASD were able to meet the prerequisites of using CVEs by recognizing emotions displayed by avatar representations in the SVE, thus demonstrating the feasibility of the CVE context for developing social skills (Moore, Cheng, McGrath, & Powell, 2005). The success of the CVE itself in improving empathy among children with ASD has also been demonstrated (Cheng, Chiang, Ye, & Cheng (2010). Research with Tito, the robot, identified two crucial results that will be integral to shaping robotic social skills interventions. First, robots are more effective for some children than others. Although children exposed to Tito showed reduced repetitive play with their favorite toy and no repetitive or stereotyped behavior toward the robot, non-verbal children demonstrated less interest and participation than the pre-verbal children. This finding is particularly salient for research with individuals with disabilities whose needs are vastly heterogeneous. Second, although interactive technologies may be particularly motivating tools for individuals with disabilities, increased motivation is likely not the sole contributor accounting for the change in children's behaviors and/or abilities. Rather, there may need to be bi-directional interactions that are attuned to individualized needs. CHARLIE, the Robot, represents a step in this direction, since researchers studying CHARLIE have demonstrated the proof-of-concept of a robot capable of bi-directional interactions that may be coordinated with the child's actions. Future trends will involve understanding characteristics of avatars and robots that maximize their efficacy, and continue to make virtual environments and robotic interactions as natural as possible.

Physical and Motor Abilities

Based on the physical and motor impairments consistent with many types of developmental disabilities, there have been several attempts to utilize virtual reality to improve motion among children with CP (Rostami et al., 2012; Sandlund, Lindh Waterworth, & Hager (2011) and developmental delay (Salem, Gropack, Jaffee, Coffin, & Godwin, 2012).

Videogame Interventions

Researchers have explored the feasibility of using a low-cost interactive virtual game as a four-week home-based intervention for children (ages 6-16) with CP (Sandlund, Lindh Waterworth, & Hager, 2011). This study was designed to test participants' motivation for practice and compliance of training, the impact on physical activity and the feasibility of using activity monitors to assess energy expenditure in children with CP. The virtual system used a video-capture technique that allowed children to watch themselves on the screen and interact with the games without having to wear any technical equipment. The games typically involved whole body movements with elements of hitting or avoiding virtual objects displayed on the screen, as well as requiring the user to jump, balance, or run on the spot. Researchers have also tested the potential for preschool children with developmental disabilities to improve their physical abilities by using Wii™ videogames (i.e., Wii Sports™ and Wii Fit™) that include games focused on balance, strength training, and aerobics (Salem, Gropack, Jaffee, & Godwin, 2012). Forty children with developmental delay (age 39 to 58 months) were randomly assigned to an experimental (Wii Sports™ and Wii Fit™) group (n = 20) or to a control group (n = 20). In the experimental group, children participated in two weekly sessions for 10 weeks using Wii Sports™ and Wii Fit™.

Findings

There were three main findings from the aforementioned studies. First, some children may need more assistance engaging with the technology than others. For example, one child with CP experienced difficulty coping with the motion interactive game and needed help, particularly with the fast rhythmic movements and balance while playing in a standing position (Sandlund, Lindh Waterworth, & Hager, 2011). These results indicate that simply having such videogames in the home may not be sufficient to see improvements in children's physical or motor abilities, and a greater level of assistance or supervision may be necessary. Second, virtual reality in-home rehabilitation (i.e., video game intervention contexts, such as Wii™) is both feasible and safe (Salem, Gropack, Jaffee, & Godwin, 2012), although more research needs to be conducted on the efficacy of such interventions. In the Wii™ study, there were no adverse effects or injuries reported over 267 training sessions. Moreover, children who used Wii™ showed more improvements than the control group in the single leg stance test, right grip strength, and left grip strength. However, despite the positive effects, findings from this study did not reach statistical significance, indicating that improvements in children's physical abilities may not be due to a more than chance occurrence. Thus, these benefits should be interpreted with caution. Third, children report enjoying participating in such interactive technologies, indicating that motivation may be higher to engage in virtual reality or robots therapies than more traditional therapies. Researchers identified the need to conduct further studies to validate the potential benefits of low-cost commercially available gaming systems as treatment strategies.

Play

Virtual reality and robot researchers have investigated the potential for interactive technologies to improve children's play skills among children with ASD and ID, specifically focusing on observing children in both free and structured play (Herrera et al., 2008). Children with physical disabilities have also been able to utilize robotic systems to facilitate play (Cook, Howery, Gu & Meng, 2000; Prazak, Kronreif, Hochgatterer & Furst, 2004).

Virtual Supermarket

Herrera et al. (2008) investigated pretend play skills in two children with ASD (age 8 and 15) who engaged with a virtual reality environment that aimed to improve symbolic and imagination understanding. The study employed touch-screen technology that features a virtual supermarket, which includes "supermarket exploration" and "functional use" of objects within the virtual environment. Of primary interest in the study was an "imaginary play" stage that followed the initial exploration stage. This stage consisted of three aspects: 1) a set of videos where the play of the protagonist is no longer functional but symbolic, (e.g., acting as if a piece of clothing were a pair of trousers) 2) an imaginary transformation is shown explicitly (e.g., the pair of trousers is transformed into a road) and the transformation is framed in a think bubble and 3) the same set of transformations are shown, but this time without the think bubble, illustrating that this kind of situation can occur "magically" (Herrera et al., 2008, p. 146-147).

Robots Supporting Play

Researchers have studied the potential for three children (age 9-11) with physical disabilities, such as tetra paresis and transverse spinal cord syndrome, to use a toy robot system for autonomous playing (Prazak, Kronreif, Hochgatterer & Furst, 2004). In this study, a robot developed by the IROMEC group was embedded in traditional play therapy and this was compared with the effects of traditional play therapy without a robot. Other such studies have allowed children with physical disabilities to independently manipulate real objects in the context of a play activity through a robot (Cook, Howery, Gu & Meng, 2000). Such studies have evaluated the ways in which children play with adults when a robot is integrated into the play session.

Findings

First, findings from the aforementioned studies suggest the potential for virtual reality and robots interventions have far reaching effects on children's play skills, including fostering imagination and understanding, as well as allowing children to physically participate in play. For example, following the virtual supermarket intervention, children experienced significant advances in their play skills during both structured and free play (Herrera et al., 2008). Second, children both enjoy playing with robots (Prazak, Kronreif, Hochgatterer & Furst, 2004) and are able to more effectively play with adults through the use of robots (Cook, Howery, Gu & Meng, 2000). However, children with multiple impairments may have difficulty in understanding the robotic system (Prazak, Kronreif, Hochgatterer & Furst, 2004). Therefore, there is a clear need to both understand the effects these interventions have on children's play skills as they develop over time, and understand the circumstances (i.e., specific factors in children's disabilities) under which robots are effective in facilitating children's play.

Cognitive Processes

Researchers have demonstrated the immense potential of virtual reality to improve cognitive processes (e.g., spatiality, spatial rotation; mathematics abilities) for children who are blind, deaf or hard-of-hearing, or have ASD (Bouck, Satsangi, Doughty, & Courtney, 2012; Passig & Eden, 2000; Sanchez & Saenz, 2006). In these efforts, the researchers have explored the concepts of three-dimensional sound and physical objects.

Virtual Objects and Sounds

AudioChile is a virtual environment that can be navigated through three-dimensional sound to enhance spatiality and immersion throughout the environment (Sanchez & Saenz, 2006). The virtual environment in AudioChile represents three major Chilean cities. The user navigates through these cities searching for cues and information to solve a posed problem. Interaction occurs through actions (e.g., take, give, open, push, pull, look, speak, use, travel, check the backpack), movements, and turns (90 and 180 degrees). Both the joystick and keyboard are involved in navigating the virtual environment. An additional area of inquiry pertains to elementary mathematics education among students with ASD. Elementary school students often learn mathematical concepts by manipulating physical objects that can be used for counting and mathematical operations (i.e., manipulatives). One study investigated academically based mathematics instruction for three elementary school students with ASD (age 6-10-years-old) included in general education classes (Bouck, Satsangi, Doughty, & Courtney, 2012). The authors explored the effectiveness of using either concrete (physical objects that can be manipulated) or virtual (three-dimensional objects from the internet that can be manipulated) manipulatives to teach subtraction skills. Researchers have also investigated the potential for rotating virtual reality three-dimensional objects (e.g., in the context of a Tetris game) to assist deaf and hard-of hearing-children in using inductive reasoning (Passig & Eden, 2000).

Findings

Findings from these studies suggest that three-dimensional objects and sounds may be important tools in assisting learners who do not hear or see, as well as highly effective tools in teaching elementary school mathematics concepts. In AudioChile, blind learners are able to clearly identify and discriminate environmental sounds to solve everyday problems (Sanchez & Saenz, 2006). Findings have also revealed that virtual reality objects for teaching math contribute to children demonstrating greater accuracy and faster independence with the virtual manipulatives as compared to the concrete manipulatives. Moreover, students were able to generalize their learning of subtraction to more real-world applications (Bouck, Satsangi, Doughty, & Courtney, 2012). Additional virtual three-dimensional object paradigms have improved deaf and hard-of-hearing users' flexible thinking (Passig & Eden, 2000). Further research has found that three-dimensional virtual reality significantly improved the children's performance of spatial rotation, which enhanced their ability to better perform sign language (Passig & Eden, 2001). There is limited evidence that these effects generalize, but future research is needed.

VIRTUAL REALITY AND ROBOTS IN ADOLESCENCE

The applications of virtual reality and robots in adolescence have not been tested as extensively as in childhood. However, with the continued development of innovations, the scope of the use of virtual reality and robots in adolescence has been steadily expanding to address the needs of adolescents with disabilities and their families. This section will focus on the use of virtual reality and robots in adolescence in the following three domains: 1) assessment 2) social skills interventions and 3) efforts to improve adolescents' physical and motor abilities.

Assessment

Research on virtual reality as an assessment tool in adolescence has sought to investigate the extent to which adolescents with disabilities navigate the world in the domains of social behavior (Parsons, Mitchell, & Leonard, 2004), as well as driving behavior (Clancy, Rucklidge, & Owen, 2006; Cox et al., 2006).

Virtual Café

Researchers have explored the potential for a computer-based and joystick-controlled virtual café to serve as an assessment context for adolescents with ASD (Parsons, & Mitchell, & Leonard, 2004). In the virtual café, there are both textual and verbal prompts at different points within the users' experience.

For example, when the user moves close to a table, he/she hears a voice in the program say, "Would you like to sit here?" Following this prompt, two text boxes appear on the screen showing the words "yes" and "no". The user is required to respond to these prompts before being able to progress further. The user progresses through a number of tasks, including sitting at a table and ordering food and drink. Each task involves communication (i.e., the computer asks the user a question), interaction (i.e., the participant uses the mouse to interact with part of the screen), and navigation (i.e., the participant uses the joystick to move from one area to the next within the virtual environment).

Virtual Traffic and Driving Scenarios

Research on the application of virtual reality for adolescents with ADHD has focused on assessing participants in real-world traffic and driving simulations. One study compared the potential accident-proneness of 24 adolescents with and without ADHD (aged 13-17) in a hazardous road-crossing environment, using an immersive virtual reality task (Clancy, Rucklidge, & Owen, 2006). Participants wore a head-mounted display of a realistic traffic environment and were instructed to safely cross the virtual road when an approaching van was at varying distances away from the participant. Participants had to choose when and how fast to cross the lane to avoid being hit by the approaching vans. Previous research found inattention to be a major contributor to driving mishaps among adolescent drivers with ADHD. Studies have suggested that manual transmission is associated with driver arousal. Researchers tested the hypothesis that manual transmission, compared to automatic transmission, is associated with better attention and performance on a driving simulator among ten adolescent drivers with ADHD (Cox et al., 2006).

Findings

Findings show the validity of utilizing virtual reality as an assessment context for both social skills among adolescents with ASD as well as for traffic-and driving-based decision-making and attention among adolescents with ADHD. First, results from the Virtual Café underscored the already burgeoning potential to use virtual reality as a context for social skills training for adolescents with ASD. Adolescents with ASD were significantly more likely to bump into or walk between other people in the virtual cafe, compared to their paired matches. The authors could not explain this difference by executive dysfunction or general motor difficulty; rather, they attributed this difference to a sign that understanding personal space is impaired in individuals with ASD. Second, virtual reality traffic and driving scenarios serve as viable assessment contexts for adolescents with ADHD (Clancy, Rucklidge, & Owen, 2006). Participants with ADHD had a lower margin of safety, walked slower, underutilized the available gap in incoming traffic, showed greater variability in road-crossing behavior and evidenced twice as many collisions as compared to their typically-developing peers. Cox et al. (2006) found that participants reported being more attentive while driving manual transmission and drove more safely in the manual transmission mode. Taken together, findings from adolescents with ADHD suggest the potential for virtual reality to effectively identify adolescents who may be at risk for dangerous traffic situations, as well as to assist adolescents with ADHD in understanding car characteristics that may help them drive most effectively.

Social Skills

An important goal of virtual reality as an intervention tool for adolescents with disabilities has been in improving social skills of adolescents with ASD. Researchers have demonstrated the potential to use virtual reality as a means of improving social skills through simulations of real-world environments (e.g., virtual café and virtual bus). While exploration into the potential for robots to serve as an effective intervention context for children with ASD is increasing, there remains very limited research on the potential uses for robots with adolescents with ASD.

Virtual Café and Virtual Bus

As previously mentioned, a virtual café environment was able to discern impairments in adolescents with ASD (Parsons, Mitchell, & Leonard, 2004). A later study tested the feasibility of using a virtual reality café (as previously described) and bus environment as an intervention context to improve social judgments and explanations among six teenagers aged 14-16-years-old with ASD (Mitchell, Parsons & Leonard, 2007). In the virtual reality paradigm, built with Superscape Virtual Reality Toolkit® and accessed via a laptop computer, the user views video clips of a real café and the interior of a bus. Users maneuver around, activate objects, or initiate interactions within the environment (e.g., clicking on the person the participant wished to speak to) through both a joystick and mouse. A facilitator scaffolds sessions (i.e., provides necessary support to assist participants) by adapting to participants' individual needs through questions and discussions. Participants progress through a series of four levels, with the virtual environment and learning objectives becoming increasingly complex over the course of six weeks. The program provides corrective feedback on behaviors that were considered social errors, such as sitting at a full table when an empty table was available or sitting at a table without asking. In this study, participants' social understanding was inferred from their descriptions and explanations of how they would behave in a scene shown in the video.

Robotics Summer Camp

Kaboski et al. (2014) published a brief report on a pilot study that evaluates the efficacy of a weeklong robotics summer camp in reducing social anxiety and improving social and vocational skills among adolescents with ASD and typically developing adolescents. The researchers recruited eight adolescents with ASD and eight typically developing adolescents (ages 12-17). During the camp, individuals worked in pairs (1 ASD: 1 TD) on a programming project that culminated in a presentation in front of campmates and family.

Findings

Findings from utilizing virtual reality and robots as social skills intervention contexts for adolescents with ASD suggest that gains may generalize into varying virtual contexts, although the aforementioned studies do not guarantee that gains experienced during the intervention can be observed in the real world. In the virtual café and bus scenarios, there were several instances of significant improvements in judgments and explanations about where to sit, both in the videos of the café and bus. The most notable finding from this study was that participants' learning was not only confined to a particular context of application (café), but was generalized to another context (bus). After the robotics camp, the ASD group showed a significant decrease in social anxiety and both groups showed an increase in robotics knowledge, although neither group showed a significant increase in social skills. Therefore, although there is potential for inclusive settings with motivating tasks to serve as important intervention contexts, there is currently no evidence that it improves social skills. The authors note that there is a need to implement similar programs with a larger and more diverse sample and to use multiple levels of analysis of behavioral change (i.e., assess gains or improvements from the intervention in different ways).

Physical and Motor Abilities

As is the case for interventions for children with physical and motor disabilities, interventions for adolescents with physical and motor disabilities associated with Cerebral Palsy (CP) or Down syndrome (DS) have also focused on in-home rehabilitation programs (Golomb et al., 2010), some of which are embedded in videogames, such as Wii™ games (Berg, Becker, Martian, Danielle, & Wingen, 2012; Deutsch, Borbely, Filler, Huhn, & Guarrera-Bowlby, 2008).

Videogame Interventions

A three-month proof-of-concept pilot study with three adolescents (aged 13-15) with hemiplegic CP, investigated whether an in-home, remotely monitored, virtual reality videogame-based tele-rehabilitation can improve hand function and forearm bone health, as well as demonstrate alterations in motor circuitry activation (Golomb et al., 2010). In this study, videogame-based rehabilitation systems were installed in the homes of three participants and networked via secure Internet connections to a collaborating engineering school and children's hospital. Participants were asked to exercise the plegic hand 30 minutes a day, 5 days a week, using a sensor glove fitted to the plegic hand and attached to the game console installed in the home. Games were custom-developed, focused on finger movement, and included a screen avatar of the hand. Another study examined motor outcomes following an 8-week intervention period of family-supported Wii™ by a 12-year-old child with a diagnosis of Down syndrome (DS). Under the supervision of physical therapy students, the child played four different games, four times per week for 20 minutes each session for 8 weeks, with a particular emphasis on a snowboarding game (Berg et al., 2012). A third study described the feasibility and outcomes of using a low-cost, commercially available gaming system (Wii™) to augment the rehabilitation of an adolescent with CP (Deutsch et al., 2008). This particular study was school-based, and the adolescent was treated during a summer session. Wii™ games included boxing, tennis, bowling, and golf that were executed in both standing and sitting positions.

Findings

Research findings point to the potential for videogame interventions to have a beneficial impact on physical disabilities that accompany both CP and DS. Studies on adolescents with CP demonstrate that the use of remotely monitored virtual reality videogame tele-rehabilitation produces improved hand function and forearm bone health, in adolescents who practiced regularly (Golomb et al., 2010). Improved hand function also appeared to be associated with functional brain changes in motor circuitry activation. In the case study of the adolescent with CP who participated in a Wii™ intervention program, there were positive outcomes at the impairment and functional levels (Deutsch et al., 2008). Results were also positive for an adolescent with DS, as there were improvements in the child's postural stability, limits and stability, balance, upper-limb coordination, manual dexterity and postural control (Berg et al. 2012). Future research with larger samples is necessary to ascertain these findings.

VIRTUAL REALITY AND ROBOTS IN ADULTS

As was the case for adolescents with disabilities, the applications of virtual reality and robots in adulthood have not been tested as extensively as in childhood. However, with the continued advent of innovations in technology, the scope of the use of virtual reality and robots in adulthood has been steadily expanding to address the needs of adults with disabilities and their families. Specifically, research has shifted virtual reality and robotic interventions to promoting independent living and job interview skills among adults with disabilities. This section will focus on the use of virtual reality and robots in adulthood in the following four domains: 1) assessment, 2) social skills interventions, 3) efforts to improve physical and motor abilities, and 4) promoting independent living skills.

Assessment

As in adolescents, virtual reality assessment for adults with disabilities has shifted towards assessing practical abilities, including driving performance and perceived driving performance among adults with ADHD (Knouse, Bagwell, Barkley, & Murphy, 2005). Researchers have also assessed the effects of alcohol on driving performance among adults with ADHD (Barkley, Murphy, O'Connell, Anderson, & Connor, 2006).

Virtual Driving Scenarios

One study examined the accuracy of self-evaluation in clinic-referred adults diagnosed with ADHD as pertaining to driving in both naturalistic and virtual reality settings (Knouse, Bagwell, Barkley, & Murphy, 2005). In this study, adults with ADHD engaged in virtual simulations of driving, as well as evaluated their own driving in a self-assessment. Another study compared 50 adults with ADHD and 40 control adults on the effects of alcohol on driving performance (Barkley et al., 2006). This study used a virtual reality simulator to evaluate attention and inhibition and adults were randomized to either low or high dose alcohol treatment groups.

Findings

Two important findings emerge from research on assessing driving ability among adults diagnosed with ADHD. First, virtual reality simulations of driving serve as valid contexts for differentiating adults with ADHD from their typically developing counterparts. When compared with a community comparison group, the group diagnosed with ADHD had a higher rate of collisions, speeding tickets, and total driving citations in their driving history. They also reported less use of safe driving behaviors in naturalistic settings and used fewer safe-driving behaviors in the virtual reality simulator (Knouse, Bagwell, Barkley, & Murphy, 2005). Results from the other study demonstrate that alcohol may have a greater detrimental effect on some aspects of driving performance in ADHD than adult controls (Barkley et al., 2006). Second, findings highlight that self-awareness may be an important skill to foster in this age group in future intervention work, particularly pertaining to safety. While adults with ADHD exhibited poorer driving on these measures compared to the community sample, they provided similar driving self-assessments. Given that adults with ADHD present with poorer driving but similar self-assessments to their peers, adults with ADHD may not see a need to seek assistance with driving and may have difficulties anticipating consequences while driving. Virtual reality has the potential to serve as an effective conduit to bridge the gap between self-awareness and driving behaviors.

Social Skills

As in childhood and adolescence, virtual reality and robots research has focused on social skills training interventions within the ASD population (Kandalaft et al., 2013), with a particular focus on social skills necessary for successful job interviews (Smith et al., 2014; Strickland, Coles, & Southern, 2013).

Social Cognition Training

One study investigated the feasibility of engaging in a Virtual Reality Social Cognition Training intervention focused on enhancing social skills, social cognition, and social functioning (Kandalaft et al., 2013). The virtual reality technology was developed using Second Life® (as previously described) and included a wide range of virtual environments, including an office, a fast food restaurant and a school. Avatars representing the user in the virtual world were modeled to resemble each participant and the coach involved in the study. Eight young adults diagnosed with high-functioning ASD completed 10 sessions across 5 weeks. Social scenarios were aligned with individualized learning objectives, including meeting new people, dealing with a roommate or negotiating financial or social decisions.

Virtual Reality Job Interview Training

Smith et al. (2014) tested the feasibility and efficacy of virtual reality job interview training (VR-JIT) in a single-blinded randomized controlled trial. VR-JIT is a computerized virtual reality simulation that can be used as computer software or via the Internet. VR-JIT is unique in its "non-branching logic," which means it is equipped to accommodate variation in users' responses. Interviewers are able to display a wide range of emotions, personality, and memory. VR-JIT offers in-the-moment feedback and displays scores on key dimensions of interviewees' performance (Smith et al., 2014, p. 2452). JobTIPS, produced by Do2Learn™, is another job interview training delivered via virtual reality (Strickland, Coles, & Southern, 2013). JobTIPS provides practice sessions for teaching appropriate job interview skills to individuals with high functioning ASD or Asperger's Disorder. In a randomized study, 22 participants were asked to practice their job interview skills in the virtual world so as to prepare for a real-world, mock job interview. The virtual world practice session was conducted via a computer monitor in a basic office environment at Emory University. A clinician at a different physical location led 30-minute interview practice simulations remotely. The clinician assumed the role of interviewer, and the treatment group participant assumed the role of interviewee.

Findings

Virtual reality social skills training for adults with ASD have demonstrated potential. First, following social cognition training, adults experienced significant increases in social cognitive measures of theory of mind and emotion recognition, as well as in real life social and occupational functioning (Kandalaft et al, 2013). Second, participants not only reported that VR-JIT was enjoyable and easy to use, but was also more successful during live, standardized job interview role-play than for participants randomized to the comparison group. Participants in the experimental group also reported greater self-confidence (Smith et al., 2014). Youth who completed the JobTIPS employment program demonstrated significantly more effective verbal content skills than those who did not (Strickland, Coles, & Southern, 2013). The benefit of randomized controlled designs allows us to attribute a greater amount of confidence to these findings than would be possible if the technology had only been tested on a few individuals without a comparison group. The continued development of job interview training for individuals with disabilities is currently underway. For example, Vocational Interview Training Agents (VITA) is an interactive virtual reality job interview practice system that is currently undergoing testing (USC Institute for Creative Technologies, 2014). VITA aims to build competence and reduce anxiety in young adults with ASD. VITA affords the unique advantage of creating interviewers with different behavior disciplines (i.e., soft-touch, neutral, and hostile) so as to more effectively simulate real-life job interviews.

Physical and Motor Abilities

There is limited research on improving physical and motor abilities with interactive technologies among adults with disabilities. One study tested the effectiveness of an in-home virtual reality-based exercise program aimed at improving the physical fitness of adults with Intellectual Disability (ID) (Lotan, Yalon-Chamovitz, & Weiss, 2009). Forty-four men and women between the ages of 21 and 60 were recruited for participation in this study. The system employed was GestureTek™ single camera-based video capture virtual reality, which responds in real time to participants' movements. An advantage of GestureTek™ is that it allows for the grading of the level of difficulty (based on direction and speed of virtual objects that the participant needs to control).

Findings

Findings revealed significant improvements in physical fitness for the intervention program, suggesting virtual reality technology might be a feasible method for improving physical fitness levels among adults with disabilities. There is a clear need for further investigation into promoting physical fitness among adults with disabilities using interactive technology, particularly given the success of the limited available research. Results point to the need to choose virtual systems based on the particular needs of the population.

Independent Living Skills

Research on the potential for virtual reality to foster independent living skills among adults with Learning Disabilities (LD) and ID has been particularly far-reaching. A wide range of independent living skills among adults with LD has been fostered through virtual environments, including teaching horticulture-related employment, leisure, travel, public presentation skills (Brown, Standen, Proctor, & Sterland, 2001) and even assisting vulnerable witnesses to prepare for their attendance in court (Cooke, Laczny, Brown, & Francik, 2002). This research has also investigated the potential for a more diverse range of individuals with LD to benefit from learning through technology. It tested the feasibility of integrating tutors to assist adults with LD to utilize virtual environments as a means to acquire independent living skills (Standen, Brown, Horan, & Proctor, 2002).

As our nation's health care system continues to change, of particular importance is research that assesses the acceptability, usability, and potential utility of a virtual reality experience as a means of providing health care-related information to people with ID (Hall, Conboy-Hill, & Taylor, 2011). Using Second Life®, the researchers designed a prototype multimodal experience based on a hospital scenario. The virtual reality simulations replicated both the exterior and interior of hospital buildings, which came equipped with programmed nurses. Participants were recorded while they navigated through the virtual environment. Participants were interviewed one week after the virtual experience; they were asked to recount as much as possible from the experience and were subsequently shown screenshots of the exposure and asked questions aimed at further prompting memory.

Findings

Virtual reality interventions to promote independent living skills foster a wide range of skills, including vocational skills, serving as witnesses in court, and navigating the health care system. Participants with ID not only enjoyed receiving health care-related information from the virtual reality context, but also showed potential for experiential learning to aid retention of knowledge (Hall, Conboy-Hill, & Taylor, 2011). These findings are increasingly important in the context of the need to navigate continuous reforms in the United States health care system.

KEY QUESTIONS

Does Improved Performance with Virtual Reality and Robots Equate to Improved Performance in the Real World?

Several of the aforementioned studies report that gains observed from virtual reality and robots interventions can be observed in the real world (Hall, Conboy-Hill, & Taylor, 2011; Kandalaft et al., 2013). While these studies certainly demonstrate that virtual reality and robots are promising intervention approaches for individuals with disabilities, it is important to consider the difficulties and limitations of assessing real world performance. For example, Kanadlaft et al. (2013) measured real world performance on a follow-up survey that measured social skills and cognition, as well as if participants felt that social, academic, and occupational functioning were directly and positively impacted by the intervention. While follow up measures such as this one offer researchers valuable information that should be taken into consideration when designing further interventions, they also reflect participants' perceived benefits from the intervention, which may be biased by a wide range of factors that are out of the researchers' control. Therefore, while numerous studies report that treatment effects generalize to the real world, it is important to consider the ways in which researchers define this generalization and decide the extent to which this definition is meaningful in light of the goals of the particular user. In addition to the limitation of studying real world experiences, the majority of the aforementioned studies did not study long-term impacts. While there is considerable evidence of some short-term changes in either participants' behaviors or knowledge, real world impact cannot be understood until researchers follow up with participants over time, after an extended period of time without the intervention.

Are Virtual Reality and Robot Technologies More Effective than Existing Traditional Therapeutic Procedures?

Select studies have found that interactive technologies may serve as more effective interventions than traditional therapies. For example, a recent study by Krishnaswamy, Shriber, & Srimathveeravalli (2014) investigated the effects of a robot-mediated visual motor program on improving the visual motor skills of children (aged 5-11-years) with LD and visual motor delays. This study employed a randomized experimental design to test the efficacy of the robotic device integrated with a computer device that engaged the child and provided feedback. This technology was compared in relation to traditional occupational therapy. The children who received the robotic program, as opposed to traditional occupational therapy, demonstrated significant gains in visual motor performance.

While interactive technology interventions clearly show great promise among the studies mentioned in the current chapter, the majority of the current research suggests that there is insufficient evidence to determine that virtual reality and robot technologies are more effective than existing therapies. A randomized controlled trial with the Mandala® GestureXtreme™ (i.e., a system with virtual applications such as virtual drums, paint, and volleyball) was conducted with 31 children (ages 8-10) diagnosed with CP who were also receiving occupational and/or physical therapy (Reid & Campbell, 2006). The authors compared results with those from standard occupational or physical therapy. While there was some evidence that participants receiving virtual reality may have felt more accepted by their peers and felt more competent as a result of experiencing virtual reality, results suggested that virtual reality might not be more effective than traditional occupational therapy or physical therapy intervention for children with CP.

However, there is some evidence that utilizing interactive technologies to supplement existing treatment may be more effective than treatment alone. Rostami et al. (2012) implemented a four-week 18-hour randomized controlled trial with 32 children (ages 6-11) with spastic hemiparetic CP. The researchers investigated three different groups: virtual reality modified constraint-induced movement therapy and a combination group. The virtual reality environment was a comprehensive evaluation and exercise system, in which exercises were in the form of games such as soccer or throwing balls in a bucket. Visual aspects of the environment were presented to children on a large flat screen through a projector, while auditory feedback was delivered through speakers. In the modified constraint-induced movement therapy group, one day before the intervention, the unaffected hand was immobilized by a volar resting splint extending from the finger tips to the proximal forearm to prevent administering daily activities with the unaffected side. Children wore the splint every day for at least five waking hours. The intervention included daily activities such as reaching, grasping, manipulating objects or toys, dressing and undressing, eating, and grooming, all according to the child's age and abilities. Children in the third group received a combination of virtual reality and modified constraint-induced movement therapy. Findings revealed significantly stronger gains in the combination therapy for the amount of limb use, quality of movement, speed and dexterity. Significantly, the training effects were preserved after a three-month follow-up period.

There is a need for further research to investigate the circumstances under which virtual reality and robots may be more or less effective than traditional therapeutic techniques, as well as the extent to which interactive technology interventions can effectively supplement existing treatment.

How Strong is the Evidence on the Virtual Reality and Robots as Intervention Approaches?

When researchers determine if there is evidence to support particular types of interventions or treatments, there are several factors that are considered in making this determination. Research design is an important determinant of the extent to which a research study provides evidence of an intervention approach. Research design is a particularly critical factor to consider when researchers evaluate the contribution of individual studies.

Several of the aforementioned studies are case studies, which typically assess only one or a few individuals and study these individuals in depth (Deutsch et al., 2008; Herrera et al., 2008). The strength of the case study is that it affords researchers the opportunity to study one or more individuals in depth. The limitation of this design is that the findings may not be representative of how others may experience the intervention. This is particularly the case in studying individuals with disabilities, where there is variability within each disability.

Numerous single subject designs have also been discussed (Bouck, Satsangi, Doughty, & Courtney, 2012; Ke & Im, 2013). Studies that employ a single subject design typically also assess only a few individuals, but often implement rigorous testing before the intervention (i.e., multiple baseline design). As in case studies, the advantage of a single subject design is the opportunity to study a few individuals in depth. An additional advantage is that assessing individuals multiple times before the intervention allows researchers to more conclusively determine that changes observed after the intervention were indeed due to the contribution of the intervention. As in case studies, these studies are also limited in the extent to which they apply to other individuals, even individuals with the same disabilities.

While the vast majority of virtual reality and robot research with individuals with disabilities includes case and single subject studies, there has been an increasing body of research involving randomized trials over the past few years (Krishnaswamy, Shriber, & Srimathveeravalli, 2014; Rostami et al., 2012; Smith et al., 2014; Strickland, Coles, & Southern, 2013). While there is variation in the types of randomized designs, a key feature of this design type is that participants are randomly assigned to participate in the intervention or either another intervention or no intervention. This type of design affords researchers the capacity to compare the effects of the intervention to other interventions or to no intervention. Since groups are randomly assigned, the assumption in randomized design is that the groups do not differ on any other characteristics before the intervention; thus the effects observed after the intervention can be attributed to the treatment. A disadvantage is that often the information collected on participants may not be as in-depth as in the case of a single subject study design. There is a general consensus that randomized designs are the gold standard, and that studies with this design represent a more credible degree of evidence.

How Can Individuals with Disabilities Access Virtual Reality and Robots Technologies at Home?

The advent of videogame (e.g., Wii™) and desktop (e.g., Superscape Virtual Reality Toolkit®) virtual environments provides individuals with disabilities the option of pursuing potentially beneficial interventions in their homes. Wii™ has demonstrated potential benefits with improving physical abilities in preschoolers with developmental delay (Salem, Gropack, Jaffee, & Godwin, 2012), in adolescents with DS (Berg et al., 2012), as well as functional abilities in an adolescent with CP (Deutsch et al., 2008). Desktop options include Superscape Virtual Reality Toolkit®, which has yielded improvements in social understanding in adolescents with ASD (Mitchell, Parsons, & Leonard, 2007), and Second Life®, which has yielded effects in communication and social interaction in children (Ke & Im, 2013) and adults (Kandalaft et al., 2013).

While these resources offer substantial potential for individuals with disabilities, the lack of professional monitoring and inconsistent engagement in virtual environments may contribute to highly variable results in treatment effects. An alternative would be to pursue interventions that are controlled by professionals remotely but are accessible in the home such as iSocial™ (Stichter, Laffey, Flaven, & Herzog, 2014), a three dimensional virtual learning environment that was developed based on support from the University of Missouri Research Board, the Thompson Center for Autism and Neurodevelopmental Disorders, Autism Speaks, and the Institute of Education Sciences (IES). iSocial™ is a 31-lesson social competence intervention for adolescents. iSocial™ includes a social space, a social competence curriculum and a networked community, allowing learners to participate in a social space, develop skills, and interact with others. The premise behind iSocial™ is steeped in the increasing need to provide qualified teachers with evidence-based practices in rural areas that are in need of support. iSocial™ was implemented across three small cohorts totaling 11 students, over a period of 4 months (Stichter, Laffey, Galyen, & Herzog, 2014). Results demonstrated that the social competence curriculum was delivered with fidelity in the three-dimensional virtual learning environment. Moreover, learning outcomes suggest that the iSocial™ approach shows promise for social competence benefits for youth.

CONCLUSION

Virtual reality and robots have enormous potential for individuals with disabilities across the lifespan. This chapter has shed light on the numerous technological breakthroughs over the last fifteen years that have shaped our understanding of how interactive technologies can improve the lives of individuals with disabilities. The research shows potential for interactive technologies to transform educational, assessment, and therapeutic contexts. At the same time, our current understanding and capabilities are largely in flux, and many questions remain unanswered. As virtual reality and robots begin to be become more accessible options for assessment and intervention, it is critical to equip potential users and professionals with the knowledge to make informed decisions based on individualized needs.

REFERENCES

Adams, R., Finn, P., Moes, E., Flannery, K., & Rizzo, A. (2009). Distractibility in Attention/Deficit/ hyperactivity disorder (ADHD): The virtual reality classroom. *Child Neuropsychology*, *15*(2), 120–135. doi:10.1080/09297040802169077 PMID:18608217

Austin, D. W., Abbott, J. A. M., & Carbis, C. (2008). The use of virtual reality hypnosis with two cases of autism spectrum disorder: A feasibility study. *Contemporary Hypnosis*, *25*(2), 102–109. doi:10.1002/ ch.349

Barkley, R. A., Murphy, K. R., O'Connell, T., Anderson, D., & Connor, D. F. (2006). Effects of two doses of alcohol on simulator driving performance in adults with attention-deficit/hyperactivity disorder. *Neuropsychology*, *20*(1), 77–87. doi:10.1037/0894-4105.20.1.77 PMID:16460224

Berg, P., Becker, T., Martian, A., Danielle, P. K., & Wingen, J. (2012). Motor control outcomes following Nintendo Wii use by a child with Down syndrome. *Pediatric Physical Therapy*, *24*(1), 78–84. doi:10.1097/PEP.0b013e31823e05e6 PMID:22207475

Boccanfuso, L., & O'Kane, J. M. (2011). CHARLIE: An adaptive robot design with hand and face tracking for use in autism therapy. *International Journal of Social Robotics*, *3*(4), 337–347. doi:10.1007/ s12369-011-0110-2

Bouck, E. C., Satsangi, R., Doughty, T. T., & Courtney, W. T. (2014). Virtual and Concrete Manipulatives: A Comparison of Approaches for Solving Mathematics Problems for Students with Autism Spectrum Disorder. *Journal of Autism and Developmental Disorders*, *44*(1), 180–193. doi:10.1007/s10803-013-1863-2 PMID:23743958

Braddock, D., Rizzolo, M. C., Thompson, M., & Bell, R. (2004). Emerging technologies and cognitive disability. *Journal of Special Education Technology*, *19*(4), 49–56.

Brown, D. J., Standen, P. J., Proctor, T., & Sterland, D. (2001). Advanced design methodologies for the production of virtual learning environments for use by people with learning disabilities. *Presence (Cambridge, Mass.)*, *10*(4), 401–415. doi:10.1162/1054746011470253

Chantry, J., & Dunford, C. (2010). How do computer assistive technologies enhance participation in childhood occupations for children with multiple and complex disabilities? A review of the current literature. *British Journal of Occupational Therapy*, *73*(8), 351–365. doi:10.4276/030802210X12813483277107

Cheng, Y., & Chen, S. (2010). Improving social understanding of individuals of intellectual and developmental disabilities through a 3D-facial expression intervention program. *Research in Developmental Disabilities*, *31*(6), 1434–1442. doi:10.1016/j.ridd.2010.06.015 PMID:20674267

Clancy, T. A., Rucklidge, J. J., & Owen, D. (2006). Road-crossing safety in virtual reality: A comparison of adolescents with and without ADHD. *Journal of Clinical Child and Adolescent Psychology*, *35*(2), 203–215. doi:10.1207/s15374424jccp3502_4 PMID:16597216

Cook, A., Howery, K., Gu, J., & Meng, M. (2000). Robot enhanced interaction and learning for children with profound physical disabilities. *Technology and Disability*, *13*(1), 1.

Cook, A. M., Meng, M. Q. H., Gu, J. J., & Howery, K. (2002). Development of a robotic device for facilitating learning by children who have severe disabilities. *IEEE Transactions on Neural Systems and Rehabilitation Engineering: A Publication of the IEEE Engineering in Medicine and Biology Society, 10*(3), 178-187.

Cooke, P., Laczny, A., Brown, D. J., & Francik, J. (2002). The virtual courtroom: A view of justice. Project to prepare witnesses or victims with learning disabilities to give evidence. *Disability and Rehabilitation, 24*(11), 634–642. doi:10.1080/10.1080/09638280110111414 PMID:12182804

Cox, D. J., Punja, M., Powers, K., Merkel, R. L., Burket, R., Moore, M., & Kovatchev, B. et al. (2006). Manual Transmission Enhances Attention and Driving Performance of ADHD Adolescent Males Pilot Study. *Journal of Attention Disorders, 10*(2), 212–216. doi:10.1177/1087054706288103 PMID:17085632

Dautenhahn, K., & Werry, I. (2004). Towards interactive robots in autism therapy: Background, motivation and challenges. *Pragmatics & Cognition, 12*(1), 1–35. doi:10.1075/pc.12.1.03dau

Deutsch, J. E., Borbely, M., Filler, J., Huhn, K., & Guarrera-Bowlby, P. (2008). Use of a low-cost, commercially available gaming console (Wii) for rehabilitation of an adolescent with cerebral palsy. *Physical Therapy, 88*(10), 1196–1207. doi:10.2522/ptj.20080062 PMID:18689607

Duquette, A., Michaud, F., & Mercier, H. (2008). Exploring the use of a mobile robot as an imitation agent with children with low-functioning autism. *Autonomous Robots, 24*(2), 147–157. doi:10.1007/s10514-007-9056-5

Goldsmith, T. R., & LeBlanc, L. A. (2004). Use of Technology in Interventions for Children with Autism. *Journal of Early and Intensive Behavior Intervention, 1*(2), 166–178. doi:10.1037/h0100287

Golomb, M. R., McDonald, B. C., Warden, S. J., Yonkman, J., Saykin, A. J., Shirley, B., . . . Nwosu, M. E. (2010). In-home virtual reality videogame telerehabilitation in adolescents with hemiplegic cerebral palsy. *Archives of Physical Medicine and Rehabilitation, 91*(1), 1-8. e1.

Gutiérrez-Maldonado, J., Letosa-Porta, À., Rus-Calafell, M., & Peñaloza-Salazar, C. (2009). The assessment of attention deficit hyperactivity disorder in children using continous performance tasks in virtual environments. *Anuario de Psicología, 40*(2), 211–222.

Hall, V., Conboy-Hill, S., & Taylor, D. (2011). Using virtual reality to provide health care information to people with intellectual disabilities: Acceptability, usability, and potential utility. *Journal of Medical Internet Research, 13*(4), e91. doi:10.2196/jmir.1917 PMID:22082765

Herrera, G., Alcantud, F., Jordan, R., Blanquer, A., Labajo, G., & De Pablo, C. (2008). Development of symbolic play through the use of virtual reality tools in children with autistic spectrum disorders: Two case studies. *Autism, 12*(2), 143–157. doi:10.1177/1362361307086657 PMID:18308764

Hodson, H. (2014). The first family robot. *New Scientist, 223*(2978), 21. doi:10.1016/S0262-4079(14)61389-0

IROMEC. (2015, March 31). Retrieved from http://www.iromec.org/6.0.html

Kaboski, J. R., Diehl, J. J., Beriont, J., Crowell, C. R., Villano, M., Wier, K., & Tang, K. (2014). Brief Report: A Pilot Summer Robotics Camp to Reduce Social Anxiety and Improve Social/Vocational Skills in Adolescents with ASD. *Journal of Autism and Developmental Disorders*, 1–8. PMID:24898910

Kandalaft, M. R., Didehbani, N., Krawczyk, D. C., Allen, T. T., & Chapman, S. B. (2013). Virtual reality social cognition training for young adults with high-functioning autism. *Journal of Autism and Developmental Disorders*, *43*(1), 34–44. doi:10.1007/s10803-012-1544-6 PMID:22570145

Ke, F., & Im, T. (2013). Virtual-reality-based social interaction training for children with high-functioning autism. *The Journal of Educational Research*, *106*(6), 441–461. doi:10.1080/00220671.2013.832999

Kim, E. S., Berkovits, L. D., Bernier, E. P., Leyzberg, D., Shic, F., Paul, R., & Scassellati, B. (2013). Social robots as embedded reinforcers of social behavior in children with autism. *Journal of Autism and Developmental Disorders*, *43*(5), 1038–1049. doi:10.1007/s10803-012-1645-2 PMID:23111617

Kim, E. S., Paul, R., Shic, F., & Scassellati, B. (2012). Bridging the research gap: Making HRI useful to individuals with autism. *Journal of Human-Robot Interaction*, *1*(1).

Kirshner, S., Weiss, P. L., & Tirosh, E. (2011). Meal-maker: A virtual meal preparation environment for children with cerebral palsy. *European Journal of Special Needs Education*, *26*(3), 323–336. doi:10.1080/08856257.2011.593826

Knouse, L. E., Bagwell, C. L., Barkley, R. A., & Murphy, K. R. (2005). Accuracy of self-evaluation in adults with ADHD evidence from a driving study. *Journal of Attention Disorders*, *8*(4), 221–234. doi:10.1177/1087054705280159 PMID:16110052

Krishnaswamy, S., Shriber, L., & Srimathveeravalli, G. (2014). The design and efficacy of a robot-mediated visual motor program for children learning disabilities. *Journal of Computer Assisted Learning*, *30*(2), 121–131. doi:10.1111/jcal.12025

Life, S. ® (2003). Available from http://secondlife.com (Retrieved March 31, 2015).

Lotan, M., Yalon-Chamovitz, S., & Weiss, P. L. T. (2009). Improving physical fitness of individuals with intellectual and developmental disability through a Virtual Reality Intervention Program. *Research in Developmental Disabilities*, *30*(2), 229–239. doi:10.1016/j.ridd.2008.03.005 PMID:18479889

Mitchell, P., Parsons, S., & Leonard, A. (2007). Using virtual environments for teaching social understanding to 6 adolescents with autistic spectrum disorders. *Journal of Autism and Developmental Disorders*, *37*(3), 589–600. doi:10.1007/s10803-006-0189-8 PMID:16900403

Moore, D., Cheng, Y., McGrath, P., & Powell, N. J. (2005). Collaborative virtual environment technology for people with autism. *Focus on Autism and Other Developmental Disabilities*, *20*(4), 231–243. doi:10.1177/10883576050200040501

Nintendo® *Wii™* (2006). Available from http://wii.com (Retrieved March 31, 2015).

Parsons, S., & Mitchell, P. (2002). The potential of virtual reality in social skills training for people with autistic spectrum disorders. *Journal of Intellectual Disability Research*, *46*(5), 430–443. doi:10.1046/j.1365-2788.2002.00425.x PMID:12031025

Parsons, S., Mitchell, P., & Leonard, A. (2004). The use and understanding of virtual environments by adolescents with autistic spectrum disorders. *Journal of Autism and Developmental Disorders, 34*(4), 449–466. doi:10.1023/B:JADD.0000037421.98517.8d PMID:15449520

Parsons, T. D., Bowerly, T., Buckwalter, J. G., & Rizzo, A. A. (2007). A controlled clinical comparison of attention performance in children with ADHD in a virtual reality classroom compared to standard neuropsychological methods. *Child Neuropsychology, 13*(4), 363–381. doi:10.1080/13825580600943473 PMID:17564852

Passig, D., & Eden, S. (2000). Improving flexible thinking in deaf and hard of hearing children with virtual reality technology. *American Annals of the Deaf, 145*(3), 286–291. doi:10.1353/aad.2012.0102 PMID:10965592

Passig, D., & Eden, S. (2001). Virtual reality as a tool for improving spatial rotation among deaf and hard-of-hearing children. *Cyberpsychology & Behavior, 4*(6), 681–686. doi:10.1089/109493101753376623 PMID:11800175

Passig, D., & Eden, S. (2003). Cognitive intervention through virtual environments among deaf and hard-of-hearing children. *European Journal of Special Needs Education, 18*(2), 173–182. doi:10.1080/0885625032000078961

Pollak, Y., Shomaly, H. B., Weiss, P. L., Rizzo, A. A., & Gross-Tsur, V. (2010). Methylphenidate effect in children with ADHD can be measured by an ecologically valid continuous performance test embedded in virtual reality. *CNS Spectrums, 15*(2), 125–130. PMID:20414157

Prazak, B., Kronreif, G., Hochgatterer, A., & Fürst, M. (2004). A toy robot for physically disabled children. *Technology and Disability, 16*(3), 131–136.

Reid, D., & Campbell, K. (2006). The use of virtual reality with children with cerebral palsy: A pilot randomized trial. *Therapeutic Recreation Journal, 40*(4), 255–268.

Reid, D. T. (2002). The use of virtual reality to improve upper-extremity efficiency skills in children with cerebral palsy: A pilot study. *Technology and Disability, 14*(2), 53–61.

Rizzo, A. A., Buckwalter, J. G., Bowerly, T., Van, D. Z., Humphrey, L., Neumann, U., & Sisemore, D. et al. (2000). The virtual classroom: A virtual reality environment for the assessment and rehabilitation of attention deficits. *Cyberpsychology & Behavior, 3*(3), 483–499. doi:10.1089/10949310050078940

Robins, B., Dautenhahn, K., & Dubowski, J. (2006). Does appearance matter in the interaction of children with autism with a humanoid robot? *Interaction Studies: Social Behaviour and Communication in Biological and Artificial Systems, 7*(3), 509–542. doi:10.1075/is.7.3.16rob

Rostami, H. R., Arastoo, A. A., Nejad, S. J., Mahany, M. K., Malamiri, R. A., & Goharpey, S. (2012). Effects of modified constraint-induced movement therapy in virtual environment on upper-limb function in children with spastic hemiparetic cerebral palsy: A randomised controlled trial. *NeuroRehabilitation, 31*(4), 357–365. PMID:23232158

Salem, Y., Gropack, S., Coffin, D., & Godwin, E. M. (2012). Effectiveness of a low-cost virtual reality system for children with developmental delay: A preliminary randomised single-blind controlled trial. *Physiotherapy*, *98*(3), 189–195. doi:10.1016/j.physio.2012.06.003 PMID:22898574

Sánchez, J., & Sáenz, M. (2006). 3D sound interactive environments for blind children problem solving skills. *Behaviour & Information Technology*, *25*(4), 367–378. doi:10.1080/01449290600636660

Sandlund, M., Lindh Waterworth, E., & Häger, C. (2011). Using motion interactive games to promote physical activity and enhance motor performance in children with cerebral palsy. *Developmental Neurorehabilitation*, *14*(1), 15–21. doi:10.3109/17518423.2010.533329 PMID:21241174

Smith, M. J., Ginger, E. J., Wright, K., Wright, M. A., Taylor, J. L., Humm, L. B., & Fleming, M. F. et al. (2014). Virtual Reality Job Interview Training in Adults with Autism Spectrum Disorder. *Journal of Autism and Developmental Disorders*, 1–14. PMID:24803366

Standen, P. J., Brown, D., Horan, M., & Proctor, T. (2002). How tutors assist adults with learning disabilities to use virtual environments. *Disability and Rehabilitation*, *24*(11), 570–577. doi:10.1080/09638280320179244 PMID:12182796

Stichter, J. P., Laffey, J., Galyen, K., & Herzog, M. (2014). iSocial: Delivering the social competence intervention for adolescents (SCI-A) in a 3D virtual learning environment for youth with high functioning autism. *Journal of Autism and Developmental Disorders*, *44*(2), 417–430. doi:10.1007/s10803-013-1881-0 PMID:23812663

Strickland, D. C., Coles, C. D., & Southern, L. B. (2013). JobTIPS: A transition to employment program for individuals with autism spectrum disorders. *Journal of Autism and Developmental Disorders*, *43*(10), 2472–2483. doi:10.1007/s10803-013-1800-4 PMID:23494559

Strickland, D. C., McAllister, D., Coles, C. D., & Osborne, S. (2007). An evolution of virtual reality training designs for children with autism and fetal alcohol spectrum disorders. *Topics in Language Disorders*, *27*(3), 226–241. doi:10.1097/01.TLD.0000285357.95426.72 PMID:20072702

USC Institute for Creative Technologies. (2014). *VITA: Virtual Interactive Training Agent*. Available from http://ict.usc.edu/prototypes/vita/

KEY TERMS AND DEFINITIONS

Collaborative Virtual Environments: Two forms of virtual environment can be distinguished: a single user virtual environment (SVE) and a multiuser, collaborative virtual environment (CVE). In the SVE, the user is restricted to interacting the environment and possibly with other avatars, response from which may need to be preprogrammed. In a CVE, there can be more than one user and users can communicate with each other via their avatars.

IROMEC: Interactive Robotic Social Mediators as Companions (IROMEC) is an interdisciplinary imitative that combines the field of robots with other disciplines such as cognitive science and developmental psychology with the aim "to empower children with disabilities to prevent dependency and isolation, develop their potential and learn new skills by development of a robot-supported play environment which meets the users' expectations for a safe and reliable, versatile and tailorable, ready to use and affordable system" (IROMEC, 2015).

Nintendo® Wii™: Nintendo® Wii™ is a videogame console that allows users to engage with virtual reality in the home. A wide range of games that promote physical fitness, such as Wii Fit™ and Wii Sports™, are available. These games include virtual sports such as soccer, boxing, and snowboarding. The current chapter discusses the success of using Wii™ as an intervention for children and adolescents with physical or motor disabilities, such as those consistent with CP, developmental delay, DS, or ID (Berg et al., 2012; Deutsch et al., 2008; Salem, Gropack, Jaffee, & Godwin, 2012).

Robots/Robotic Systems: Robots are technologies that "can interact with humans and show aspects of human-style social intelligence" (Dautenhahn & Werry, 2004, p. 2). Robots can also take a wide range of forms, from "humanoids" (i.e., robots that resemble humans), to animal-resembling figures. Robotic systems are robots that do not resemble an interactive agent like a human or animal; rather they are interactive configurations that may consist of gripper systems, switches, and buttons that a user can engage with during play (Prazak, Kronreif, Hochgatterer, & Furst, 2004).

Second Life®: Second Life® is a three-dimensional virtual world software available to the public. Examples of Second Life® settings are virtual schools (including a playground and school cafeteria) and house parties (Second Life, 2013).

Virtual Reality/Virtual Environments: Virtual reality or a virtual environment is three-dimensional computer-based world, in which users can interact with objects or "avatars" (i.e., figures that resemble humans). These environments can be modified to resemble a wide range of environments, including classrooms, offices, and cafes. The extent to which the user is embedded in the scene is also highly variable, as some users may be able to watch themselves through a camera interacting in the scene, whereas other users may be represented by an avatar within a scene. Virtual reality affords users the opportunity to practice skills repeatedly in a "safe" environment. Depending on the particular set-up within a virtual environment, users may also be able to receive direct feedback on performance, or interact with real people also using the program. Virtual reality can be accessed through a wide range of mediums, including videogames, head-mounted displays, or desktop computers (Parsons & Mitchell, 2002).

Chapter 9
Microswitch–Based Programs (MBP) to Promote Communication, Occupation, and Leisure Skills for Children with Multiple Disabilities:
A Literature Overview

Fabrizio Stasolla
University of Bari, Italy

Viviana Perilli
Lega del Filo d'Oro Research Center, Italy

ABSTRACT

This chapter provides a literature overview concerning microswitch-based programs (MBP) to promote communication, occupation and leisure skills for children with multiple disabilities. The first aim of the chapter is to present an overview of the empirical studies about the use of MBP, published in the last decade (i.e. period from 2004 to 2014) to emphasize the most recent strategies for children with developmental disabilities, providing a general picture of the different options available. The second goal is to underline strengths and weaknesses of the various studies included in the overview. Finally, the third purpose is to outline issues and questions to be addressed in the future and discuss their implications for research and practice.

INTRODUCTION

Children with severe to profound multiple disabilities (PMD) (i.e., intellectual, motor and sensory disabilities) may be quite passive and isolated from the outside world due to their clinical conditions (e.g. medical, breath, postural abnormalities, lack of speech, unawareness of their off-task or chal-

DOI: 10.4018/978-1-4666-8395-2.ch009

lenge behaviors) and may consequently experience serious challenges across their many environments (Borg, Larson, & Ostenberg, 2011; Lontis & Struijk, 2010). In addition to needing physiotherapy and pharmacological treatments, those children need specific help to: (a) interact and engage constructively and independently with surrounding preferred items and to (b) increase positive opportunities for communication, occupation and leisure. Moreover, they present incapacities to develop request and choice responses autonomously, although they have learning skills concerning adaptive responses (Kagohara et al., 2011; Reichle, 2011). The aforementioned conditions may have negative consequences on their quality of life (Felce & Perry, 1995).

One way of enabling that children with severe to profound multiple disabilities achieve the dual objective of reducing challenging behaviors and increasing the performance maintenance and generalization of adaptive responses is to use microswitches-based programs (mbp) combined with motivational strategies based on learning principles (i.e. the causal association between behavioral responses and environmental consequences) (Lancioni & Singh, 2014). A microswitch is a basic form of assistive technology (AT) that allows persons with a very limited behavioral repertoire to access and interact positively with their environment. Thus, a child can activate toys, music, lights, and vibratory stimulation through the exhibition of small behavioral responses. For example, depending on individual learning perspectives, (i.e. participant's characteristics and/or skills) one may envisage a rehabilitative intervention with a microswitch enabling a child to turn on a brief period of stimulation by a small hand closure (Lancioni, Singh, O'Reilly, & Oliva, 2005). Alternatively, one may design a two microswitch program that provides a choice between two different categories of stimuli (e.g. visual and auditory) by performing two behavioral responses (e.g. hand closure and eye blinking) (Lancioni, Sigafoos, O'Reilly, & Singh, 2012).

In addition, practitioners can encourage a microswitch and Voice Output Communication Aid (VOCA) strategy that allows the individual to choose between access to preferred stimuli independently and social contact with a caregiver (Lancioni et al., 2009; Schlosser & Sigafoos, 2006). Furthermore, matched with a personal computer, a microswitch may supply a participant with a request and choice opportunity concerning preferred options (e.g., video, music, food, beverage, personal or physical needs) (Stasolla, Caffò, Picucci, & Bosco, 2013). Moreover, a microswitch cluster pursues the dual goal of promoting an adaptive behavior with the simultaneous reduction of a challenging behavior (Lancioni et al., 2008). Finally, a microswitch program with contingent stimuli may foster ambulation responses and fluency (Stasolla & Caffò, 2013).

For persons without intellectual disabilities who have extensive motor impairments, (e.g., children with cerebral palsy), a microswitch program linked to a keyboard emulator may enhance literacy. In addition, it may promote self-monitoring of on-task behavior during academic activities (Chiapparino, Stasolla, De Pace, & Lancioni, 2011; Stasolla, Perilli, & Damiani, 2014). Next to the importance of reducing passivity and encouraging an active role by those persons, professionals are dealing with improving their appearance and status and, consequently, their quality of life (Ivancic & Bayley, 1996).

The main aspect of quality of life is happiness, which includes three basic components: personal well-being, pleasure and contentment. Those components are particularly difficult to detect among individuals with developmental disabilities, especially if those persons are *non-verbal individuals*. To overcome this barrier, researchers refer to behavioral responses connected with happiness, labeling them as *indices of happiness* (e.g. smiling, laughing, excited body movements with or without vocalizations). Those indices are commonly recorded in a MBP or in a learning principles strategy in order to assess their effects on positive mood concerning the participants involved (Lancioni, Singh, O'Reilly, Oliva, & Basili, 2005).

The first aim of the chapter is to present an overview of the empirical studies about the use of MBP, published in the last decade (i.e. period from 2004 to 2014) in line to emphasize the most recent strategies for children with developmental disabilities, providing a general picture of the different options available. The second goal is to underline strengths and weaknesses of the various studies included in the overview. Finally, the third purpose is outline issues and questions to be addressed in the future and discuss their implications for research and practice.

1. BACKGROUND

AT (Assistive Technology) defines 'any item, piece of equipment, product or system, whether acquired commercially, off the shelf, modified or customised, that is used to increase, maintain or improve functional capabilities of individuals with cognitive, physical or communication disabilities' (Assistive Technology Act, 2004). More commonly, the term AT refers to a variety of electronic or computerized devices aimed at helping persons with disabilities to function more easily and independently within their daily context and achieve a higher quality of life (Lancioni, Sigafoos, O'Reilly, & Singh, 2013).

Assistive technology-based interventions for individuals with multiple disabilities relying on the use of technological supports, overcome the limits of other rehabilitative programs, because they do not only enrich participants' sensory systems aimed at increasing their vigilance and alertness but also attempt to emphasize their active role (i.e. self determination) by seeking and managing such inputs by themselves. The final purpose is to facilitate learning and promote consolidation of small behavioral responses necessary to control and to access to environmental stimulation or to ask for a caregiver mediation (Lancioni & Singh, 2014).

2. METHOD

A computerized search was conducted using the SCOPUS, ERIC, PubMed, and PsychInfo databases for journal articles from 2004 to 2014, inserting combinations of the following keywords: "developmental disabilities," "multiple disabilities," "autism spectrum disorders," "attention deficits hyperactivity disorders," "Rett syndrome," "cerebral palsy," "indices of happiness," "quality of life," "communication impairments," "rehabilitative interventions," "assistive technologies," "microswitches". A manual search of journal was added as a supplement to identify empirical studies in this area. Inclusion criteria for studies, included: (a) at least one child or an adolescent (range age 3-18 years) with developmental disabilities, multiple disabilities, Rett syndrome, autism spectrum disorders, cerebral palsy or attention deficit hyperactivity disorders, (b) a MBP intervention, and (c) the presentation of individual or some group evidence regarding the effects or results of the intervention. The excluding criteria regarded (a) Snoezelen rooms, environmental enrichment and/or sensorial stimulation unique approaches; and (b) studies involving adults (age more than 18 years) only, as their inclusion would exceed the goals of the present chapter. According to the aforementioned criteria, 40 studies were included in this overview. For practical reasons, they were divided into eight different categories, according to the type and level of technology they used: (a) one microswitch, (b) two microswitches, (c) a combination of microswitch and VOCA, (d) microswitches and contingent stimuli to promote ambulation, (e) microswitch-cluster programs to promote an adaptive response and simultaneously reduce a challenge behavior, (f) a microswitch connected to a computer system to allow request and choice of preferred items with caregiver mediation or automatically delivered by the system, and (g) a microswitch connected to a computer system ensuring children with extensive motor impairments and without any intellectual disabilities access to a literacy process. Moreover, within each section, following a brief explanation concerning the objectives and the principles of the rehabilitative intervention, two representative studies will be described (i.e. with the pursued goals, the participants involved, the adopted procedures and the empirical results), irrespective of the number of the studies included in each category (see Table 1).

2.1 One Microswitch

Six studies, involving ten participants, used a single microswitch. In two cases, the microswitch was an optic sensor monitoring an eyelid response (Lancioni et al., 2010a, 2011). Three studies incorporated a microswitch that consisted of a pair of optic sensors controlling lip and/or chin movements (Lancioni et al., 2005, 2006, 2009), and one study included tilt sensors (Lancioni et al., 2004). For example, Lancioni et al. (2004a) adapted a grid into a microswitch to detect the hand movements of a girl, in a supine position, with profound multiple disabilities. The grid, suspended above the girl's face, was equipped with two mercury devices, i.e., small sealed ampules containing a mercury drop, and ending with conductive leads. A lateral or forward movement of the grid would make the mercury drop shift along the conductive leads and activate the device. During the intervention, the activation of one of the two devices on either side of the grid (activation that occurred when participants hit the grid) produced the same preferred stimulation. Analysis showed that the girl increased the frequency of hand movements and microswitch activations during the intervention phases compared to the baseline phases (when her favorite stimuli were not available). The increase of adaptive responses was consolidated during a post-intervention check which occurred one month after the end of intervention phase.

Lancioni et al. (2006) conducted two studies that supported two children with multiple disabilities and minimal motor behavior to use chin movements to operate microswitches in order to obtain preferred stimuli. Each study was carried out using an ABAB design. A two-month post-intervention check also occurred. The data revealed that both children increased the frequency of the chin response, thus increasing the level of environmental stimulation during the intervention phases. This performance was retained at the post-intervention check.

2.2. Two Microswitches

Four studies, involving seven participants, have been carried out for this purpose, in which two responses with two adapted microswitches were retained for each participant for various stimulation opportunities (Lancioni et al., 2007a, 2014a; Lancioni, et al., 2004b; Stasolla, Damiani, et al., 2014). Eventually, request and choice opportunities were provided, ensuring participants with the opportunity to exhibit different behavioral responses. Furthermore, one may envisage request and choice intervention programs, ensuring participants' access to preferred items independently.

For example, Lancioni et al. (2007a) carried out two single-case studies using different procedural and technological approaches to enable two adolescents with multiple disabilities to choose among environmental stimuli. The first study focused on replicating a previous developed procedure, which relied on samples of the auditory stimuli available as cues for choice responses. The second study assessed a new procedural and technical setup relying on the use of pictorial representations of the stimuli

Table 1. Studies grouped according to the rehabilitative intervention applied.

Studies	Participants	Age Ranges	Responses	Outcomes
One ms				
Lancioni et al., 2004	1	7.06	Push with hands or legs	One Positive
Lancioni et al., 2005	1	8.05	Eye blinking	One Positive
Lancioni et al., 2006	2	6.3-9.4	Chin movements	Two Positive
Lancioni et al., 2009	2	9.6-9.7	Lip and chin movements	Two Positive
Lancioni et al., 2010	2	8.7-9.2	Eye blinking	One Negative
Lancioni et al., 2011	2	9.5-9.8	Ee blinking	Two Positives
Two ms				
Lancioni, et al., 2004b	2	15-17	Select a preferred item	One negative
Lancioni et al., 2007	2	14-16	Select a preferred item	Two Positives
Lancioni et al., 2014a	1	13	Insert an object in a container	One Positive
Stasolla, Damiani, et al., 2014	2	8.7-9.7	Insert an object in a container	Two Positives
Ms and VOCA				
Lancioni et al., 2008a	1	13	Hand/head movements	One Positive
Lancioni et al., 2008b	2	16-18	Legs/head movements	One Positive
Lancioni et al., 2008c	3	12-16	Hand/head movements	Three Positives
Lancioni et al., 2009a	1	14	Vocalization/hand movement	One Positive
Lancioni et al., 2009b	11	5-8	Head/hand movements	Two Negatives
Lancioni et al., 2009c	3	10-15	Head/trunk movements	Three Positives
Lancioni et al., 2012	1	16	Head/hand movements	One Positive
Ms and Ambulation				
Lancioni et al., 2005a	1	10.08	Forward step	One Positive
Lancioni et al., 2005b	1	16	Forward step	One Positive
Lancioni et al., 2007b	1	11	Forward step	One Positive
Lancioni et al., 2007c	2	6-9	Forward step	Two Positives
Lancioni et al., 2010b	5	5-10	Forward step	Five Positives
Lancioni et al., 2013a	3	8-15	Forward step	Three Positives
Stasolla & Caffò, 2013	2	12-17	Four forward steps within 3 s	Two Positives
Ms-Clusters				
Lancioni et al., 2007d	2	9-12	Head/Hand movements	Two Positives
Lancioni et al., 2008d	3	7-16	Foot/hands	Three Positives
Lancioni et al., 2009d	1	14	head/hand	One Positive
Lancioni et al., 2009e	2	10-14	hand/head	Two Positives
Lancioni et al., 2013b	2	10-12	touch/head	Two Positives
Stasolla et al., 2014	3	8-10	manipulation/mouthing	Three Positives

continued on following page

Table 1. Continued

Studies	Participants	Age Ranges	Responses	Outcomes
Ms and Computer				
Lancioni et al., 2011b	1	12	Select a preferred item	One Positive
Lancioni et al., 2012b	1	11	Select a preferred item	One Positive
Stasolla et al., 2013	3	6-9	Select a preferred item	Three Positives
Stasolla, Caffò, et al., 2015	3	9-12	Select a preferred item	Three Positives
Stasolla & De Pace, 2014	2	8-9	Select a preferred item	Two Positives
Ms and Literacy				
Chiapparino et al., 2011	1	17	Select rows/letters	One Positive
Lancioni et al., 2007d	1	18	Select rows/letters	One Positive
Lancioni et al., 2009f	2	10-13	Select rows/letters	Two Positives
Lancioni et al., 2010c	2	9-12	Select rows/letters	Two Positives
Stasolla, Caffò, et al., 2015	3	9-12	Select rows/letters	Three Positives

for choice responses. The auditory samples and the pictorial representations were presented through computer systems. The participants' choice responses relied on microswitches connected to the computer systems. Supporting previous findings with the same procedural approach, the participant learned to choose preferred stimuli and bypass non preferred ones. Data from the second study showed that the participant learned to address his choice responses on a few stimuli, suggesting that these stimuli were actually preferred and that responding was purposeful.

Lancioni, Singh, O'Reilly, and Oliva (2004) examined two students with multiple disabilities with two or three request microswitches and one choice microswitch. Activation of a request microswitch triggered the verbal announcement of one of the stimulus events related to it. The student could choose such an event through the choice microswitch or bypass it. The request microswitches were introduced individually and were made available simultaneously by the end of the intervention and the post-intervention period. Analysis showed that both students learned to use the microswitches. Transfer of the microswitch program into the students' home was very successful with one student and presented some difficulties with the other.

2.3. Microswitch and VOCA

Seven studies including a total of 22 participants have been carried out, in which the participants were provided with a combination of one microswitch and one or two VOCA(s) (Lancioni et al., 2008a, b, c, 2009a, b, c, 2012). The aim of these studies was to provide participants with active engagement and independent access to preferred stimulation with an opportunity to request social contact with their caregivers, and to choose between both aforementioned options.

For example, Lancioni, et al. (2009b) conducted two studies applying microswitch and VOCA technologies. The first of these two studies assessed whether 11 participants with multiple disabilities would succeed in combining a microswitch for accessing preferred environmental stimuli and a Voice Output Communication Aid (VOCA) for requesting social contact. Data showed that all participants learned to use the microswitch and the VOCA. Moreover, the 10 participants who received a 1-month post-intervention check largely maintained their responses.

Lancioni et al. (2008c) assessed the possibility of enabling three participants (two children and one adolescent) to combine two microswitches (for accessing environmental stimuli) and a VOCA, which allowed them to ask for a caregiver's attention. Initially, the participants were required to use each of the two microswitches individually and then together. Thereafter, they were taught to use the VOCA. Eventually, the VOCA was available together with the microswitches, and the participants could use any of the three. The results, which support preliminary data on this topic, showed that all participants (a) were able to operate the two microswitches as well as the VOCA; and (b) used all three consistently when they were simultaneously available. The authors stated that teaching individuals with multiple disabilities to combine a VOCA with conventional microswitches may enrich their general input, emphasize their active social role and eventually enhance their social image.

2.4. Microswitch and Contingent Stimuli to Promote Ambulation Responses

Children with severe or profound intellectual and motor disabilities often present problems of balance and ambulation and often spend much of their time sitting or lying down, with negative consequences to their development and social status. Recent research has shown the possibility of using a walker (support) device and microswitches with preferred stimuli to promote ambulation with these children. Seven studies (Lancioni et al., 2005a, b, 2007b, c, 2010b, 2013a; Stasolla & Caffò, 2013) are included in this section, with fifteen participants involved. Those intervention strategies may represent an integration/supplement to traditional forms of physiotherapy.

For example, Lancioni et al. (2010) assessed a study which replicated the aforementioned research featuring five children with multiple disabilities. For four children, the study involved an ABAB design. For the fifth child, only an AB sequence was used. All children succeeded in increasing their frequencies of step responses during the intervention phase(s) of the study, although the overall frequencies of those responses varied largely. These findings support the positive evidence already available about the effectiveness of this intervention approach in motivating and promoting children's ambulation.

Stasolla and Caffò (2013) assessed a study aimed at promoting fluency in the locomotor behavior of two girls with Rett syndrome and severe to profound developmental disabilities. Both girls were ambulatory in their walkers. By using optic sensors (i.e. photocells) and contingent stimuli, participants were provided with three seconds of pleasant stimulation automatically delivered by the system when they performed four steps within three seconds (i.e. fluency criterion). Results showed that both participants increased their performance during intervention phases.

2.5. Microswitch-Clusters

Microswitch-cluster programs are aimed at pursuing the dual goal of promoting an adaptive response and reducing a challenge behavior. Typically, in a microswitch-cluster based program protocol, following an initial baseline where both behaviors are recorded without any environmental consequences, a first intervention phase occurs in which the adaptive behavior is followed by contingent positive stimulation, even if at the same time a challenge behavior occurs. Finally, the cluster-intervention phase is carried out, where the adaptive response is positively reinforced only if it occurs with the simultaneous absence of the problem behavior. Additionally, positive stimulation is interrupted if a challenge behavior is exhibited during its supply. Eight studies are included in this section (Lancioni et al., 2007d, 2008d, 2009d, e, 2013b, Stasolla et al., 2014), involving thirteen participants.

For example, Stasolla et al. (2014) carried out a microswitch-cluster aimed at promoting object manipulation and reducing hand mouthing (i.e. put his hands near or in to the mouth) for three boys with severe autism spectrum disorders and profound intellectual disabilities. The adaptive response was monitored through a wobble microswitch fixed on the table in front of the participants involved (that would be pulled, pushed or moved sideways), and the challenging behavior was recorded through an optic sensor fixed on participants' chin with an adaptive frame. Both devices constituted the cluster. The study was carried out through an ABB^1AB^1 experimental sequence, where A represented baseline phases, and B represented intervention phases with the enhancement of adaptive behavior regardless of the challenging behavior. B^1 indicated the cluster-intervention phases, with the object manipulation positively reinforced (only if exhibited with the absence of hand mouthing) (see above). Indices of happiness as an outcome measure of quality of life were also coded. Results showed that all participants learned to use the cluster technology, increased their adaptive responses and decreased their challenging behaviors. Furthermore, all participants seemed to enjoy the sessions, since their indices of happiness improved during intervention phases, compared to baseline.

Lancioni et al. (2007c) assessed the viability of using microswitch-cluster plus contingent stimulation to promote adaptive responding and to reduce aberrant behavior for two children with multiple disabilities. The results revealed that both children increased their adaptive responses, learned to perform these responses free of aberrant behavior, and maintained this level of performance three months later (i.e. during follow-up phase).

2.6. Microswitch Connected to a Computer System

In this section, we presented microswitch devices connected to computer systems through an interface, enabling persons with multiple disabilities to request and choose preferred items, directly delivered from the system or with the mediation of a caregiver. Broadly speaking, the system provides various categories of stimuli (e.g. encircled pictures matched with verbal cues), selected through a formal preference screening (Crawford & Schuster, 1993) automatically scanned by the system. By responding (i.e. by activating the microswitch), participants are encouraged to request (and choose) the selected item. Typically, the first response let the system open a second page, which presents different items within the previous category. The second response is necessary to request and choose the selected item. A final confirmation response may be required, inquiring as to whether participants really desired the selected item. Consequently, if a positive response occurred, the item would be available to participants for 8-20 seconds, depending on the requested item. Five studies are included in this section (Lancioni et al., 2011b, 2012b, Stasolla, Caffò, et al., 2014; Stasolla, Caffò, Picucci, & Bosco, 2013; Stasolla & De Pace, 2014), with ten participants involved.

For example, Stasolla, Caffò, Picucci, & Bosco (2013) worked with three participants with cerebral palsy and severe communication impairments, presenting them with a pressure sensor (circular button) connected to a computer system introducing three categories (i.e. food, beverage, leisure) including, each of them, four items. Participants were requested to respond (i.e. activate the pressure sensor) three times to perform a selection of a requested item. With a first activation, they would select a category, with a second response-item and finally they would confirm their choice, in order to assure the item's availability through the mediation of the caregiver. Indices of happiness were additionally recorded. A post-intervention check phase occurred 15 days after the end of the second intervention phase (sequence ABABC). Results showed that all participants increased their request and choices of preferred items during intervention phases and consolidated their performance during the post- intervention phase. Indices of happiness rose during intervention and post intervention phases, compared to baseline, for all the participants.

Stasolla and De Pace (2014) worked on two post-coma children who emerged from a minimal conscious state and presented extensive motor disabilities. The participants were presented with a new set-up aimed at promoting constructive engagement and self-determination to access the preferred stimuli. Specifically, both children were equipped with a two membrane sensor embedded in a small box-like structure inside the participant's right hand. The outer membrane of the sensor (i.e. the one facing to the fingers) was a touch-sensitive layer and was activated by a simple contact of the fingers. The inner membrane was applied with a 20 g pressure handled by the participants. The microswitch was connected to a computer system through an interface. The first page of the system presented four boxes, automatically encircled and scanned. That is, a boy who was singing, a boy who was watching a video, a boy who was getting cold and a boy who was asking for his mother. Selecting the song box (i.e. by responding and consequently activating the microswitch) a new window (page) with five different songs was consequently open. By selecting one of them, participants were then provided with a new page asking them to confirm (that is YES and NO responses available) their choice. Finally, the preferred item was available for 10 seconds. Results showed that both participants increased their performance during the intervention phase and the effectiveness of the rehabilitative program was formally endorsed by 60 raters in a social validation assessment.

2.7. Microswitch and Literacy Process

This section deals with the opportunity to provide access to the literacy process for those children who have no intellectual disabilities but are confined to a bed or wheelchair, due to their extensive motor impairments. They are unable to produce understandable verbal utterances, as a consequence, for example, of a tracheotomy practiced for medical reasons. The prerequisite is that the individual has previously acquired literacy skills before the intervention program, since the latter one does not teach the literacy but enables the individual to access the process (Lancioni et al., 2007). Usually, the technology includes a microswitch depending on the behavioral response that needs to be detected, a computer system with a word processor, a keyboard emulator and an interface connecting the microswitch to the computer. Typically, in the upper panel of a monitor provided in front of the participant, a word page is available to write down desired words, while in the lower panel of the monitor a keyboard emulator is also available, with rows and letters automatically encircled and scanned, according to a predefined time (e.g. 2 seconds), depending on participant's skills. That is, to write down a word, the participant is requested to activate the microswitch by exhibiting the behavioral response. Five studies are included in this section (Chiapparino, Stasolla, De Pace, & Lancioni, 2011; Lancioni er al., 2007d, 2009f, 2010c, Stasolla, Caffò, et al., 2015), with nine participants involved.

For example, Lancioni et al. (2009f) assessed the use of a voice-detecting sensor interfaced with a scanning keyboard emulator to allow two boys with extensive motor disabilities to write. Specifically, the study (a) compared the effects of the voice-detecting sensor with those of a familiar pressure sensor on the boys' writing time, (b) checked which of the sensors the boys preferred, and (c) conducted a social validation assessment of the boys' performance with the two sensors, employing psychology students as raters. The difference in the boys' overall mean writing time per letter across sensors was, by the end of the study, about 1.5 s. This difference favored the pressure sensor for one of the boys and the voice-detecting sensor for the other boy. Both boys showed preferences for the voice- detecting sensor. Moreover, the psychology students involved in the social validation assessment indicated that such sensors were more satisfactory, suitable, and educationally relevant than the pressure sensor, and represented the solution that they, as raters, supported more.

Lancioni et al. (2010b) assessed the effectiveness and acceptability of microswitch technology and a keyboard emulator to enable a girl with extensive neuro-motor disabilities to write words. The participant, aged 12, used the sliding movement and panel and a vocalization response with a voice-detecting microswitch. The sliding movement allowed her to light up the keyboard and select the letters and the vocalization to perform the scanning. The girl showed better performance (i.e. shorter writing time) and less tiring performance with the new technology, instead of the traditional available to her before the beginning of the study. Furthermore, she preferred using such technology and its effectiveness was corroborated by a social validation assessment involving students as raters.

DISCUSSION

3.1. Empirical Results

The positive outcomes of the studies reviewed and of most of the studies using microswitches and related forms of technology such as VOCAs, microswitch-clusters, and microswitch combined with computer systems, in general, point out the importance of such forms of assistive technology for children with severe/profound developmental disabilities (Lancioni, Singh, O'Reilly, & Sigafoos, 2011; Shih, Chang, & Shih, 2010; Sigafoos et al., 2009). The possibilities of positive results of a rehabilitative intervention such as those described in this overview are definitely higher when (a) the response is in the individual's behavioral repertoire and requires a fairly low level of effort to be performed, (b) the stimulus events are powerful and motivating, and (c) the intervention time is carefully designed and sufficiently protracted to meet the person's learning conditions (Kazdin, 2001; Lancioni et al., 2011; Saunders et al., 2003).

Selecting a suitable response may have different meanings for different participants. For some participants, one may successfully identify fairly simple (typical) movements that do not need to be particularly precise spatially, do not involve any remarkable physical effort, and can provide some obvious types of feedback (e.g., swaying a grid above one's face with small hand movements). For other individuals, one may need to resort to less conventional forms of behavior that may including, vocalizations, eyelid movements, or chin and lip movements (Lancioni, Sigafoos, O'Reilly, & Singh, 2012; Lancioni & Singh, 2014). Selecting the stimulus events that the child can access directly through microswitch responses and the VOCA-mediated events is a crucial step. The selection of stimuli occurs through indirect and direct strategies, such as through observations of the persons within their regular environment, interviews with parents, staff and caregivers, and stimulus preference screening procedures (Crawford & Schuster, 1993; Stasolla et al., 2014). Two cautionary measures that could help maximize the chance of success are represented by (a) the selection and use of more than one event so as to avoid satiation risks, and (b) repetitions of the selection procedures over time to ensure that the events are related to the person's current interest (Kazdin, 2001; Kennedy, 2005; Lancioni & Singh, 2014; Saunders et al., 2003).

The aforementioned overview and comments primarily emphasize the importance of targeting single, non-typical responses for successful microswitch-based programs. The studies adopting those responses have provided a new level of evidence that is quite encouraging as to the possibility of helping children with very minimal motor behavior learn to control their surrounding environment. These persons would be most unlikely to benefit from intervention programs involving typical motor responses and traditional microswitches (Lancioni et al., 2005; Lancioni & Singh, 2014). Providing these children with the opportunity to be active and to decide about their environmental stimulation effectively and autonomously can be considered highly relevant, in terms of improving the individuals' quality of life as well as from a technical standpoint (Felce & Perry, 1995; Lachapelle et al., 2005; Petry, Maes, & Vlaskamp, 2005; Stasolla et al., 2014). Indeed, the possibility of being constructively engaged and of determining independently the level of stimulation, may increase the person's overall satisfaction, improve his or her general mood, and enhance his or her social image and status (Browder, Wood, Test, Karvonen, & Algozzine, 2001; Karvonen, Test, Wood, Browder, & Algozzine, 2004; Petry et al., 2005; Wehmeyer & Schwartz, 1998; Zekovic & Renwick, 2003).

From a technical point of view, one can underline the relevance of having isolated and successfully targeted small, non-typical responses and having developed viable interfaces (i.e., microswitch devices) to ensure that responses control relevant environmental stimuli. The non-typical responses used in the studies include vocalization, chin and lip movements, eyelid and eyebrow movements, small hand-closure movements, and forehead skin movements. Additional responses or response variations should be examined in order to provide practical alternatives to those mentioned above and thus allow a wider applicability of this approach (i.e., make it suitable to a larger number of participants with different characteristics). For example, one could assess the suitability of full/protracted eyelid closures as target responses for participants for whom such behaviors may be more reliable than double blinks or looking up. Such closures could be monitored with simple adaptations of the optic-microswitch technology previously used for eyelid responses. Similarly, one could target small hand opening movements for participants who tend to have their hands clenched (i.e., keeping the fingers against the palms of their hands). Technically, one could resort to a modified version of the microswitch now available for the hand-closure responses. The new adapted microwsitch would be activated as the person decreases the pressure applied on it or ends the contact with it.

The use of multiple responses through multiple microswitches represents a critical issue in the application of microswitch-based programs. Multiple responses/microswitches enable a child to increase the range of his or her engagement and the variety of sensory input (preferred stimulation) that he or she can access. Various responses are generally matched to different sets of stimuli, and this stimulus differentiation constitutes a useful condition to limit the risks of satiation and saturation. In addition to enjoying the variation of environmental events, the child may also gratify his or her possible preferences for some of the stimuli available by performing the response(s) which are instrumental in accessing them more frequently than the other responses (Cannella, O'Reilly, & Lancioni, 2005; Lancioni et al., 2011; Stafford, Alberto, Fredrick, Heflin, & Heller, 2002). Choice opportunities and self-determined access to the most preferred stimuli may enhance a sense of personal fulfillment, pleasure (expressed in indices of happiness), and strong engagement motivation (Dillon & Carr, 2007; Green & Reid, 1999; Hoch, McComas, Johnson, Faranda, & Guenther, 2002; Kazdin, 2001; Lancioni et al., 2005, 2011; Ross & Oliver 2003).

3.2. Future Perspectives Research

Despite the high potential of programs involving multiple responses with multiple microswitches, one can argue that they do not allow the participant to ask for social contact with the caregiver. With regard to this point, two comments may be appropriate. First, the objection could be realistic when the program includes (a) participants who are used to and obviously enjoy social contact and (b) parents and caregivers who integrate the provision of social contact within their daily schedule. Second, whenever the aforementioned conditions (for participants, parents and caregivers) apply, interventions with multiple microwitches may be modified into programs with combinations of microswitches and VOCAs (Lancioni et al., 2008, 2009; Schlosser & Sigafoos, 2006; Sigafoos et al., 2009). Combining a VOCA to request caregiver attention, mediation or social contact with regular microswitches that allow direct access to environmental stimuli, may be considered a fairly straightforward strategy, as indicated by the studies reviewed earlier (Lancioni et al., 2008, 2009; Lancioni & Singh, 2014). Programs offering the participant the option of asking for caregiver or parent attention/mediation parallel to independent access to preferred stimuli could also justify longer occupational sessions as compared to programs involving only the use of microswitches (and thus excluding contact with the caregiver).

With regard to the microswitch clusters, one may argue that they represent a most constructive and positive approach to helping children with severe/profound multiple disabilities advance in their development. In fact, the use of microswitch clusters serves to integrate the intervention conditions to increase adaptive responding and to reduce problem behavior/posture within the same program. The technology to realize such an approach may be considered reasonably accessible both in terms of complexity and costs.

The studies summarized earlier in this overview were concerned with basic adaptive responses and specific forms of problem behavior or inadequate posture (e.g., hand mouthing, eye poking, and head forward tilting) (Stasolla et al., 2014). Other adaptive responses and other problem behaviors/postures may also be targeted to extend the applicability and relevance of the approach. More extensive forms of the program may also be considered. . For example, one may envision a situation in which the cluster involves two or more microswitches linked to different adaptive responses and one microswitch linked to a problem behavior/posture.

With regard to intervention strategies, connecting a microswitch to a computer system, enabling a child with developmental disabilities and extensive motor impairments, one may argue that these strategies foster communication opportunities for those children. Their passivity, isolation and deprivation hamper their social image, and desirability is significantly reduced, while self-determination, personal active role, and constructive engagement are enhanced. Thus, participants may choose whether to select a preferred item automatically delivered by the system (e.g., a video or a song), to ask for the mediation of parents or caregivers (e.g. when he or she is in pain), or to record his/her personal needs in a word file and to access the literacy process, eventually within the same rehabilitative program. All of these foster the children's communicative potential (Lancioni & Singh, 2014; Stasolla et al., 2014).

Summarizing, this brief/selective overview emphasizes that forms of assistive technology such as microswitches, VOCAs, microswitch clusters, and microswitches combined with computer systems may represent crucial educational and rehabilitative resources for the implementation of behavioral programs for children with severe to profound developmental disabilities in daily contexts. The different applications of the aforementioned forms of technology, while already practical and beneficial, could be advanced profitably. For example, one may envision research initiatives to extend and upgrade the microswitches for monitoring minimal, non-typical responses, namely, to adapt such microswitches to different response situations and make them work with minimal invasion/contact (i.e., realizing devices that do not need to be fixed onto the person's body) (Lancioni et al., 2011; Leung & Chau, 2010). Similarly, one could develop microswitch-cluster programs suitable to help reduce posture problems and the physical deterioration of persons with extensive motor disabilities. These programs could become an effective supplement to physiotherapy and ergonomics (Begnoche & Pitetti, 2007; Leyshon & Shaw, 2008). Moreover, one may enhance the communicative repertoire by proposing combinations of microswitches and computer systems, allowing a child with extensive motor disabilities to request, choose and/or write his/her personal needs.

CONCLUSION

The studies reviewed identify eight intervention approaches to improve the success of children who present with developmental disabilities with various levels of functioning. The outcomes of the studies were largely positive. However, readers should cautiously interpret some of these findings. Indeed, questions emerged about (a) some of the measures used to determine the effects of the intervention and some of the evidence available about them, (b) the lack of control over the time variable characterizing some of the studies, and (c) the absence of direct emphasis on the participants' acquisition of a constructive engagement role. Given the aforementioned criticisms and the consequent caution necessary to interpret part of the available literature, the need to extend the research activity seems necessary. Furthermore, it is indeed crucial to analyze the studies reviewed in terms of (a) their size, (i.e., the quantitative relevance of the changes observed) and (b) their credibility/reliability based on the methodological conditions underlying the programs (Barlow, Nock, & Hersen, 2009; Kazdin, 2001; Kennedy, 2005).

With regard to the first point, one may argue that there were substantial differences among the studies. Many of the studies reported statistically and functionally significant changes in the participants' behavior, which were measured through specific scales or by means of response frequencies (Schiff et al., 2007). Other studies (a) reported changes which were not specifically related to scales or response frequencies but rather to behavioral ratings expressed by professionals involved in the intervention program and other representative figures and/or (b) presented partial, inconclusive or negative statistical evidence on formal measures (Barreca et al., 2003). The outcomes of the studies using single-subject designs could be taken as more solid and reliable, because these designs allow for control over the time (history) variable (Kennedy, 2005). Quantitative relevance and credibility are the two important criteria on which to judge the outcomes. A supplementary criterion could be the practical relevance of changes observed in terms of participants' environmental engagement and interaction involvement. With regard to this criterion, it might be noted that not all the studies code for this outcome, but it is becoming more common.

FUTURE RESEARCH

In line with the above, the following perspectives for future research could be considered. A first research effort could be aimed at evaluating the extension of assistive technologies, such as microswitches for other children with developmental disabilities. Those efforts should take the following into account (a) the extensive literature on the use of this intervention approach in other rehabilitation trades, such as in the area of acquired or congenital pathology; (b) the ethical considerations related to whether and when the participants' legal representatives have the right to decide on the use of such an approach; and (c) the need for methodological sophistication so as to ensure that the contribution of this approach to any performance improvement can be detected beyond doubt. Furthermore, rehabilitative interventions through MBP should consider the individual's involvement in the decision making and his/her positive interaction with the outside world (Lancioni & Singh, 2014).

A second extension may concern the settings, the generalization and the maintenance over time. With respect to the first point, one may design intervention programs in different settings, involving school, home, or community. With respect to the second point, one may consider different tasks, caregivers, research assistants, parents or teachers concerned in the intervention programs. With respect to the third point, one may design maintenance, generalization, and/or post intervention phases systematically within those studies.

A third extension may relate to the technologies. One may project new devices and new technological solutions and options responding to participants' characteristics on the one hand and to contexts' resources on the other. With respect to participants' characteristics, one may examine new technologies that ensure that participants can interact actively with minimal effort while developing new behavioral responses. With respect to the second point, one should consider the financial resources available to families and to rehabilitative centers.

REFERENCES

Assistive Technology Act of 2004, H.R. 4278, 108th Cong. 2004.

Barlow, D. H., Nock, M., & Hersen, M. (2009). *Single case experimental designs: Strategies for studying behavior change* (3rd ed.). New York: Allyn and Bacon.

Barreca, S., Velikonja, D., Brown, L., Williams, L., Davis, L., & Sigouin, C. S. (2003). Evaluation of the effectiveness of two clinical training procedures to elicit yes/no responses from patients with a severe acquired brain injury: A randomized single-subject design. *Brain Injury: [BI]*, *17*(12), 1065–1075. doi:10.1080/0269905031000110535 PMID:14555365

Begnoche, D., & Pitetti, K. H. (2007). Ef- fects of traditional treatment and partial body weight treadmill training on the motor skills of children with spastic cerebral palsy: A pilot study. *Pediatric Physical Therapy*, *19*(1), 11–19. doi:10.1097/01.pep.0000250023.06672.b6 PMID:17304093

Borg, J., Larson, S., & Ostenberg, P. O. (2011). The right to assistive technology: For whom, for what, and by whom? *Disability & Society*, *26*(2), 151–167. doi:10.1080/09687599.2011.543862

Browder, D. M., Wood, W. M., Test, D. W., Karvonen, M., & Algozzine, B. (2001). Reviewing resources on self-determination: A map for teachers. *Remedial and Special Education*, *22*(4), 233–244. doi:10.1177/074193250102200407

Cannella, H. I., O'Reilly, M. F., & Lancioni, G. E. (2005). Choice and preference assessment research with people with severe to profound developmental disabilities: A review of the literature. *Research in Developmental Disabilities*, *26*(1), 1–15. doi:10.1016/j.ridd.2004.01.006 PMID:15590233

Chiapparino, C., Stasolla, F., de Pace, C., & Lancioni, G. E. (2011). A touch pad and a scanning keyboard emulator to facilitate writing by a woman with extensive motor disability. *Life Span and Disdability*, *14*, 45–54.

Crawford, M. R., & Schuster, J. W. (1993). Using microswitches to teach toy use. *Journal of Developmental and Physical Disabilities*, *5*(4), 349–368. doi:10.1007/BF01046391

Dillon, C. M., & Carr, J. E. (2007). Assessing indices of happiness and unhappiness in individuals with developmental disabili- ties: A review. *Behavioral Interventions*, *22*(3), 229–244. doi:10.1002/bin.240

Felce, D., & Perry, J. (1995). Quality of life: Its definition and measurement. *Research in Developmental Disabilities*, *16*(1), 51–74. doi:10.1016/0891-4222(94)00028-8 PMID:7701092

Green, C. W., & Reid, D. H. (1999). A behavioral approach to identifying sources of happiness and unhappiness among individuals with profound multiple disabilities. *Behavior Modification*, *23*(2), 280–293. doi:10.1177/0145445599232006 PMID:10224953

Hoch, H., McComas, J. J., Johnson, L., Faranda, N., & Guenther, S. L. (2002). The effects of magnitude and quality of reinforcement on choice responding during play activities. *Journal of Applied Behavior Analysis*, *35*(2), 171–181. doi:10.1901/jaba.2002.35-171 PMID:12102136

Ivancic, M. T., & Bailey, J. S. (1996). Current limits to reinforcer identification for some persons with profound multiple disabilities. *Research in Developmental Disabilities*, *17*(1), 77–92. doi:10.1016/0891-4222(95)00038-0 PMID:8750077

Kagohara, D. M., Sigafoos, J., Achmadi, D., van der Meer, L., O'Reilly, M. F., & Lancioni, G. E. (2011). Teaching students with developmental disabilities to operate an iPod Touch to listen to music. *Research in Developmental Disabilities*, *32*(6), 2987–2992. doi:10.1016/j.ridd.2011.04.010 PMID:21645989

Karvonen, M., Test, D. W., Wood, W. M., Browder, D., & Algozzine, B. (2004). Putting self-determination into practice. *Exceptional Children*, *71*(1), 23–41. doi:10.1177/001440290407100102

Kazdin, A. E. (2001). *Behavior modification in applied settings* (6th ed.). New York: Wadsworth.

Kennedy, C. (2005). *Single case designs for educational research*. New York: Allyn & Bacon.

Lachapelle, Y., Wehmeyer, M. L., Haelewyck, M. C., Courbois, Y., Keith, K. D., Schalock, R., & Walsh, P. N. et al. (2005). The relationship between quality of life and self-determination: An international study. *Journal of Intellectual Disability Research*, *49*(10), 740–744. doi:10.1111/j.1365-2788.2005.00743.x PMID:16162119

Lancioni, G. E., Antonucci, M., De Pace, C., O'Reilly, M. F., Sigafoos, J., Singh, N. N., & Oliva, D. (2007). Enabling two adolescents with multiple disabilities to choose among environmental stimuli through different procedural and technological approaches. *Perceptual and Motor Skills*, *105*(2), 362–372. doi:10.2466/pms.105.2.362-372 PMID:18065057

Lancioni, G. E., Bellini, D., Oliva, D., Singh, N. N., O'Reilly, M. F., Lang, R., & Didden, R. (2011). Camera-based microswitch technology to monitor mouth, eyebrow, and eyelid responses of children with profound multiple disabilities. *Journal of Behavioral Education*, *20*(1), 4–14. doi:10.1007/s10864-010-9117-2

Lancioni, G. E., Bellini, D., Oliva, D., Singh, N. N., O'Reilly, M. F., & Sigafoos, J. (2010). Camera-based microswitch technology for eyelid and mouth responses of persons with profound multiple disabilities: Two case studies. *Research in Developmental Disabilities, 31*(6), 1509–1514. doi:10.1016/j.ridd.2010.06.006 PMID:20598501

Lancioni, G. E., O'Reilly, M., Singh, N., Green, V., Chiapparino, C., De Pace, C., & Stasolla, F. et al. (2010c). Use of microswitch technology and a keyboard emulator to support literacy performance of persons with extensive neuro-motor disabilities. *Developmental Neurorehabilitation, 13*(4), 248–257. doi:10.3109/17518423.2010.485596 PMID:20629591

Lancioni, G. E., O'Reilly, M. F., Singh, N. N., Buonocunto, F., Sacco, V., Colonna, F., & Bosco, A. et al. (2009). Technology-based intervention options for post-coma persons with minimally conscious state and pervasive motor disabilities. *Developmental Neurorehabilitation, 12*(1), 24–31. doi:10.1080/17518420902776995 PMID:19283531

Lancioni, G. E., O'Reilly, M. F., Singh, N. N., Green, V. A., Oliva, D., Campodonico, F., & Buono, S. et al. (2013a). Technology-aided programs to support exercise of adaptive head responses or leg-foot and hands responses in children with multiple disabilities. *Developmental Neurorehabilitation, 16*(4), 237–244. doi:10.3109/17518423.2012.757661 PMID:23323848

Lancioni, G. E., O'Reilly, M. F., Singh, N. N., Oliva, D., Coppa, M. M., & Montironi, G. (2005). A new microswitch to enable a boy with minimal motor behavior to control environmental stimulation with eye blinks. *Behavioral Interventions, 20*(2), 147–153. doi:10.1002/bin.185

Lancioni, G. E., O'Reilly, M. F., Singh, N. N., Sigafoos, J., Didden, R., Oliva, D., & Groeneweg, J. et al. (2009b). Persons with multiple disabilities accessing stimulation and requesting social contact via microswitch and VOCA devices: New research evaluation and social validation. *Research in Developmental Disabilities, 30*(5), 1084–1094. doi:10.1016/j.ridd.2009.03.004 PMID:19361954

Lancioni, G. E., O'Reilly, M. F., Singh, N. N., Sigafoos, J., Oliva, D., Alberti, G., & Lang, R. et al. (2013). Technology-based programs to support adaptive responding and reduce hand mouthing in two persons with multiple disabilities. *Journal of Developmental and Physical Disabilities, 25*(1), 65–77. doi:10.1007/s10882-012-9303-3

Lancioni, G. E., O'Reilly, M. F., Singh, N. N., Sigafoos, J., Oliva, D., Baccani, S., & Stasolla, F. et al. (2004b). Technological aids to promote basic developmental achievements by children with multiple disabilities: Evaluation of two cases. *Cognitive Processing, 5*(4), 232–238. doi:10.1007/s10339-004-0030-2

Lancioni, G. E., O'Reilly, M. F., Singh, N. N., Sigafoos, J., Oliva, D., & Severini, L. (2008b). Enabling two persons with multiple disabilities to access environmental stimuli and ask for social contact through microswitches and a VOCA. *Research in Developmental Disabilities, 29*(1), 21–28. doi:10.1016/j.ridd.2006.10.001 PMID:17174529

Lancioni, G. E., O'Reilly, M. F., Singh, N. N., Sigafoos, J., Oliva, D., & Severini, L. (2008c). Three persons with multiple disabilities accessing environmental stimuli and asking for social contact through microswitch and VOCA technology. *Journal of Intellectual Disability Research, 52*(4), 327–336. doi:10.1111/j.1365-2788.2007.01024.x PMID:18339095

Lancioni, G. E., O'Reilly, M. F., Singh, N. N., Sigafoos, J., Oliva, D., Smaldone, A., & Chiapparino, C. et al. (2009c). Persons with multiple disabilities access stimulation and contact the caregiver via microswitch and VOCA technology. *Life Span and Disability, 12,* 119–128.

Lancioni, G. E., O'Reilly, M. F., Singh, N. N., Sigafoos, J., Oliva, D., Smaldone, A., & Chirico, M. et al. (2011b). Technology-assisted programs for promoting leisure or communication engagement in two persons with pervasive motor or multiple disabilities. *Disability and Rehabilitation. Assistive Technology, 6*(2), 108–114. doi:10.3109/17483107.2010.496524 PMID:20545564

Lancioni, G. E., O'Reilly, M. F., Singh, N. N., Sigafoos, J., Tota, A., Antonucci, M., & Oliva, D. (2006). Children with multiple disabilities and minimal motor behavior using chin movements to operate microswitches to obtain environmental stimulation. *Research in Developmental Disabilities, 27*(3), 290–298. doi:10.1016/j.ridd.2005.02.003 PMID:16005183

Lancioni, G. E., O'Reilly, M. F., Singh, N. N., Stasolla, F., Manfredi, F., & Oliva, D. (2004a). Adapting a grid into a microswitch to suit simple hand movements of a child with profound multiple disabilities. *Perceptual and Motor Skills, 99*(2), 724–728. doi:10.2466/pms.99.2.724-728 PMID:15560365

Lancioni, G. E., Olivetti Belardinelli, M., Stasolla, F., Singh, N. N., O'Reilly, M. F., Sigafoos, J., & Angelillo, M. T. (2008a). Promoting engagement, requests and choice by a man with post-coma pervasive motor impairment and minimally conscious state through a technology-based program. *Journal of Developmental and Physical Disabilities, 20*(4), 379–388. doi:10.1007/s10882-008-9104-x

Lancioni, G. E., Sigafoos, J., O'Reilly, M. F., & Singh, N. N. (2012). *Assistive Technology, Interventions for Individuals with Severe/Profound and Multiple Disabilities.* New York: Springer.

Lancioni, G. E., Sigafoos, J., O'Reilly, M. F., & Singh, N. N. (2012). *Assistive technology: interventions for individual with severe/profound and multiple disabilities.* New York: Springer.

Lancioni, G. E., & Singh, N. N. (2014). *Assistive technologies for people with diverse abilities.* New York: Springer. doi:10.1007/978-1-4899-8029-8

Lancioni, G. E., Singh, N. N., O'Reilly, M. F., Campodonico, F., Oliva, D., & Vigo, C. M. (2005b). Promoting walker-assisted step responses by an adolescent with multiple disabilities through automatically delivered stimulation. *Journal of Visual Impairment & Blindness, 99,* 109–113.

Lancioni, G. E., Singh, N. N., O'Reilly, M. F., Campodonico, F., Piazzolla, G., Scalini, L., & Oliva, D. (2005a). Impact of favorite stimuli automatically delivered on step responses of persons with multiple disabilities during their use of walker devices. *Research in Developmental Disabilities, 26*(1), 71–76. doi:10.1016/j.ridd.2004.04.003 PMID:15590239

Lancioni, G. E., Singh, N. N., O'Reilly, M. F., Green, V. A., Oliva, D., Buonocunto, F., & Di Nuovo, S. et al. (2012b). Technology-based programs to support forms of leisure engagement and communication for persons with multiple disabilities: Two single-case studies. *Developmental Neurorehabilitation, 15*(3), 209–218. doi:10.3109/17518423.2012.666766 PMID:22582852

Lancioni, G. E., Singh, N. N., O'Reilly, M. F., & Oliva, D. (2005). Microswitch programs for persons with multiple disabilities: An overview of the responses adopted for microswitch activation. *Cognitive Processing, 6*(3), 177–188. doi:10.1007/s10339-005-0003-0 PMID:18231820

Lancioni, G. E., Singh, N. N., O'Reilly, M. F., Oliva, D., & Basili, G. (2005). An overview of research on increasing indices of happiness of people with severe/profound intellectual and multiple disabilities. *Disability and Rehabilitation, 27*(3), 83–93. doi:10.1080/09638280400007406 PMID:15823988

Lancioni, G. E., Singh, N. N., O'Reilly, M. F., Oliva, D., Smaldone, A., Tota, A., & Groeneweg, J. et al. (2006). Assessing the effects of stimulation versus microswitch-based programmes on indices of happiness of students with multiple disabilities. *Journal of Intellectual Disability Research, 50*(10), 739–747. doi:10.1111/j.1365-2788.2006.00839.x PMID:16961703

Lancioni, G. E., Singh, N. N., O'Reilly, M. F., & Sgafoos, J. (2011). Assistive technology for behavioral interventions for persons with severe/profound multiple disabilities: A selective overview. *European Journal of Behavior Analysis, 12*, 7–26.

Lancioni, G. E., Singh, N. N., O'Reilly, M. F., Sigaffos, J., Chiapparino, C., Stasolla, F., & Oliva, D. (2007d). Using an optic sensor and a scanning keyboard emulator to facilitate writing by persons with pervasive motor disabilities. *Journal of Developmental and Physical Disabilities, 19*(6), 593–603. doi:10.1007/s10882-007-9073-5

Lancioni, G. E., Singh, N. N., O'Reilly, M. F., Sigafoos, J., Alberti, G., Perilli, V., & Groeneweg, J. et al. (2014a). People with multiple disabilities learn to engage in occupation and work activities with the support of technology-aided programs. *Research in Developmental Disabilities, 35*(6), 1264–1271. doi:10.1016/j.ridd.2014.03.026 PMID:24685943

Lancioni, G. E., Singh, N. N., O'Reilly, M. F., Sigafoos, J., Buonocunto, F., Sacco, V., & De Pace, C. et al. (2009a). Two persons with severe post-coma motor impairment and minimally conscious state use assistive technology to access stimulus events and social contact. *Disability and Rehabilitation. Assistive Technology, 4*(5), 367–372. doi:10.1080/17483100903038584 PMID:19565377

Lancioni, G. E., Singh, N. N., O'Reilly, M. F., Sigafoos, J., Didden, R., & Oliva, D. (2009d). A technology-based stimulation program to reduce hand mouthing by an adolescent with multiple disabilities. *Perceptual and Motor Skills, 109*(2), 478–486. doi:10.2466/pms.109.2.478-486 PMID:20038002

Lancioni, G. E., Singh, N. N., O'Reilly, M. F., Sigafoos, J., Didden, R., & Oliva, D. (2009e). Two boys with multiple disabilities increasing adaptive responding and curbing dystonic/spastic behavior via a microswitch-based program. *Research in Developmental Disabilities, 30*(2), 378–385. doi:10.1016/j.ridd.2008.07.005 PMID:18760566

Lancioni, G. E., Singh, N. N., O'Reilly, M. F., Sigafoos, J., Didden, R., Oliva, D., & Cingolani, E. (2008d). A girl with multiple disabilities increases object manipulation and reduces hand mouthing through a microswitch-based program. *Clinical Case Studies, 7*(3), 238–249. doi:10.1177/1534650107307478

Lancioni, G. E., Singh, N. N., O'Reilly, M. F., Sigafoos, J., Green, V., Chiapparino, C., & Oliva, D. et al. (2009f). A voice detecting sensor and a scanning keyboard emuloator to support word writing by two boys with extensive motor disabilities. *Research in Developmental Disabilities, 30*(2), 203–209. doi:10.1016/j.ridd.2008.03.001 PMID:18417320

Lancioni, G. E., Singh, N. N., O'Reilly, M. F., Sigafoos, J., Oliva, D., & Basili, G. (2012). New rehabilitation opportunities for persons with multiple disabilities through the use of microswitch technology. In S. Federici & M. J. Scherer (Eds.), *Assistive technology assessment handbook* (pp. 399–419). New York: CRC Press.

Lancioni, G. E., Singh, N. N., O'Reilly, M. F., Sigafoos, J., Oliva, D., Piazzolla, G., & Manfredi, F. et al. (2007c). Automatically delivered stimulation for walker-assisted step responses: Measuring its effects in persons with multiple disabilities. *Journal of Developmental and Physical Disabilities*, *19*(1), 1–13. doi:10.1007/s10882-006-9030-8

Lancioni, G. E., Singh, N. N., O'Reilly, M. F., Sigafoos, J., Oliva, D., Scalini, L., & Di Bari, M. et al. (2007b). Promoting foot-leg movements in children with multiple disabilities through the use of support devices and technology for regulating contingent stimulation. *Cognitive Processing*, *8*(4), 279–283. doi:10.1007/s10339-007-0179-6 PMID:17680286

Lancioni, G. E., Singh, N. N., O'Reilly, M. F., Sigafoos, J., Oliva, D., & Severini, L. et al.. (2007d). Microswitch technology to promote adaptive responses and reduce mouthing in two children with multiple disabilities. *Journal of Visual Impairment & Blindness*, *101*, 628–636.

Lancioni, G. E., Singh, N. N., O'Reilly, M. F., Sigafoos, J., Oliva, D., Smaldone, A., & Groeneweg, J. et al. (2010a). Promoting ambulation responses among children with multiple disabilities through walkers and microswitches with contingent stimuli. *Research in Developmental Disabilities*, *31*(3), 811–816. doi:10.1016/j.ridd.2010.02.006 PMID:20207105

Leung, B., & Chau, T. (2010). A multiple camera tongue switch for a child with severe spastic quadriplegic cerebral palsy. *Disability and Rehabilitation. Assistive Technology*, *5*(1), 58–68. doi:10.3109/17483100903254561 PMID:19941441

Leyshon, R. T., & Shaw, L. E. (2008). Using the ICF as a conceptual framework to guide ergonomic intervention in occu- pational rehabilitation. *Work (Reading, Mass.)*, *31*, 47–61. PMID:18820420

Lontis, E. R., & Struijk, L. N. (2010). Design of inductive sensors for tongue control system for computers and assistive devices. *Disability and Rehabilitation. Assistive Technology*, *5*(4), 266–271. doi:10.3109/17483101003718138 PMID:20307253

Petry, K., Maes, B., & Vlaskamp, C. (2005). Domains of quality of life of people with profound multiple disabilities: The perspective of parents and direct support staff. *Journal of Applied Research in Intellectual Disabilities*, *18*(1), 35–46. doi:10.1111/j.1468-3148.2004.00209.x

Reichle, J. (2011). Evaluating assistive technology in the education of persons with severe disabilities. *Journal of Behavioral Education*, *20*(1), 77–85. doi:10.1007/s10864-011-9121-1

Ross, E., & Oliver, C. (2003). The assess- ment of mood in adults who have severe or profound mental retardation. *Clinical Psychology Review*, *23*(2), 225–245. doi:10.1016/S0272-7358(02)00202-7 PMID:12573671

Saunders, M. D., Timler, G. R., Cullinan, T. B., Pilkey, S., Questad, K. A., & Saunders, R. R. (2003). Evidence of contingency awareness in people with profound multiple impairments: Response duration versus response rate indicators. *Research in Developmental Disabilities*, 24(4), 231–245. doi:10.1016/S0891-4222(03)00040-4 PMID:12873657

Schiff, N. D., Giacino, J. T., Kalmar, K., Victor, J. D., Baker, K., Gerber, M., & Rezai, A. R. et al. (2007). Behavioural improvements with thalamic stimulation after severe traumatic brain injury. *Nature*, 448(7153), 600–603. doi:10.1038/nature06041 PMID:17671503

Schlosser, R., & Sigafoos, J. (2006). Augmentative and alternative communication interventions for persons with developmental disabilities: Narrative review of comparative single-subject experimental studies. *Research in Developmental Disabilities*, 27(1), 1–29. doi:10.1016/j.ridd.2004.04.004 PMID:16360073

Shih, C. H., Chang, M. L., & Shih, C. T. (2010). A new limb movement detector enabling people with multiple disabilities to control environmental stimulation through limb swing with a gyration air mouse. *Research in Developmental Disabilities*, 31(4), 875–880. doi:10.1016/j.ridd.2010.01.020 PMID:20381996

Sigafoos, J., Green, V. A., Payne, D., Son, S. H., O'Reilly, M. F., & Lancioni, G. E. (2009). A comparison of picture exchange and speech-generating devices: Acquisition, preference, and effects on social interaction. *Augmentative and Alternative Communication*, 25(2), 99–109. doi:10.1080/07434610902739959 PMID:19444681

Stafford, A. M., Alberto, P. M., Fredrick, L. D., Heflin, L. J., & Heller, K. W. (2002). Preference variability and the instruction of choice making with students with severe intellectual disabilities. *Education and Training in Mental Retardation and Developmental Disabilities*, 37, 70–88.

Stasolla, F., & Caffò, A. O. (2013). Promoting adaptive behaviors by two girls with Rett Syndrome through a microswitch-based program. *Research in Autism Spectrum Disorders*, 7(10), 1265–1272. doi:10.1016/j.rasd.2013.07.010

Stasolla, F., Caffò, A. O., Damiani, R., Perilli, V., Di Leone, A., & Albano, V. (2015). Assistive technology-based programs to promote communication and leisure activities by three children emerged from a minimal conscious state. *Cognitive Processing*, 16(1), 69–78. doi:10.1007/s10339-014-0625-1 PMID:25077461

Stasolla, F., Caffò, A. O., Picucci, L., & Bosco, A. (2013). Assistive technology for promoting choice behaviors in three children with cerebral palsy and severe communication impairments. *Research in Developmental Disabilities*, 34(9), 2694–2700. doi:10.1016/j.ridd.2013.05.029 PMID:23770888

Stasolla, F., Damiani, R., Perilli, V., Di Leone, A., Albano, V., Stella, A., & Damato, C. (2014). Technological supports to promote choice opportunities by two boys with fragile X syndrome and severe to profound developmental disabilities. *Research in Developmental Disabilities*, 35(11), 2993–3000. doi:10.1016/j.ridd.2014.07.045 PMID:25118066

Stasolla, F., & De Pace, C. (2014). Assistive technology to promote leisure and constructive engagement by two boys emerged from a minimal conscious state. *NeuroRehabilitation*, 35, 253–259. PMID:24990021

Stasolla, F., Perilli, V., Damiani, R., Caffò, A. O., Di Leone, A., Albano, V., & Damato, C. et al. (2014). A microswitch-cluster program to enhance object manipulation and to reduce hand mouthing by three children with autism spectrum disorders and intellectual disabilities. *Research in Autism Spectrum Disorders, 8*(9), 1071–1078. doi:10.1016/j.rasd.2014.05.016

Wehmeyer, M. L., & Schwartz, M. (1998). The relationship between self-determina-tion, quality of life, and life satisfaction for adults with mental retardation. *Education and Training in Mental Retardation and Developmental Disabilities, 33*, 3–12.

Zekovic, B., & Renwick, R. (2003). Quality of life for children and adolescents with developmental disabilities: Review of conceptual and methodological issues relevant to public policy. *Disability & Society, 18*(1), 19–34. doi:10.1080/713662199

ADDITIONAL READING

De Pace, C., & Stasolla, F. (2013). Promoting environmental control, social interaction and leisure/academyengagement among people with severe/profound multiple disabilities through assistive technology. In G. Kouroupetroglou (ed.) Assistive technologies and computer access for motor disabilities (pp. 285-319). Hershey: Medical Information Science Reference (IGI Global).

Lancioni, G. E., Comes, M. L., Stasolla, F., & Manfredi, F. (2005). A microswitch cluster to enhance arm-lifting responses without dystonic head Tilting by a child with multiple disabilities. *Perceptual and Motor Skills, 100*(3), 892–894. doi:10.2466/PMS.100.3.892-894 PMID:16060461

Lancioni, G. E., O'Reilly, M. F., Singh, N. N., Sigafoos, J., Oliva, D., Montironi, G., & Bosco, A. et al. (2005). Extending the evaluation of a computer system used as microswitch for word utterances of persons with multiple disabilities. *Journal of Intellectual Disability Research, 49*(9), 639–646. doi:10.1111/j.1365-2788.2005.00698.x PMID:16108981

Lancioni, G. E., Singh, N. N., O' Reilly, M. F., la Martire, M. L., Stasolla, F., Smaldone, A., & Oliva, D. (2006). Microswitch-based programs as therapeutic recreation interventions for students with profound multiple disabilities. *American Journal of Recreation Therapy, 5*, 15–20.

Lancioni, G. E., Singh, N. N., O'Reilly, M. F., & Oliva, D. (2004c). A microswitch program including words and choice opportunities for students with multiple disabilities. *Perceptual and Motor Skills, 98*(1), 214–222. doi:10.2466/pms.98.1.214-222 PMID:15058884

Lancioni, G. E., Singh, N. N., O'Reilly, M. F., Sigafoos, J., Didden, R., Manfredi, F., & Basili, G. et al. (2009). Fostering locomotor behavior of children with developmental disabilities: An overview of studies using treadmills and walkers with microswitches. *Research in Developmental Disabilities, 30*(2), 308–322. doi:10.1016/j.ridd.2008.05.002 PMID:18573637

Lancioni, G. E. O., Reilly, M. F., Singh, N. N., Sigafoos, J., Chiapparino, C., Stasolla, F., & Oliva, D. et al. (2007). Enabling a Young man with minimal motor behavior to manage indipendently his leisure television engagement. *Perceptual and Motor Skills, 104*(1), 47–54. doi:10.2466/pms.105.1.47-54 PMID:17918548

KEY TERMS AND DEFINITIONS

Assistive Technology: is an umbrella term that includes assistive, adaptive, and rehabilitative devices for people with disabilities and also includes the process used in selecting, locating, and using them. Assistive technology promotes greater independence by enabling people to perform tasks that they were formerly unable to accomplish, or had great difficulty accomplishing, by providing enhancements to, or changing methods of interacting with, the technology needed to accomplish such tasks.

Autism Spectrum Disorders: Group of pervasive developmental disabilities that can cause significant social, communication and behavioral challenges, added to intellectual disabilities and stereotypies.

Cerebral palsy: Disorder of the development of movement and posture, causing activity limitations attributed to nonprogressive disturbances of the fetal or infant brain that may also affect sensation, perception, cognition, communication, and behavior.

Coma: State of unconsciousness lasting more than six hours, in which a person: cannot be awakened; fails to respond normally to painful stimuli, light, or sound; lacks a normal sleep-wake cycle; and, does not initiate voluntary actions.

Indices of Happiness: Behavioral expressions of happiness (i.e., smiling, laughing, energized body movements with or without vocalizations) detected among non verbal individuals as outcome measure of quality of life within a microswitch-based program.

Microswitches: Technological Devices (e.g. optic, pressure, tilt) ensuring an individual with multiple disabilities to access independently and autonomously to environmental preferred stimuli, through a control system unit.

Multiple Disabilities: Combination of intellectual, motor, communication, and/or sensory disabilities (impairments). A person with multiple disabilities has a very low behavioral repertoire, minimal independent responses and is totally dependent from others (e.g. parents and caregivers).

Quality of Life: Multidimensional construct categorized within five dimensions. That is, physical wellbeing, material wellbeing, social wellbeing, emotional wellbeing, and development and activity.

Rett syndrome: Progressive Neuro-developmental disorder, due to genetic mutations, that can cause severe to profound multiple and/or developmental disabilities.

Chapter 10
Improving Students' Academic Learning by Helping Them Access Text

Michael Ben-Avie
SCSU Center of Excellence on Autism Spectrum Disorders, USA

Régine Randall
Southern Connecticut State University, USA

Diane Weaver Dunne
Connecticut Radio Information System, USA

Chris Kelly
Connecticut Radio Information System, USA

ABSTRACT

Conventional methods of addressing the needs of students with print disabilities include text-to-speech services. One major drawback of text-to-speech technologies is that computerized speech simply articulates the same words in a text whereas human voice can convey emotions such as excitement, sadness, fear, or joy. Audiobooks have human narration, but are designed for entertainment and not for teaching word identification, fluency, vocabulary, and comprehension to students. This chapter focuses on the 3-year pilot of CRISKids; all CRIS recordings feature human narration. The pilot demonstrated that students who feel competent in their reading and class work tend to be more engaged in classroom routines, spend more time on task and demonstrate greater comprehension of written materials. When more demonstrate these behaviors and skills, teachers are better able to provide meaningful instruction, since less time is spent on issues of classroom management and redirection. Thus, CRISKids impacts not only the students with print disabilities, but all of the students in the classroom.

DEFINITION OF A PRINT DISABILITY

The definition of a print disability is a condition that prevents individuals from gaining information from printed materials, at anticipated levels, and requires the use of alternative access methods or specialized formats such as Braille, large print, audio, or digital text to access that information. This definition includes individuals with a visual, physical, perceptual, developmental, cognitive, or learning disability (Kerscher, 2002). The Higher Education Opportunity Act defines "print disabled" as "a student with

DOI: 10.4018/978-1-4666-8395-2.ch010

a disability who experiences barriers to accessing instructional material in non-specialized formats, including an individual described in Title 17 of the Copyright Act" (H.R. 4137: Higher Education Opportunity Act," 110th Congress, 2007-2009). The definition includes physical limitations that could be the result of a spinal cord injury, cerebral palsy, traumatic brain injury, a neurological condition, etc. (e.g., students who cannot physically hold or manipulate a book).

The 2004 reauthorization of IDEA (Section CFR 300.172) added the requirement that states and local education agencies must ensure that **"accessible instructional materials"** are provided to students with print disabilities in a timely manner. The Chafee Amendment (Public Law 104-197) allows authorized entities to reproduce recordings of previously published nondramatic literary works in specialized formats for those who are blind or have print-disabilities without the need to pay royalties (i.e., the recordings are not an infringement on copyright). Using the most *conservative* estimate of the number of K-12 students in the U.S. with print disabilities based on the "copyright exemption" and the number who qualify for accessible instructional materials, last year there were 2,004,000 students (this estimate was based on figures provided by Connecticut's Bureau of Special Education). **The number is most likely far higher because students present multiple disabilities**. For example, last year in Connecticut 4,941 students with learning disabilities also qualified as having a print disability so there is an overlap in who may need certain accommodations. Annually, the American Printing House for the Blind (APH) polls each state for data on the number of legally blind children (through age 21) enrolled in elementary and secondary schools in the U.S. eligible to receive free reading materials in Braille, large print, or audio format. This is used to develop a "quota" of federal funds to be spent in each state for materials in each alternative format. Based on the APH polls and the above data, the range of students with print disabilities is from 2,004,000 to 3,500,000.

In schools, a "reading disability" is generally conceptualized in three ways: word-based/dyslexia, specific comprehension, and mixed (Allington & McGill-Franzen, 2009). In word-based or dyslexic-type disability, students can understand age-appropriate text when it is read aloud but continue to have severe difficulties with decoding even after evidence-based instruction/intervention. Other characteristics of this type of disability include but are not limited to difficulty with spelling, writing (dysgraphia), orientation, organization, mathematical operations, and learning a foreign language; yet, despite these difficulties, individuals who experience word-specific disability may also have highly developed memory skills, creative abilities, originality, intuition, and good "people skills." (IDEA, 2014). Students identified with specific comprehension disability can read accurately and fluently but still have difficulty constructing meaning from text. These students are unable to use text to develop their own abilities, improve content area knowledge, solve problems, or apply new learning. They are also less likely to read for pleasure. The last group of students with reading disabilities has both difficulty with word recognition and comprehension.

CRISKIDS™ FOR SCHOOLS, A SCHOOL-BASED INITIATIVE OF CRIS RADIO

As Bill Haberman stuffed envelopes for the Connecticut Radio Information System, Inc. (CRIS), a 36-year-old nonprofit that provides audio recordings for people who are blind or cannot read print materials due to a disability, he made a suggestion that would set the organization on a new path. Haberman, a retired special education teacher, is one of the 300 CRIS volunteers, most of whom provide the voice talent for the audio recordings of articles featured in more than 70 newspapers and magazines.

Teachers struggle to provide timely access to print materials for students facing the challenges of a print disability, said Haberman. While acknowledging that CRIS had achieved an important milestone by becoming the only service in the nation to provide an extensive line-up of on-demand audio versions of children's magazines—all featuring human narration—he explained that teachers also needed recordings of specific curriculum materials. If CRIS could also offer custom recordings and turn them around in a prompt and suitable manner, teachers would be thrilled, he suggested. Further, current teacher evaluation models are, in part, based on the identification of student learning objectives that are specific to progress toward a grade level goal or content area standards. Students with special needs often experience considerable difficulty meeting criteria that were conceptualized based on general academic competencies. In fact, the use of reading, writing, and critical thinking rubrics in place at many schools does have many students with individualized education plans for language-based disability performing at the lowest levels because these measures do not take into account the special needs of these learners. Rubrics of this sort assume that certain skills are already in place and do not necessarily show growth for students who are making progress in a variety of skills although they are still below grade level when compared to their classmates. Making the growth of these students with disability "invisible" because they fall short of grade-level expectations or benchmarks articulated in the Common Core State Standards is at odds with the spirit of IDEA and best practice. To that end, CRIS allows teachers to differentiate materials for students whose reading abilities may interfere with their achievement of specific academic goals; yet, this is only the first step. Teachers must become accustomed to using digital texts as teaching tools. It is the considered and thoughtful combination/application of both adaptive technology and instructional practices that facilitate student achievement.

CRIS Radio

Volunteers at CRIS broadcast 24 hours a day, seven days a week in a state-of-the-art digital broadcast center located near Hartford, Connecticut. CRIS was incorporated in 1978 and broadcasted its first program in 1979, featuring two hours of news featured in *The Hartford Courant*, the state's newspaper of record, on the subcarrier frequency of WJMJ, the radio station operated by the Roman Catholic Diocese of Hartford. CRIS has consistently expanded its service throughout its history. In 1983, it extended its two-hour daily broadcast into a 14-hour broadcast, and also extended its reach with the addition of another subcarrier service provided by WPKN, a Bridgeport, Connecticut radio station. In 1984, CRIS began broadcasting 24 hours a day, seven days a week. It continued to expand its reach throughout Connecticut, adding additional radio subcarrier services. In 1988, CRIS added cable TV channels through the second audio program (SAP) channels as a way to increase access to CRIS programs. In 2002, CRIS converted its broadcasts from analog to digital, and in 2009 it began to stream its broadcasts via the Internet. In 2011, CRIS began to offer on-demand programming for a modest subscription fee.

Throughout CRIS Radio's 36-year history, CRIS broadcasts with the help of volunteers who are blind. Among its visually disabled volunteers, some produce live, one-hour broadcasts. They control the microphones for the two, on-air voice talents, cue up the station identification announcements and public service announcements every 15 minutes, and announce the weather forecasts by reading them in Braille during the live broadcast. Other volunteers who are blind also provide their services to CRIS, including serving on the Board of Directors as well as providing customer service and outreach to new listeners.

Expanding CRIS Radio's Services to Schools

Bill Haberman, the CRIS volunteer described above, suggested expanding CRIS Radio's services to schools by offering custom recordings to teachers. Based on Haberman's recommendation, CRIS staff explored the audio services currently available to educators. They evaluated various audio services that provide computerized text-to-speech recordings, as well as those that offer human narration. One of the major drawbacks of current audio services is the lengthy time it takes to record a text. In contrast, CRIS, with its extensive roster of volunteers including many voice-over, radio, and television on-air professionals, could make the recordings available quickly. This quick turn-around would ensure that both students who qualify for special services and students with print disabilities would have the opportunity to access the same classroom materials made available to their classmates within a timely manner. A byproduct is the more meaningful inclusion in regular classes of students who qualify for special services.

Haberman's suggestion shaped the development of CRISKids™ for Schools. Launched in November 2012, CRISKids provides custom recordings requested by classroom teachers in addition to its extensive line-up of children's magazines. The custom recordings also can be shared by and with educators from other schools and school districts. CRIS Radio's goal regarding custom recordings is to create an extensive audio library of classroom materials that provides instant access in the classroom. The CRISKids for Schools Audio Library was made available on-demand from any Internet accessible computer or mobile device.

Participating teachers now have the opportunity to receive custom recordings featuring human narration, of academic print materials such as curricular units within 10 business days, a dramatic improvement over the lengthy delay provided by other services offering human narration. Teachers participating in the current CRISKids three-year pilot generally download the recordings from a computer onto an MP3 player (in the future, tablets may be used).

A few months following the official launch of CRISKids™ for Schools, in Spring 2013, Justin Gussy, assistive technology director for Vernon Public Schools, made yet another suggestion that would also shape the development of children's programming. He advised CRIS Radio to record the text exemplars identified in the K-12 Common Core State Standards resulting in the creation of another unique addition to the CRISKids Audio Library that includes the Common Core State Standards. Within a few months, CRIS had completed recordings of nearly 75 percent of the Language Art component of the Common Core, creating the only extensive audio library of educational materials of the Common Core in the nation that features human voice. Supported by its recent construction in 2009 of a state-of-the-art digital broadcast center and the dedication and talent of more than 300 volunteers, CRIS was able to ramp up its children's programming within 10 months. Expansion of children's programming is allowing CRIS Radio to increase its service while keeping true to its mission of providing high quality audio access for people who are blind or print disabled. Within 15 months from launching CRISKids for Schools, the new program had attracted more than 20 schools to participate in its pilot.

In 2012, with the ability to create an extensive audio library for children easily accessible through an Internet connection and the fast adoption of smartphones and tablets, CRIS received two, three-year foundation grants – The Gibney Family Foundation and the Hartford Foundation for Public Giving – to develop its CRISKids for Schools program. It also received several smaller foundation grants to support various components of the program, such as the purchase of MP3 players and sponsorships of CRISKids for Schools' subscriptions for schools.

During the initial introduction of CRISKids for Schools, teachers integrated the service into their classroom in different ways. Some used it for required classroom assignments while others used it for independent reading assignments within the classroom and at home. Others also utilized the service as part of their summer reading program. Teachers also differed in how they utilized the MP3 recordings: in the classroom, in the special education room and in a combination of general and special education classrooms as well as at home.

In 2013, two additional CRISKids streams were made available for medically vulnerable populations who were not attending school for either short or long periods due to their conditions of care and treatment. The first stream was for elementary-aged patients and the second was for secondary school-aged students; both direct streams were made available from the CRIS Broadcast Center to televisions in each patient room at Connecticut Children's Medical Center, making CRISKids available to 6,800 patients annually. Having some level of continuity in content and materials common to different grade levels is one factor that supports medically fragile students when they, as appropriate, enter or re-acclimate to school settings.

THEORETICAL AND EMPIRICAL SUPPORT, AND THEORY OF CHANGE

Review of Literature

Access to education, as well as the expectation that all students progress in their learning, serve as bedrock principles of the Individuals with Disabilities Education Improvement Act (2004, 1995, 1997). Over time, research has consistently shown that literacy achievement is highly correlated with overall academic success and positive learner outcomes (Hernandez, 2011; Kern & Friedman, 2008; Butler, Marsh, Sheppard, & Sheppard, 1985; Sénéchal & Lefevere, 2002; Stainthorpe & Hughes, 2004). In fact, Snow (2001) considers literacy to be the cornerstone of all other school achievement. Yet, a variety of disabilities (including but not limited to, dyslexia, visual impairment, and attention-deficit) can impede students' ability to acquire literacy skills – the ability to learn to read and then, later, the ability to read to learn (Chall, 1983). Increasing students' access to the texts that they can and want to read, while also providing high quality instruction in the classroom and within intervention settings, has been shown to improve reading achievement in all grade levels, because these supports allow elementary and secondary students to routinely experience high success reading (Allington, 2012; Guthrie, 2000). In light of these findings, understanding what scaffolds are necessary for high success reading undoubtedly includes bringing together students and texts in such a way that every child can contribute to the intellectual work of a classroom and meet the standards for different content areas and technical subjects (Buehl, 2011).

The adoption of the Common Core State Standards across most states in the country has led many schools to realign curriculum, re-evaluate the type of texts students use to learn content, reconsider traditional teaching methods, and offer additional professional development for teachers (Walpole & McKenna, 2013). Although not met with applause by all, the Common Core does underscore the need for children to have multiple literacies in the 21st century and an ability to operate in a world where printed text is only one modality associated with mixed media (Leu et al., 2013; Richards & McKenna, 2003; Biancarosa & Snow, 2006; Kamil, 2003; McKeown, Beck, & Blake, 2009; Vacca, 2002; Bean, 2000; Brozo & Hargis, 2003). Because of this, the use of digital and audio texts is becoming more common for all students – not just those with disability. In fact, performance measures linked to the Common Core actually require students to access, among other things, audio texts in the assessment of comprehension. Perhaps of more importance is that opportunities to use technology often factor into motivation and a student's willingness to engage in the content of a class (Snow, Porche, Tabors & Harris, 2007).

The goal to raise reading achievement and allow students to continually develop as literate thinkers is largely dependent on three areas that can be controlled from within the classroom: ensuring student growth in basic reading skills (word identification, fluency, vocabulary, comprehension), helping students develop a positive reading affect (confident attitude, motivation, self-efficacy), and maintaining ongoing reading support for struggling readers and writers beyond the primary grades (McKenna & Robinson, 2009; ACT, 2008 & 2012; Balfanz, 2009; Darche & Stem, 2013; Snow, Porche, Tabors & Harris, 2007). Reading support begins by assuring that students can access and understand the texts used in their classrooms. The use of books on tape and text-to-speech programs are among the important accommodations offered to students over the last thirty years (Hecker, Elkind, Elkind, & Katz, 2002). Yet, they are not without their limitations. While many text-to-speech programs also offer study features to students (highlighting, bookmarking, annotation), these options only work for students who already have the skills to identify main ideas, supporting details, and other key information—skills learned, generally, through explicit instruction in the classroom. Finally, how something is read impacts what is understood (Rasinski, 2004; 2006; Fox, 2010) and most elements of fluency are best captured through voice narration. In some earlier discussions of fluency, reading rate and reading accuracy were paramount (Wiederholt & Bryant, 2001). Yet, more recent conversations around fluency and comprehension skills highlight tone, prosody, and emphasis--features associated with how "natural language" sounds and the exact features that are most difficult to capture with computerized speech (Rasinski, 2004; 2006). Beyond reading skills and reading scores, however, a very real issue is whether voice narration increases the pleasure that should be part of any student's reading experience (Newkirk, 2012).

On-task and productive reading requires sustained attention, something that is difficult to accomplish if students lack the skills necessary to decode and interpret text (Kupietz, 1990). Students who have undeveloped decoding skills or have other disabilities that interfere with their capacity to manage grade-level print tasks may also have more difficulty following academic routines, engaging in text-dependent conversations, completing assignments, and learning requisite content necessary for advanced study (Gunning, 2014). Ensuring that all students, regardless of ability and past achievement, have access to the same texts as their grade-level peers is one step toward meeting the letter and spirit of the IDEA, and achieving grade-level standards.

Theory of Change

To improve educational outcomes among students who have a print disability due to physical/mobility impairments, sensory/perceptual limitations, or mental/psychological limitations (The Advisory Commission on Accessible Instructional Materials in Postsecondary Education for Students with Disabilities, 2011), an intervention is needed that promotes academic achievement as well as their cognitive, communicative, behavioral, and social development. An intervention of this nature is of particular relevance to students who are unable to decode texts without audio intervention; students who find reading too daunting because they cannot connect words they know only in speech to written texts; and students who experience reading as hard work and, therefore, are less motivated to read.

Offering multiple technology options to access text removes one more obstacle for students with print disabilities. When this use of technology is paired with such best practices as differentiation in materials and explicit reading instruction, students have a better chance to fully participate in the classroom and expand their potential. Students with stronger academic records are more likely to demonstrate the competencies outlined in the Standards for College and Career Readiness and, no small feat, are more likely to possess the requisite skills for admission to more selective colleges and universities.

The intervention developed by the Connecticut Radio Information System (CRIS) is comprised of print and audio components that are offered simultaneously. In this way, CRISKids helps students to identify difficult words that would be an impediment to their progress, enables students to associate sounds with the written word and blocks out external sensory distractions (McKenna, 1998). The human voice is able to convey emotion, proper articulation, and the rhythm of language, which are all necessary components to engage students and promote their cognitive development.

Instead of requiring a teacher to read texts aloud to them (a common practice in schools), students will be able to access written texts in a non-stigmatizing way that promotes their autonomy. While guided reading activities and think-alouds are considered best practice, there is a distinction between teachers simply reading aloud so students get through texts and the interactive read-aloud and questioning strategies that are part of sound instructional practice.

As a result, students' comprehension will improve as they gain competence in reading (word identification, fluency, vocabulary), increase their independence in learning, sharpen their focus on academics, catch up or stay at level with their classmates, and engage in text-dependent classroom discussions. Since students who feel competent in their reading and class work tend to be more engaged and less disruptive in class, CRISKids will impact not only the students who are unable to access written texts, but the learning environment of all the students in the classroom.

Description of CRISKids in Action

A focus group discussion was held on March 20, 2014 with educators and related-service providers to learn more about the benefits of using CRISKids with students. The focus group was comprised of educators and providers who are currently using CRISKids with students in their schools. A salient theme that emerged addressed the limitations of text-to-speech and the advantage of human narration. Samantha Grayeck, a speech pathologist with CT Regional School District 13 who participated in the focus group, pointed out that reading interventions teach students to pay attention to inflection and punctuation (which are not always or clearly present in text-to-speech). For instance, students are instructed to read passages aloud and note that they tend to naturally pause between sentences (hence the need for periods at the end of sentences; semi-colons between independent clauses or simply commas used within a variety of sentence constructs). Students listening to texts that describe the emotions of characters are asked to indicate how they know that the characters are mad, sad, happy, surprised, etc. Students are taught to pay attention to indicators in the characters' speech that may reveal how they are feeling (e.g., if characters say something in a louder voice and pause between words, this may reveal that the characters feel very strongly about the point they are making).

An additional theme was that schools use CRISKids to increase students' motivation to read. Students who have print disabilities tend to feel a lack of connection to printed material and a fear of humiliation. When they cannot read independently while all the other students are able to do so or when the teacher singles them out by reading aloud only to them, students are placed in a stressful situation. Stress of this nature decreases their motivation to try to read. By way of contrast, there is a "cool factor" to using MP3 players in the classroom. Moreover, students are able to utilize CRISKids at their desks like the other students because they are not tethered to computers. Students are rewarded at some schools for time-on-task behavior: If they are diligent and complete their schoolwork in a timely manner, then they can listen-and-read one of the children's magazines that CRIS Radio records.

Another focus group participant, Brooke Doyon, a special education intern who based her master's thesis on a study of students attending Kennelly School, a neighborhood school in Hartford, Connecticut, said that by grade three, her students have "no relationship with print in that they can't read it." Those students tell her, "I don't get it," and they are well aware that their classmates are moving forward. With CRISKids, accessing the audio versions on an MP3 player of the same materials as their classmates, they can keep up. Said Doyon, students who use CRISKids tell her "Now, I look cool and I'm reading."

Doyon and Greg Eckbolm, who works for Vernon Public Schools, both describe how CRISKids can help students with emotional disorders or Attention Deficit Hyperactivity Disorder. Doyon described how some students with ADHD or emotional disorders can't sit at their desks. But when using CRISKids, they are better able to stay on task.

Eckbolm stated that the frustration becomes a barrier to learning, noting that some of his students "shut down all the time." At the Vernon, Connecticut school where he teaches, CRISKids is used not only as a reward, but also as an alternative activity that helps students work independently at their desk. "It's better than having [a student] put his head down and refuse to participate," Eckbolm said.

Teri Faucher, a reading teacher at Clover Street School in Windsor, Connecticut, explained that CRISKids was used specifically with fifth graders identified with special needs or reluctant readers. The teachers downloaded a number of audio versions of children's magazines and some Common Core exemplars onto the MP3 players, letting students select what they want to read. "CRISKids really helps with the fluency for students who struggle to learn to read and [work] so hard to get the words. Something like [CRISKids] really models for them, especially if they are not read to at home. Students unanimously like the MP3 players and don't feel stigmatized, but rather "cool" with them," Teri said.

Grayeck, the Durham schools' speech pathologist, emphasized that while CRISKids is a motivator for students who have print disabilities, it is much more than that. The audio readers help students with print disabilities to contribute to class discussions, allowing them to read at their grade level and access the same materials read by their classmates. "We can ask them pointed questions," Grayeck said. "This is on your [grade] level. You can read to yourself now. They had been stuck [before CRISKids].

Based on student-tests before and after using CRISKids, Doyon, the special education teacher working with Grade 7 students in Hartford, Connecticut, found that the audio versions improved reading comprehension. Students would not understand the main ideas of text after they read it. "I would ask if they understood it, and they would say 'yes,'" Doyon explained. Before using CRISKids, results of the student comprehension tests showed their complete lack of awareness of the main ideas in the story because they were so busy decoding. "I would ask a question, and they knew nothing," she said. When the students listened while following along in the text using CRISKids, their comprehension improved significantly, Doyon said.

John Pryor, an educator with the Wethersfield Public Schools and also a participant in the CRISKids focus group, explained how the custom audio recordings assisted a student with special needs to do well on his mid-term exams.

In 2014, the ten schools currently using CRISKids were asked to complete a survey which the authors of this chapter developed on the impact of CRISKids on students' learning and development. Of the ten schools:

- 90% agreed that "CRISKids contributes to the reading ability of the students with whom I work."
- 80% agreed that "CRISKids contributes to my students' motivation to read."
- 80% agreed that "CRISKids contributes to improve on-task and appropriate behavior of students."

CRISKids may be used by both educational professionals and families. Schools may provide families with access to recordings of Common Core text exemplars, which students may use at home as part of homework reinforcement. This is particularly critical in families in which English is not spoken or families in which the adults tend to be unfamiliar with words typically contained in Common Core text exemplars. Since the students are able to listen-and-read texts using CRISKids, their independence in completing their homework increases, which provides them with a sense of competency. Another factor that increases students' motivation to read is having the choice of which texts to listen-and-read. With CRISKids, some teachers allow students to choose what they want to read during the school day and listen-and-read these written materials at home.

Instruction to Increase Students' Fluency and Comprehension

CRISKids increases students' fluency and comprehension. Sometimes students with print disabilities expend all of their focus and energy on decoding texts at the cost of gaining fluency in reading or understanding the main ideas in a selection. The teachers reported that CRISKids helps students complete and better comprehend their assignments. Students who struggle with their reading assignments can complete them successfully by listening and following along, using the recordings as a mechanism to help them recognize words they cannot decipher in written text. The key here is to pair the audio text with a print version and for the teacher to provide direct instruction in target areas – word identification, vocabulary, comprehension, and/or response before, during, and after reading. In terms of growth in fluency, teachers must also target instruction around *how* something is read in addition to heeding what is actually said. Finally, whole group instruction in the classroom must be evaluated before tier 2 & 3 interventions or special education services are put into place.

Questions for teachers to consider include:

- Do I have up-to-date data and reliable information on the reading levels of all the students in my classrooms?
- For students who struggle, do I know what areas are most problematic? Are the problems academic or behavioral or some combination of both? What supports are already in place for these students; are they used regularly throughout the school day; and, to what extent have they been effective?
- How experienced am I in teaching the different components of reading? Regardless of how units/readings are organized, do *all* of my lessons include word study (vocabulary & identification) and comprehension activities?
- In what ways do I teach my students to read and respond to text strategically?

- Can I articulate how any text read in the class or assigned as homework is linked to both curricular and student learning objectives? Do all students read the same text all the time? Or, do I plan lessons using an anchor text as well as supplemental materials in a media (graphics, audio, film, websites, etc.)?
- Do I teach with the text or simply assign reading in my class? Are the texts that I ask students to read of interest and of importance to me?
- What importance do I place on the use of technology in the classroom? How experienced am I in the use of instructional technology? Does the technology support in my building or district actually meet the needs I have? Does professional development in the use of technology change my teaching or impact classroom environment in ways that clearly benefit students?
- What percent of classroom instruction involves whole group, small group, partner, or individual work?
- If success is defined as continuing growth in academic skills and personal competencies (understanding and following routines, demonstrating autonomy, positive interactions with others), how much success does each student experience in my classroom?
- Other than asking questions about the reading, what other techniques do I use to have students show what they know about a text and what we're studying in class?
- What might a guest in my classroom notice about its environment and my work with students?

Like the instructional "non-negotiables" identified by the National Reading Panel at the beginning of the 21st century (2000), these questions provide a core framework for teachers to evaluate their own practices around the use of text in the classroom as well as more general instructional routines, professional knowledge, and developmental perspectives. This type of reflection ideally leads to praxis and should be a prerequisite to the adoption of any type of technology that is intended to support students because, in isolation, the technology does not automatically lead to improved reading skills in any student. Although teaching effectiveness, teacher efficacy, student learning, and greater academic achievement can be positively impacted with the thoughtful and targeted integration of technology, the technology – the hardware itself – is not sufficient in ensuring any of these outcomes.

CRISKids not only benefits students who are unable to independently access written material, but also all the students in the classroom. During sustained silent reading, teachers who read aloud to only those who cannot access written material cannot circulate among the rest of the students. In many classrooms, teachers may become overly focused on work with only one or two students. Students who have print disabilities who also exhibit disruptive behavior pull teachers' attention away from the curriculum and distract other students. The three-year pilot of CRISKids demonstrated that students who feel competent in their reading and classroom tend to be less disruptive, thereby benefiting all of the students in the classroom.

Opportunities to improve all students' participation, engagement, and learning depend upon skillful instruction that is characterized by differentiation as well as specific instructional routines. For instance, teachers who ask students to repeat directions in their own words can clarify or correct misunderstandings for all students in the class. Using graphic organizers or cue cards to help students remember the steps in an assignment or identify what on-task behavior looks like helps students identify key information without necessarily waiting for a prompt or redirection from the teacher. Using a variety of materials simultaneously (Smartboard, handouts, audio texts, etc.) can reinforce learning for many students. Teaching and reviewing key vocabulary and academic language from the readings throughout a lesson, as well as having students use these terms and phrases in classroom conversation and writing, promotes word consciousness, conceptual understanding, and retention. Most importantly, vocabulary and spelling instruction that is based on the materials students are actually reading in class (as opposed to workbooks) is a more authentic learning experience. A quick, daily review of readings and previous learning through activities such as entrance/exit slips or Hot Seat (Zwiers, 2008) where students identify – ideally using the vocabulary of the discipline – what they have learned, why it matters, and to whom it is most important provide vital connections between prior knowledge and new information.

CRISKids in the Classroom

The following description of CRISKids in the classroom was written by Sara Gutis, Head Teacher of ED students at an alternative school in Connecticut, and a Ph.D. student:

Working with students who have print disabilities is never easy for a teacher. Reading and writing are skills needed in all curriculum areas. When there is a deficit in these areas, all subjects can become extra challenging to young people and the staff (teachers, assistants) working with them. If you also add other difficulties to the list (e.g., behavioral struggles), what was once just a hurdle now can seem like a mile long race full of hurdles, but assistive technologies can help.

At the beginning of the year, I had a class filled with eight students of varied abilities. The one commonality they shared was their special education designation of Emotional Disability (ED). Two of the students were proficient readers – at grade level. Three of the students had some fluency/decoding difficulties but could read efficiently enough to read aloud in class and be understood (but they would not necessarily remember the details of what they were reading). The remaining students would either refuse to read, resulting in some sort of oppositional behavior such as leaving the room or throwing the book, or their reading level was so far below grade level that it was too much of a struggle for them to decode most words.

As a teacher of students—students whose first reaction to almost anything is to cause a disruption (at a minimum) to a violent outburst (at the worst)—I have looked for ways to make reading and writing more engaging. I have tried changing up the reading materials to high interest short stories with surprise endings or more modern literature selections my students are more likely to identify with (e.g. Piri Thomas's <u>Down These Mean Streets</u> *and Walter Dean Meyers's* <u>Monster</u>*). I have integrated other subject areas into the reading including history topics and episodes in America's past (lynching in the context of* <u>To Kill a Mockingbird</u>*). I have modified work, read aloud, chunked, differentiated input and production. As a special education teacher, I have tried it all. Unfortunately, for some students, there was still a block.*

In my search for anything and everything new and technological, I met Chris Kelly from CRIS Radio at a professional development workshop. I made arrangements for him to come to the school and present CRISKids to the staff. I thought with the non-readers in my room as well as the rest of the school, this would be a great opportunity for something new and different!

I introduced CRISKids into the classroom quickly after Kelly visited. The students had many options for magazines that we could listen to as a class, or they could listen to individually when they were in the computer lab. The students had an interest in the new "thing" and wanted to check it out. Admittedly, some of the magazines were a little "younger" than my students. However, they looked at those, too. After clicking around here and there, I decided to use one of the magazines on the website.

We were already using the weekly current events magazine, The Week, in class. The students were reading small bits and only what was assigned for class discussion. Now, we had an audio version of the magazine. I started to see a difference in some of the students. Instead of balking and wincing when I handed out the magazines, they were more apt to open to the article and engage. They knew they were not going to be called on to read, and they no longer had to hear the same old voice (mine) when they no longer wanted to participate. It was different to them. The magazine being read to them also let the students who did the lion's share of the reading, off the hook, relieving them of some resentment and anxiety.

Overall, CRISKids has had a positive impact on the classroom. Taking the fear out of reading for students who struggle makes their attending to the tasks easier. Providing them with variety relieves boredom. Both together, make for a more engaged class, an easier lesson, and a happier classroom.

Anticipated Challenges and Limitations

Reviewing national data trends can often provide some insight into levels of academic performance. For instance, the 2013 Nation's Report Card showed that students' reading scores in fourth and eighth grades have improved since the early 1990s. Fewer students are in the basic or below basic bands, and more students are scoring at or above proficient; the growth in these scores from1992 to 2013 is statistically significant.

While certainly encouraging, the actual numbers tell something of a different story and speak to the continued need for high quality reading instruction and diverse reading experiences for all children. In 2013, only 35% of the nation's fourth graders were at or above proficient in reading and only 36% of the nation's eighth graders were at or above proficient. When considered along with the increasing demands for multiple literacies in the 21st century, these relatively low levels of performance have generated some urgency in rethinking reading instruction and best practices as well as what constitutes access to diverse reading materials (McKeown, Beck, & Blake, 2009).

The last thirty years have shown that implementing and sustaining a model of literacy instruction that consistently supports the acquisition of good reading skills in order to ground subject matter learning and prepare students to become informed citizens has been difficult or even nonexistent for the majority of classrooms in grades 4-12 (Durkin, 1978, 1979; Taylor & Pearson, 2002). Along with this, however, comes the challenge of helping teachers who may or may not be "digital immigrants" discover more ways to actively use assistive technology as part of day-to-day instruction (Prensky, 2006; Asselin, 2001). Although there is clear evidence that explicit instruction in reading comprehension is associated with higher achievement among students beyond the primary grades, studies indicate that as little as 3% of classroom time is designated for teaching strategic approaches to text and fewer than 15% of teachers regularly employed such techniques (Pearson, Roehler, Dole, & Duffy; 1992; Duffy, 2002; Langer, 2001; Ness, 2007; Ness, 2009). To that end, projects pairing technology with professional development in literacy must ensure that: 1) teacher training in technology and literacy increases students' access to and engagement with texts in and out of the classroom; 2) technology tools are used in conjunction with high quality content and/or reading instruction; and 3) support for teachers is job-embedded, on-going, and reflects the specific needs of individual classrooms (Hsu and Malkin, 2013).

By acknowledging such challenges, CRISKids is actually looking beyond how we can improve students' access to text by creating a unique model of professional development for the projects' teachers. This model addresses issues related to fidelity of implementation among teachers who bring different levels of technological and reading experience to the classroom. Also, it lessens concerns about how to help students who have print disabilities learn from text because curricular materials are made readily available through audio recordings using different devices, e.g. tablet, MP3 player, etc. Finally, the model helps every teacher become more fluent in their use of assistive technology while also enabling them to gain experience in providing age-appropriate and discipline-specific literacy instruction (Stewart & O'Brien, 1989; McConachie, Hall, Resnick, Ravi, Bill, Bintz, & Taylor, 2006; Deshler, Schumaker, Lenz, Bulgren, Hock, Knight, & Ehren, 2001).

CONCLUSION

To improve educational outcomes among students who are blind or unable to access printed texts, a reading intervention is needed that promotes their academic achievement as well as their cognitive, communicative, behavioral, and social development. An intervention of this nature is of particular relevance to students who are unable to decode texts without audio intervention, students who find reading too daunting because of uneven development in receptive and expressive language and, finally, students who find nearly every reading experience laborious and, therefore, are less motivated to read.

Instead of requiring a teacher or paraprofessional to read texts aloud to them (a common practice in many schools), students using CRISKids are able to access written texts in a non-stigmatizing way that promotes their autonomy. While guided reading activities and think-alouds should be part of teachers' routine instruction, there is a distinction between simply reading aloud so students get through texts and interactive read-aloud and questioning activities that are part of best practice. When teachers pull them aside only so a text can be read aloud to them, they tend to feel stigmatized and humiliated. As mobile devices and tablets become increasingly more common in classrooms, students using those devices as an assistive technology "tool" no longer report feeling stigmatized or different from their classmates who are able to read at grade level. Teachers often report that this is a very important component that translates into a successful intervention when using assistive technology with their students with print disabilities. Teachers report that students prefer human narration because digital speech does not convey such human emotions as excitement, sadness, fear, or joy. Teachers found that human narration promotes student motivation, helps students decode difficult words, improves reading comprehension, and allows students to "read" at a reading level similar to that of their classmates. Students who feel competent in their reading and class work tend to be more engaged in classroom routines, spend more time on task, and demonstrate greater comprehension of materials within a curricular unit. When more (or all students) demonstrate these behaviors and skills, teachers are better able to provide meaningful instruction as less time is spent on issues of classroom management and redirection. Thus, CRISKids impacts not only the students with print disabilities, but all the students in the classroom.

CRISKids is currently partnering with the IDEAL Group to develop new technologies. IDEAL has 20 years of experience developing systems and software that enhances the independence, quality-of-life, and employability of individuals with disabilities. The technologies will enable students with print disabilities to independently transform, access, read, and acquire knowledge from inaccessible digital content, particularly through the generation of visual supports based on the text they are studying (students who are blind will be provided with human-narrated recordings synchronized with their underlying texts and text-to-speech supports). Technologies include:

- CRISKids E-Book Reader DAISY Functionality – this enhanced version of IGR (IDEAL Group Reader) will enable students with print disabilities to navigate and listen to human narrated audio books in a completely accessible manner
- CRIS Radio Knowledge Discovery Infrastructure – IDEAL Group's improved knowledge-discovery infrastructure (KDI) will enable students, teachers, parents, and all other educative professionals to submit digital content in a wide range of formats to be processed by the software
- Visual Knowledge Map (Mind Map) Editor – this feature adds editing capabilities to the KDI along with other additional usability functions
- Mobile Software Development Kit (SDK) Including APIs – this development will allow content owners, educators, managers, and administrators to generate mind-maps from an easy-to-use resource
- MathML Extraction Module for STEM Documents – this deliverable will create a method for extracting MathML strings from digital content in order to make STEM subject content more accessible

As a result of current and new technologies paired with targeted instruction and intervention, CRISKids students will comprehend better, gain competence in reading (word identification, fluency, vocabulary), increase their independence in learning, sharpen their focus on academics, catch up or stay at level with their classmates, and engage in text-dependent classroom discussions.

ACKNOWLEDGMENT

The authors wish to thank Ben Brown for his contributions to the editing of this chapter.

REFERENCES

Allington, R. L. (2012). *What really matters for struggling readers* (3rd ed.). Boston, MA: Pearson.

Allington, R. L., & McGill-Franzen, A. (2009). Comprehension difficulties among struggling readers. In S. E. Duffy & G. G. Duffy (Eds.), *Handbook of research on reading comprehension* (pp. 551–568). New York, NY: Routledge.

Asselin, M. (2001). Literacy and technology. *Teacher Librarian, 28*(3), 49–51.

Balfanz, R. (2009). *Putting middle grades students on the graduation path: A policy and practice brief.* Westerville, OH: National Middle School Association.

Bean, T. W. (2000). Reading in the content areas: Social constructivist dimensions. In M. L. Kamil, P. B. Mosenthal, P. D. Pearson, & R. Barr (Eds.), *Handbook of reading research* (Vol. 3, pp. 629–654). Mahwah, NJ: Erlbaum.

Biancarosa, G., & Snow, C. E. (2006). *Reading next — A vision for action and research in middle and high school literacy: A report to Carnegie Corporation of New York* (2nd ed.). Washington, DC: Alliance for Excellent Education.

Brozo, W. G., & Hargis, C. H. (2003). Taking seriously the idea of reform: One high school's efforts to make reading more responsive to all students. *Journal of Adolescent & Adult Literacy, 47*(1), 14–23. doi:10.1598/JAAL.47.1.3

Buehl, D. (2011). *Developing readers in the academic disciplines.* Newark, DE: International Reading Association.

Butler, S. R., Marsh, H. W., Sheppard, M. J., & Sheppard, J. L. (1985). Seven-year longitudinal study of the early prediction of reading achievement. *Journal of Educational Psychology, 77*(3), 349–361. doi:10.1037/0022-0663.77.3.349

Chall, J. (1983). *Learning to Read: The Great Debate.* New York, NY: McGraw-Hill.

Coughtrey, K. (2014). Connected Mind [Mind Mapping]. *Google.* Retrieved, February 4, 2014, from http://www.connected-mind.appspot.com

Davis, V. (2012). *Does electronic versus paper book experience result in differences in level of emergent literacy development in young children?* Retrieved July 25, 2014, from http://www.uwo.ca/fhs/csd/ebp/reviews/2011-12/Davis.pdf

Denhart, H. (2008). Deconstructing barriers: Perceptions of students labeled with learning disabilities in higher education. *Journal of Learning Disabilities, 41*(6), 483–497. doi:10.1177/0022219408321151 PMID:18931016

Deshler, D. D., Schumaker, J. B., Lenz, B. K., Bulgren, J. A., Hock, M. F., Knight, J., & Ehren, B. J. (2001). Ensuring content-area learning by secondary students with learning disabilities. *Learning Disabilities Research & Practice, 16*(2), 96–108. doi:10.1111/0938-8982.00011

Duffy, G. G. (2002). The case for direct explanation of strategies. In C. Block & M. P. Pressley (Eds.), *Comprehension instruction: Research-based best practices* (pp. 28–41). New York: Guilford Press.

Durkin, D. (1978/1979). What classroom observations reveal about reading comprehension instruction. *Reading Research Quarterly, 14*(4), 481–533. doi:10.1598/RRQ.14.4.2

Editorial Projects in Education Research Center. (2011). Issues A-Z: Achievement Gap. *Education Week.* Retrieved, July 24, 2014, from, http://www.edweek.org/ew/issues/achievement-gap/

Fox, B. J. (2010). *Fluency contributes to comprehension.* Retrieved, 27 May 2014, http://www.education.com/reference/article/fluency-contributes-comprehension/

Freeplane. (2007). Freeplane (v1.3.11) [Free mind mapping and knowledge management software]. *MediaWiki*. Retrieved, February 4, 2014, from http://www.freeplane.org./wiki/index.php/Main_Page

Gerber, P. J., Reiff, H. B., & Ginsberg, R. (1996). Reframing the learning disabilities experience. *Journal of Learning Disabilities*, *29*(1), 98–101. doi:10.1177/002221949602900112 PMID:8648281

Greenbaum, B., Graham, S., & Scales, W. (1995). Adults with learning disabilities: Educational and social experiences during college. *Exceptional Children*, *61*, 460–471.

Gunning, T. G. (2012). *Creating literacy instruction for all students* (8th ed.). Boston, MA: Allyn and Bacon.

Guthrie, J. T. (2000). Contexts for engagement and motivation in reading. In M. L. Kamil, P. B. Mosenthal, P. D. Pearson, & R. Barr (Eds.), *Handbook of reading research* (Vol. 3, pp. 629–654). Mahwah, NJ: Erlbaum.

Hall, L. A. (2004). Comprehending expository text: Promising strategies for struggling readers and students with reading disabilities? *Reading Research and Instruction*, *44*(2), 75–95. doi:10.1080/19388070409558427

Hecker, L., Burns, L., Elkind, J., Elkind, K., & Katz, L. (2002). Benefits of assistive reading software for students with attention disorders. *Annals of Dyslexia*, *52*(1), 244–272. doi:10.1007/s11881-002-0015-8

Helfgott, D., & Westhaver, M. (1982). *Inspiration Software (v9.0.3)*. Portland, OR: Inspire.

Hernandez, D. J. (2011). *How third-grade reading skills and poverty influence high school graduation*. Annie E. Casey Foundation.

Hess, S. (2014). Digital media and student learning: Impact of electronic books on motivation and achievement. *New England Reading Association Journal*, *49*(2), 35–39.

Hollauf, M., & Vollmer, T. (2006). *MindMeister* (Web 2.0) [From MeisterLabs]. Munich, Germany: MeisterLabs. Retrieved, February 4, 2014, from http://www.mindmeister.com

Hsu, A., & Malkin, F. (2013). Professional development workshops for student teachers: An issue of concern. *Action in Teacher Education*, *35*(5-6), 354–371. doi:10.1080/01626620.2013.846165

International Dyslexia Association. Promoting Literacy through Research, Education and Advocacy. (2014). Retrieved June 2, 2014, from http://www.interdys.org/SignsofDyslexiaCombined.htm

Jetter, B., & Jetter, M. (1998). MindManager (v9) [Product of Mindjet]. *Mindjet*. Retrieved, February 4, 2014, from http://www.mindjet.com/mindmanager

Kamil, M. L. (2003). *Adolescents and literacy: Reading for the 21st century*. Washington, DC: Alliance for Excellent Education.

Kern, M. L., & Friedman, H. S. (2008). Early educational milestones as predictors of lifelong academic achievement, midlife adjustment, and longevity. *Journal of Applied Developmental Psychology*, *30*(4), 419–430. doi:10.1016/j.appdev.2008.12.025 PMID:19626128

Kerscher, G., & Fruchterman, J. (2002). The soundproof book: Exploration of rights conflict and access to commercial ebooks for people with disabilities. *First Monday, 7*(6). doi:10.5210/fm.v7i6.959

Kupietz, S. S. (1990). Sustained attention in normal and in reading-disabled youngsters with and without ADDH. *Journal of Abnormal Child Psychology, 18*(4), 357–372. doi:10.1007/BF00917640 PMID:2246429

Laitusis, C. (2010). Examining the impact of audio presentation on tests of reading comprehension. *Applied Measurement in Education, 23*(2), 153–167. doi:10.1080/08957341003673815

Lamb, A., & Callison, D. (2011). Graphic inquiry for all learners. *School Library Monthly, 28*(3), 18-22. Retrieved, February, 4, 2014 from, http://search.proquest.com/docview/1018179930?accountid=1060

Langer, J. A. (2001). Beating the odds: Teaching middle and high school students to read and write well. *American Educational Research Journal, 38*(4), 837–880. doi:10.3102/00028312038004837

Larson, L. C. (2009). e-Reading and e-Responding: New tools for the next generation of readers. *Journal of Adolescent & Adult Literacy, 53*(3), 255–258. doi:10.1598/JAAL.53.3.7

Leu, D. J., Kinzer, C. K., Coiro, J., Castek, J., & Henry, L. A. (2013). New literacies: A dual level theory of the changing nature of literacy, instruction, and assessment. In D. E. Alvermann, N. J. Unrau, & R. B. Ruddell (Eds.), *Theoretical models and processes of reading* (6th ed.; pp. 1150–1181). Newark, DE: International Reading Association. doi:10.1598/0710.42

Lisle, K. (2011). *Identifying the negative stigma associated with having a learning disability.* (Thesis for honors in psychology). Retrieved, March 20, 2014, from, http://digitalcommons.bucknell.edu/cgi/viewcontent.cgi?article=1021&context=honors

McConachie, S., Hall, M., Resnick, L., Ravi, A., Bill, V., Bintz, J., & Taylor, J. (2006). Task, text, and talk: Literacy for all subjects. [theses]. *Educational Leadership, 64*(2), 8–14.

McKenna, M. C. (1998). Electronic texts and the transformation of beginning reading. In D. R. Reinking, M. C. McKenna, L. D. Labbo, & R. D. Kieffer (Eds.), *Handbook of literacy and technology: Transformations in a posttypographic world* (pp. 45–59). Hillsdale, NJ: Lawrence Erlbaum.

McKenna, M. C., Reinking, D., Labbo, L. D., & Kieffer, R. D. (1999). The electronic transformation of literacy and its implications for the struggling reader. *Reading & Writing Quarterly, 15*, 111–126. doi:10.1080/105735699278233

McKenna, M. C., & Robinson, R. D. (2009). *Teaching through text: Reading and writing in the content areas.* New York, NY: Pearson.

McKeown, M., Beck, I., & Blake, R. (2009). Reading comprehension instruction: Focus on content or strategies? *Perspectives on Language and Literacy, 35*(2), 28.

McNulty, M. A. (2003). Dyslexia and the life course. *Journal of Learning Disabilities, 36*(4), 363–381. doi:10.1177/00222194030360040701 PMID:15490908

MediaWiki. (2014). *MediaWiki, The Free Wiki Engine.* Retrieved, February 4, 2014, from http://www.mediawiki.org/w/index.php?title=MediaWiki&oldid=740803

Melzi, G., & Caspe, M. (2005). Variations in maternal narrative styles during book reading interactions. *Narrative Inquiry, 15*(1), 101–125. doi:10.1075/ni.15.1.06mel

MindGenius, Ltd. (2001). *MindGenius* (v5) [Part of Gael Group]. MindGenius, Ltd. Retrieved, February 4, 2014, from http://www.mindgenius.com

Moody, A. K. (2010). Using electronic books in the classroom to enhance emergent literacy s skills in young children. *Journal of Literacy and Technology, 11*(4), 22–52.

Mullenweg, M. (2005). *Wordpress.com* (v3.9.1) [state-of-the-art semantic personal publishing platform]. San Francisco, CA: Automattic. Retrieved, February 4, 2014, from http://www.wordpress.com

Müller, J. (2011). FreeMind (v0.9.0). *MediaWiki*. Retrieved, July 29, 2014, from http://www.freemind.sourceforge.net/wiki/index.php/Main_Page

National Reading Panel. (2000). *Teaching children to read: An evidence-based assessment of the scientific research literature on reading and its implications for reading instruction*. Retrieved January 25, 2014, from http://www.nichd.nih.gov/publications/nrp/report.cfm

Ness, M. (2007). Reading comprehension strategies in secondary content-area classrooms. *Phi Delta Kappan, 89*(3), 229–231. doi:10.1177/003172170708900314

Ness, M. (2009). Reading comprehension strategies in secondary content area classrooms: Teacher use of and attitudes towards reading comprehension instruction. *Reading Horizons, 49*(2), 143–166.

Newkirk, T. (2012). *The art of slow reading: Six time-honored practices for engagement*. Portsmouth, NH: Heinemann.

Nielsen, J., Clemmensen, T., and Yssing, R. (2002). *Getting Access to What Goes on in People's Heads – Reflections on the Think-Aloud Technique*. NordiCHI, 2002.

Pearson, P. D., Roehler, L. R., Dole, J. A., & Duffy, G. G. (1992). Developing expertise in reading comprehension. In S. J. Samuels & A. E. Farstrup (Eds.), *What research has to say about reading instruction* (pp. 145–199). Newark, DE: International Reading Association.

Po, S., Howard, S., Vetere, F., & Skov, M. (2004). Heuristic evaluations and mobile usability: Bridging the realism gap. In S. Brewster & M. Dunlop (Eds.), MobileHCI (LNCS), (pp. 49-60). Berlin: Springer.

Prensky, M. (2006). *Don't bother me, mom, I'm learning*. St. Paul, MN: Paragon House.

Rasinski, T. V. (2004). *Assessing reading fluency*. Honolulu, HI: Pacific Resources for Education and Learning.

Rasinski, T. V. (2006). Reading fluency instruction: Moving beyond accuracy, automaticity, and prosody. *The Reading Teacher, 59*(7), 704–706. doi:10.1598/RT.59.7.10

Richards, J., & McKenna, R. (2003). *Integrating multiple literacies in K-8 classrooms: Cases, commentaries, and practical applications*. Mahwah, NJ: Lawrence, Erlbaum.

Roer-Strier, D. (2002). University students with learning disabilities advocating for change. *Disability and Rehabilitation, 24*(17), 914–924. doi:10.1080/09638280210148611 PMID:12519487

Ruffin, T. M. (2012). Assistive technologies for reading. *Reading Matrix: An International Online Journal, 12*(1), 98–101.

Scott, C. (2008). *iThoughts.* Retrieved February 4, 2014, from http://www.ithoughts.co.uk/_iThoughtsHD/Welcome.html

Segal-Drori, O., Korat, O., Shamir, A., & Klein, P. S. (2010). Reading e-books and printed books with and without adult instruction: Effects on emergent reading. *Reading and Writing, 23*(8), 913–930. doi:10.1007/s11145-009-9182-x

Sénéchal, M., & LeFevre, J.-A. (2002). Parental involvement in the development of children's reading skill: A five-year longitudinal study. *Child Development, 73*(2), 445–460. doi:10.1111/1467-8624.00417 PMID:11949902

Shirky, C. (2008). *It's not information overload. It's filter failure.* Lecture presented at Web Expo 2.0 2008 in New York, New York. Retrieved January 31, 2014, from http://www.mascontext.com/issues/7-information-fall-10/its-not-information-overload-its-filter-failure/

Snow, C. E. (2001). *Improving reading outcomes: Getting beyond third grade.* Washington, DC: The Aspen Institute.

Snow, C. E., Porche, M. V., Tabors, P. O., & Harris, S. R. (2007). *Is literacy enough? Pathways to academic success for adolescents.* Baltimore, MD: Paul H. Brookes.

Software, Inc. (n.d.). Retrieved, July 29, 2014, from http://www.inspiration.com

Stainthorp, R., & Hughes, D. (2004). What happens to precocious readers' performance by the age eleven? *Journal of Research in Reading, 27*(4), 357–372. doi:10.1111/j.1467-9817.2004.00239.x

Stewart, R. A., & O'Brien, D. G. (1989). Resistance to content area reading: A focus on pre-service teachers. *Journal of Reading, 32*(5), 396–401.

Taylor, B. M., & Pearson, D. P. (Eds.). (2002). *Teaching reading: Effective schools, accomplished teachers.* Mahwah, NJ: Lawrence Erlbaum.

The Advisory Commission on Accessible Instructional Materials in Postsecondary Education for Students with Disabilities. (2011). *AIM commission report.* Retrieved, from https://www.library.cornell.edu/research/citation/apa

The Nation's Report Card. (2013). *Mathematics and Reading.* Retrieved August 13, 2014, from http://www.nationsreportcard.gov/reading_math_2013/#/

Topping, K.J., Bircham, A., & Shaw, M. (1997). Family electronic literacy: Home-school links through audiotaped books. *Reading, 31*(2), 7-12.

Vacca, R. T. (2002). Making a difference in adolescents' school lives: Visible and invisible aspects of *content area reading.* In A. E. Farstrup & S. J. Samuels (Eds.), *What research has to say about reading instruction* (3rd ed.). Newark, DE: International Reading Association. doi:10.1598/0872071774.9

Van Rijmenam, M. (2014). *Seven big data trends for 2014.* [Big data startup]. Retrieved, February 4, 2014, from http://www.bigdata-startups.com/big-data-trends-2014/

Walpole, M., & McKenna, S. (2013). *The literacy coach's handbook*. New York, NY: The Guilford Press.

Wiederholt, J. L., & Bryant, B. R. (2001). *Gray oral reading test-IV examiner's manual*. Austin, TX: Pro-Ed.

Williams, E. (2004). *Blogspot.com* [Blogger]. Retrieved February 4, 2014, from http://www.blogger.com

XMind, Ltd. (2008). *XMind 2013* (v3.4.1) [The world's most popular mind mapping tool]. Hong Kong, People's Republic of China: XMind, Ltd. Retrieved February 4, 2014, from http://www.xmind.net

Zwiers, J. (2008). Building academic language: Essential practices for content classrooms, grades 5-12. San Francisco, CA: Jossey-Bass.

ADDITIONAL READING

Cummins, J., Brown, K., & Sayers, D. (2007). *Literacy, Technology, and Diversity: Teaching for Success in Changing Times*. Boston: Pearson/Allyn & Bacon.

Passey, D. (2014). *Inclusive technology enhanced learning: Overcoming cognitive, physical, emotional, and geographic challenges*. New York: Routledge.

Shirley, D. (2013). Mindful teaching with technology: steps toward harmonization. In H. Malone (Ed.), *Leading educational change: global issues, challenges, and lessons on whole-system reform*. New York: Teacher's College Press.

KEY TERMS AND DEFINITIONS

Assistive Technology: Refers to devices that promote independence of individuals who, because of disability, would be unable to complete or participate in certain tasks.

Audio Learning: Refers to situations where successful completion of tasks and/or an understanding of concepts depends on hearing information as opposed to having it presented in other modalities, e.g. print.

Print Disability: Refers to individuals who are unable to read or access print because of any number (or combination) of disabilities including visual, learning, physical, perceptual, cognitive, etc.

Reading Intervention: Refers to a program or special instruction to support students experiencing difficulty in any area of reading; supplements existing instruction.

Voice Narration: The use of actual voice (live; recorded) to read or explain content, not computer or digitally generated.

Chapter 11
Video Modeling for Learners with Developmental Disabilities

Peggy J. S. Whitby
University of Arkansas, USA

Christine R. Ogilvie
FSU CARD, USA

Krista Vince Garland
SUNY Buffalo State, USA

ABSTRACT

Video modeling is an evidence-based practice for learners with autism spectrum disorders (ASD). However, the use of video modeling interventions for learners with other developmental disabilities has received less applied attention in home, community, and classroom settings. This is unfortunate since the research literature supports the use of video modeling interventions for all learners with developmental disabilities. The purpose of this chapter is to introduce the research literature and make suggestions for implementing video modeling with learners who have developmental disabilities other than autism.

INTRODUCTION

Video modeling involves the use of videos to teach or modify behaviors. Short videos can be used to provide instruction in social skills, functional or daily living skills, and many other areas. Creating video models involves identifying a target behavior, developing a task analysis of the target, assessing content validity of the target behavior by observing typical peers implementing the task, and adjusting task analysis based upon the findings. Next, a type of video modeling intervention is selected based upon the needs of the learner, and differentiating the intervention begins.

The use of video modeling as an effective intervention for learners with autism spectrum disorders (ASD) has gained much attention recently as the National Autism Center (2014) has identified it as a research-based practice. The majority of research focuses on video self-modeling and video modeling with others as models for learners with ASD. While these two types of video modeling are effective

DOI: 10.4018/978-1-4666-8395-2.ch011

interventions for learners with ASD, there are other types of video modeling that have garnered less attention and may be more appropriate for learners with developmental disabilities that include comorbid intellectual disabilities. Since roughly 33% of those diagnosed with an ASD also have a comorbid intellectual disability (Centers for Disease Control, 2014), inclusion of other types of video modeling for both learners with ASD and related developmental disabilities is quite important. Models such as video modeling and video self-modeling, in particular, have led to a base of evidence-based practices for learners with ASD; however, point-of-view modeling for learners with other developmental disabilities has received less attention despite still being appropriate interventions. This is unfortunate, since video modeling for learners with differing abilities is an appropriate intervention that is well supported by the research literature (Bellini, Peters, Benner, & Hopf, 2007; Gresham, 2002; Hart & Whalon, 2012; Mechling & Collins, 2012). One purpose of this chapter is to present the different types of video modeling interventions, accompanied by a review of relevant literature. The second purpose of this chapter is to provide strategies to determine which type of video modeling procedure is appropriate for teaching skills to children with developmental disabilities while providing guidelines in using point-of-view video modeling for learners with developmental disabilities.

Case Study-Karen: Throughout the chapter, you will see vignettes about Karen, a young woman with Down syndrome. The purpose of the vignette is to provide you with a real-life example of when and how to use video modeling for learners with developmental disabilities.

Karen is a 15-year-old with Down Syndrome. She attends public school and participates in resource room classes for reading and math. She is an active, friendly young woman who enjoys spending time with her friends and participates on the local swim team. Karen will be turning 16 in a few months and it is her wish, as well as her parents' and teachers', to get a job during summer break. Her IEP team will be meeting soon to determine what type of interventions would be appropriate for teaching Karen specific job-related tasks.

What are Developmental Disabilities?

According to the Centers for Disease Control and Prevention (CDC) (2014), the term "developmental disability" refers to a group of conditions that reflect impairments in physical, language, behavioral and learning abilities that begin during the developmental period, generally last throughout the individual's lifetime, and may impact day-to-day functioning. Among the conditions housed under the CDC's definition are Autism Spectrum Disorders, Cerebral Palsy, Fetal Alcohol Syndrome, Fragile X Syndrome, Intellectual Disabilities, and others. In 2008, the CDC reported that the prevalence of any developmental disability from 1997-2008 was 13.87% with developmental delays having a specific prevalence of 3.65%. For the purpose of this chapter, the term "developmental disability" will refer to learners with limitations in their ability to learn at an expected level as well as those who are struggling with day-to-day independent functioning.

What is Video Modeling?

Video modeling is an antecedent-based intervention that uses video recording and display equipment to provide a visual model of a targeted behavior or skill (Bellini & Akullian, 2007; National Autism Center, 2014). Types of video modeling include basic video modeling with other as model (VM), video self-modeling (VSM), point-of-view video modeling (POV), and video prompting (VP) (Bellini et al, 2007; Shukla-Mehta, Miller, & Callahan, 2010). The specific type of video modeling employed in the intervention is determined by the specific skill levels and needs of individual for which the intervention is being designed and the type of behavior / task to be modified / introduced.

Video modeling with other (i.e. – peer, adult, etc.) as model (VM) involves the use of a recording of a peer or adult implementing a target behavior (Bellini, 2008). Once the video is recorded, the student views the video prior to performing the activity. Video models can be made for the individual student, or commercially made videos can be purchased (Bellini & Akullian, 2007). Video modeling with other as model incorporates modeling strategies first introduced in the 1970s by Bandura (1977). Bandura demonstrated that children acquire skills through observing other learners performing the skills (1977).

Video self-modeling (VSM) is a specific application of VM in which the learner observes him or herself accurately and independently performing the target behavior (Dowrick, 1999). VSM is a form of observational learning in which learners view themselves performing a task at a more advanced level than they typically perform the skill (Buggey, Toombs, Gardener, & Cervetti, 1999; Burton, Anderson, Prater, & Dyches, 2013). This is achieved by editing out prompts for task and reinforcement for completion of each step in the task. Video self-modeling is used to record the learner displaying the target skill or behavior and is reviewed later (Franzone & Collet-Klingenberg, 2008). VSM is also based on observational learning theories (Bandura, 1977). Dowrick (1999) suggested that utilizing the "self" as model is the most powerful model and should be considered a learning mechanism on its own, since it increases the likelihood of the behavior occurring in the future. Video self-modeling allows the student to not only see the task being completed, but may increase the students' belief that they can perform the task (Dowrick, 1999).

Point-of-view (POV) video modeling is when the target behavior or skill is recorded from the perspective of the learner (Franzone & Collet-Klingenberg, 2008). Third-person perspective, currently the most common modality for recording, allows the viewer to see the video as if he/she is an onlooker. Point-of view video modeling, however, involves recording the video from the vantage point of the person carrying out the task. Point-of-view modeling offers advantages over the typical third-person perspective. From a production standpoint, POV requires limited preparation and editing. Since the video is recorded from the visual perspective of the model, it depicts what the individual would see (Rayner et al, 2009), thus minimal time is allocated to preparing the scene or the model. In addition, given the nature of the visual perspective, extraneous stimuli are not included in the video, naturally directing attention to the steps necessary to complete the desired task or to demonstrate the appropriate behavior (Shukla-Mehta et al., 2010).

For some learners, watching the entire skill being performed at once does not lead to skill acquisition. These learners may require the task to be broken down into steps that are more manageable. When a video model of a complex task is broken down into smaller units and each unit is viewed individually as a cue for the behavior, the process is called video prompting (Horn, Miltenberger, Weil, Mowery, Conn, & Sams, 2008). Video prompting is a teaching method versus an antecedent intervention. Many times other techniques are embedded into the procedure, such as various prompting hierarchies, feedback, time delay, and/or reinforcement (Franzone & Collet-Klingenberg, 2008; Horn et al. 2008).

Why Use Video Modeling?

Sturmey (2003) suggested that video technology is a useful tool for modeling behavior, providing feedback, teaching children to discern their own behavior, and for presenting basic instruction. Technology is highly reinforcing and a preferred activity for many learners, including those with developmental disabilities (Bellini & Akullian, 2007; Sherer, Pierce, Paredes, Kisacky, Ingersoll, & Schreibman, 2001).

The role of technology in society is becoming commonplace as increasing numbers of professionals, family members and learners with developmental disabilities have access to technology including Smart Phones and other handheld devices (Shane, Laubscher, Schlosser, Flynn, Sorce, & Abramson, 2011). Video technology is a cost-effective, readily available technology that can be used across settings (i.e. school, home, and community) (Nikopoulos, Canavan, & Nikopoulou-Smymi, 2009).

Video modeling helps learners by directing attention to relevant stimuli in a learning task. This is accomplished by using a highly preferred mode of instruction; thereby increasing motivation, carefully designing the model to include only relevant stimuli, and removing the distractions in the environment by editing the content. Video modeling is more efficient than live modeling since it simplifies the process in terms of ease of repetition (i.e., pressing play for video is much faster than getting the same group together to replay the desired behavior). The ease of repetition allows intervention teams to use the video model as a prime as priming consists of previewing the behavior in less demanding settings before the behavior should occur (Alberto & Troutman, 2006).

LITERATURE REVIEW

The following section provides an overview of the literature on the different types of video modeling for learners with developmental disabilities other than ASD. For more information on video modeling specific to ASD, see Video Modeling for Individuals with Autism Spectrum Disorders in *Innovative Technologies for Teaching Students with Autism Spectrum Disorders* edited by Silton (Ogilvie & Whitby, 2013).

Contemporary Research on Video Modeling

Research on Video Modeling Interventions

Video modeling with other as model has been used to teach a variety of skills to learners with developmental disabilities. Table 1 provides examples of skills addressed in the research literature across four domains.

Video Modeling with other as model has been shown to be effective in teaching many self-care, independent living skills, and vocational tasks. The majority of studies addressing both self-care and vocational tasks focused on adolescents or adults with developmental disabilities. However, Mason, Ganz, Parker, Burke, & Carmago (2012) suggest that video self-modeling may not be the most effective video modeling intervention for learners with developmental disabilities, compared to learners with ASD. More research is needed on video modeling with other as model for learners with developmental disabilities. No studies were identified that addressed younger children with developmental disabilities other than ASD.

Table 1. Video Modeling with other as model

Skill Type	Example Target Behaviors
Self-Care Skills	iPhone Use (Walser, Ayres, & Foot, 2012) Cooking (Mechling & Collins, 2012) Simple Meal Preparation (Rehfeldt, Dahman, Young, Cherry, & Davis, 2003) Making coffee (Bidwell and Rehfeldt, 2004) Set Table (Cannella-Malone et al., 2006) Put away groceries (Cannella-Malone et al., 2006) Dental Procedures (Conyers et al., 2004) Purchasing (Haring, Kennedy, Adams, and Pitts-Conway, 1987) Making a sandwich (Rehfeldt, Dahman, Young, Cherry, & Davis, 2003) Change batteries (Van Laarhoven, Zurita, Johnson, Grider, & Grider, 2009) Clean Sink (Van Laarhoven, Zurita, Johnson, Grider, & Grider, 2009) Make a hotdog (Van Laarhoven, Zurita, Johnson, Grider, & Grider, 2009) Domestic Skills (Rehfeldt, 2004) Cleaning (Mechling et al., 2014) ATM Use (Scott, Collins, Knight, Kleinert, 2013)
Academic Skills	N/A
Social Skills	N/A
Vocational and Leisure Skills	Kitchen Related Vocational Tasks (Laarhoven, Winiarski, Blood, & Chan, 2012) Furniture Assembly (Martin et al., 1992) Library Skills (Taber-Doughty & Brennan, 2008) Watching movies on IPOD touch (Kagohara, 2010) Responding on computer to fast food questions (Mechling, Pridgen, & Cronin, 2005) Physical Activities (Cannella-Malone et al., 2013)

Research on Video Self-Modeling Interventions

Video Self-Modeling (VSM) has fewer research studies documented in the literature for teaching students with developmental disabilities other than autism. Table 2 provides examples of studies utilizing VSM across four domains.

Even though VSM may be a powerful intervention (Dowrick, 1999), few studies have addressed teaching learners with developmental disabilities other than ASD. VSM has been used to teach academic skills to students with developmental disabilities (Burton et al, 2013; Hart & Whalon, 2012). Both studies focused on adolescents with intellectual disabilities and/or autism.

Table 2. Video Self-Modeling

Skill Type	Example Target Behaviors
Self-Care Skills	Managing clothing during toilet use (Ohtake, Takeuchi, & Watanabe, 2014) First-Aid (Ozkan, 2013)
Academic Skills	Functional Math (Burton, Anderson, Prater, & Dyches, 2013) Academic Responding (Hart & Whalon, 2012)
Social Skills	N/A
Vocational and Leisure Skills	N/A

Table 3. Point of View Video Modeling

Skill Type	Example Target Behaviors
Self-Care Skills	Independent Living Skills (Alberto, Cihak, Gama, 2005; Cannella-Malone et al., 2011; Hammond, Whatley, Ayres, & Gast, 2010; Mechling & Collins, 2012: Mechling, Gast, & Barthold, 2003; Norman, Collins, & Schuster, 2001: Van Laarhoven, Zurita, Johnson, Grider, & Grider, 2009) Fire Extinguisher Use (Mechling, Gast, & Gustafson, 2009)
Academic Skills	N/A
Social Skills	N/A
Vocational and Leisure Skills	N/A N/A

Research on Point-of-View Video Modeling Interventions

Point-of-view video modeling has been used extensively to teach independent living and self-care skills to learners with developmental disabilities. Table 3 provides examples of research literature across domains.

Point-of-view video modeling has been shown to be highly effective for teaching independent living and self-care skills to adolescents and adults with developmental disabilities (Mason, Davies, Boyles & Goodwyn, 2013). Interestingly, the use of POV video modeling, though very effective, has not been assessed with skills other than independent living and self-care for learners with developmental disabilities other than ASD.

Research on Video Prompting Interventions

Video prompting (VP) has been used extensively to teach independent living and self-care to learners with developmental disabilities. Table 4 provides a variety of examples of studies using VP to teach learners with developmental disabilities other than ASD.

Again, much of the research literature focused on teaching independent living skills and self-care. Two studies assessed video prompting to teach leisure skills. One study extended the skill (making coffee) into the social-skill arena (serving coffee to friends) (Bidwell & Rehfeldt, 2004). Independent living

Table 4. Video Prompting

Skill Type	Example Target Behaviors
Self-Care Skills	Independent Living skills (Cannella-Malone et al., 2011; Mechling, Gast, Barthold, 2003; Norman, Collins, & Schuster, 2001) Microwave oven skills (Sigafoos et al., 2005) Cleaning Sunglasses, zipping, putting on a wrist watch (Norman, Collins, & Schuster (2001) Laundry Skills (Horn, Miltenberger, Weil, Conn, & Sams, 2008) Dental Care (Conyers et al. 2004) Coffee Making (Bidwell & Rehfeldt, 2004) Cooking (Mechling, Gast, & Seid, 2010
Academic Skills	N/A
Social Skills	Serving coffee in a social setting (Bidwell & Rehfeldt, 2004)
Vocational and Leisure Skills	Painting, listening to music, and photography (Chan et al., 2013) Photography (Edrisinha, O'Reilly, Choi, Sigafoos, & Lancioni, 2011)

Table 5. Matching Methodologies to the Needs of the Learner

Type and Definition	Good for Learners Who:
Video Modeling with other as model – Creating a video of another person completing a task. Student watches the video prior to completing the task.	-can complete part of the task but may not be proficient in all of the task. -can attend to a whole task. -can discriminate between relevant and irrelevant stimuli in the environment. -can generalize the skill from the model to self.
Video Self-Modeling- Creating a video of the person completing the task and editing out all prompts so that the final product is a video of the person proficiently completing the task. Student then watches the video prior to completing the task.	-can complete part of the task but may not be proficient in all of the task. -can attend to a whole task. -need more support in directing their attention as seeing themselves on video may increase attention. -will be reinforced by seeing themselves successfully complete the task.
Point of View Video Modeling- Creating a video from the perspective of the person completing the task. Student then watches the video prior to completing the task.	-can complete part of the task but may not be proficient in all of the task. -can attend to a whole task. -need more direction to relevant stimuli - become distracted easily by environmental distractors
Video Prompting- Breaking down each step of the video model into discrete steps, infusing prompts into the video, and pausing the video after each step until the student completes the step.	-can complete very little of the task if any. -Cannot attend to the entire task. -Need more direction and reinforcement within the task. -require prompting to complete each step.

and self-care may be the most pressing concern for learners with developmental disabilities in terms of long-term outcomes. However, this intervention could be extended to other skill areas, as these areas are important for long-term happiness and self-determination.

Issues and Perspectives

Access to technology and relatively inexpensive devices available (iPods, iPads, Smart Phones, MP3 players, etc.) have provided a way to integrate video models into students' school days and across the community (Carnahan, Basham, Christman, & Hollingshead, 2012). Much focus has been given to the use of video modeling and video self-modeling for teaching social skills to learners with ASD. Less attention has been given to teaching learners with developmental disabilities other than ASD. However, research supports the use of video modeling interventions to teach a variety of skills to learners with differing abilities. For many who need an increased break-down of learning tasks and additional focus on relevant stimuli, video point-of-view modeling and video prompting may be an ideal intervention choice based upon the individual learner's needs. Table 4 provides an overview of the video modeling types and considerations for matching the intervention to the learner's needs.

Video modeling interventions for learners with developmental disabilities has focused mainly on self-care/independent living skills with adolescents and adults. However, these interventions have the potential to address other skills, which can have a great impact on quality of life (social, leisure, vocational and functional academics skills). There is the possibility of using these interventions with younger children, which may have a greater impact on outcomes across the lifespan.

SOLUTION

The use of video modeling is not new and should be considered a staple in teaching all children with developmental disabilities. Given the learning issues of learners with developmental disabilities who have intellectual disabilities, point of view and video prompting should be considered as viable methods of intervention.

With guidance from her Individualized Education Program (IEP) team, Karen has decided that she would like to apply for a job in the local supermarket as a cashier. Karen is familiar with the supermarket from shopping there with her family and attending community-based field trips with her class. Karen and her IEP team have decided to create video models of the tasks that will be required for her to successfully obtain and keep a job as a bagger. Karen's job coach meets with the grocery store to secure a summer job and the store agrees to allow training to occur during the school year.

Karen and her IEP team decided to use the video-prompting method (with Karen as the model) to facilitate her acquiring and mastering the skills needed to be a bagger at the supermarket. First, the team met to decide which skills would be most important for Karen to master. They decided to work on clocking in, greeting costumers, and bagging items.

Creating video models involves identifying a target behavior, developing a task analysis of the target, assessing content validity of the target behavior by observing typical peers implementing the task, and adjusting task analysis based upon the findings. Next, a type of video modeling intervention is selected based upon the needs of the learner, and differentiating the intervention begins.

If video modeling with other as model (VMO) is selected, the model should be identified. If video self-modeling (VSM) is selected, the student will perform each step of the task with prompts. The model or student should then practice the skill based on the task analysis and receive feedback on the implementation of each step. If using VMO, once the task can be performed with precision and fluidity, the task can be recorded. If using VSM, the task is recorded and prompts are edited out of the video.

With point-of-view (POV) modeling and video prompting (VP), identification of a model is not necessary since the person performing the task is generally not present in the video. The person who is creating the intervention can perform the task and only the steps in the task are recorded from the first person point of view. However, it is important to record each step from the learner's viewpoint; therefore, the person completing the task for the recording should be similar in height and size to the learner. Once the video is recorded, a plan for how and when the person will access the video should be developed (Laarhoven, Winiarski, Blood, & Chan, 2012).

Accessing the video model depends upon whether or not the intervention includes priming or prompting. When using priming, it is important that the person view the video in a less demanding situation *before* he/she is expected to perform the activity. Depending on the type of skill being taught (high frequency, such as greeting friends; or low frequency, such as a morning transition into school), the video can be viewed more than once per day. For example, when teaching greetings, the video can be viewed at several set times per day. When teaching how to transition into school, the video may be watched at home prior to getting in the car and again at school before entering school (Bellini, 2008).

Prompting is the use of stimuli presented immediately before a behavior to cue the learner to display a specific behavior (Alberto & Troutman, 2006). When using video prompting, the video is viewed and paused during the activity. How long and how often to pause the video is initially determined by the task analysis and by baseline data on how many steps the student has acquired, whether or not the intervention is using forward or backward chaining, and whether or not a time-delay procedure is in place to fade the prompts. Table 6 provides 10 steps on implementing point-of-view video modeling (Mason et al, 2013).

Table 6. Steps for Implementing Point-of-View Video Modeling

Step	Description
1. Identify the target behavior	Get input from all stakeholders: parents, teachers, the child (depending on the age), paraprofessionals, extra service providers, etc. Focus on skills that can be used at home, in school, and in the community.
2. Complete task analysis	Break the task down into teachable components (task analysis). Observe a typical peer completing the task. Adjust the task analysis based upon typical peer performance (if needed).
2. Collect baseline data	Use the task analysis. Identify which steps (if any) the student can perform. Collect data until stable. Determine if the intervention is needed; if needed, proceed.
3. Prepare to create the video	Make sure to complete each step of the task. Practice until no within-task prompting is needed to complete the skill.
4. Record the video	Record in the same environment in which the task will need to be performed. Remove extra stimuli from the recording environment. Record the video from the eye view of the person completing the task (film over the shoulder of the person from behind).
5. Use the video as a prime	Determine when the learner will watch the video. Determine how many times a day the learner needs to watch the video. Make sure the video is viewed in a low demand situation before the task needs to be completed.
6. Collect data	Use the task analysis to collect data on each step of the task. If the target skill is a high frequency behavior, data can be collected on the first attempt of the day (first probe data). Set criteria for mastery (90% for 3 consecutive days).
7. Analyze effectiveness	Is there an immediate increase in percent completed from baseline to intervention? Is there an increase in trend and slope? Is the student approaching mastery? If yes, continue with step. Does student performance stabilize at low percent completed? If yes, step back to video prompting.
8. Fade the Use	If using as a prime more than one time per day, decrease the number of times per day the student watches the video. Have the student watch only part of the video (first part or last part depending on whether forward or backward chaining is appropriate. Remember to fade the use of the intervention slowly.
9. Check for Maintenance	Collect data using the task analysis three weeks after the intervention has been faded. If data indicates the student has maintained the skill, check again in three weeks. If student has lost skill, the video can be reintroduced periodically for procedural facilitation.
10. Choose the next target skill	Meet with stakeholders to determine the appropriateness of targeting a new skill. Only target one behavior at a time. Choose skills that have social validity and will be reinforced naturally across environments.

The team completes a task analysis of each skill and breaks down the steps of the skill into measurable increments. The tasks, completed by another worker at the grocery store, are then observed for validity and the task analysis is adjusted. When the task analyses are completed, Karen goes to the grocery store and is videotaped completing each step with prompting.

After taping each task, the prompts and extraneous stimuli are edited out of the video. The team's vision is that Karen can watch the videos before going to work and can view and pause each video on her smart phone during the task for prompting. Once the skill is acquired, prompting will be faded.

It is important to remember that video modeling is an antecedent intervention. Antecedent interventions used to evoke behavior should always be used in conjunction with reinforcement of the target behavior. Without reinforcement, the targeted behavior will not increase or be maintained. By choosing skills that will be naturally reinforced and pairing the intervention with positive reinforcement procedures, an intervention team can increase the likelihood that the behavior will increase and be maintained over time.

FUTURE RESEARCH DIRECTIONS

There are three areas that should be addressed in future research on using video modeling interventions for learners with developmental disabilities other than ASD: 1) assess the use of video modeling interventions in social skills and functional academic skills; 2) assess the use of video modeling interventions in younger children with developmental disabilities other than autism; and, 3) further assess the variables—both student and intervention characteristics—that contribute to effective video modeling interventions for children with developmental disabilities.

The majority of research on video modeling for learners with disabilities other than ASD has focused on self-care and vocational skills. For this population, self-care and vocational skills are probably the most pressing concern for self-sufficiency. However, social skills, functional academic skills, and leisure skills are equally important and may play an equally important role in self-determination and happiness. The efficacy of different types of video modeling should be further assessed in the aforementioned domains.

The majority of video modeling research across the above mentioned domains focused on adolescents and adults with developmental disabilities. Given the evidence base of this intervention, it would be interesting to determine if the same effects would be demonstrated in younger learners. If skills can be developed at an earlier age and address pivotal skills or behavioral cusps, the intervention may have a greater impact on long-term outcomes for people with developmental disabilities.

While several studies have addressed the variables of both characteristics of the learner and intervention components, more research is needed in this area (Mason et al, 2013; Mason et al, 2013). If learner characteristics can be matched to a type of video modeling intervention, application will prove easier for teachers, families, and other practitioners. Furthermore, the likelihood of the intervention working in the applied setting may increase as the intervention matches learner needs. Video modeling is frequently packaged with behavior analytic teaching techniques such as prompting hierarchies, forward or backward chaining, schedules of reinforcement, fading procedures, and error-correction procedures. It is important to understand which independent variables are necessary to change behaviors so that practitioners are not burdened with trial and error.

CONCLUSION

Video modeling is an effective intervention. It can serve as a motivator for many students since technology and video are a preferred activity, thereby increasing the likelihood for a successful intervention (Bellini & Akullian, 2007; Sherer et al., 2001). Like any good intervention, video modeling is only effective if implemented with fidelity. Video modeling interventions require careful planning, assessment, progress monitoring and the inclusion of the learner, family members, and school supports to increase the social validity and to problem solve any stumbling blocks until the intervention can be faded (Carnahan et al., 2012).

The characteristics and needs of the learner should be assessed and matched with the type of video modeling intervention selected. If a video modeling intervention is not working, the intervention team can easily adapt the video into a video prompting intervention. Video modeling can be paired with simple behavior analytic principles such as positive reinforcement, or be part of a behavior-analytic package. Some researchers highly recommended that video models include instructional components embedded into the video to increase support for those with developmental disabilities (Mason et al., 2013).

With the advances in technology, the intervention is portable and can be accessed in any teaching site (Carnahan et al, 2012). This allows for the intervention to be delivered in authentic settings, and in multiple settings, when appropriate. Portability increases the opportunities for implementation of the intervention across settings (home, school and work), thereby increasing the likelihood of generalization.

In conclusion, video modeling is an evidence-based practice involving the use of videos to teach or modify behaviors. Video modeling may include video modeling with another person as the model, video self-modeling, point-of-view modeling or video prompting. While there is a large research base on the use of video modeling with learners with ASD, there is less research on the use of video with learners with other developmental disabilities outside the area of self-care. Extending the use of video modeling interventions to areas other than self-care and to younger children with developmental disabilities, may have a great impact on quality of life and self-determination across the life span. To be fully self-determined and have a high quality of life, are goals that everyone hope to achieve.

After the successful completion of the video prompts, Karen and her school job coach completed the job application and participated in an interview with the manager at the supermarket. The manager agreed to hire Karen on a temporary basis in order to make sure the position was right for her, and that she was right for the position.

After two weeks at the supermarket, Karen had mastered the tasks of clocking in, greeting costumers, and bagging items. Karen was struggling with problem solving if a costumer asked a question and she did not know the answer. The team decided to make a video of Karen asking for help or directing the costumer to the cashier.

Karen continued to work at the supermarket throughout the summer on a part-time basis. While most days were without incident, Karen sometimes required extra assistance from the senior cashier with whom she worked. The team reconvened once more during the summer to update the video prompts according to Karen's needs. Karen wants to continue working at the supermarket during the school year on a part-time basis.

REFERENCES

Alberto, P., Cihak, D., & Gama, R. (2005). Use of static picture prompts versus video modeling during simulation instruction. *Research in Developmental Disabilities*, *26*(4), 327–339. doi:10.1016/j.ridd.2004.11.002 PMID:15766627

Alberto, P. A., & Troutman, A. C. (2006). *Applied behavior analysis for teachers* (7th ed.). Upper Saddle River, NJ: Pearson.

Bandura, A. (1977). *Social learning theory*. Englewood Cliffs, NJ: Prentice Hall.

Bellini, S. (2008). *Building social relationship: A systematic approach to teaching social interaction skills to children and adolescents with autism spectrum disorders and other social difficulties*. Shawnee Mission, KS: Autism Asperger Publishing.

Bellini, S., & Akullian, J. (2007). A meta-analysis of video modeling and video self-monitoring interventions for children and adolescents with autism spectrum disorders. *Exceptional Children*, *73*(3), 264–287. doi:10.1177/001440290707300301

Bellini, S., Peters, J. K., Benner, L., & Hopf, A. (2007). A meta-analysis of school-based social skills interventions for children with autism spectrum disorders. *Remedial and Special Education*, *28*(3), 153–162. doi:10.1177/07419325070280030401

Bidwell, M., Biederman, G. B., & Freedman, B. (2007). Modeling skills, signs and lettering for children with down syndrome, autism, and other severe developmental delays by video instruction in classroom setting. *Journal of Early and Intensive Behavior Intervention*, *4*(4), 736–743. doi:10.1037/h0100403

Bidwell, M. A., & Rehfeldt, R. A. (2004). Using video modeling to teach a domestic skill with an embedded social skill to adults with severe mental retardation. *Behavioral Interventions*, *19*(4), 263–274. doi:10.1002/bin.165

Buggey, T., Toombs, K., Gardener, P., & Cervetti, M. (1999). Using videotaped self-modeling to train response behaviors in students with autism. *Journal of Positive Behavior Interventions*, *1*, 205–214. doi:10.1177/109830079900100403

Burton, C. E., Anderson, D. H., Prater, M. A., & Dyches, T. T. (2013). Video self-modeling on an iPad to teach functional math skills to adolescents with autism and intellectual disability. *Focus on Autism and Other Developmental Disabilities*, *28*(2), 67–77. doi:10.1177/1088357613478829

Cannella-Malone, H. I., Mizrachi, S. B., Sabielny, L. M., & Jimenez, E. D. (2013). Teaching physical activity to students with significant disabilities using video modeling. *Developmental Rehabilitation*, *16*(3), 145–154. PMID:23477636

Cannella-Malone, H. I., Sigafoos, J., O'Reilly, M., De La Cruz, B., Edrisinha, C., & Lancioni, G. E. (2006). Comparing video prompting to video modeling for teaching daily living skills to six adults with developmental disabilities. *Education and Training in Developmental Disabilities*, *41*, 344–356.

Carnahan, C. R., Basham, J. D., Christman, J., & Hollingshead, A. (2012). Overcoming challenges: Going mobile with your video models. *Teaching Exceptional Children*, *45*, 50–59.

Centers for Disease Control and Prevention. (2014). *Developmental Disabilities Homepage*. Retrieved from: http://www.cdc.gov/ncbddd/developmentaldisabilities/specificconditions.html

Chan, J. M., Lambdin, L., Van Laarhoven, T., & Johnson, J. W. (2013). Teaching leisure skills to an adult with developmental disabilities using a video prompting intervention. *Education and Training in Autism and Developmental Disabilities*, *48*(3), 412–420.

Collins, S., Higbee, T. S., & Salzberg, C. L. (2009). The effects of video modeling on staff implementation of a problem-solving intervention with adults with developmental disabilities. *Journal of Applied Behavior Analysis*, *42*(4), 849–854. doi:10.1901/jaba.2009.42-849 PMID:20514193

Conyers, C., Miltenberger, R. G., Peterson, B., Gubin, A., Jurgens, M., Selders, A., & Barenz, R. et al. (2004). An evaluation of in vivo desensitization and video modeling to increase compliance in dental procedures in persons with mental retardation. *Journal of Applied Behavior Analysis*, *37*(2), 233–238. doi:10.1901/jaba.2004.37-233 PMID:15293644

Davies, D., Stock, S., & Wehmeyer, M. L. (2004). A palmtop computer-based intelligent aid for individuals with intellectual disabilities to increase independent decision-making. *Research and Practice for Persons with Severe Disabilities*, *28*(4), 182–193. doi:10.2511/rpsd.28.4.182

Dowrick, P. W. (1999). A review of self-modeling and related interventions. *Applied & Preventive Psychology*, *8*(1), 23–39. doi:10.1016/S0962-1849(99)80009-2

Edrisinha, C., O'Reilly, M. F., Choi, H. Y., Sigafoos, J., & Lancioni, G. (2011). "Say cheese": Teaching photography to adults with developmental disabilities. *Research in Developmental Disabilities*, *32*(2), 636–642. doi:10.1016/j.ridd.2010.12.006 PMID:21227636

Franzone, E., & Collet-Klingenberg, L. (2008). Overview of video modeling. Madison, WI: The National Professional Development Center on Autism Spectrum Disorders, Waisman Center, University of Wisconsin. Retrieved from http:// autismpdc.fpg.unc.edu/sites/autismpdc .fpg.unc.edu/files/Video-Modeling _Overview_1.pdf

Gresham, F. M. (2002). Best practices in social skills training. In A. Thomas & J. Grimes (Eds.), *Best practices in school psychology* (4th ed.). Bethesda, MD: NASP.

Hammond, D. L., Whatley, A. D., Ayres, K. M., & Gast, D. L. (2010). Effectiveness of video modeling to teach iPod use to students with moderate intellectual disabilities. *Education and Training in Autism and Developmental Disabilities*, *45*(4), 525–538.

Haring, T. G., Kennedy, C. H., Adams, M. J., & Pitts-Conway, V. (1987). Teaching generalization of purchasing skills across community settings to autistic youth using videotape modeling. *Journal of Applied Behavior Analysis*, *20*(1), 89–96. doi:10.1901/jaba.1987.20-89 PMID:3583966

Hart, J. E., & Whalon, K. J. (2012). Using video self-modeling via iPads to increase academic responding of an adolescent with autism spectrum disorder and intellectual disability. *Education and Training in Autism and Developmental Disabilities*, *47*(4), 438–446.

Horn, J. A., Miltenberger, R. G., Weil, T., Mowery, J., Conn, M., & Sams, L. (2008). Teaching laundry skills to individuals with developmental disabilities using video prompting. *International Journal of Behavioral and Consultation Therapy*, *4*(3), 279–286. doi:10.1037/h0100857

Kagohara, D. M. (2011). Three students with developmental disabilities are taught to operate an iPod to access age appropriate entertainment videos. *Journal of Behavioral Education*, *20*(1), 33–43. doi:10.1007/s10864-010-9115-4

Laarhoven, T. V., Winiarski, L., Blood, E., & Chan, J. M. (2012). Maintaining vocational skills of individuals with autism and developmental disabilities through video modeling. *Education and Training in Autism and Developmental Disabilities*, *47*(4), 447–461.

Martin, J. E., Mithaug, D. E., & Frazier, E. S. (1992). Effects of picture referencing on PVC chair, love seat, and settee assemblies by students with mental retardation. *Research in Developmental Disabilities*, *13*(3), 267–286. doi:10.1016/0891-4222(92)90029-6 PMID:1626083

Mason, R. A., Davies, H. S., Boyles, M. B., & Goodwyn, F. (2013). Efficacy of Point of View Video Modeling: A Meta-Analysis. *Remedial and Special Education*, *34*(6), 333–345. doi:10.1177/0741932513486298

Mason, R. A., Ganz, J. B., Parker, R. I., Burke, M. D., & Camargo, S. P. (2012). Moderating factors of video modeling with other as model: A meta-analysis of single-case studies. *Research in Developmental Disabilities*, *33*(4), 1076–1086. doi:10.1016/j.ridd.2012.01.016 PMID:22502832

Mechling, L., Gast, D., & Gustafson, M. (2009). Use of video modeling to teach extinguishing of cooking related fires to individuals with moderate intellectual disabilities. *Education and Training in Developmental Disabilities*, *44*(1), 67–79.

Mechling, L., Gast, D. L., & Seid, N. H. (2010). Evaluation of a personal digital assistant as a self-prompting device for increasing multi-step task completion by students with moderate intellectual disabilities. *Education and Training in Autism and Developmental Disabilities*, *45*(3), 422–439.

Mechling, L. C., Ayres, K. M., Bryant, K. J., & Foster, A. L. (2014). Continuous video modeling to assist with completion of multi-step home living tasks by young adults with moderate intellectual disability. *Education and Training in Autism and Developmental Disabilities*, *49*(3), 368–380.

Mechling, L. C., & Collins, T. S. (2012). Comparison of the effects of video models with and without verbal cueing on task completion by young adult s with moderate intellectual disabilities. *Education and Training in Autism and Developmental Disabilities*, *47*(2), 223–235.

Mechling, L. C., Gast, D. L., & Barthold, S. (2003). Multimedia computer-based instruction to teach students with moderate intellectual disabilities to use a debit card to make purchases. *Exceptionality*, *11*(4), 239–254. doi:10.1207/S15327035EX1104_4

Mechling, L. C., Pridgen, L. S., & Cronin, B. A. (2005). Computer-based video instruction to teach students with intellectual disabilities to verbally respond to questions and make purchases in fast food restaurants. *Education and Training in Developmental Disabilities*, *40*, 47–59.

National Autism Center. (2014). *National standards project: Addressing the need for evidence-based practice guidelines for autism spectrum disorders*. Randolph, MA: National Autism Center.

Nikopoulos, C. K., Canavan, C., & Nikopoulou-Smyrni, P. (2009). Generalized effects of video modeling on establishing instructional stimulus control in children with autism: Results of a preliminary study. *Journal of Positive Behavior Interventions, 11*(4), 198–207. doi:10.1177/1098300708325263

Norman, J., & Collins, B. (2001). Using an instructional package including video technology to teach self-help skills to elementary students with mental disabilities. *Journal of Special Education Technology, 16*(3), 5–18.

Norman, J. M., Collins, B., & Schuster, J. (2001). Using an instructional package including video technology to teach self-help skills to elementary students with mental disabilities. *Journal of Special Education Technology, 16*, 5–18.

Ogilvie, C. R., & Whitby, P. (2014). Video Modeling for Individuals with Autism Spectrum Disorders. In N. Silton (Ed.), *Innovative Technologies to Benefit Children with Autism*. New York, NY: IGI Global. doi:10.4018/978-1-4666-5792-2.ch013

Ohtake, Y., Takeuchi, A., & Watanabe, K. (2014). Effects of video self-modeling on eliminating public undressing by elementary-aged students with developmental disabilities during urination. *Education and Training in Autism and Developmental Disabilities, 49*(1), 32–44.

Ozkan, S. Y. (2013). Comparison of peer and self-video modeling in teaching first aid skills to children with intellectual disabilities. *Education and Training in Autism and Developmental Disabilities, 48*(1), 88–102.

Rayner, C., Denholm, C., & Sigafoos, J. (2009). Video-based intervention for individuals with Autism: Key questions that remain unanswered. *Research in Autism Spectrum Disorders, 3*(2), 291–303. doi:10.1016/j.rasd.2008.09.001

Rehfeldt, R. A. (2004). Using video modeling to teach a domestic skill with an embedded social skill to adults with severe mental retardation. *Behavioral Interventions, 19*(4), 263–274. doi:10.1002/bin.165

Rehfeldt, R. A., Dahman, D., Young, A., Cherry, H., & Davis, P. (2003). Teaching simple meal preparation skills to adults with moderate and severe mental retardation using video modeling. *Behavioral Interventions, 18*(3), 209–218. doi:10.1002/bin.139

Riffel, L., Wehmeyer, M., Turnbull, A., Lattimore, J., Davies, D., Stock, S., & Fisher, S. et al. (2005). Promoting independent performance of transition-related tasks using a palmtop PC based self-directed visual and auditory prompting system. *Journal of Special Education Technology, 20*(2), 5–14.

Scott, R., Collins, B., Knight, V., & Kleinert, H. (2013). Teaching adults with intellectual disability ATM use via the iPod. *Education and Training in Autism and Developmental Disabilities, 48*(2), 190–199.

Shane, H. C., Laubscher, E. H., Schlosser, R. W., Flynn, S., Sorce, J. F., & Abramson, J. (2011). Applying technology to visually support language and communication in individuals with autism spectrum disorders. *Journal of Autism and Developmental Disorders, 42*(6), 1228–1235. doi:10.1007/s10803-011-1304-z PMID:21691867

Sherer, M., Pierce, K. L., Paredes, S., Kisacky, K. L., Ingersoll, B., & Schreibman, L. (2001). Enhancing conversation skills in children with autism via video technology: Which is better, "self" or "other" as a model? *Behavior Modification, 25*(1), 140–158. doi:10.1177/0145445501251008 PMID:11151482

Shukla-Mehta, S., Miller, T., & Callahan, K. J. (2010). Evaluating the effectiveness of video instruction on social and communication skills for children with autism spectrum disorders: A review of the literature. *Focus on Autism and Other Developmental Disabilities, 25*(1), 23–26. doi:10.1177/1088357609352901

Sigafoos, J., O'Reilly, M., Cannella, H., Edrisinha, C., de la Cruz, B., Upadhyaya, M., & Young, D. et al. (2007). Evaluation of a video prompting and fading procedure for teaching dish-washing skills to adults with developmental disabilities. *Journal of Behavioral Education, 16*(2), 93–109. doi:10.1007/s10864-006-9004-z

Sigafoos, J., O'Reilly, M., Cannella, H., Upadhyaya, M., Edrisinha, C., Lancioni, G., & Young, D. et al. (2005). Computer presented video prompting for teaching microwave oven use to three adults with developmental disabilities. *Journal of Behavioral Education, 14*(3), 189–201. doi:10.1007/s10864-005-6297-2

Sturmey, P. (2003). Video technology and persons with Autism and other developmental disabilities: An emerging technology for PBS. *Journal of Positive Behavior Interventions, 5*(1), 3–4. doi:10.1177/10983007030050010401

Taber-Doughty, T., & Brennan, S. (2008). Simultaneous and delayed video modeling: An examination of system effectiveness and student preferences. *Journal of Special Education Teaching, 23*(1), 1–18.

Van Laarhoven, T., Kraus, E., Karpman, K., Nizzi, R., & Valentino, J. (2010). A comparison of picture and video prompts to teach daily living skills to individuals with autism. *Focus on Autism and Other Developmental Disabilities, 25*(4), 1–14. doi:10.1177/1088357610380412

Van Laarhoven, T., Zurita, L. M., Johnson, J. W., Grider, K. M., & Grider, K. L. (2009). Comparison of self, other, and subjective video models for teaching daily living skills to individuals with developmental disabilities. *Education and Training in Developmental Disabilities, 44*, 509–522.

Van Laarhoven, T. V., Winiarski, L., Blood, E., & Chan, J. M. (2012). Maintaining vocational skills of individuals with autism and developmental disabilities through video modeling. *Education and Training in Autism and Developmental Disabilities, 47*(4), 447–461.

Walser, K., Ayres, K. M., & Foot, E. (2012). Effects of a video model to teach students with moderate intellectual disability to use features of an iPhone. *Education and Training in Autism and Developmental Disabilities, 47*(2).

Yakubova, G., & Taber-Doughty, T. T. (2013). Brief report: Learning via the electronic interactive whiteboard for two students with autism and a student with moderate intellectual disability. *Journal of Autism and Developmental Disorders, 43*(6), 1465–1472. doi:10.1007/s10803-012-1682-x PMID:23080208

ADDITIONAL READING

Buggey, T. (2007). A picture is worth . . . Video self-modeling applications at school and home. *Journal of Positive Behavior Interventions, 9*(3), 151–158. doi:10.1177/10983007070090030301

Carnahan, C. R., Basham, J. D., Christman, J., & Hollingshead, A. (2012). Overcoming challenges: Going mobile with your video models. *Teaching Exceptional Children, 45,* 50–59.

Clark, E., Kehle, T. J., Jenson, W. R., & Beck, D. E. (1992). Evaluation of parameters of self-modeling interventions. *School Psychology Review, 21,* 246–254.

Dowrick, P. W. (1999). A review of self-modeling and related interventions. *Applied & Preventive Psychology, 8*(1), 23–39. doi:10.1016/S0962-1849(99)80009-2

Dowrick, P. W., Tallman, B. I., & Connor, M. E. (2005). Constructing better futures via video. *Journal of Prevention & Intervention in the Community, 29*(1-2), 131–144. doi:10.1300/J005v29n01_09

Franzone, E., & Collet-Klingenberg, L. (2008). *Overview of video modeling.* Madison, WI: The National Professional Development Center on Autism Spectrum Disorders, Waisman Center, University of Wisconsin.

Graetz, J. E., Mastropieri, M. A., & Scruggs, E. (2006). Show time: Using video self-modeling to decrease inappropriate behavior. *Teaching Exceptional Children, 38,* 43–48.

LaCava, P. (2008). *Video modeling: An online training module.* (Kansas City, KS: University of Kansas, Special Education Department). In *Ohio Center for Autism and Low Incidence (OCALI), Autism Internet Modules, www.autisminternet modules.org.* Columbus, OH: OCALI.

Ogilvie, C. R. (2011). Ten steps to creating video models for students with autism spectrum disorders. *Teaching Exceptional Children, 43,* 8–19.

Quill, K. A. (1997). Instructional considerations for young children with autism: The rationale for visually cued instruction. *Journal of Autism and Developmental Disorders, 27*(6), 697–714. doi:10.1023/A:1025806900162 PMID:9455729

Rayner, C., Denholm, C., & Sigafoos, J. (2009). Video-based Intervention for individuals with autism: Key questions that remain unanswered. *Research in Autism Spectrum Disorders, 3*(2), 291–303. doi:10.1016/j.rasd.2008.09.001

Sigafoos, J., O'Reilly, M., & de la Cruz, B. (2007). *How to use video modeling and video prompting.* Austin, TX: Pro-Ed.

KEY TERMS AND DEFINITIONS

Antecedent-Based Interventions: Proactive interventions that are based upon anticipated behaviors and circumstances. These interventions are implemented prior to the behavior occurring (Alberto & Troutman, 2006).

Backward Chaining: A procedure that begins by teaching and reinforcing the last step in the task chain. All steps prior are prompted. When the student learns the last step, the second to the last step is taught, followed by the last step and then reinforced (Alberto & Troutman, 2006).

Developmental Disability: A group of conditions that reflect impairments in physical, language, behavioral and learning abilities that begin during the developmental period, generally last throughout the individual's lifetime, and may impact day-to-day functioning (Centers for Disease Control and Prevention, 2014).

Forward Chaining: A procedure that begins with teaching and reinforcing the first element in the chain and progresses to the last element in the task chain (Alberto & Troutman, 2006).

Point-of-View Video Modeling (POV): Filming from the point of view of the person who will be required to complete the task; the participant viewing the video sees the actions from the perspective (point of view) of the person performing the task (Bellini & Akullian, 2007).

Priming: A research supported intervention; its purpose is to preview activities or information with a student before the student participates in that activity (Alberto & Troutman, 2006).

Prompts / Prompting: Prompts are stimuli that are presented immediately before or after a behavior to cue the learner to display a specific behavior. Prompting can occur after an inappropriate response is given in terms of error correction (Alberto & Troutman, 2006).

Reinforcement: Any stimulus that will increase the likelihood of a behavior reappearing (Alberto & Troutman, 2006).

Task Analysis: Breaking a skill down into a series of distinct steps (Alberto & Troutman, 2006).

Video Modeling (VM): An established intervention that can be used to increase communication, cognitive functions, personal responsibility and play/social skills and decrease problem behaviors and sensory/emotional difficulties (Bellini & Akullian, 2007).

Video Modeling with Other as Model (VMO): Video modeling with other as model involves the use of a recording of a peer or adult implementing a target behavior. Once the video is recorded, the student views the video prior to performing the activity (Bellini & Akullian, 2007).

Video Prompting (VP): Creating a video displaying specific steps of a task to be completed by an individual (Bellini & Akullian, 2007).

Video Self-Modeling (VSM): Creating a video, using the student in need of a desired and using it as all or part of an intervention (Bellini & Akullian, 2007).

Chapter 12
Assistive Technologies at the Edge of Language and Speech Science for Children with Communication Disorders:
VocalID™, Free Speech™, and SmartPalate™

Joséphine Anne Geneviève Ancelle
Teachers College Columbia University, USA

ABSTRACT

About two million individuals in the United States use augmentative and alternative communication (AAC) devices with text-to-speech (TTS) synthesis to speak on their behalf. In this chapter, two specific systems are introduced and evaluated as potentially significant emerging tools for children with communication disorders. The VocalID™ project was developed to provide unique voices for children who otherwise speak through standard adult voices. Free Speech™ is an image-based system designed to address grammatical concepts perceived as abstract by children with language disorders. This chapter also reviews the latest developments in electropalatography (EPG): biofeedback technology, which enables the visualization of tongue to palate contact during speech production. SmartPalate™ has developed cutting-edge hardware and software technology to make EPG more intuitive and more accessible in the therapy room and at home.

INTRODUCTION

Imagine a young girl who is not able to speak with her own voice, but instead speaks with the voice of a grown man. How would she feel when trying to communicate with other girls she is trying to befriend? Imagine a boy who is not able to understand anything that is abstract; how could he use language to communicate? Imagine a child having to receive occupational therapy, whereby the therapist cannot

DOI: 10.4018/978-1-4666-8395-2.ch012

show him the movements and cannot manipulate his body because the fine motor skills that he struggles with are in a part of his body that is hidden: his mouth. How would he be able to learn? The following chapter will introduce three developing technologies that are attempting to help children who encounter these difficulties, because of various communication disorders. Starting with a brief introduction on the classification, forms, and causes of communication disorders in children, each of the three assistive technologies presented will then be introduced and reviewed.

1. COMMUNICATION SCIENCES AND DISORDERS: AN OVERVIEW

The field of speech language pathology and audiology is now also becoming known by its more inclusive appellation of communication sciences and disorders (CSD), as its breadth and depth of research and practice are continuously expanding to include the wide variety of elements that comprise human communication. In 1925, a few teachers of theater, debate, and rhetoric founded a scientific organization to study "speech correction" (American Speech-Language-Hearing Association, 1997-2014). Today this organization, The American Speech-Language-Hearing Association (ASHA), studies not only speech, but also language, hearing, and swallowing disorders. ASHA also explores the underlying mechanisms of all forms of communication and is involved in developing alternate modes of communication when typical mechanisms fail. Before delving into the description of three different assistive technologies (AT) that could revolutionize the lives of children with communication disorders, a brief overview of the various branches of the field will clarify the discussion to follow.

a. A Few Words about Communication

It is estimated that 40 million Americans have a communication disorder (Ruben, 2000). While the hallmark of human communication is the use of this organized system of arbitrary symbols we call language, people also use non-linguistic forms of communication. Communication includes all information transmitted between a sender and a receiver of a message, and, therefore, can include facial expressions, gestures, body language, etc. (Plante & Beeson, 2013). For the majority of people, language is transmitted through speech, which involves the vocalization and articulation of the message we wish to transmit. When using speech, it is usually necessary that the sender and receiver of the message be able to hear in order to code and decode that message appropriately. Language can, however, also be written, or signed in the form of sign language.

It is not until we find ourselves struggling to express or comprehend a thought that we realize we take our ability to communicate for granted; human language and speech are nothing short of miraculous. Communication disorders are either acquired after an injury or illness, or are developmental, caused by congenital conditions such as genetic syndromes, childbirth-related complications, autism, or idiopathic etiologies. A breakdown in communication can occur at any of the various stages of message transmission, starting from the formulation of the thought in the sender's mind to the decoding of that message in the receiver's cortex, passing by the use of our vocal folds and articulators, among other processes.

b. Language Disorders in Children

Children who are born with genetic conditions, illnesses, or disabilities that hinder development are at risk for language impairment. Some disorders that impact normal language development include attention deficit disorders (ADD), autism spectrum disorders (ASD), and intellectual disability (ID) (Plante & Beeson, 2013). However, many children suffer from language deficits in the absence of any other handicapping conditions. These children are said to have specific language impairment (SLI). SLI can affect the production and/or the comprehension of language, impacting vocabulary, syntax, or phonology. Pragmatic language impairment (PLI) has recently made its appearance in the fifth edition of the Diagnostic and Statistical Manual of Mental Disorders (DSM-5) under the subcategory of Social Communication Disorders (American Psychiatric Association, 2013). PLI is differentiated from SLI and from high functioning autism (HFA) (Gibson, Adams, Lockton, & Green, 2013). Children with PLI struggle with the social and functional aspects of language development (the pragmatics of language), however, they do not "reveal evidence of restricted/repetitive patterns of behavior, interests, or activities" (American Psychiatric Association, 2013, p. 49).

Regarding acquired language impairments, children can suffer from aphasia, a loss of language after a traumatic brain injury, after a stroke, or due to seizures that cause damage to the brain. Compared to adults, children with aphasia are more likely to regain their language abilities, thanks to the high plasticity of the child's brain, capable of re-organizing itself more efficiently (Zipse, Norton, Marchina, & Schlaug, 2012).

In conclusion, language disorders in children can impact the form of language (syntax, phonology), the content of language (semantics), and the use of language (pragmatics). Childhood language impairments can be overcome or can persist into adulthood. Approximately 6 to 8 million Americans suffer from a form of language impairment (NIDCD, 2010b).

c. Speech Sound Disorders in Children

By the time children enter first grade, five percent of them have a noticeable speech disorder (NIDCD, 2010b). Although it is typical for young children acquiring language to make speech sound errors (e.g., "wabbit" instead of "rabbit" – "tuck" instead of "truck"), articulation and phonological errors qualify as speech sound disorders when they persist past the typical ages of mastery of the sounds of their language (Plante & Beeson, 2013). In other words, a child who pronounces the phoneme "r" with difficulty at 3 years old will be said to make speech sound errors. However, since, on average, typically developing children acquire the ability to pronounce the "r" sound appropriately by the age of 5, a child who is still unable to correctly say "r" at the age of 7 might be diagnosed with an articulation disorder, a type of speech sound disorder.

Speech sound disorders can have several causes, ranging from chronic otitis media (a child with repetitive ear infections may have temporary hearing loss that prevents him from getting the appropriate feedback for typical pronunciation of the sounds of his language), to neuro-motor impairments (e.g., cerebral palsy, childhood apraxia of speech), structural abnormalities (e.g., cleft palate), or hypotonia (e.g., developmental dysarthria, Down syndrome) (Plante & Beeson, 2013). Additionally, some children make persistent speech sound errors with no apparent cause. Speech sound disorders range in severity, causing a child to be highly unintelligible, or making the child feel embarrassed when speaking, as could be the case for a child with a mild lisp.

d. Fluency Disorders in Children

Although every speaker experiences disruptions in their flow of speech, fluency disorders are recognized as such when the regular disruptions of the speech flow become such that they impede communication (Plante & Beeson, 2013). Developmental stuttering is the principal disorder of fluency, although cluttering and acquired stuttering are also included in the fluency disorder umbrella. More than three million Americans stutter (NIDCD, 2012). Stuttering is usually identified before the age of 5 and can persist into adulthood although most children who stutter (about 80%) will outgrow it by puberty. It is estimated that less than one percent of adults stutter (NIDCD, 2010b; Plante & Beeson, 2013). Stuttering is three times more prevalent in boys than in girls, and although there is a genetic component to developmental stuttering (three genes were linked to stuttering in 2010), the etiology of this phenomenon is still poorly understood. Most researchers and speech language pathologists, however, now agree that stuttering is not caused by a psychological disturbance (NIDCD, 2012; Plante & Beeson, 2013). Stuttering and other dysfluency disorders can cause anxiety or other negative psychological effects in the individual because of associated negative experiences or embarrassment, but in the majority of cases, it is not the anxiety or other psychological factors that cause the individual to be dysfluent, contrary to earlier perceptions.

e. Voice Disorders in Children

Voice disorders concern abnormal pitch, loudness, vocal quality, or resonance, and can range from mild hoarseness to a complete loss of voice. Vocal misuse (e.g., excessive talking or yelling resulting in vocal nodules or polyps), aging, neurological disorders (e.g., myasthenia gravis), disease (e.g., laryngeal cancer), congenital defects, injury, or toxins (e.g., cigarettes, alcohol) can all cause disorders of the voice (Hooper, 2004; Plante & Beeson, 2013). Voice disorders can also stem from psychological or emotional factors, such as stress or personality disorders. Although estimates vary, the National Institute on Deafness and Other Communication Disorders (2010b) reports that about 2 to 3 percent of the United States' population suffers from voice disorders (about 7.5 million people). According to a variety of studies, the prevalence of voice disorders in children ranges between 6 and 9 percent (Hooper, 2004). The majority of voice disorders in children are hyperfunctional, meaning that they are due to the misuse or abuse of the voice resulting in hoarseness, vocal nodules, or traumatic laryngitis. Although a speech language pathologist will always refer an individual with a voice disorder to a physician first, hyperfunctional voice disorders are frequently reversible with appropriate therapy, and a majority of otolaryngologists will prefer voice therapy as the sole treatment (Hooper, 2004). Children who suffer with a neurological impairment or another form of injury may have more permanent vocal difficulties.

Speech and vocal production are overlaid functions onto our breathing and swallowing mechanisms. Because of its expertise in speech production, the field of communication sciences and disorders includes the study and treatment of dysphagia (i.e., swallowing disorder).

f. Hearing Disorders in Children

Out of 1000 children born in the United States, two to three children will be born deaf or hard of hearing, and nine out of ten of those children who are deaf will be born to hearing parents (NIDCD, 2010a). About 40% of children with hearing loss have an additional disability (Gallaudet Research Institute, 2011). Since hearing loss affects the development of language and speech, audiologic habilitation is recommended to begin as early as possible in cases of permanent hearing loss (Plante & Beeson, 2013). Audiologists work with the families of the child to counsel and educate parents on hearing loss, and participate in the application of hearing technology, such as hearing aids or cochlear implants. Speech language pathologists intervene to help develop language and speech if possible, as well as alternate modes of communication (e.g., augmentative and alternative communication) if speech is insufficient or cannot be developed.

Hearing loss ranges from mild to profound, and is classified as conductive (affecting the outer or middle ear), sensorineural (affecting the inner ear or auditory nerve), or mixed (a combination of conductive and sensorineural hearing loss) (Plante & Beeson, 2013). As for other communication disorders, hearing loss can be congenital or acquired. About 50% of congenital hearing loss is genetic (i.e., syndromic or the parents are gene carriers for hearing loss) and the other half is a result of environmental factors, such as prematurity or gestational diabetes.

Additionally, many children will experience temporary hearing loss due to middle ear infections (approximately 80% of children under four years of age) (NIDCD, 2010a). Chronic otitis media can hinder normal language and speech development if left untreated.

g. Technology in Communication Sciences and Disorders

In a 2006 article of the ASHA Leader, ASHA's (American Speech-Hearing Language Association) monthly journal, clinical professor of audiology, Robert E. Novak, wrote: "There is ... a merging of physics, biology, chemistry, and engineering, with tremendous potential for application to the disciplines of speech, language, and hearing science" (Novak, 2006, p. 3). As technology is exponentially developing and as devices have now become a part of our daily routines, it has become necessary and much easier for speech language pathologists and audiologists to tap into these technological advancements for therapeutic and assistive purposes. Smart phone and tablet 'apps' have entered the therapy rooms, as well as new software, devices, or even video games developed specifically for therapists or individuals with communication disorders. The second part of this chapter will present three tools that are being developed to enhance the lives of or to provide more efficient therapy to individuals with speech, voice, hearing, or language impairments.

2. INDIVIDUALIZED VOICES FOR AAC DEVICES: VOCALID™

Nowadays, who knows what Stephen Hawking's original voice sounded like? When thinking of the astrophysicist, we also undeniably think of the voice he now has: the voice of his speech-generating device (SGD). As we have been hearing Hawking speak more frequently on the Internet, on the radio, or in television shows, we have grown to recognize the synthesized voice he uses as his. However, Hawking is not the only individual who uses the voice of his SGD. His "voice" is one of the few standard voices integrated in text-to-speech (TTS) software, a voice that is likely used by many other individuals who rely on a speech-generating device to communicate. In fact, it would not be unlikely to hear a young girl use the same voice while she is having a conversation with her friends or to answer a question in her classroom.

a. What are Augmentative and Alternative Communication and Speech-Generating Devices?

ASHA describes augmentative and alternative communication (AAC) as including "all forms of communication (other than oral speech) that are used to express thoughts, needs, wants, and ideas" (ASHA, 2014). People with severe speech or language impairments use AAC to supplement (i.e., augmentative communication) or replace (i.e., alternative communication) their communicative abilities. AAC systems are categorized as either unaided communication systems or aided communication systems. Unaided communication systems are those that rely on the individual's body to convey the desired message, such as facial expressions, sign language, or simple gestures. Aided communication systems are those that require additional tools to supplement the user's body. These tools can range from a simple pencil and piece of paper, known as low-tech devices, to high-tech devices, such as a computer, tablet, or smart phone with integrated TTS software (Wolowiec Fisher & Shogren, 2012).

Children who may benefit from AAC include children with cerebral palsy who suffer from dysarthria, those with autism who are non-verbal, children with intellectual disabilities who have difficulty acquiring language, children with severe childhood apraxia of speech who are highly unintelligible when speaking, children with voice disorders who cannot rely on their own voice, children who are deaf, etc. In the past thirty years, a significant increase of individuals with communication disorders requiring AAC has been recorded (Light & McNaughton, 2012). A number of reasons have been identified for this escalating need for AAC. The ever-growing incidence of children with Autism Spectrum Disorder (ASD; estimated in 2014 by the Centers for Disease Control at 1 in 68 children compared to 1 in 150 children in 2000) has largely contributed to a larger need for AAC devices, since approximately 30 to 50 percent of children with ASD do not develop functional speech (CDC, 2014; Light & McNaughton, 2012). Also, thanks to medical advances, more children born with developmental disabilities are surviving, the consequences of which are that many of these children survive while experiencing lifelong disabilities. Cerebral palsy (CP) is one such disability for which the prevalence has been increasing (today evaluated at 1 in 323 children in the United States) thanks to advances in medicine (CDC, 2013). It is estimated that 95 percent of children with CP who have a speech and/or language impairment would benefit from using AAC systems (Light & McNaughton, 2012). Similarly, the aging population is living longer, often surviving despite acquired disabilities (for example, stroke survivors or individuals with degenerative diseases such as amyotrophic lateral sclerosis [ALS] are populations that survive longer and can benefit from AAC intervention). Finally, professionals and users alike have now become more accepting of using AAC, as more research is demonstrating its benefits, as awareness is growing, and as new technologies are making devices more accessible and user-friendly.

Speech generating devices belong to the category of high-tech AAC systems; they translate text or images into a spoken output from a synthesized voice. Voice synthesis is capable of, either producing an infinite number of words as it generates its output from single or composed sound units (phones or diphones), or from a set of pre-recorded whole words (NIDCD, 2014). Pre-recorded words make for clearer speech but limited vocabulary. Synthesized voices based on smaller sound units are often less intelligible but enable the TTS user to compose more complex sentences and thus provides more freedom of expression.

b. Vocal Identity and the Lack of Voices for TTS Users

Just like the unique patterns of our fingerprints or irises, our voice benefits from its own unique sound (Barzilay & Hasharon, 2006). In fact, biometrics authentication relies on vocal parameters to identify individuals. The voice's uniqueness is dependent on what speech scientists call the source-filter theory. The source is the vocal folds' vibration; their speed of vibration depends on the size and length of the individual's vocal folds (Ryalls & Behrens, 2000). For example, men usually have longer and thicker vocal folds than women or children; their vocal folds, therefore, vibrate more slowly, causing them to have a lower pitched voice in general. The filter is the vocal tract's shape, which defines the various features of the voice, such as the tone of the speaker. Researchers have described the human voice as an "auditory face" (Badcock & Chhabra, 2013, p. 2), since an individual's voice has been shown to provide clues to his personality, regional origins, socio-economic status, approximate age, gender, size, and even attractiveness (Badcock & Chhabra, 2013; Schweinberger, Walther, Zäske, & Kovács, 2011). Studies have also demonstrated that listeners perceive others' voices on a dual dimension of warmth and competence. Further, unique voices enable people to discriminate among simultaneous interlocutors, a quality that is considered evolutionarily advantageous to distinguish familiar from unfamiliar speakers when other senses might be obstructed (Nass & Gong, 2000). Clearly, a voice is much more than a tool for communication. A voice does not only match our physical and biological features to create a consistent whole, it is a part of our identity and demonstrates our uniqueness.

Currently, only a small set of voices is available to speech synthesis users (Patel & Roden, 2008). Indeed, few speech synthesis programs offer child or adolescent voices, and the choice of adult voices is limited. An Internet search for speech synthesizers yields a list of multiple websites for available speech synthesis programs, most of which enable a sampling of their synthesized voices. Among these samples, it is rare to find a child's voice or a teenager's voice. The most commonly used and programmed voice is the voice of an adult male, because it has proven to be the most intelligible according to adult and young listeners (Drager & Finke, 2012; Von Berg, Panorska, Uken, & Qeadan, 2009). This would explain why one should not be surprised to hear a large group of SGD users communicating with the exact same voice, whether adult or child, female or male.

However, to be able to relate a voice with a physique is important to users of SGDs and to people interacting with speech synthesis users. Recent studies surveyed users, non-users, and professionals' perceptions towards synthesized voices. Judge and Townend (2013) found that 65% of users felt that they did not have a range of voices to choose from. Regardless of age and gender, Von Berg, Panorska, Uken, & Qeaden (2009) found non-users' voice preferences depended on the natural sounding qualities of the voice rather than intelligibility. Further, multiple studies have demonstrated that listeners' perceptions and attitudes towards synthesized voices that appeared to be more closely related in age and gender to the user were more favorable (Patel & Roden, 2008). For example, Nass and Gong (2000), who studied *Speech interfaces from an evolutionary perspective*, suggested that humans' reactions to speech are "automatic and unconscious" (p.38) and thus, "individuals behave toward and make attributions about voice systems using the same rules and heuristics they would normally apply to other humans" (p.38). This suggests that someone who interacts with an individual who uses a synthesized voice that is too robotic and unpleasant to listen to might unconsciously negatively judge the SGD user. The authors also add that if synthesized speech users were able to "select voices that match their own personalities, fit gender stereotypes, or express the appropriate emotional tone," they would be more satisfied (p.41). In other words, individuals who use speech generating devices would feel more comfortable if they could use a more personalized voice, which would also encourage individuals who converse with SGD users to interact with them in a more natural manner.

c. VocalID™: Making Synthesized Voices More Human

Rupal Patel's TED talk went viral when it was published on YouTube in February 2014 (Patel, 2014). The talk, entitled "Synthetic Voices: As Unique as Fingerprints" describes Patel's research to create unique voices for speech synthesis users. As a speech scientist with a doctorate in speech language pathology and in biomedical engineering, Patel first became interested in customizing voices at an assistive technology conference. While she was there, she was surprised to hear dozens of people relying on SGDs that were programmed with the exact same voice. She asks in her talk, "we wouldn't dream of fitting a little girl with the prosthetic limb of a grown man, so why, then, the same prosthetic voice?" (Patel, 2014). She set out to change that, in order to give children who are not able to speak a voice that is truly theirs.

Customized voices are not new. For a few years now, researcher Timothy Bunnel has been creating personal synthetic voices for individuals who are at risk of losing their ability to speak, such as those with ALS, by pre-recording these individuals speaking multiple utterances, before converting those into a synthetic voice (Bunnell, Pennington, Yarrington, & Gray, 2005). What Patel is doing that is groundbreaking, is the custom crafting of voices for individuals who never had the ability to speak or who lost their ability to speak after an accident. As a reminder, dysarthria is an acquired or developmental motor speech disorder that causes a weakening of the mouth, face, and respiratory system; children with cerebral palsy, for example, often have dysarthria. Through her research, Patel established that individuals who suffer from severe dysarthria are still able to produce sounds and control some of the prosodic qualities of those sounds, such as loudness, duration, and pitch (Patel, 2002). Placing this information through the lens of the source-filter theory, this means that the source (i.e., the production of sound by the vocal folds) is still functional, whereas the filter (i.e., the vocal tract, which is responsible for the articulation of those sounds into distinct phones or phone combinations) is not. Although the vocal tract is partly involved in creating a unique vocal quality for an individual by providing a uniquely shaped resonating chamber (even slight variations in people's vocal tract's shape and size affect how the sound resonates), as previously mentioned, the thickness and length of an individual's vocal folds are responsible for an individual's fundamental frequency or average pitch (Ryalls & Behrens, 2000). With this in mind, Patel thought that by using the source of the individual who is unable to speak but can still produce sounds, and the filter of a donor who would be as close as possible in age, size, and gender to provide a similar filter, she could craft a voice that would befit the speech synthesis user (Jreige, Patel, & Bunnell, 2009). Thus, with a team of experts, she developed a system of speech synthesis that she called VocalID™ (for vocal identity).

When building a customized voice, the researchers begin by recording a target speaker with a speech impairment vocalizing on a vowel for about 2 to 3 seconds. In order to obtain the sound as it is at the source (before it is distorted by the vocal tract), the vowel is inverse-filtered. Then, the age, size, and gender matched healthy speaker is recorded speaking 1050 utterances (words and sentences). Each combination of sounds is segmented and variations in pitch are labeled to collect prosodic information (e.g., the end syllable of a same word will be labeled as rising in pitch for ending a yes/no question, as descending for ending a statement, etc.). Once both source and filter are collected, the two are blended to create a voice that retains the vocal quality of the target speaker's original pitch but uses the qualities of resonance of the voice donor. The target speaker can then use the database to generate unlimited text-to-speech utterances with his or her own unique voice.

Once they had created a few prototypical customized voices, Patel and her team proceeded to test the voices' intelligibility (Jreige et al., 2009). Twenty-four monolingual listeners were accurate between 94% and 97.6% of the time when transcribing 220 synthetic sentences from eight transformed children's voices. Participants found no significant difference of intelligibility between male and female voices. Listeners also rated naturalness at 3.5 on a scale from 0 to 5, 5 being the most natural. Finally, listeners were asked to establish if pairs of sentences were from the same synthetic voice or from two different synthetic voices. The average accuracy for voice similarity was at 79.5%.

In a previous study that compared a child's customized synthetic voice and a generic adult male synthetic voice, Patel and Roden (2008) had found that the adult voice was significantly more intelligible than the child's customized voice. This is not surprising, since research has demonstrated that adult male voices are usually more intelligible (Drager & Finke, 2012; Von Berg et al., 2009). However, the customized voices presented by Jreige, Patel, and Bunnel in 2009 demonstrated sufficiently high intelligibility, and although intelligibility is essential, to have a voice that is representative of one's identity is non-negligible.

Samantha Grimaldo is an adolescent girl who was interviewed with Patel for a *Huffington Post* video about VocalID™ (2013). Grimaldo has a disorder called perisylvian syndrome, which causes her to have severe speech impairment. She uses her smart phone to speak, but explains that the adult female voice she uses "sounds weird." In the video, her mother tells the interviewer that Samantha is reluctant to use the phone in public in order to avoid embarrassment, but the young girl agrees that she would use her device more frequently if it sounded more like her. Samantha's mother adds that as you get older, your voice becomes your identity. The video has Patel describe the VocalID™ story and process, and shows, at the end of the interview, Samantha's radiating smile as she hears her new voice for the first time. Then, with a grin on her face and a twinkle in her eye, Samantha is shown experimenting with her new voice on her tablet; she "says:" "My favorite food is pizza!"

Patel is still working on developing the VocalID™ project. Her goal is to provide customized voices for anyone who would like to have one. She is currently accumulating large databases of voices from donors around the world. Donors need to vary in gender, age, and size, but also speak different languages and dialects, and have various accents, since all of these factors contribute to shaping our vocal identity. Furthermore, Patel is taking the personalization of AAC devices a step further, by advocating for research to develop "more intelligent and personalized AAC" (Wiegand & Patel, 2014). According to Wiegand and Patel (2014), AAC devices should be user-specific (customized), adaptive (based on user's changing behavior), and context-sensitive (varying according to the location or time of day).

In conlusion, VocalID™'s main limitation is the reduced intelligibility for customized voices, compared to the standard adult male voices. Another limitation is the current lack of donated voices in their database to fit the needs of the wide variety of possible users. However, these limitations are likely to decrease with time, as the technology improves and the database expands. On the other hand, Patel's technology also fulfills a few significant needs of those who rely on SGDs to communicate. First, VocalID™'s customized voices enable more natural interactions by making the user and listener more comfortable, which in turn is likely to increase communication of SGD users in general, as well as with a larger variety of people. Further, the customized voices provide TTS users with the ability to choose a voice that they find satisfying. Finally, thanks to VocalID™, individuals with severe communication disorders could regain a part of their identity. To feel unique makes us feel human. There are millions of individuals who depend on an AAC device in the world. On a grand scale, Patel's work is likely to have powerful repercussions.

3. TRANSFORMING MAPS OF IMAGES INTO LANGUAGE: FREE SPEECH™

Are "a venetian blind" and "a blind Venetian" the same thing? Do the following sentences convey the same idea: "The boy loves the dog" or "The dog loves the boy"? These sentences are built with the exact same words, but the word order, the syntax of the sentence, is changed, making all the difference in meaning. Children with severe language impairment often rely on AAC devices that use pictorial representations of items and actions, rather than words to communicate. However, without an understanding of the importance of word (or image) order, some of these children might regularly express something they did not mean. Ajit Narayanan (2014a) experienced this phenomenon first hand after he had created Avaz, a picture-based app for children with communication disorders. Since then, Narayanan has been working on developing a new app that he calls Free Speech™, that would enable children who struggle with language to express exactly what they want through more complex sentences.

a. Language and Language Impairment

Every language is composed of a lexicon and of a grammar (Fernandez & Smith Cairns, 2011). Grammar itself is made up of three rule systems: phonological rules, morphological rules, and syntactic rules. Phonological rules pertain to the sound patterns of language, for example describing which sounds can follow another for a particular language. Morphological and syntactical rules describe the structure of words and sentences; they are responsible for creating a relationship between words and phrases, and thus form a coherent whole with the various units that compose a sentence. Morphemes are the smallest units of language that carry meaning, and morphology describes the rules for their combinations. For example, a morpheme can be the root of a word, such as "play" in "*play*ed." A morpheme can also be an affix such as "_ed" in "play*ed*." By adding the suffix for the regular past tense to a verb in a sentence, the meaning of that sentence is changed. Syntactic structure, although an essential aspect of language, is not represented in the symbolic signal (written, spoken, or signed) of language; it is abstract. It is syntax that is responsible for changing the meaning of the phrases "a venetian blind" and "a blind Venetian." A person may be able to convey some meaning with single words, but his or her communicative abilities would be very limited. Anyone who has attempted (or succeeded!) to learn a second language after the critical period for language acquisition will understand and remember how limiting and frustrating it can be to only have a few words or a meager understanding of grammar to convey ideas.

Indeed, for some, language does not develop in a typical way. Unfortunately, neuroscientists and psycholinguists have only scratched the surface as to what might cause this atypical development. What is now understood, however, is that there is a particular processing order for the encoding and decoding of a message. Starting with a thought, an individual then selects words out of his lexicon, continues to create a syntactic representation of what he or she is trying to convey, builds a phonological representation, and sends the information to his articulatory system (Fernandez & Smith Cairns, 2011). The decoding of a message occurs in the exact opposite way, although it starts with the auditory system. This all happens, of course, in a few milliseconds. Language impairments can be caused by a breakdown at any of these stages. For example, children with SLI usually struggle with lexical and morphological aspects of language (Plante & Beeson, 2013). Children with intellectual disability (ID) can be slow to acquire all aspects of language (Hill & Flores, 2014; Keskinen, Heimonen, Turunen, Rajaniemi, & Kauppinen, 2012). Some children with ASD have been shown to have unevenly developed morphological and syntactic skills, meaning that some skills are on par with typical peers, and others are not (Park, Yelland, Taffe, & Gray,

2012). Children with ASD also have difficulties with the pragmatics of language, like children who are diagnosed with pragmatic language impairment (PLI) (American Psychiatric Association, 2013). The pragmatics of language (i.e., its appropriate use in varying social contexts) add to the complexity of what language involves cognitively. As for all disorders of communication, language impairments can range from mild difficulties to a complete inability to use language to express thoughts (American Psychiatric Association, 2013; Plante & Beeson, 2013). For example, children with autism have a high risk of never developing language. More specifically, about 25 percent of children with autism are non-verbal and will never develop language in their lifetime (Tek, Mesite, Fein, & Naigles, 2014). Depending on the severity of their linguistic impairment, some children might require an AAC device to communicate effectively.

b. Picture-Based AAC Devices and Their Linguistic Limitations

Like those who suffer from speech impairments, many children whose language is severely impaired rely on AAC devices to express their wants and needs. However, for some of these children, AAC devices that are language-based (e.g., offering letters, words, or pre-programmed phrases) are too complex and/ or abstract. Children with severe language impairments may use low-tech or high-tech picture-based AAC systems instead. These systems use drawings, pictograms, or symbols with varying correspondence to language (Keskinen et al., 2012). For example, a child could select images that correspond to single words or to actions. If capable, the child could put a few images together to create a sentence. For example, one image would symbolize "I," another image would symbolize "want," and yet another image would represent a glass of juice; if the child puts all three images in the correct order, he can create the sentence "I want juice." A high-tech AAC device would then speak the sentence through text-to-speech synthesis. Previous research has demonstrated that certain individuals with autism think in pictures, or visually (Kunda & Goel, 2011). These findings support the selection of a picture-based AAC device for a non-verbal or linguistically limited child with autism. Similarly, a child with ID might also rely on a picture-based AAC system if his language delays are severe.

A number of image-based software and applications are available for AAC devices. The most common ones have a one-to-one relationship between a word or action and a picture (Narayanan, 2014b). Although it is easy to understand, one challenge for such a system is that a large number of words needs to be stored to give the individual who uses the device enough choices of things to say (usually, at least 3000). Due to the large number of images that need to be stored, a system of organization of words and concepts needs to be established. For children with a low IQ, to understand the categorization system can be challenging. Another difficulty can stem from having to organize pictures in a particular order to be able express a syntactically correct, and thus, meaningful sentence.

Another type of image-based AAC system is called semantic compaction. Invented by Bruce Baker in the 1980s, this system is based on the idea that one item or image could represent multiple concepts (Baker, 2009). For example, the image of a bed can express the word bed, as well as the concepts of sleeping, being tired, furniture, saying goodnight, or underneath. By putting various icons together, the user can code for the word desired (Semantic Compaction Systems, 2009). For example, the image of bed next to an image that represents a verb (a man that looks like he is going somewhere, called the "Action Man"), the concept becomes 'to sleep.' There is an icon to represent a noun and an adjective as well. The software that was built for semantic compaction is called Minspeak™. Minspeak™ is useful in that it works independently of the language being spoken, and that it reduces the number of images that need to be stored and organized on the device, making them easier to access. However, a limitation that has been noted is that the concepts that can be expressed by one image can be culturally biased (van der Merwe & Alant, 2004). Further, the difficulty of such a system is that it requires that the user memorize sequences of icons to form the various meanings, at least to get started (Semantic Compaction Systems, 2009). Also, the user needs to have a certain understanding of grammar. The structure of image sequencing matters in order to convey the right meaning, and even though the icons to form verbs, nouns, and adjectives are represented by imagery (i.e., Mr. action man for action words, Mother Hubbard for thing words, and the paintbrush for describer words, respectively), an understanding of the difference between parts of speech is still necessary. For certain children with language impairment, this can be too abstract. For example, it has long been documented that a large number of children with autism across the spectrum of disorders have a deficit in abstract reasoning (Minshew, Meyer, & Goldstein, 2002). Since language requires the ability to think in abstract terms, any form of AAC that requires the individual to use an advanced level of abstract thinking to communicate will pose a challenge to more concrete thinkers.

c. Free Speech™: Expressing Grammar through Maps of Images

Ajit Narayanan invented his app Free Speech™ in order to help children with autism who are non-verbal communicate in an efficient way (Narayanan, 2014a). The app is still in the process of being developed and no research has been published yet (although it is undergoing research trials) to demonstrate that children with autism can use the app in a meaningful way (Avaz Free Speech, 2014). However, the idea behind Free Speech™ is worth exploring.

Narayanan (2014a) explains that he came up with the idea for Free Speech™ because of an interaction he witnessed between a mother and her child with autism. The child suddenly said "eat" to his mother. Because there was no context to help the mother know exactly what her son meant, the mother proceeded to ask him a series of questions to make sure that she could fulfill his need appropriately. Therefore, she asked him questions such as: "eat what? Do you want ice cream? Do *you* want to eat? Does *somebody else* want to eat? Do you want to eat ice cream now? Do you want to eat later?" (Narayanan, 2014a). Narayanan explains that by asking questions such as "What? When? Who? Where?" the mother had been able to communicate with her child in an accurate way without the use of a grammatical sentence from the child. This is when Narayanan had his light bulb moment; he realized that if he could find a way to create an app that asks the right questions and then translates the answers to form a complete sentence, he could enable children who struggle with the grammar of language to communicate effectively.

Free Speech™ functions in the following way. Instead of having to organize words in a particular order, words are related to each other through questions and answers and end up forming a type of map. As previously mentioned, it is believed that the meaning of what we want to say is retrieved in our mind before the sentence is structured; lexical retrieval is the first major step before syntactic structure. It could therefore be easier for a child to retrieve vocabulary words than to arrange them in the right order to convey the desired meaning. If the child provides one word in the form of a picture, the Free Speech™ app would then suggest the right questions to help the child retrieve more words and to relate each word to the others to convey the intended meaning. In the patent's description of this mechanism called 'questioning,' Narayanan (2014b) explains that by asking the right questions, the app could reconstruct the original intended meaning and translate it into a grammatical sentence. The author affirms, "All sentences, however complex, can be decomposed as a cascading set of answers to a set of questions. This generates a data structure that looks like a tree" (Narayanan, 2014b, p. 8). He adds that this structure also needs to contain back-references and inter-links, such as referents for pronouns, as well as inflections. These are added in the form of filters or descriptors that specify negation, interrogation, tense, aspect, gender, or number information. Various icons represent different filters. The filter set varies depending on the part of speech it is connected with (e.g., the past tense icon is not offered with an icon representing a noun). For example, to transform the tree of images that represents the sentence "I want to" into "I didn't want to," icons that represent the past (a clock with an arrow going backward) and negation (a backslash) would be selected for the icon representing "want." In other words, Free Speech™ would be capable of helping the AAC user specify morphology as well as syntax.

Like most other picture-based apps, Free Speech™ requires the storage of thousands of pictures and icons for the user to have a wide range of available vocabulary. However, depending on the user's cognitive and linguistic abilities, the image database can be reduced or expanded (Narayanan, 2014b). Also, in order to make the system easier to navigate, various topics and related words are grouped into what the inventor calls ontologies. A main list of ontologies is first displayed in the form of pictures, and by selecting each list, a new list of related branches of ontologies appear. The main list can be tailored to the user or can simply be comprised of commonly used branches such as 'school,' 'home,' 'food,' 'actions,' or 'things.' The app also uses predictive technology to facilitate the selection of pictures by displaying high frequency images first. Predictive technology is also used to ask the most common questions when relating words with one another. For example, if the icon for "eat" is selected, the first suggested questions would be 'who' and 'what,' rather than 'where' and 'when.' Once all questions have been asked to relate all the words with each other, the app transforms the map of images into an English sentence that can be spoken through TTS synthesis. Narayanan has developed a set of rules, which he calls the Free Speech Engine, to translate Free Speech™ into English. Thanks to this system, children with severe language impairments that affect the grammar of language would be able to communicate in English clearly with their caregivers and friends.

Some limitations, however, need to be pointed out. First, the user of Free Speech™ would still need to have at least some basic understanding of grammar and word relationships. For example, the following sentence is provided to illustrate Free Speech™'s mechanism: "I told my father that I did not want to eat food" (Avaz Free Speech, 2014). In order to express the relationship between the sender and receiver of the message in the sentence, the following stream of questions and answers are shown in a demonstration video: "*Who told?* I told (answers are expressed by linking icons representing "I" and "tell;" in this case, the verb is connected to the past tense filter) – *Whom did I tell?* I told the father – *Whose father?* My father." Questions like "whose" and "whom" already express complex grammatical relationships of possessive and objective case. A child who struggles with grammar might find it difficult to answer these questions. Further, Narayanan's presentation of his invention focuses on expressive language. Receptive language can also be affected by language impairment; it would be interesting to investigate if Free Speech™ could also help decode spoken or written language. Additionally, since every word relationship needs to be established with a question and answer, this system would make rapid communication impossible. Still, in situations when specificity is important, Free Speech™ could provide the support needed to those who struggle with grammar, so that they can express exactly what they mean to express. Clearer communication would thus reduce the guessing and frustration that might go on between a child who has language impairment and his or her caregiver. Furthermore, children with language disorders could also interact effectively with people who are not familiar with their wants and needs. Finally, by communicating with more complex sentences, these children could more easily interact to develop relationships outside of their immediate circle of care.

Overall, Narayanan's project is worth monitoring since it could open up a whole new world of communication to many individuals who are isolated because of their linguistic limitations. Indeed, Narayanan (2014a) not only sees this system as a form of augmentative and alternative communication, but also as a possible tool to help second language learners around the world. Until we fully understand how language is produced in the human brain, no machine could pretend to emulate human language. However, Free Speech™ could provide linguistic support to those who lack this intrinsically human quality, and thus help these individuals regain some of their humanity.

4. A SMARTPALATE™ TO ASSESS AND TREAT SPEECH SOUND DISORDERS: NEW DEVELOPMENTS IN ELECTROPALATOGRAPHY

Who could imagine, only about a century ago, that we would one day be able to see inside people's bodies without having to cut them open? Nowadays, healthcare professionals can not only see what is going on under our flesh while we are completely conscious, via scans like ultrasonography, radiography, or magnetic resonance imaging (MRI), they can also visualize movements within our oral cavity in real time, thanks to electromagnetic articulography (EMA) or cineradiography (Preuß, Neuschaefer-Rube, & Birkholz, 2013). Electropalatography (EPG) enables healthcare professionals, but also the people they treat, to see the invisible. Thanks to EPG, a person can get a sense of what is going on in his or her mouth while he/she is speaking. For individuals with speech impairments, to learn how to produce sounds can be akin to being taught a complicated dance only through oral descriptions, without being able to see someone demonstrating it, and without being able to see their own movements in a mirror to compare. Thanks to EPG, these individuals can now see the "dance teacher's choreography" (i.e., the SLP's articulatory movements) and look at their own "moves in the mirror" (i.e., their own articulatory movements) to attempt to learn the complicated dance that is speech production.

a. Background on the Production of Speech Sounds

In order to understand what electropalatography is and how it functions, a short lesson on the anatomy and physiology of the speech mechanism is necessary. A slow but sufficiently strong exhale causes the adducted vocal folds in the larynx to vibrate, thus producing a sound (Small, 2012). The articulators are the speech organs involved in shaping that sound into phonemes - when referring to a speech sound, linguists, SLPs, and other speech scientists refer to a phoneme. A phoneme is the basic unit of sound for a particular language. It is differentiated from a letter or grapheme, because in many languages, a letter is pronounced in various ways depending on its surrounding letters. Each phoneme has a corresponding symbol in the International Phonetic Alphabet (IPA). For example, /i/ is the sound of the two "e"s in "bee;" /I/ is the sound of the "i" found in "bit." Each phoneme is classified according to its position of articulation in the mouth. Most of the major articulators are located in the oral cavity (i.e., the mouth). Articulation means "joining together," therefore, the articulators are the organs that come together to produce speech sounds. The main articulators for English sounds include *the lips* (e.g., the lips come together to make the /p/, /b/, and /m/ sounds); *the teeth* (e.g., the top front teeth and lower lip come together to produce /f/ and /v/); *the alveolar ridge*, which is the bony ridge at the roof of the mouth between the teeth and the palate (e.g., the /t/ sound is produced by placing the tip of the tongue against the alveolar ridge); *the palate* (e.g., the tongue touches the sides of the palate to produce a sound like "sh" as in "shoe"); *the velum* is also known as the soft palate and is the muscular structure located at the back of the palate that lowers for the production of nasal sounds (e.g., /n/ or /m/); *the glottis*, the opening between the vocal folds when they are not vibrating (e.g., the glottis is used to make the /h/ sound as in "hat"); and *the tongue*, which is the major articulator, since most sounds are produced with a part of the tongue coming together with another articulator (e.g., the tip of the tongue comes between the teeth to make the "th" sound; the body of the tongue is high and towards the front of the oral cavity when producing a /i/ as in "key" and low and towards the back of the oral cavity when producing a /a/ as in "cod."

Individuals who have a speech impairment, such as dysarthria, apraxia of speech, a lisp, or other speech sound disorders have a hard time coordinating or controlling the movements of their articulators, either due to muscle weakness, to neuromotor damage, to physical abnormalities, to hearing loss, or to unknown causes. The movements of the articulators are very precise and are performed very rapidly. Furthermore, most of these movements cannot be seen. For these reasons, it is often difficult to teach someone how and when to place the articulators for the production of a certain sound, or to assess their sound production (Gibbon & Lee, 2007). Speech language pathologists and researchers have used various methods over the years in order to provide or acquire feedback of articulators' placement; these methods included the use of a mirror or placing cocoa powder an charcoal on the tongue, or peanut butter on the palate to get a sense of where the tongue is or to teach where to place it (Articulate Instruments, 2013b). However, these methods are not very accurate, and the more typical perceptual auditory judgments are subjective (Gibbon & Wood, 2010). Electropalatography provides visual feedback of the tongue's movements, providing objective support for assessment and therapy. EPG is not new; however, it has lately been developing to combine its improving technology with engaging apps for children, and user-friendly designs, giving articulation biofeedback a makeover that is likely to entice children and adults alike.

b. What Is Electropalatography?

Electropalatography is a procedure that enables the recording of the position and timing of the tongue's contact with the hard palate while someone is speaking (Gibbon & Lee, 2007). It consists of a customized artificial palate, sometimes called a palatometer, molded and fitted for the individual who is going to use it (Articulate Instruments, 2013a; Complete Speech, 2013). This palate is embedded with electrodes (between 62 and 124 depending on the manufacturer) that transmit the information of tongue-palate contact to a microprocessor, which itself connects to a computer through a USB port. The information is then processed and displayed on the screen through software, enabling the user to see in real time his tongue movements in relation to his palate, or rather, to the many sensors distributed all over the artificial palate, which, depending on the manufacturer, represent some or most of the various places of articulation, from bilabial to velar. For example, the production of the /t/ phoneme should provide the user of EPG with a horseshoe shape image if produced correctly, since the tongue will connect with the palate on both sides and in the front, by the alveolar ridge, but not in the center or back of the oral cavity. In Figure 1, electrodes are represented by each dot. The larger dots are those with an established contact between the tongue and palate. These images represent appropriate tongue placement for the sounds /s/, /t/, and /k/, as well as inappropriate tongue placement in the case of a lateralized lisp.

Software that accompanies the EPG hardware can prompt for target words, as well as display a synchronized acoustic recording (Articulate Instruments, 2013a; Complete Speech, 2013). It is also possible for the therapist to connect his/her own artificial palate at the same time his/her client does, through a dual screen display that enables the child to immediately compare his speech production to his therapist's. Software also provides a library of palatal shapes for appropriate phoneme production, and feedback and analysis of production.

Figure 1. Tongue-Palate contact as displayed in SmartPalate™ software for the sounds /s/, /s/ with a lateralized lisp, /t/, and /k/. © 2014 SmartPalate International, LLC. Used with permission.

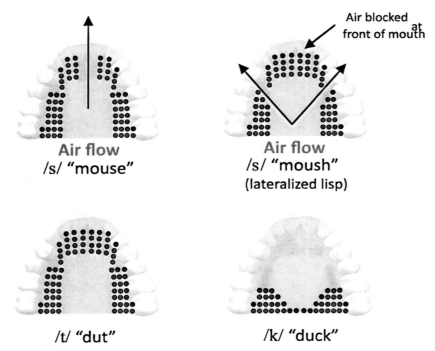

EPG dates back to 1938, invented at the College of Iowa State by graduate student Herbert Koepp-Baker (Articulate Instruments, 2013b). The original palatometer consisted of a thick artificial palate that contained only 10 electrodes; the acquired measurements were recorded on a paper chart. Starting from the late 1960's, professors Hardcastle and Fletcher, each in Edinburgh and Utah respectively, developed the basic instrument design; they have been responsible for its main developments. Although a few companies emerged to make the instruments available for commercial use, three main companies remain: Articulate Instruments, Ltd. and Rose Medical Solutions, Ltd., both located in the United Kingdom, and Complete Speech, LLC., located in the United States (Articulate Instruments, 2013b; Complete Speech, 2013; Gibbon & Lee, 2007; Rose Medical Solutions, 2014). The companies differ in the way they manufacture the artificial palates (e.g., using a different number of electrodes), and each has developed their own hardware and software.

Originally, EPG therapy was only used as a last resort when traditional therapy had failed, due to its costly and hard to access nature (Gibbon & Wood, 2010). In the past ten to fifteen years, EPG has become more accessible to speech therapists and their clients, since the equipment is becoming slightly more affordable and available (Gibbon & Lee, 2007). Still, few speech therapists are equipped to provide EPG therapy compared to the large population of children (and adults) who could potentially benefit from it (Gibbon & Wood, 2010). Despite a small number of EPG laboratories in the world, EPG research dates back to the early days of its invention, with the intent to demonstrate its use in speech pathology, phonetic research, or even for swallowing therapy (Chi-Fishman & Stone, 1996; Hardcastle, 1972). Studies from multiple countries, such as Japan, Sweden, Great Britain, Canada, or the United States support its use in speech therapy for children with hearing impairments, children with cerebral palsy, children with repaired cleft palate, or other children with speech impairments that concern lingual articulation (EPG provides visual biofeedback only for lingual-palatal phonemes) (Bacsfalvi & Bernhardt, 2011; Gibbon & Wood, 2010; Lohmander, Henriksson, & Havstam, 2010; Nordberg, Carlsson, & Lohmander, 2011; Preuß et al., 2013). Still, more adequate research is needed to demonstrate the efficacy of EPG in the treatment of speech impairments. There is a lack of studies with large numbers of participants and with control groups; most studies are case studies or case reports (Gibbon & Wood, 2010). However, recent developments of EPG technology are likely to enable studies on a larger scale. In the United Kingdom, Articulate Instruments, Ltd. has made available Portable Training Units (PTUs) that do not need to be connected to a computer. The feedback is limited to the tongue-palate contact information, but it allows children to practice on their own at home, thus enabling more regular and intensive practice (Gibbon & Lee, 2007). In the United States, Complete Speech, LLC. has been updating EPG technology to catch-up with twenty-first century interfaces and to give their product a brand new look and additional tools, making the therapy process with EPG more attractive and playful for children and their therapists.

c. SmartPalate™: Newest Developments in EPG Technology

Professor Samuel G. Fletcher founded Complete Speech in 2008 with the idea to make his newest version of the palatometer, the SmartPalate™, widely available for use and to advance research (Complete Speech, 2010-2014). His team of engineers and developers have been working on reducing costs, providing training, and improving the hardware and software to make EPG more user-friendly and accessible. Although few research studies have been conducted with the SmartPalate™ technology as of yet, some of its features already appear advantageous over other EPG technology. First, the visual display is more concrete. Whereas other EPG software displays the electrodes as squares on the screen, SmartPalate™ software shows electrodes' placement within a representation of a mouth that can be adapted to the user, such as by displaying the correct number of teeth, for example. This anatomically accurate visual is likely to help children have a clearer understanding of what they are looking at. Further, SmartPalate™ uses a high number of sensors for increased precision (124 compared to 64 in other palatometers), and it also includes two lip closure sensors, which can thus monitor bilabial sounds (/p/, /b/, and /m/) as well. Also, the software offers various types of practice settings, including a simple display of the sensors and acoustic waves for practice with a therapist, oral coordination training involving the tip of the tongue touching specific sensors that light-up on the screen, or templates of appropriate tongue placement for the production of specific sounds to reproduce (Complete Speech, 2013). Additionally, produced sounds can be recorded and re-played at a slower speed in order to see patterns of pronunciation clearly. Also, SmartPalate™ software allows for baseline recordings of the tongue placement and rate of speech before therapy begins for comparative purposes throughout and after therapy ends. It enables the SLP to test the child's oral coordination and muscle tone through games. Further, the SLP can create tongue targets that are specific to the client they are working with, either by building the targets from scratch, or by capturing them during live speech recordings. These targets can be exported so that a client can continue to practice them in between therapy sessions, provided they have the equipment at home. Finally, SmartPalate™ allows for specific sounds to be monitored within sentences, or provides progress reports since all of the data can be recorded and saved. Other qualities of the SmartPalate™ software include its more modern interface and its ability to have multiple students work simultaneously during a session by splitting the screen display. In other words, the software can provide support to the SLP during evaluation, during treatment, and to encourage generalization (the ability to reproduce what is learned in the therapy room in every day interactions). All of these qualities make the SmartPalate™ an attractive tool to work with, for clients and therapists alike.

In conclusion, although EPG technology has been over fifty years in the making, recent developments have given it a makeover that could potentially impact the lives of many of the children who suffer from speech sound disorders. However, EPG technology is still relatively costly, thus preventing its widespread use. It also involves complicated procedures, since it requires the fabrication of a customized synthetic palate for each user. Furthermore, systematic studies with large groups of participants and controls need to be conducted to establish the validity of such a tool, such as in its therapeutic use for improved intelligibility of children with speech sound disorders. Anecdotal evidence seems to point to not only better and faster results, but also to increased enthusiasm from the children who work with SmartPalate™. Many speech language pathologists know that a motivated child is essential for success. Additionally, children who improve their speech production skills have been shown to build their confidence level (Thomas-Stonell, Oddson, Robertson, & Rosenbaum, 2009). Therefore, future EPG research involving SmartPalate™ is worthy of investigation, since it could accelerate a child's improvement in speech production, and with it, his ability to interact with others with more self-assurance.

CONCLUSION

Our linguistic abilities, whether expressed through speech, through written text, or through sign language, are paramount to making us feel human, because language is a uniquely human ability. Any assistive tool that can help an individual who struggles with communication skills, will not only improve this person's linguistic interactions, but also his quality of life. Throughout this chapter, we investigated three developing technologies that have the potential of truly making a difference for those with various communication disorders. By creating unique voices, VocalID™ could provide a sense of identity and an increased desire to communicate for children who rely on text-to-speech synthesis to communicate their thoughts. Free Speech™ could give the gift of grammar to children who can only rely on their lexicon, and thus enable them to finally express exactly what they mean to say. And the latest EPG technology in the form of SmartPalate™ could help children spend less time in speech therapy, and more time socializing with their friends with renewed confidence. Since all of these products are quite relatively new on the market, they are all in need of testing via large randomized research studies. Researchers are beginning to conduct these studies and it will be useful to assess their findings.

VocalID is a registered trademark of Vocal ID Inc., located in Boston, MA, USA.
Minspeak is a registered trademark of Semantic Compaction Systems, located in Pittsburgh, PA, USA
Free Speech is a registered trademark of Avaz Inc., located in Chennai, India.
SmartPalate is a registered trademark of Smart Palate International, LLC, located in Orem, UT, USA.

REFERENCES

American Psychiatric Association. (2013). *Diagnostic and statistical manual of mental disorders* (5th ed.). Arlington, VA: American Psychiatric Association.

American Speech-Language-Hearing Association. (1997-2014). *History of ASHA*. Retrieved 08/04/2014, 2014, from http://www.asha.org/about/history/

Articulate Instruments, Ltd. (2013a). *EPG Products*. Retrieved 08/08/2014, 2014, from http://www.articulateinstruments.com/epg-products/

Articulate Instruments, Ltd. (2013b). *A History of EPG*. Retrieved 08/07/2014, 2014, from http://www.articulateinstruments.com/a-history-of-epg/

ASHA, American Speech Language Hearing Association. (2014). *Augmentative and Alternative Communication (AAC)*. Retrieved 08/01/2014, 2014, from http://www.asha.org/public/speech/disorders/AAC.htm

Avaz Free Speech. (2014). *Avaz Free Speech*. Retrieved 08/12/2014, 2014, from http://avazapp.com/freespeech/

Bacsfalvi, P., & Bernhardt, B. M. (2011). Long-term outcomes of speech therapy for seven adolescents with visual feedback technologies: Ultrasound and electropalatography. *Clinical Linguistics & Phonetics*, *25*(11/12), 1034–1043. doi:10.3109/02699206.2011.618236 PMID:22106893

Badcock, J. C., & Chhabra, S. (2013). Voices to reckon with: Perceptions of voice identity in clinical and non-clinical voice hearers. *Frontiers in Human Neuroscience*, *7*. doi:10.3389/fnhum.2013.00114 PMID:23565088

Baker, B. R. (2009). *MinspeakTM History*. Retrieved 08/15/2014, 2014, from http://www.minspeak.com/HistoryofMinspeak.php#.U-yIylYivuc

Barzilay, Z., & Hasharon, R. (2006). United States Patent No. 0259304A1.

Bunnell, H. T., Pennington, C., Yarrington, D., & Gray, J. (2005). *Automatic personal synthetic voice construction*. Paper presented at the Eurospeech 2005, Lisbon, Portugal.

CDC, Centers for Disease Control and Prevention. (2013). *Cerebral Palsy, Data and Statistics*. Retrieved 08/04/2014, 2014, from http://www.cdc.gov/ncbddd/cp/data.html

CDC, Centers for Disease Control and Prevention. (2014). *Autism Spectrum Disorders - Data and Statistics*. Retrieved 08/04/2014, 2014, from http://www.cdc.gov/ncbddd/autism/data.html

Chi-Fishman, G., & Stone, M. (1996). A new application for electropalatography: Swallowing. *Dysphagia*, *11*(4), 239–247. doi:10.1007/BF00265208 PMID:8870350

Complete Speech, L. L. C. (2013). *What is a SmartPalate*. Retrieved 08/08/2014, 2014, from http://www.completespeech.com/speech/smartpalate1/what_is_a_smartpalate/

Complete Speech, L. L. C. (2010-2014). *Complete Speech Blog*. Retrieved 08/10/2014, 2014, from http://www.completespeech.com/speech/blog/P20

Drager, K. D. R., & Finke, E. H. (2012). Intelligibility of Children's Speech in Digitized Speech. *AAC: Augmentative & Alternative Communication*, *28*(3), 181–189. doi:10.3109/07434618.2012.704524 PMID:22946993

Fernandez, E. M., & Smith Cairns, H. (2011). *Fundamentals of Psycholinguistics*. Hoboken, NJ: Wiley-Blackwell.

Gallaudet Research Institute (GRI). (2011). Regional and National Summary Report of Data from the 2009-10 Annual Survey of Deaf and Hard of Hearing Children and Youth. Washington DC: Gallaudet University.

Gibbon, F. E., & Lee, A. (2007). Electropalatography as a Research and Clinical Tool. *SIG 5 Perspectives on Speech Science and Orofacial Disorders, 17*, 7-13.

Gibbon, F. E., & Wood, S. E. (2010). Visual feedback therapy with electropalatography. In A. L. Williams, S. McLeod, & R. J. McCauley (Eds.), *Interventions for Speech Sound Disorders in Children* (pp. 509–536). Baltimore, MD: PH Brooks Publishing Company.

Gibson, J., Adams, C., Lockton, E., & Green, J. (2013). Social communication disorder outside autism? A diagnostic classification approach to delineating pragmatic language impairment, high functioning autism and specific language impairment. *Journal of Child Psychology and Psychiatry, and Allied Disciplines, 54*(11), 1186–1197. doi:10.1111/jcpp.12079 PMID:23639107

Hardcastle, W. J. (1972). The use of electropalatography in phonetic research. *Phonetica, 25*(4), 197–215. doi:10.1159/000259382 PMID:4565321

Hill, D., & Flores, M. (2014). Comparing the Picture Exchange Communication System and the iPad™ for Communication of Students with Autism Spectrum Disorder and Developmental Delay. *TechTrends: Linking Research & Practice to Improve Learning, 58*(3), 45–53. doi:10.1007/s11528-014-0751-8

Hooper, C. R. (2004). Treatment of Voice Disorders in Children. *Language, Speech, and Hearing Services in Schools, 35*(4), 320–326. doi:10.1044/0161-1461(2004/031) PMID:15609635

Huffington Post (Producer). (2013). Cutting-Edge Tech Gives a Synthetic Voice to the Voiceless. *Huff Post Tech*. [Video] Retrieved from http://www.huffingtonpost.com/2013/09/13/vocalid_n_3915829.html?utm_hp_ref=tw

Jreige, C., Patel, R., & Bunnell, H. T. (2009). Vocal ID: Personalizing Text-to-Speech Synthesis for Individuals with Severe Speech Impairment. *Proceedings of the 11th international ACM SIGACCESS conference on Computers and Accessibility*, 259-260.

Judge, S., & Townend, G. (2013). Perceptions of the design of voice output communication aids. *International Journal of Language & Communication Disorders, 48*(4), 366–381. doi:10.1111/1460-6984.12012 PMID:23889833

Keskinen, T., Heimonen, T., Turunen, M., Rajaniemi, J.-P., & Kauppinen, S. (2012). SymbolChat: A flexible picture-based communication platform for users with intellectual disabilities. *Interacting with Computers, 24*(5), 374–386. doi:10.1016/j.intcom.2012.06.003

Kunda, M., & Goel, A. K. (2011). Thinking in Pictures as a Cognitive Account of Autism. *Journal of Autism and Developmental Disorders, 41*(9), 1157–1177. doi:10.1007/s10803-010-1137-1 PMID:21103918

Light, J., & McNaughton, D. (2012). The Changing Face of Augmentative and Alternative Communication: Past, Present, and Future Challenges. *AAC: Augmentative & Alternative Communication, 28*(4), 197–204. doi:10.3109/07434618.2012.737024 PMID:23256853

Lohmander, A., Henriksson, C., & Havstam, C. (2010). Electropalatography in home training of retracted articulation in a Swedish child with cleft palate: Effect on articulation pattern and speech. *International Journal of Speech-Language Pathology, 12*(6), 483–496. doi:10.3109/17549501003782397 PMID:20602582

Minshew, N. J., Meyer, J., & Goldstein, G. (2002). Abstract reasoning in autism: A disassociation between concept formation and concept identification. *Neuropsychology, 16*(3), 327–334. doi:10.1037/0894-4105.16.3.327 PMID:12146680

Narayanan, A. (Producer). (2014a). Ajit Narayanan: A word game to communicate in any language. *TED Talks*. [Video] Retrieved from http://www.ted.com/talks/ajit_narayanan_a_word_game_to_communicate_in_any_language

Narayanan, A. (2014b). *Systems and methods for picture based communication: Google Patents.*

Nass, C., & Gong, L. (2000). Speech interfaces from an evolutionary perspective. *Communications of the ACM, 43*(9), 36–43. doi:10.1145/348941.348976

NIDCD, National Institute on Deafness and Other Communication Disorders. (2010a). *Quick Statistics - Hearing Loss*. Retrieved 07/31/2014, 2014, from http://www.nidcd.nih.gov/health/statistics/Pages/quick.aspx

NIDCD, National Institute on Deafness and Other Communication Disorders. (2010b). *Quick Statistics - Statistics on Voice, Speech, and Language*. Retrieved 07/30/2014, 2014, from http://www.nidcd.nih.gov/health/statistics/vsl/Pages/stats.aspx

NIDCD, National Institute on Deafness and Other Communication Disorders. (2012). *Stuttering*. Retrieved 07/30/2014, 2014, from http://www.nidcd.nih.gov/health/voice/pages/stutter.aspx

NIDCD, National Institute on Deafness and Other Communication Disorders. (2014). *Assistive Devices for People with Hearing, Voice, Speech, or Language Disorders*. Retrieved 08/04/2014, 2014, from http://www.nidcd.nih.gov/health/hearing/pages/assistive-devices.aspx

Nordberg, A., Carlsson, G., & Lohmander, A. (2011). Electropalatography in the description and treatment of speech disorders in five children with cerebral palsy. *Clinical Linguistics & Phonetics, 25*(10), 831–852. doi:10.3109/02699206.2011.573122 PMID:21591933

Novak, R. E. (2006). New Technology and Changing Demographics: Part One of a Two-Part Series on Challenges to our Professions Over the Next 10 Years, *The ASHA Leader*. Retrieved from http://www.asha.org/publications/leader/2006/060117/f060117a.htm

Park, C. J., Yelland, G. W., Taffe, J. R., & Gray, K. M. (2012). Morphological and syntactic skills in language samples of pre school aged children with autism: Atypical development? *International Journal of Speech-Language Pathology, 14*(2), 95–108. doi:10.3109/17549507.2011.645555 PMID:22390743

Patel, R. (2002). Phonatory Control in Adults with Cerebral Palsy and Severe Dysarthria. *AAC: Augmentative & Alternative Communication, 18*(1), 2.

Patel, R. (2014). *Rupal Patel: Synthetic Voices, As Unique as Fingerprints*. YouTube.

Patel, R., & Roden, A. (2008). Intelligibility and attitudes toward a speech synthesizer vocoded using dysarthric vocalizations. *Journal of Medical Speech-Language Pathology, 16*(4), 243–249.

Plante, E., & Beeson, P. M. (2013). *Communication & Communication Disorders: A Clinical Introduction*. Pearson Education, Inc.

Preuß, S., Neuschaefer-Rube, C., & Birkholz, P. (2013). Prospects of EPG and OPG sensor fusion in pursuit of a 3D real-time representation of the oral cavity. *Studientexte zur Sprachkommunikation: Elektronische Sprachsignalverarbeitung*, 144-151.

Rose Medical Solutions, Ltd. (2014). *Electropalatography*. Retrieved 08/08/2014, 2014, from http://www.rose-medical.com/electropalatography.html

Ruben, R. J. (2000). Redefining the survival of the fittest: Communication disorders in the 21st century. *Laryngoscope, 110*(2 I), 241-245.

Ryalls, J., & Behrens, S. J. (2000). *Introduction to Speech Science: From Basic Theories to Clinical Applications*. Needham Heights, MA: Allyn & Bacon.

Schweinberger, S. R., Walther, C., Zäske, R., & Kovács, G. (2011). Neural correlates of adaptation to voice identity. *British Journal of Psychology, 102*(4), 748–764. doi:10.1111/j.2044-8295.2011.02048.x PMID:21988382

Semantic Compaction Systems. (2009). *AAC Core Vocabulary Communication Device - What is Minspeak*. Retrieved 08/15/2014, 2014, from http://www.minspeak.com/what.php#.U_B3w1Yivuc

Small, L. H. (2012). *Fundamentals of Phonetics: A practical guide for students*. Upper Saddle River, NJ: Pearson Education, Inc.

Tek, S., Mesite, L., Fein, D., & Naigles, L. (2014). Longitudinal Analyses of Expressive Language Development Reveal Two Distinct Language Profiles Among Young Children with Autism Spectrum Disorders. *Journal of Autism and Developmental Disorders, 44*(1), 75–89. doi:10.1007/s10803-013-1853-4 PMID:23719855

Thomas-Stonell, N., Oddson, B., Robertson, B., & Rosenbaum, P. (2009). Predicted and Observed Outcomes in Preschool Children Following Speech and Language Treatment: Parent and Clinician Perspectives. *Journal of Communication Disorders, 42*(1), 29–42. doi:10.1016/j.jcomdis.2008.08.002 PMID:18835607

van der Merwe, E., & Alant, E. (2004). Associations with Minspeak™ icons. *Journal of Communication Disorders, 37*(3), 255–274. doi:10.1016/j.jcomdis.2003.10.002 PMID:15063146

Von Berg, S., Panorska, A., Uken, D., & Qeadan, F. (2009). DECtalk™ and VeriVox™: Intelligibility, Likeability, and Rate Preference Differences for Four Listener Groups. *AAC: Augmentative & Alternative Communication, 25*(1), 7–18. doi:10.1080/07434610902728531 PMID:19280420

Wiegand, K., & Patel, R. (2014). *Towards More Intelligent and Personalized AAC*. Paper presented at the CHI 2014, Toronto, Canada. http://homepage.cs.uiowa.edu/~hourcade/workshops/complexcommunicationneeds/papers/wiegand.pdf

Wolowiec Fisher, K., & Shogren, K. A. (2012). Integrating Augmentative and Alternative Communication and Peer Support for Students with Disabilities: A Social-Ecological Perspective. *Journal of Special Education Technology*, *27*(2), 23–39.

Zipse, L., Norton, A., Marchina, S., & Schlaug, G. (2012). When right is all that is left: Plasticity of right-hemisphere tracts in a young aphasic patient. *Annals of the New York Academy of Sciences*, *1252*(1), 237–245. doi:10.1111/j.1749-6632.2012.06454.x PMID:22524365

KEY TERMS AND DEFINITIONS

Augmentative and Alternative Communication (AAC): Refers to any form of communication other than speech that can be used to communicate wants, needs, feelings, thoughts, or anything else that could typically be communicated through speech. AAC supplements or replaces communicative abilities for some individuals with speech, language, voice, or hearing disorders.

Electropalatography (EPG): A technique that enables real-time visual feedback of tongue to palate contact. A customized artificial palate that contains multiple electrodes sends the signal to a processing unit when contact occurs. Electrodes are displayed on a computer screen or on a portable unit. Electrodes light up on the screen when the tongue makes contact with the artificial palate to indicate tongue placement during speech production.

Morpheme: The smallest unit of language that carries meaning. A morpheme can either stand alone (e.g., cat), or it can be bound to another morpheme (e.g., '-s' in cat*s*). Bound morphemes can mark tense, gender, number, or case; they can also change the meaning or part of speech of the root it is affixed to (e.g., the prefix 'un-' changes 'kind' into 'unkind,' thus changing the meaning of the root).

Palatometer: The device used in electropalatography. It consists of three elements: an artificial palate lined with electrodes (between 64 and 124 depending on the manufacturer); a microprocessor that sends the signal from the electrodes to the computer; and a computer software that provides the visual feedback of tongue to palate contact during speech.

Speech Generating Device (SGD): A type of high-tech AAC device that speaks out words or sentences from a written sentence or from symbolic representations of items or actions. The spoken output can be generated from speech synthesis or from digitized pre-recorded whole words or phrases.

Speech Synthesis: The artificial production of speech stemming from the concatenation of small units of pre-recorded speech. Speech synthesis allows for the creation of an unlimited number of words and sentences.

Syntax: The rules that determine the structures of sentences in a language. It is responsible for creating a sentence's basic structure, for combining basic sentences into complex ones, and for establishing how elements of a sentence can be moved. Syntax contributes to determining meaning.

Text-to-Speech (TTS) system: A system that enables written text to be spoken out loud by a device with a speech synthesizer.

Chapter 13
Telehealth Technology and Pediatric Feeding Disorders

Taylor A. Luke
University of Texas – Austin, USA

Rebecca R. Ruchlin
Monmouth University, USA

ABSTRACT

Ongoing advances in technology have provided a platform to extend the accessibility of services for children with developmental disabilities across locations, languages and the socioeconomic continuum. Teletherapy, the use of video-conferencing technology to deliver therapy services, is changing the face of healthcare by providing face-to-face interactions among specialists, parents and children. The current literature has demonstrated success in utilizing teletherapy as a modality for speech-language intervention and for social-behavioral management, while research on feeding therapy remains scarce. The current chapter discusses the prevalence of feeding disorders among infants, toddlers and children with developmental disorders. Using evidence from the current literature, a rationale for the utilization of teletherapy as a means of feeding therapy is presented.

INTRODUCTION

Video-conferencing technology (i.e. Skype ™, Google Hangouts ™, etc.) emerged for personal recreational use in face-to-face correspondence with family and friends, but soon this powerful tool was introduced into the workplace, due to its communicative effectiveness. This technology has given us the power to communicate visually and audibly from worldwide locations. With the power of the internet and video conferencing technology, we no longer have the barrier of distance when communicating with clients or associates in the workplace or with distant friends and family. As technology advances and the potential uses for videoconferencing are discovered, the use of this tool grows and expands opportunities for all who utilize it.

DOI: 10.4018/978-1-4666-8395-2.ch013

In addition to traditional workplace and at-home usage of video conferencing technology, the medical field has swiftly taken notice of its serviceable nature and has been increasingly utilizing this technology. With the medical field taking advantage of this tool to better serve their patients, other health and behavior-related fields have experimented with video conferencing technology due to its potential to be a powerful tool for providing individualized and diagnosis-specific therapy services. As a low-cost and accessible option, teletherapy is now a viable source for speech-language, psychological, behavioral and feeding therapies.

Historically, teletherapy has been used more regularly in the treatment of acute medical cases. However, recent developments in technology have made teletherapy systems more economical and user-friendly. Due to these improvements, there has been a significant increase in the number of teletherapy programs catering to non-acute cases within the past decade (McCullough, 2001). The present chapter will discuss the current and potential uses of video conferencing technology as a viable means of treatment for children with developmental disabilities focusing on its usage for feeding and swallowing disorders.

BACKGROUND

Children with developmental disabilities such as Down syndrome, cleft lip and/or palate, autism spectrum disorder, central nervous system disorders (e.g. cerebral palsy, meningitis, etc.), Pierre Robin Sequence (PRS), Williams Syndrome, Prader Willi Syndrome, Rett Syndrome, and weak musculature of the face and neck, commonly experience feeding and swallowing disorders (American Speech-Language-Hearing Association, 2014; Cooper-Brown et al., 2008). Feeding disorders encompass a broad range of eating activities that may or may not be accompanied by difficulty with swallowing food and liquid. Feeding disorders may be characterized by food behavior, rigid food preferences, less than optimal growth and failure to master self-feeding skills expected for developmental levels. The incidence of feeding disorders is estimated to be 25-40% in typically developing children and up to 80% for children with developmental disabilities (Arvedson, 2008). In addition, children with delayed speech and motor milestones have an increased risk for feeding difficulties (Hutchinson, 1999).

Treatment of feeding and swallowing disorders that are found in cases of genetic and developmental disabilities often require a multidisciplinary effort by a team of specialists including, but not limited to, speech-language pathologists, occupational therapists, and medical specialists such as gastroenterologists, cardiologists, geneticists, pediatricians, endocrinologists, psychologists, and nutritionists. Due to the range of professionals who treat children with feeding and swallowing difficulties, there is a broad spectrum of treatment and diagnostic options to be explored (Cooper-Brown et al., 2008).

In current practice, there is not a widely accepted classification system for childhood feeding disorders in place. However, it should be noted that the DSM-V (Diagnostic and Statistical Manual of Mental Disorders) defines a feeding disorder using several heterogeneous diagnostic criteria including: 1.) Failure to eat adequately, 2.) Absence of another condition that interferes with feeding, 3.) Absence of a mental disorder or lack of food, 4.) Onset of problems with feeding must occur before age three, and lastly, 5.) Avoidance of food due to sensory characteristics such as texture, color, and/or temperature (Kenney et. al., 2013; Williams et. al., 2009).

Due to the complex nature of feeding disorders, the professionals who specialize in child feeding therapy and their facilities are, unfortunately, not readily accessible to the growing number of children presenting with feeding difficulties. However, technology used for video-conferencing has become readily available and a staple in most homes across the country and abroad. Utilizing this technology to provide services has the potential to provide comprehensive care while saving time and money.

Telepractice has been used successfully in other disciplines that provide treatment and trainings, but its use in pediatric care and services has been lagging behind. According to the Individuals with Disabilities Education Act (2004), there are strict standards for providing care for children in government funded school-based intervention and home-based early intervention programs. However, due to the lack of resources and accessibility, being in compliance with these standards for treatment can be difficult. In sum, to better serve children in need of feeding services, the implementation of videoconferencing as a means of domestic and school-based treatment has the potential to expand the opportunities for quality and consistent rehabilitation for families across the continuum of accessibility (Olsen et al., 2008).

TELETHERAPY FOR INFANTS AND TODDLERS

Children with developmental disabilities, who are between birth and early childhood, typically receive services domestically, through early intervention services or in a clinical setting exclusively or in combination. It can be a challenge to provide consistent and quality treatment for individuals who are in need of feeding intervention services in rural or remote areas. In these cases, challenges for both parents and interventionists can include travel distance, weather conditions and the shortage of qualified pediatric early interventionists (Olsen et al., 2008).

Feeding-related concerns are among the most common issues in preschool children who are brought to primary health care professionals by parents (Arvedson, 2008). In a 2001 study, 79 preschool-aged children with neurodevelopmental disabilities who presented with suspected feeding disorders were examined. It was found that 56% exhibited gastro-esophageal reflux, 27% presented with oropharyngeal dysphagia, and 18% of the children showed aversive feeding behaviors. These results demonstrate the large scope of feeding difficulties that can occur in infancy and early childhood and strongly suggest the need for individualized, diagnosis-specific treatment for children with feeding disorders (Schwarz et al., 2001).

Comparing a child's feeding behavior problem with that of a typically developing child's feeding behavior is crucial in identifying the severity of the feeding problem. Immediately after birth, typically developing babies will feed on breast milk or formula. Within a few weeks, their sucking response should strengthen, as they grow accustomed to and learn how to coordinate the suck-swallow-breathe pattern. After about four to six months, the infants are typically introduced to baby foods. They are able to consume mashed table foods and even small bites of regular, textured food at twelve months, once their dental development progresses (Piazza, 2008).

However, children with feeding difficulties do not progress with food intake in the same way as their typically developing peers. Problematic feeders have poor coordination with the suck-swallow-breathe pattern after birth, and no progression occurs over time. Some children consistently reject breast or bottle feedings, which is especially concerning when continuous and persistent rejection prevents weight gain. Some children with feeding problems feed on the bottle or breast successfully but have an extremely difficult time transitioning to baby, mashed, or table food (Piazza, 2008). The ability to transition from breast milk or formula to food is important to strengthen oral motor skills and to prepare for chewing solids (Throughton et al., 2001).

One of the most straightforward, most quantifiable ways to detect a feeding problem is via weight gain. Children should gain weight consistently and not lose weight. Key indications of a feeding problem that needs treatment are weight loss over a three month period, a decrease in expected rate of growth, or crossing more than two major weight percentiles downward (Piazza, 2008). Children with developmental disorders are more prone to feeding disorders and are at high risk for experiencing such problematic feeding difficulties that can impact growth rate. One of the most crucial periods of growth is during infancy. When growth rate and weight gain are compromised due to problems with feeding, professional intervention is crucial to promote the infants' ability to thrive.

Although not all difficulty with early feeding is a predictor of developmental impairment in the pre-school years, a 2001 study by Motion et al. predicts that children with persistent feeding difficulties that occur from birth through fifteen months of age would experience significant motor, behavioral, speech and language impairments in early childhood. Results were yielded by 14,138 parent-response questionnaires that reflected the prevalence rates of feeding difficulties based on age in infancy. In addition to feeding difficulty prevalence rates, it was found that infants who presented with persistent feeding difficulties in the first fifteen months were more likely to be born preterm. Infants in this category were also less likely to have been breast-fed after four weeks of age and more likely to use a pacifier. Lastly, infants presenting with feeding difficulties within the first fifteen months were more likely to have received assessment by a specialist in a hospital setting (Motion et al., 2001).

UTILIZING TELETHERAPY TECHNOLOGY TO ASSIST BREASTFEEDING

Video-conferencing technology has been shown to be useful in consulting with new mothers, who are experiencing problems with breastfeeding their infants. As modern mothers are more commonly taking their infant-related questions to the Internet, whether it be on a search engine, forum, or social media site, they are becoming increasingly more comfortable with using the latest forms of technology, such as video-conferencing, to receive counsel from family members, friends and professionals (Macnab et al., 2012).

Research and professional practice has indicated that video-conferencing technology has a place in the field of lactation support for mothers and their infants. Costs and inconvenience of travelling with a small infant to a private practice or hospital are some of the largest barriers for mothers in need of assistance with feedings. While there are deterrents to this form of therapy, the costs of technology are decreasing and mothers' familiarity with video-conferencing tools make this form of consultation viable and accessible across the continuum of mothers experiencing difficulties with nursing (Macnab et al., 2012).

A prime example of the successful use of telehealth technologies for lactation consultation is evident in its use by the Texas Women, Infants and Children Program (WIC), a government-funded program that provides nutrition and breastfeeding assistance to low-income women and their children. Texas terrain can pose challenges due to its highly congested metropolitan cities as well as its extremely rural communities. In addition to the difficulty of commuting to, from and within these areas, the WIC program has limited resources of professionals who are available to provide lactation consults to the many mothers who qualify for the program. The proven solution to these challenges lies in the low-cost and convenient option of using video-conferencing technology that allows lactation specialists to reach a wide scope of mothers in need. Typically, WIC offices are located near the areas in which participating mothers live. To receive breastfeeding assistance, mothers visit their local WIC office and teleconference with a lactation specialist in the presence of a trained remote assistant who supports mother-infant positioning and offers technical support (Macnab, 2012).

Telehealth technology has proven to be successful in providing an opportunity for mothers to receive the nursing assistance that might not otherwise be available to them. This powerful tool has demonstrated the ability to promote breastfeeding, an act that has exponential benefits for mothers and their infants.

Another vast opportunity for the use of teletherapy as a means of lactation consultation lies in mothers who are experiencing a language barrier. Circumstances of all kinds can lead mothers to relocate to another region or country in which they are not fluent or comfortable with the language spoken, especially in terms of nursing vocabulary. Mothers in these particular situations experience limited to no professional assistance that is required to best care for their infant. Video-conferencing technology offers the lactation professional a view of mother-infant positioning and feeding behaviors. It can then assist with recommendations and modifications. Conversely, the ability for a mother to view the lactation professional demonstrate positioning and modifications eases these processes for the mother and infant.

UTILIZING TELETHERAPY IN EARLY CHILDHOOD

Telehealth-based therapy programs have been shown to be beneficial for nursing mothers who elect to participate due to distance, language barriers and availability of qualified professionals (Macnab, 2012). This same level of success has been translated to infants who are no longer nursing through early childhood (Clawson et al., 2008). Awareness of normal feeding and swallowing development is crucial to understanding atypical feeding and swallowing behavior patterns in children from birth through childhood (Shakashita et al., 2004). In order to accurately diagnose atypical feeding behaviors, a standard reference for typical feeding patterns from birth through childhood must be established, based on empirically-driven findings.

In a 2004 study by Shakashita et al., a randomized sample of 1,400 children aged birth to six years were studied via parent-response questionnaires regarding their child's feeding patterns. The study was aimed at establishing a standard reference for age of the transition between milk to solid foods, using the transitional food process (TFP) scale. The value of the standard reference of transitioning from milk to solid foods lies in the diagnosis of feeding behaviors that fall below the mean age range and as an instructional tool for introducing foods at appropriate stages of development.

The parent-response questionnaires revealed major trends in feeding behaviors among the 1,400 children studied. Results showed that infants were found, on average, to no longer have dependence on milk at 11.9 +/- 1.5 months. In addition, infants were successfully introduced to rice gruel, a cream of wheat textured substance, at six months or below and accepted "pulp-like" gruel (oatmeal texture) at 5.1+/- 1.5 months. Interestingly, the transitional process from milk to solid foods was found to be faster for breast-fed infants and infants using chewing-type nipples than for infants that used typical round-hole nipples. Regarding typical patterns of food acceptance, survey results demonstrated that the number of accepted foods most rapidly increased between the ages of six months and one year and at 2.5 years. In general, toddlers were found to accept most foods that were introduced. However, after 2.5 years, it was found that the rate of accepted foods decreased (Shakashita et al., 2004). This suggests that early childhood is a particularly sensitive time for food intake among other experiences.

At around 18 months of age, children may begin to develop food selectivity or a strong preference for certain foods only. The food preferences may be unpredictable from day to day or week to week. Selectivity can also be a major problem when the child's diet is limited to nutritionally deficient foods. Selectivity can also be a problem when it is accompanied by dramatic, emotional responses such as long lasting temper tantrums, or, in extreme cases, self-injury (Piazza, 2008).

Findings from these studies inform feeding interventionists and diagnosticians in their efforts to evaluate and treat children with developmental disorders who present with feeding difficulties. However, these feeding interventionists and diagnosticians are not accessible to all locations, languages and socioeconomic statuses. In order to provide the most frequent, thorough and professional care to children in need of feeding intervention, telehealth-based feeding programs have demonstrated the potential to serve understaffed communities effectively (Clawson et al., 2008).

A 2008 pilot study performed by the Feeding Disorders Program at the Children's Hospital in Richmond, Virginia has demonstrated the efficacy of utilizing teletherapy for feeding interventions and offers potential for the continued success of teletherapy for this purpose. The Feeding Disorders Program houses a multidisciplinary team of feeding specialists who provide treatment for children who exhibit mild, moderate and severe feeding disorders. Due to the program's specialization, families of children with feeding disorders outside of the Richmond area, travel great distances to seek out their professional care (Children's Hospital of Richmond at VCU, 2014). In order to provide cost-effective services from the Feeding Disorders Program to families in remote locations, both in the United States and abroad, the Children's Hospital of Richmond began developing a pilot teletherapy program for the treatment of children with feeding disorders (Clawson et al., 2008).

The pilot teletherapy feeding program was implemented for 15 pediatric participants with complex feeding disorders, ranging in age from 8 months to 10 years (80% under the age of 5). All participants lived in remote areas in the United States and in England ranging from 300 to 3,500 miles in distance from Richmond, Virginia. The children, their families and the feeding specialist team at the Children's Hospital of Richmond worked collaboratively, using video-conferencing technology to deliver feeding interventions. The participating families and children attended teletherapy sessions at their nearest collaborating hospital or university. Outcomes of the pilot teletherapy intervention, derived from family responses on a survey following the program, demonstrated that families of the participating children were highly satisfied with the care their child was receiving. Moreover, the children exhibited less reliance on present feeding tubes and more nutritional intake after the 26 month treatment period (Clawson et al., 2008). The following are goals for the pilot feeding teletherapy study:

Goal 1: Offer a resource to community-based physicians to provide necessary care after local resources have been exhausted.

Goal 2: Provide sufficient information to recommend the next steps in the child's feeding treatment, whether community-based or center-based.

Goal 3: Minimize costs for families.

Goal 4: Maximize generalization and effective medical follow up in the patient's home community.

Goal 5: Ensure that the treatment team is comfortable with the availability of adequate clinical information and the technology of teleconferencing.

Goal 6: Ensure that families are adequately informed about what to expect from the teleconference, both the format of the conference and the range of possible outcomes resulting from the teleconference.

Goal 7: Maximize the efficiency and effectiveness of treatment teams at both sites of the teleconference.

Goal 8: Have adequate information on the basis of a teleconference consultation to justify authorization by the insurer of the next steps of care needed.

Goal 9: Enable the child to receive effective treatment for feeding disorders as soon as possible. (Clawson et al., 2008, p.214)

Utilizing video-conferencing technology to meet the underlying goals stated above proved to be successful in facilitating the progression of feeding skills in children with complex feeding disorders. The pilot study goals provided a framework for the feeding specialists at the Children's Hospital of Richmond to be more accessible to the children who need them most. As the results of the pilot study suggests that the authors' goals were successful in facilitating teletherapy, it can be further gleaned from the study's success that these goals would serve as a successful platform in future tele-based feeding programs.

TELETHERAPY AS HUMANITARIAN RELIEF FOR SPECIAL PEDIATRIC POPULATIONS

Children and adults, in remote underserved regions around the world, often carry the burden of developmental disorders and structural abnormalities of the head and neck. Environmental factors such as limited access to health care, lack of nutrition, and behavior related risk factors increase the prevalence of these serious disorders. Unfortunately, these locations offer minimal or no opportunities for subspecialty care (i.e. speech-language pathology, otolaryngology, audiology, etc.) (Groom et al., 2011). To illustrate the immense need for subspecialty care in these developing areas, research has suggested that in 2004, for every 100,000 people in the continent of Africa, there were .11 otolaryngologists. In the United States, there were 3.1 otolaryngologists for every 100,000 people (Fagan & Jacobs, 2009). For over ten years, professionals have considered using teletherapy to remedy the lack of subspecialty medical services. In 1997, the World Health Organization (WHO) Director General Dr Hiroshi Nakajima, stated, "Developing an adequate and affordable telecommunication infrastructure can help to close the gap among the haves and the have-nots in health care." (Groom et al., 2011, p. 1252). Since he made that statement, immense progress has been made in telecommunication and video-conferencing technologies. However, while large strides are being made in technological advancement, the utilization of teletherapy for humanitarian relief is still lagging behind. As research continues to investigate the varying uses for teletherapy, its potential as a modality for treating underserved domestic and remote locations remains to be seen (Groom et al., 2011).

The range of head and neck abnormalities and disorders is wide-ranging in underdeveloped countries, due to environmental factors that have an adverse effect on overall health and wellness. If untreated, one of the prevalent developmental disorders that has profound effects on children, adolescents and adults is cleft lip and/or palate (CL/P). Cleft lip and/or palate are congenital craniofacial abnormalities wherein a child is born with an opening in the lip, the palate or both. These openings have significant effects on speech production, feeding and often on hearing ability. CL/P can often be observed during preterm ultrasounds, however, medically underserved mothers are less likely to have access to these important screenings. If a CL/P is not observed during ultrasounds before the time of birth, signs of the cleft lip will be observed at birth. Cleft palate, if not observed at the time of birth examination, will be evident during feedings. A child with cleft palate does not have sufficient closure between the mouth and the nose, causing food or liquid to come out through the nose. Furthermore, children with cleft palate have problems with speech and hearing as a result of their craniofacial abnormalities. Children with a cleft palate often need multiple surgeries over time to close the opening in the palate that causes feeding, speech and hearing problems (American Speech-Language-Hearing Association, 2014).

It is widely accepted across the world medical community that a multidisciplinary approach is necessary for the remediation of cleft palate. Surgery alone is not enough; pre and postoperative care are necessary for optimal recovery. However, developing countries lack the number of trained professionals to provide long-term care for those with cleft palate. These trained professionals who are involved with the treatment of cleft palate can include maxillofacial surgeons, oral surgeons, reconstructive surgeons, speech-language pathologists, audiologists and dentists. With the assistance of video-conferencing technology and the expanding availability of wireless internet, essential treatment for patients with cleft palate in remote developing locations has the potential to become more accessible (Furr et al., 2011).

A 2011 study by Furr et al. investigated the use of teletherapy to provide preoperative and postoperative speech-language therapy for patients with cleft palate in Peru. The patients ranged in age from 4 to 24 years of age and participated in 15-25 minutes of tele-based speech-language therapy sessions with the assistance of a remote healthcare assistant who coordinated appointments and aided in setting up the equipment. It was observed that the participating patients embraced the use of video-conferencing technology and those who attended multiple teletherapy sessions showed great improvement in speech intelligibility and nasality. Due to the high degree of enthusiasm and progress that patients with cleft palate made during speech-language teletherapy sessions, the authors predicted that the participants' improvements would be closely equivalent to that of face-to-face traditional therapy (Furr et al., 2011). Furthermore, the same rate of success could be applied to preoperative and postoperative consultation in other disciplines, namely, feeding therapy.

Cleft lip and cleft palate have a broad range of severity which affects the amount of feeding and swallowing therapy needed. For an infant with an isolated cleft lip, feeding problems are minimal. For an infant with cleft palate, and multiple other anomalies, feeding therapy is crucial. However, regardless of the severity of the cleft lip and/or palate, strategies to optimize growth and development are vital (Cooper-Brown et al., 2008).

Understanding the functions of an intact lip and an intact palate during feeding is necessary to understand how cleft lip and cleft palate impair feeding abilities. Infants with an intact palate create negative intraoral pressure as their lips and tongue form a seal around the nipple and the tongue produces rhythmic sucking motions. An intact soft palate elevates to seal off the nasopharynx. However, infants with a cleft palate have significant difficulty developing the negative pressure needed for nipple feeding due to the inability to seal the nasal cavity and oropharynx (Reid et al., 2007). In contrast, infants with an isolated cleft lip generally do not have much difficulty feeding. Along with difficulty in feedings, infants with cleft palate commonly ingest excess air because of the lack of separation between the nasal and oral cavities. This often leads to bloating, choking, gagging, fatigue with feeding, prolonged feeding times, and contributes to spitting up and emesis (Cooper-Brown et al., 2008).

Through humanitarian mission surgical team efforts and growing local surgeon accessibility in developing countries, patients with cleft lip and palate have the opportunity to correct the craniofacial abnormalities that they were born with. However, in cases of CL/P, surgery is just the beginning of recovering speech, hearing and feeding skills. A multidisciplinary team of subspecialists is essential to advances in recovery and ultimately quality of life (Furr et al., 2011). Through the utilization of wireless internet connectivity and video-conferencing technology, professionals have the opportunity to provide care to pediatric special populations in need of cost-effective and accessible long-term treatment.

UTILIZING TELETHERAPY IN CHILDHOOD DEVELOPMENTAL DISORDERS

Ideally, children with developmental disorders would have the opportunity to receive treatment in a private practice or clinic with the most highly qualified specialist and parent-involvement. However, due to accessibility and cost, this option is not always available. Early intervention programs or therapy provided at school are government-funded and an accessible option for children with developmental disabilities. However, flaws in these types of services can hinder a child's progress in their therapy goals (McCullough, 2001).

Since parent involvement is an essential component of their child's success in therapy, it is crucial that parents are knowledgeable and up-to-date on the skills their child is working on and their progress in therapy. However, traditional governmentally funded face-to-face services provided in the home or at school are susceptible to having a low rate of parental involvement, in both early childhood and in school-based therapy, and a lack of facilitating newly acquired skills at home.

Video conferencing technology has the potential to increase parent-involvement in the therapy process in its use during school-based therapy sessions. During these sessions, parents have the ability to utilize video conferencing technology in order to observe their child receiving therapy during school. This allows the parent to view the techniques the clinician is using, their child's progression, and the ability to ask the clinician questions. This opportunity for parent observation and participation has the potential to increase the progression of their child toward their therapy goals (McCullough, 2001).

Furthermore, in addition to utilizing teletherapy to allow parents to "televisit" their child during school-based therapy, video conferencing technology also allows clinicians to virtually visit clients and their parents in their most natural environment at home. Since the clinician and parent must work together to facilitate the therapy session for the child, the outcome is highly parent-involved which translates to parent confidence in working on learned skills at home with their child. This carry-over of new and previously acquired skills is crucial for further development and progression (McCullough, 2001).

TELETHERAPY AND AUTISM SPECTRUM DISORDER

Some individuals with developmental disorders have a greater likelihood of developing a feeding and/or swallowing disorder. One group of individuals in particular includes those with autism spectrum disorder (ASD). The diagnosis and classification of feeding disorders in children with ASD can be challenging due to the unique characteristics of each individual case in which delays and hypersensitivities manifest themselves (Keen, 2008).

It is suggested that if severe feeding problems or atypical feeding behaviors are causing failure to thrive in infancy, there is an impetus for professional evaluation for underlying ASD. Studies have suggested that feeding disorders in children with ASD can be related to vulnerabilities in biology that can cause sensory, cognitive and/or emotional deficits in combination with atypical attachment and learned behaviors. Children with ASD who present with complex and severe feeding difficulties may require a dynamic and multidisciplinary intervention (Keen, 2008).

The prevalence of feeding problems in children with ASD often occurs due to detail-oriented characteristics, perseveration, impulsive behaviors, and aversion to new experiences, food intolerance, sensory deficits and difficulties with compliance. Feeding disorders in children with ASD can be categorized as behavioral feeding disorders and sensory-based feeding disorders (Schawrz, 2003). Behavioral feeding disorders are categorized by aversive feeding behaviors such as refusal, gagging, choking and food expulsion without a medical reason. In contrast, sensory-based feeding disorders are categorized by aversions to certain textures of food.

Children with ASD have more mealtime challenges than their typically developing peers (Johnson et al., 2008). Mealtime challenges include not staying seated at mealtimes, not eating with the family, eating fewer than 20 foods, and having phases where they persistently desire the same foods (Nadon et al., 2011). These problems require long-term and intensive care and support for parents contending with these significant mealtime challenges. Literature states that providing services to children with ASD in their natural home environments with parents as the main initiators of therapy demonstrates the most success for global development. However, to reach the child's therapy goals, supervision is often required from a trained specialist to effectively initiate therapy. As expected, availability of professional care needed to meet the long-term and intense requirements that are necessary for a child with ASD is lacking. The use of video-conferencing technology has the potential to fill the gap between the professional care that is accessible to families of children with ASD and the regular, long-term, intense care which they require to make significant improvements (Baharav & Reiser, 2010).

A 2010 pilot study compared two clinical models of therapy to promote positive behavior and communicative interaction for children with ASD: 1) traditional face-to-face therapy and 2) traditional face-to-face therapy combined with teletherapy home-based sessions. Two children, ages 4 and 5 years old, clinically diagnosed with ASD, participated in the study with their respective parents. The study consisted of two 6-week treatment periods, the first being a control period wherein the participants received traditional therapy twice weekly. Following the control period, the participants were treated once weekly with traditional therapy and once weekly with teletherapy sessions in their homes for the second 6-week experimental period. During teletherapy sessions, the clinician shared lesson plans with the child's parents as well as provided them with cues to implement therapy strategies in their home (Baharav & Reiser, 2010).

By comparing the children in the experimental and control conditions, it was determined, that the participants made similar gains in social, behavioral and communicative skills, using the combined teletherapy and traditional therapy model, as they did with the traditional therapy model. Other findings included increased parent confidence in engaging their children in therapeutically meaningful interactions and an overall sense of ability to assist their children's development. Furthermore, parent questionnaires indicated overall positive experiences with the use of the technology and the teletherapy process ((Baharav & Reiser, 2010).

Feeding a child can be one of the most satisfying interactions a caregiver can have with a child. Unfortunately, feeding problems are a common occurrence among children with developmental disabilities (Palmer et al., 1978).Parents of children with developmental disabilities often become frustrated, Rather than experience pleasure, parents of children with developmental disabilities often grow frustrated when feeding becomes difficult or unmanageable. When a caregiver is unable to feed and nourish her child appropriately, she often feels inadequate.

Parents of children who have developmental disabilities and medical disorders, often have to make difficult decisions when prioritizing their child's medical and developmental needs (Guerriere et al., 2003). Sometimes feeding must be relegated to the back burner to ensure parents are contending with more serious, sometimes life threatening matters.

FEEDING DISORDERS AND PARENTAL STRESS

Adapting and coping with problems in infants and children at any age can be a source of tremendous stress for parents. When parents are ineffective at facilitating feeding for their children, increased feelings of rejection, self-doubt regarding parental capabilities, and an overall increase in stress can occur. Some parents successfully face the strenuous demands made by children with feeding disorders. However, many use unsuccessful coping strategies such as "force feeding." This type of strategy is found to only further induce negative behaviors, such as head turns, coughing, food refusal, or any other avoidant behaviors from the child, which is ultimately counterintuitive in reducing the stress of the parent. It is of utmost importance that parents monitor their own emotions to facilitate optimal feeding sessions. The development of coping mechanisms, as opposed to using force-feeding methods, may end a never-ending cycle of negative behavior and stress (Didehbani et al., 2011).

CONCLUSION

Caregivers who worry that their children will fail to thrive, face a daunting task when working with infants and children who exhibit challenging feeding disorders. The strain of feeding their child several times a day can take a significant toll on the child, primary caregiver and family as a whole. In terms of remediating feeding disorders in infants and children, the literature delineates the successes that teletherapy technology has demonstrated and provides a rationale for integration into practice and further research. Not only has the current research determined the success rate of tele-based feeding therapy, but it has revealed the wide-ranging prevalence of feeding disorders in children with developmental disabilities and has highlighted the immense need for feeding therapy services around the world.

Additionally, video conferencing technology has already begun to bridge the gap between caregivers and their children in remote areas; cost, language barriers and ongoing support that prevent the success of infants and children with feeding disorders can also be ameliorated. It can be hypothesized that with the increased availability of support that teletherapy can provide, caregivers of children with developmental disabilities, who experience feeding difficulties, will develop more effective strategies for feeding and will resort less to ineffectual methods like force-feeding. The wide-ranging uses of this rapidly advancing technology can improve the overall health and development of children with developmental disabilities who are in need of long-term intensive therapies and can potentially reduce parental stressors and increase parents' confidence levels.

REFERENCES

Arvedson, J. C. (2008). Assessment of pediatric dysphagia and feeding disorders: Clinical and instrumental approaches. *Developmental Disabilities Research Reviews*, *14*(2), 118–127. doi:10.1002/ddrr.17 PMID:18646015

Baharav, E., & Reiser, C. (2010). Using Telepractice in Parent Training in Early Autism. *Telemedicine Journal and e-Health*, *16*(6), 727–731. doi:10.1089/tmj.2010.0029 PMID:20583950

Clawson, B., Selden, M., Lacks, M., Deaton, A. V., Hall, B., & Bach, R. (2008). Complex Pediatric Feeding Disorders: Using Teleconferencing Technology to Improve Access To a Treatment Program. *Pediatric Nursing*, *34*(3), 213–216. PMID:18649810

Cleft Lip and Cleft Palate. (n.d.). Retrieved Aug 30, 2014, from http://www.asha.org/public/speech/disorders/CleftLip/

Cooper-Brown, L., Copeland, S., Dailey, S., Downey, D., Petersen, M., Stimson, C., & Van Dyke, D. C. (2008). Feeding and swallowing dysfunction in genetic syndromes. *Developmental Disabilities Research Reviews*, *14*(2), 147–157. doi:10.1002/ddrr.19 PMID:18646013

Didehbani, N., Kelly, K., Austin, L., & Wiechmann, A. (2011). Role of Parental Stress on Pediatric Feeding Disorders. *Children's Health Care*, *40*(2), 85–100. doi:10.1080/02739615.2011.564557

Fagan, J., & Jacobs, M. (2009). Survey of ENT services in Africa: Need for a comprehensive intervention. *Global Health Action*. Feeding and Swallowing Disorders (Dysphagia) in Children. *Feeding and Swallowing Disorders (Dysphagia) in Children*. Retrieved June 7, 2014, from http://www.asha.org/public/speech/swallowing/feeding-and-swallowing-disorders-in-children/

Furr, M., Larkin, E., Blakeley, R., Albert, T., Tsugawa, L., & Weber, S. (2011). Extending Multidisciplinary Management of Cleft Palate to the Developing World. *Journal of Oral and Maxillofacial Surgery*, *69*(1), 237–241-237–241.

Groom, K., Ramsey, M., & Saunders, J. (2011). Teleheal th and Humanitarian Assistance in Otolaryngology. *Otolaryngologic Clinics of North America*, *44*(6), 1251–1258. doi:10.1016/j.otc.2011.08.002 PMID:22032479

Guerriere, D. N., McKeever, P., & Llewellyn-Thomas, H. et al.. (2003). Mothers' decisions about gastrostomy tube insertion in children: Factors contributing to uncertainty. *Developmental Medicine and Child Neurology*, *45*(7), 470–476. doi:10.1111/j.1469-8749.2003.tb00942.x PMID:12828401

Keen, D. V. (2008). Childhood autism, feeding problems and failure to thrive in early infancy. *European Child & Adolescent Psychiatry*, *17*(4), 209–216. doi:10.1007/s00787-007-0655-7 PMID:17876499

Kenney, L., & Walsh, B. (2013). Avoidant/restrictive food intake disorder (ARFID) defining ARFID. *Eating Disorders Review*, *24*(3), 1.

Macnab, I., Rojjanasrirat, W., & Sanders, A. (2012). Breastfeeding and Telehealth. *Journal of Human Lactation*, *28*(4), 446–449. doi:10.1177/0890334412460512 PMID:23087193

McCullough, A. (2001). Viability and effectiveness of teletherapy for pre-school children with special needs. *International Journal of Language & Communication Disorders*, 36321–36326. PMID:11340805

Motion, S., Northstone, K., Emond, A., & Team, A. L. S. P. A. C. S. (2001). Persistent early feeding difficulties and subsequent growth and developmental outcomes. *Ambulatory Child Health*, *7*(3/4), 231–237. doi:10.1046/j.1467-0658.2001.00139.x

Olsen, S., Fiechtl, B., & Rule, S. (2012). An Evaluation of Virtual Home Visits in Early Intervention: Feasibility of "Virtual Intervention". *The Volta Review*, *112*(3), 267–281.

Piazza, C. C. (2008). Feeding disorders and behavior: What have we learned? *Developmental Disabilities Research Reviews*, *14*(2), 174–181. doi:10.1002/ddrr.22 PMID:18646017

Sakashita, R. R., Inoue, N. N., & Kamegai, T. T. (2004). From milk to solids: A reference standard for the transitional eating process in infants and preschool children in Japan. *European Journal of Clinical Nutrition*, *58*(4), 643–653. doi:10.1038/sj.ejcn.1601860 PMID:15042133

Schwarz, S. M., Corredor, J., Fisher-Medina, J., Cohen, J., & Rabinowitz, S. (2001). Diagnosis and Treatment of Feeding Disorders in Children With Developmental Disabilities. *Pediatrics*, *108*(3), 671–676. doi:10.1542/peds.108.3.671 PMID:11533334

Throughton, K. E., & Hill, A. E. (2001). Relation between objectively measured feeding competence and nutrition in children with cerebral palsy. *Developmental Medicine and Child Neurology*, *43*(3), 187–190. doi:10.1111/j.1469-8749.2001.tb00185.x PMID:11263689

Williams, K. E., Riegel, K., & Kerwin, M. (2009). Feeding Disorder of Infancy or Early Childhood: How Often Is It Seen in Feeding Programs? *Children's Health Care*, *38*(2), 123–136. doi:10.1080/02739610902813302

ADDITIONAL READING

Cornwell, S. L., Kelly, K., & Austin, L. (2010). Pediatric Feeding Disorders: Effectiveness of Multidisciplinary Inpatient Treatment of Gastrostomy-Tube Dependent Children. *Children's Health Care*, *39*(3), 214–231. doi:10.1080/02739615.2010.493770

Field, D., Garland, M., & Williams, K. (2003). Correlates of specific childhood feeding problems. *Journal of Paediatrics and Child Health*, *39*(4), 299–304. doi:10.1046/j.1440-1754.2003.00151.x PMID:12755939

Jordan, B. (2012). Therapeutic play within infant-parent psychotherapy and the treatment of infant feeding disorders. *Infant Mental Health Journal*, *33*(3), 307–313. doi:10.1002/imhj.21321

Ledford, J. R., & Gast, D. L. (2006). Feeding Problems in Children With Autism Spectrum Disorders: A Review. *Focus on Autism and Other Developmental Disabilities*, *21*(3), 153–166. doi:10.1177/10883576060210030401

Lucarelli, L., Cimino, S., D'olimpio, F., & Ammaniti, M. (2013). Feeding disorders of early childhood: An empirical study of diagnostic subtypes. *International Journal of Eating Disorders*, *46*(2), 147–155. doi:10.1002/eat.22057 PMID:23015314

Rogers, L., Magill-Evans, J., & Rempel, G. (2012). Mothers' Challenges in Feeding their Children with Autism Spectrum Disorder-Managing More Than Just Picky Eating. *Journal of Developmental and Physical Disabilities*, *24*(1), 19–33. doi:10.1007/s10882-011-9252-2

Sugayaman, S. M. M., Leone, C., & Chauffaille, M. D. L. L. F. et al.. (2007). Willams syndrome, development of a new scoring system for clinical diagnosis. *Clinics (Sao Paulo)*, *62*(2), 159–166. doi:10.1590/S1807-59322007000200011 PMID:17505701

Symon, J. (2001). Parent Education for Autism: Issues in Providing Services at a Distance. *Journal of Positive Behavior Interventions*, *3*(3), 160–174. doi:10.1177/109830070100300304

Vismara, L., Young, G., & Rogers, S. (2012). Telehealth for Expanding the Reach of Early Autism Training to Parents. *Autism Research and Treatment*, *2012*, 1–12. doi:10.1155/2012/121878 PMID:23227334

Wolf, L., & Glass, R. (1992). *Feeding and swallowing disorders in infancy: assessment and management*. San Antonio, TX: Therapy Skill Builders.

KEY TERMS AND DEFINITIONS

Autism Spectrum Disorder (Asd): A pervasive developmental disorder that affects sensory, cognitive and/or emotional deficits.

Cleft Lip And/Or Palate (Cl/P): Congenital craniofacial abnormalities wherein a child is born with an opening in the lip, the palate or both simultaneously.

Developmental Disability: Condition that can affect mental and/or physical functioning discovered early in life and persists through adulthood.

Down Syndrome: Genetic disorder that affects growth, facial structure and intellectual ability.

Feeding Disorder: A broad range of eating activities that may or may not be accompanied by a difficulty with swallowing food and liquid; may be characterized by food behavior, rigid food preferences, less than optimal growth, and failure to master self-feeding skills expected for developmental levels.

Multidisciplinary: Involving multiple professional fields.

Prader Willi Syndrome: Genetic disorder that affects growth, learning and behavior.

Rett Syndrome: Genetic disorder that causes abnormal growth characteristics, severely impaired language, mobility and behavior.

Teletherapy, Telepractice, Telehealth-Based Therapy: The use of video-conferencing technology to deliver therapy services.

Traditional Therapy Model: Client and clinician engage face-to-face in a same location during the therapy session.

Video-Conferencing Technology: Basic computer tools required to engage in telecommunication (i.e. computer, microphone, web camera etc.) and internet connection.

Williams Syndrome: Genetic disorder that causes developmental delays and learning disabilities.

Chapter 14
Music and Developmental Disabilities

Michelle Renee Blumstein
Marymount Manhattan College, USA

ABSTRACT

The following chapter presents a compilation of research about various types of technology that are employed by music therapists to benefit children with developmental delays. Music therapy can be an effective way to meet the goals of the individual. Music can also be a very powerful motivator. Previous musical skill or experience is not required for music therapy to be effective for clients with developmental disabilities or for clients more generally. Many music-based technologies are designed to create a positive, successful, and enjoyable experience for all users. Music therapy can provide a safe and confidence building environment where children are able to feel in control of a situation, possibly for the first time in their lives.

INTRODUCTION

Music therapy provides a unique opportunity, which is not necessarily present in all forms of therapy. Thanks to a wide variety of music based technologies employed during a music therapy session, the child is not only able to work on improving important skills that will benefit him/her in life, but the child is also able to participate in activities that provide happiness and enjoyment. Many children, especially those with more severe physical impairments often rely on others to perform a majority of their daily routines. During music therapy sessions, the child is in control and is able to create and accomplish tasks for him or herself; this may be the first time an opportunity of this sort has arisen. The following chapter provides a brief background on music therapy: what it is, how it is done, why it works, how its effectiveness has been tested, as well as an explanation of a wide variety of contemporary technologies that are being used to benefit children with developmental delays.

DOI: 10.4018/978-1-4666-8395-2.ch014

BACKGROUND

Music Therapy

What Is Music Therapy?

According to the American Music Therapy Association (AMTA), "Music therapy is the clinical and evidence-based use of music interventions to accomplish individualized goals within a therapeutic relationship by a credentialed professional who has completed an approved music therapy program" (AMTA). Music is used by a trained music therapist as an apparatus to help elicit a predetermined behavior or goal from the individual (Dolan, 1973, pg. 173). Music can also be used by the therapist to reinforce or prolong the determination of the individual to achieve the chosen behavior (Dolan, 1973, pg. 173).

The purpose of Music Therapy is to, "...address the physical, emotional, cognitive, and social needs of individuals" (AMTA). The main focus of the music therapist is to improve the non-musical skills of the individual such as motor skills, social skills, and educational abilities (Dolan, 1973, pg. 173). Music therapy can open an alternative means of communication for individuals who struggle with verbal expression (AMTA).

Although exposure to music through many different processes can have therapeutic effects, not all of these processes are considered clinical practices of music therapy. "Clinical music therapy is the only professional, research-based discipline that actively applies science to the creative, emotional, and energizing experiences of music for health treatment, and educational goals" (AMTA). For instance Alzheimers' patients listening to music through headphones and musicians performing at hospitals, though therapeutic experiences are not considered clinical music therapy. However, a music therapist using music to improve the communication skills of a child with autism would be an example of clinical music therapy, according to the AMTA.

Why Does Music Therapy Work?

According to an article published in The Journal of Music Therapy, there are "three basic processes" that allow music therapy to be successful (Dolan, 1973, pg. 174).

1. Structure: Music has a structure and this structure creates sound, that when heard, stimulates the aural senses of the individual. When that stimulation occurs, it requires a response. In order to elicit this response, a music therapist could use activities such as singing, creative movement and dance, playing instruments, and listening to music.
2. Self-organization: Music presents a unique approach to self-expression for many individuals. Music allows a type of communication which is completely nonverbal, allowing an individual to express his or her feelings, attitudes, and mood. Self-Organization activities can also offer a safe and efficient way for an individual to relieve tension, aggression, and to express negative feelings. The purpose of the self-organization activities should be to create, "success-oriented experiences that allow one to improve his/her self-esteem through music.
3. Communication: This is a major element of social interactions. Since music allows for communication to occur completely nonverbally, music also allows for a unique form of social interaction which affords the individual the opportunity to relate to others in new ways. Many individuals who

have sensory issues, such as those on the Autism Spectrum, can also benefit from a music therapist, using dance in this situation. Dance creates a context in which a type of physical contact that does not occur naturally is acceptable. Another benefit of music in the sense of relating to others is that it requires cooperation when conducted in a group setting. All group participants take on the responsibility of their own behavior and can see how those behaviors affect the other members of the group.

How Is It done?

Music Therapists use a variety of music-based technologies and activities to design a specific treatment plan for each individual with whom they work. According to the AMTA these activities incorporate any combination of making, listening to, and/or moving to music. Each session is customized to meet the goals and needs of each individual. Music Therapists must be flexible and able to accommodate to change very quickly based on the feelings of the individual at the time of the session.

An example of this can be seen in Bunt's (2003) case study of a young girl named Jane (a pseudonym) which was published in the British Journal of Music Education. Jane attended music therapy to address her needs in social communication. This music therapist was already familiar with Jane and had the room prepared with all of Jane's favorite instruments; organized in an easily accessible way. When Jane arrived for her session, she felt distressed and paranoid that everyone around her disliked her. The therapist recognized how upset Jane was through her body language. The therapist then began playing a melody on the piano that mirrored how Jane was feeling as he calmly told Jane that it is okay for her to display her feelings. The therapist gradually slowed the music to a more calming tempo. As Jane began to relax, she chose a small percussion instrument which she focused on while she attempts to express her feelings verbally. Jane and the therapist continued to play together throughout the forty -minute session, focusing on how Jane was feeling and how she was verbally communicating her thoughts and feelings. At the conclusion of the session, Jane expressed that she was feeling better.

An important role of the music therapist is to be receptive to Jane and to compensate for her needs (Bunt, 2003). This is true of the relationship between all individuals and their music therapists. A key factor which contributes to the success of Jane's session is trust and consistency. The sessions are always consistent in start time, location, and length. Jane and the therapist have developed a relationship over time which has created an environment in which Jane feels safe and comfortable not only exploring, but also expressing how she is feeling. Jane has developed trust not only in her therapist but also in the process and this is why it works so well for her. This trust and consistency are vital aspects which are required for the music therapy process to be successful for all individuals.

If the structure of the session is not adjusted to address a pressing issue of an individual, such as it was with Jane, the music therapist will continue as planned, working in order to attain the goals and objectives that have been set out for that individual. Goals and objectives that are focused on through music therapy can either be supported through other forms of therapy or independent of other therapies. While many other therapies explore alternative means of learning for the individual, a unique component of music therapy is that it also enables the individual to focus on, "...factors that prepare the mind and body for learning" (Berger, 2003). Berger believes that using the six elements of music, rhythm, melody, timbre (sound quality), dynamics (volume), harmony, and form will allow the brain to intake, process, and remember information more efficiently, which will improve the effectiveness of other therapies (Berger, 2003).

Keeping in mind particular aspects of the musical elements, the role of a music therapist includes observing the individual for existing problems and deciding on possible treatment methods incorporating the six elements (Berger, 2003). In order to be successful, music therapists must also have an understanding of how sensory information is processed, and the cognitive abilities and the emotional state of the individual (Berger, 2003). It is also necessary to have an understanding of how all of these aspects interact (Berger, 2003).

It is important, when establishing goals, that the music therapist arranges them in order of importance for the individual. One could consider the following modus operandi for working with a child on the spectrum: Reduce physiological stress and anxiety (possibly due to sensory misinterpretation) while limiting visual distraction with the objective that the child will undertake ten minutes of a calming and centering activity with the therapist's prompt (Berger, 2003). Music therapy goals reach beyond the academic goals often listed in an Individualized Education Plan (IEP) and are a key factor in preparing the individual to succeed in other aspects of his or her education and in his or her life.

Tools and Technologies which Help Facilitate Music Therapy

Since the 1980's, music therapists have been developing various ways, some technology-based, to track and monitor the progress of individuals with whom they work. During the late 1980's however, many of the programs being used such as, SCRIBE™, AIMSTAR™, and EMTEK™ were not developed by music therapists (Hadley et al., 2014). Now there are a variety of programs being used such as. the Individualized Music Therapy Assessment Profile (IMTAP) ™, the Music Therapy Toolbox™, MAWii™, the Music Therapy Analyzing Partitura (MAP) ™, and the Music Therapy Logbook (Hadley et al., 2014).

According to Baxter et al. (2007), the IMTAP™ computer software program was designed to be used with children and young adults. The program is able to assess the individual on many levels. After information is inputted into the system, the program is able to graph and show the progress and development of the individual's longitudinal growth over a period of time. The program will respond both to improvisational therapy activities as well as to those planned more structurally by the therapist. IMTAP has many uses in the area of tracking progress and assisting in the development of goals. IMTAP can be used, "...as a treatment plan for music therapy, as a tool to develop goals and objectives, as a means to address and assess targeted skill sets, as an indicator of overall functioning, as a baseline for treatment, as a research method and as a communication tool for parents and healthcare professionals" (Baxter et al., 2007 pg.13). IMTAP is able to assess either baseline data or to track the growth of, Gross/Fine Motor Skills, Oral Motor Skills, Sensory Skills, Receptive Communication/Auditory Perception, Expressive Communication, Cognitive Abilities, Emotional Abilities, Social Abilities, and Musicality.

Music Based Technologies

Soundbeam

Soundbeam™ was first created in 1984 by the composer Edward Williams (Swingler, 1998 pg.18). This device, which is able to create music and a variety of sounds without the need for physical touch by the user, was originally designed to be used by dancers (Swingler, 1998 pg.18). Soundbeam requires such a minimal amount of movement from the user that special education schools quickly realized the immense benefit that the device would have for their students; this is why soundbeam became used more widely

(Swingler, 1998 pg.18). The Soundbeam system uses ultrasonic ranging to detect the movement of the user (Swingler, 1998 pg.18). It allows the device to recognize, "...the distance, direction and velocity of body movements in a defined space" (SoundTree, 2014). Soundbeam then uses the movements to generate electronic music sounds (SoundTree, 2014). In order to create sound using Soundbeam, the child may simply move any part of his or her body over or across the beam. Soundbeam comes equipped with a variety of different sounds such as ocean sounds, bells, string instruments, and even choir voices (Ellis, Leeuwen, 2000 pg. 6). A major benefit of the Soundbeam system is the vast array of sounds available for the child to experiment with during each session. Not every child will be motivated by the same sounds, therefore other electronic instrument simulation systems may not work as well for each child (Ellis, Leeuwen, 2000 pg. 4). On the Soundbeam website, www.soundbeam.co.uk, there are multiple video demonstrations of the Soundbeam system being used by children with disabilities. Soundbeam is particularly beneficial for children, who require a wider range of motion since the technology can allow for this via adjusting the Soundbeam sensors (Swingler, Brockhouse, 2009, pg. 50). The beam can be set from anywhere between 0.25 and 6 meters from the sensors (Swingler, Brockhouse, 2009, pg. 50).

Before the introduction of Soundbeam, much of the music making responsibility was with the music therapist in situations where the child was profoundly disabled or had very limited mobility (Swingler, 1998 pg. 4). Soundbeam provides a unique experience for children with severe disabilities who lead a very stationary lifestyle, where they are forced to rely heavily on the care of others. Due to the limited amount of mobility required to produce sound using Soundbeam, this may be the first time an individual is able to do accomplish something for him or herself (Swingler, 1998 pg.4). This can be a much stronger motivator than many other forms of therapy.

According to Tim Swingler, Dr. Phil Ellis was the first person to examine the long- term effect of Soundbeam in the field of music therapy (1998, pg.4). Ellis concluded that the use of Soundbeam with severely disabled children was a strong motivator to encourage movement and to eventually improve posture, balance and body control (Swingler, 1998 pg.4). However, the most important part may very well be the enjoyment and strong sense of accomplishment the child feels after using Soundbeam (Swingler, 1998 pg.4). Fun and enjoyment are incredibly strong motivators, especially when working with children. This idea is supported by Jean Piaget, a well-known developmental psychologist, who believed that "play and cognitive development are inseparable" (Lane, Mistrett, 1996). Despite the differences in their theories, another well -known developmental psychologist, Lev Vygotsky, also agreed about the importance of play for children. He wrote, "When a child is engaging in play, he or she is functioning close to his or her optimal developmental level" (Lane, Mistrett, 1996).

Children with Cerebral Palsy

Children with cerebral palsy, who often experience involuntary bodily movements, may enjoy working with Soundbeam, as well. Any movement, whether voluntary or involuntary in front of the Soundbeam sensor will create a sound, therefore if a child with cerebral palsy is using the Soundbeam system in a therapy session and he/she experiences an involuntary movement, the activity will not be disrupted and he/she will still be able to create music independently.

Children with Autism

Children with autism struggle with a hallmark impairment in the area of social-emotional communication and interaction. Using Soundbeam in a group situation can help children with autism become more aware of individuals around them and can help interest them in communicating with others and participating in activities. Since Soundbeam can be used with multiple sensors, multiple children can engage in a music-making activity simultaneously. Each sensor can control a different sound, and when each child moves in front of a sensor, he/she can create a sound. In a group setting, the child will see how his/her sound fits in and he/she can learn how or when he/she should move to create a sound as a group that he/she enjoys listening to. In order for this to work, the group of children must be mindful of those around them, must communicate with one other and must work together. Soundbeam allows this to occur in a fun and natural way, where a child with autism, who may not typically engage with or pay attention to others, is now involved in the activity. Soundbeam is also equipped with a plethora of sounds, so it is not a problem to find sounds that appeal to children with autism.

Soundbeam is often used to facilitate a variation of music therapy known as Sound Therapy. In 2000, Ellis and van Leeuwen examined the effects of Sound Therapy on children with autism. Through a case study with a 13 year old boy named John, a child with severe autism, severe learning disabilities and significant developmental delays caused by his hypotonic muscles, Dr. Ellis and Dr. Leeuwen were able to show the significant benefits of using the Soundbeam system (2000 pg.11). John showed a substantial improvement in many areas after several weeks of Sound Therapy. Before the therapy, John was tense and his movements were incredibly awkward. He had an irregular breathing pattern and was unfocused; even with assistance from another person, his attention span was brief. John was rarely engaged in eye contact and only used limited vocalized speech to express negativity. John would often seem angry and upset, barely ever laughing or smiling. After Sound Therapy, John was more relaxed and was able to move more fluidly. His breathing had become more regular, his attention span greatly improved, and his eye contact was improving. John was now using speech more frequently and in a positive way, he also showed increased smiling and laughter. Soundbeam and Sound Therapy offer an alternative approach into opening up the minds of children with autism and allowing them the opportunity to learn new things across a variety of subjects and situations (Ellis, Leeuwen, 2000, pg. 21).

Soundbox™

Another way to experience sounds and music is to feel them through vibrations. Vibroacoustics is another means of music and Sound Therapy. Vibroacoustic therapy began in the 1980s (Wigram, 1996 pg. 18). A form of technology that is widely used now for vibroacoustic therapy is Soundbox, which is created by the makers of Soundbeam. Children, who experience vibroacoustics during Sound Therapy, generally use Soundbox and Soundbeam together (Ellis, Leeuwen, 2000, pg. 9). However, the Soundbox, which is generally 4 feet by 3 feet and 6 inches deep with large speakers located beneath it, will work with any other sound processor (Ellis, Leeuwen, 2000, pg.9). The child is able to feel the vibrations if they sit or stand directly on the Soundbox or through a chair or wheelchair that is placed directly on the box (Ellis, Leeuwen, 2000 pg. 9).

Vibroacoustics are centered around using the effects sounds have on the body as a stimulus (Wigram, 1996, pg. 63). Olav Skille, a therapist and teacher in Norway, suggested three overarching principles in relation to vibrations:

1. "Low frequencies can relax and high frequencies can raise tension"
2. "Rhythmic music can stimulate and non-rhythmic music can pacify"
3. "Loud music can create aggression and soft music can act as a sedative" (Wilgram, 1996, pg.64).

Soundbox can be very helpful for children with Cerebral palsy and Rett Syndrome (Wigram, 1996, pg. 75). Vibroacoustic therapy has been successful in calming muscle spasms associated with Cerebral palsy (Wigram, 1996, pg. 75). Olav Skille, discovered that vibroacoustic therapy could be used to increase relaxation and decrease restlessness in children with Rett Syndrome (Wigram, 1996, pg. 75).

Switches

Due to the nature of some developmental delays, which may cause a child to have a lack of fine or gross motor skills, using certain computer-based tools such as a mouse or keyboard can be incredibly challenging if not impossible (Magee, 2006 pg. 163). Alternative input devices, which replace the need for a mouse or keyboard, such as a single switch, can be used as a form of assistive technology (AT) to allow a child to create computer based music in new ways (Magee, 2006, pg. 163).

There are various types and sizes of switches which allow the music therapist to select the specific switch that will work best for each child (Bache, et al., 2014, pg. 64). Cook and Hussey (1995) organized the various forms of switches based on how they are triggered (1995). They use five categories: mechanical, proximity, electrical, pneumatic, and sound of voice. A mechanical switch is controlled by applying pressure to perform a physical action such as pressing a button or flipping a switch. With a proximity switch, there is no physical contact needed. In order for a proximity switch to be activated, the user must move in the near vicinity of the detector. Electrical switches are slightly more complicated; they are controlled by electrical signals that can be detected through the skin. To detect these signals, the music therapist can use either an electromyography (EMG) or an electrooculography (EOG). Air flow or air pressure by breathing, controls the pneumatic switch. The sound/voice switch is controlled through verbal speech through a microphone. However, in 1989, Nesbit and Poon had already developed a categorization for the different types of switches. The three categories are contact -target, contact-non-target, and non-contact. The contact- target switch is similar to the mechanical switch. It is activated by physical touch to the switch. The contact - non-target switch is controlled through physical contact, as well, however, through alternative movements, besides pressing or touching the switch to activate it. The non-contact switch is similar to the proximity switch, which is activated by body movement. Some switches are momentary, meaning they turn a device on when the switch is pressed, and the device will turn off when the switch is released. Another type of switch, the latched switch, turns a device on when the switch is pressed and will turn the device off when the switch is pressed again (Bache et al,. 2014, pg. 66).

Switches come in a variety of sizes, colors, and textures, making the devices much more accessible to a wide range of users. It is essential that the switch/switches chosen by the music therapist align with the abilities of the child (Bache et al., 2014, pg. 69). When a music therapist is considering using a switch with a child, it is important that there is time spent observing the child, so the music therapist can select a switch that revolves around a skill-set that best matches the child's needs and interests. However, the switch skills will still need to be practiced and developed, since the child has no previous experience with the device. Allowing children to use a switch without training them on how to activate the switch, could ultimately result in frustration for the child and could reduce the child's motivation (Bache, et al,. 2014, pg. 77). There would be little to no benefit for the child, if this were to be the case. Switches allow the child not only to control the situation at hand, but also to accomplish something entirely on his/her own. This may be a unique and invaluable opportunity for the child to experience independence and to feel that he/she is accomplishing something worthwhile. .

Switches can be particularly beneficial for child with a wide variety of abilities. A child with Down syndrome, with low muscle tone, may experience difficulty using a mechanical switch, since he/she is not able to exert the amount of force needed to activate the switch. However, a proximity switch could work very well since there is no need for force, just movement in front of the sensor. Proximity switches can also work well for children with cerebral palsy, who have low muscle tone or poor coordination, since these children might particularly struggle with pressing a button or flipping a switch. A major benefit of using a switch is that the placement of the switch is very flexible to best accommodate the abilities of the child. A mechanical switch, or any type of switch, would only work well for a child with cerebral palsy if it were placed on their dominant side.

Larger mechanical switches, as well as switches that click or make a sound when they are activated can be used to accommodate children with cerebral palsy who have poor vision or hearing. Switches can also be made from or covered in various materials and textures to accommodate children with autism, with sensory issues, who are averse to the feel of certain textures. Larger mechanical switches as well as proximity switches can also be used to help children with autism, who have poor coordination. If the child is able to communicate verbally, but has impaired coordination or motor skills, then a sound/voice switch may be the best option for them. Pneumatic and electrical switches are also an option for a child with Down syndrome or cerebral palsy whose motor skills are impaired to the extent that physical movement to activate the switch may not be possible or physical movement could be too strenuous for the child and therefore not an enjoyable experience.

Many of the skills developed through the use of music therapy using a switch device can also be applied to other areas of the child's development and learning. The skills that would be developed with the switch during music therapy sessions could also be applied to an Alternative and Augmentative Communication (AAC) device with a speech therapist or to any other therapy modality or technology which can be used with a switch (Bache, et al,. 2014, pg. 76). In a situation of this sort, music therapy could be used to teach the required skill with the switch that could then be applied to any number of communication or academic areas, and as a form of motivation, as well. The switch can be particularly useful for a child with autism who is nonverbal and is interested in or enjoys music. Using an AAC device will most likely help the child to communicate, while music can become a strong motivator for a child who may not be motivated by the desire to communicate, alone.

BIGmack and LITTLEmack are additional options that can be used as a switch. The BIGmack switch, which is battery operated and lies flat, is a round switch, 5 inches in diameter and is able to record a single recording for up to two minutes. . The LITTLEmack switch is raised and sits at an angle. The diameter of the LITTLEmack is only two and a half inches; however, it is still able to record for the same two minute interval, as the BIGmack switch. Both the BIGmack and LITTLEmack are available in red, yellow, blue, and green and can be attached to other switches or toys to encourage or expand use. BIGmack and LITTLEmack can be viewed on the following website: www.ablenetinc.com/assistive-technology/communication/BIGmack-Littlemack.

Eye Gaze

An eye gaze system uses a camera to track where the eyes of the user are looking by either moving the cursor on the screen or by making an on-screen selection or by blinking or focusing on one area for an extended period of time (Bache, et al,. 2014, pg. 78). The eye gaze system can be used independently from and/or with a switch. When used with a switch, the eye gaze system will move the cursor on the screen and the switch will be used to make a selection (Bache, et al,. 2014, pg. 78).

Banche, Derwent, and Magee (2014) discuss the three main eye gaze systems, all-in-one systems, dedicated modular devices, and add-on systems (2014, pg. 78). All-in-one devices work independently and do not need to be connected to any other device to function. . The benefits of the all-in-one system include that it is easily portable and there is never a need to worry if it will be compatible with the computer/software that it is being used in conjunction with. The one downfall of this system is that it is not possible to update or upgrade the hardware without buying an entirely new device. The dedicated modular system is easily updatable, since it is a computer based system. Dedicated modules can be used with switches or with other touch-screen devices as a secondary or as an alternative means of activation or interaction with a device. The final type of eye gaze system is the add-on system. This device can be synched with any type of computer and is portable and easily updatable. The add-on system is never updated, it is simply attached to a new/updated computer and it will continue to work. These systems are ideal for educational, work, or recreational activities. Eye gaze systems can also be used with a computer-based music creating software program to play single notes or chords as well as to use a music player to select a song that the child wants to hear (Bache, et al,. 2014, pg. 80).

Interactive Metronome

Children with autism and cerebral palsy can benefit from using a program called Interactive Metronome (IM). According to the Interactive Metronome website, IM works by improving the ability of the brain to keep time ("Interactive Metronome"). Using the time-keeping qualities of a metronome in music, the program uses interactive games and 3-D graphics to help improve: attention, coordination, language processing, fluency in reading and math, as well as in impulse and aggression control. IM can be used with a button trigger, tap mat, and with an in-motion switch.

The IM button trigger encourages movement when used; the trigger is wireless, so it can be placed anywhere. This can either be used to help improve movement, to develop fine motor skills from gross motor skills or to give access to children with very limited mobility. The button triggers are designed to respond to light touches as well as to be able to handle harder, more aggressive slapping or tapping, making it an ideal tool to use with children. Since the button trigger is wireless, the music therapist is also able to hold it and change its position while the child is playing to help improve hand-eye coordination. The tap mat is even more durable than the button trigger. While the tap mat was originally designed to be stood on and tapped or stomped on to help improve balance, the tap mat now has many more uses. The tap mat can also be used on a table to practice typing on a keyboard or playing on the keys of the piano. Children can practice typing or playing to the beat of IM and are able to improve their fine motor skills, dexterity and speed over time. Therefore, IM gives children the opportunity to develop new skills, they will then be able to use their new skills to play MIDI keyboards for other musical instruments. The IM in-motion switch is designed to facilitate the ability of the child to walk and hold a conversation at the same time, while still being mindful of the environment around him. The in-motion switch uses wireless headphones to provide immediate feedback to help the child walk at a steady and consistent pace, to help avoid falls and to develop dual concentration.

Children with autism may struggle with slower brain timing (Nicholas et al, 2007). Researchers (Nicholas et al, 2007) believe this can be seen through disrupted sleep patterns, trouble with information processing, a lack of attention, difficulty transitioning between tasks, challenged communication, disrupted processing of sensory information, and a lack of coordination in children with autism. The Interactive Metronome program could help improve brain timing and could therefore help improve some of these hallmark deficits.

Apollo Ensemble

Apollo Ensemble takes the idea of transforming movement into sound to a whole new level by incorporating the multimedia elements of light, pictures, and videos, as well. As evident through videos on their website, www.apollocreative.co.uk/apolloensemble.shtml, the Apollo system can be used to control the lights, images, and sounds projected into an entire room, using a varied array of controllers ("Apollo Creative"). Although the system may seem complex, it is designed for quick and simple access. The various themes are displayed on a single screen, intended to be touch-activated, such as an iPad or another touch-screen device. Each theme is represented by its own icon. The user must simply press an icon to get started.

Once a theme has been selected, the lights, images, and sounds are controlled by various sensors. Apollo has created a variety of wireless sensors to use with their system. The dice sensor can tell which way it is being held. Each side of the device can be assigned its own sound. As the device is moved and held in different ways, the sounds are activated. The press switch is a different option for children who have more control over their fine motor skills. The press sensor is touch-sensitive and detects changes in pressure, giving the child greater control over the sounds being created. The tilt sensor, although easier to use, does not allow for as much creative control. This device is tilted from side to side to adjust the pitch of a note or the sound and to adjust the volume up and down. The tag sensor is the only device that is not activated by movement. Sounds can be attached to tags, each of which has a unique ID. The ID is read by the tag sensor when the tag is placed in front of it, activating the desired sound. It is also possible to use game controllers, joy sticks, and just about any other type of sensor or switch with the Apollo Ensemble system. Although any game controller should work, the Microsoft Xbox 360 Wireless Controller for Windows, the Rockband Drum Kit Controller for Xbox 360, and the Logitech Freedom 2.4 Cordless Joystick have been tested with the Apollo Ensemble program.

Elin Skogdal of The SKUG Centre in Norway finds Apollo Ensemble to be more versatile than many other systems like it. The Apollo Ensemble will work with almost every type of switch; therefore all needs and accommodations can be met for all users. Mike Sissons of The Dale school uses Apollo Ensemble as well and has seen improvements not only in the mobility of some of his students, for example a child being able to move his/her wheelchair, but also affording students the ability to participate in other academic activities, as well. An example presented by Mr. Sissons is storytelling. Some children with autism or other developmental delays may not be able to participate in a storytelling activity because they do not communicate verbally. Although the child may be able to enjoy the experience of hearing the story, they are not as actively engaged. Apollo Ensemble creates an environment that brings a story to life and gives the child the opportunity to control the lights, sounds, and images that can accompany that story. This connects back to affording the child a feeling of accomplishment, a sense of having control and being able to make something happen independently.

MIDIGrid

A MIDI is a Musical Instrument Digital Interface. MIDIs are used to connect various digital or electronic instruments, such as keyboards, to a computer (Kirk et al, 2002). MIDIGrid, a computer-based system, allows the user to easily select various musical sounds using the mouse of the computer (Kirk et al, 2002). Examples of what the MIDIGrid software looks like as well as product demos can be seen on their website (www.midigrid.com). The MIDIGrid program, which looks similar to a spread sheet, can contain anywhere from one to two hundred boxes. Each box is assigned a unique sound, whether a single note, a combination of notes, or a sound created by other sounds on the MIDIGrid.

Each MIDIGrid can be preset before use. This allows each child to use a MIDIGrid that is unique to them and includes only the sounds they wish to use. The more boxes and sounds that are included in the grid, the smaller each box appears. Conversely, the fewer sounds that are featured in the grid, the larger each box appears. This can be beneficial in both ways. For a child with cerebral palsy, who has very limited use of fine motor skills and only wishes to use a few sounds, the MIDIGrid requires less dexterity to select the sound they wish to use. However, more sounds can be added and skills and dexterity can improve through practice and continuous use of the program. A child who has more control over their fine motor skills, possibly a child with autism could experiment with a wider variety of sounds and could narrow down their selection to a smaller size grid with only the sounds the child enjoys using.

MIDIGrid can be controlled in many different ways. Although commonly controlled by musicians through the mouse of the computer, any means of interaction the child can use with a computer will work, including switches, joy sticks, and MIDI keyboards. Switches and joy sticks are used to allow the child to browse through the grid boxes and to make selections of which sounds to play. MIDI keyboards can be used as well. When using a MIDI keyboard, each key is assigned to correspond to a box from the grid. It is also possible to assign multiple keys to the same grid box. This allows for easier access to a child with Down syndrome or cerebral palsy, who may have poor coordination. If the keys on the keyboard that control the same box are grouped next to each other, then the child does not have to be as precise. As children become more comfortable with the keyboard, they can use fewer keys as their motor skills improve.

Adaptive Use Music Instruments

The Adaptive Use Musical Instruments (AUMI) software is designed to accommodate all users. The AUMI system is activated by movement, just like many other systems. However, this particular system is unique because it detects movement through the forward facing camera of a computer, laptop, or other device. AUMI was developed and is supported by the Deep Listening Institute. The AUMI software can be purchased and downloaded from their website: http://deeplistening.org/site/adaptiveuse. Video demos posted on the AUMI website feature a more detailed visual explanation of how the software works.

AUMI can be played with piano, percussive, and/or prerecorded sounds. AUMI displays the image of the user from the camera onto the computer screen. On the video image there will be a tracking box, or tracking line and a tracking ball. For piano, a tracking box will be used. The color and size of the box can be adjusted as well as the thickness of the box. This is to accommodate the greatest number of users. The designers of this program believe that the software should adapt to fit the needs of the user, as opposed to having the user change to meet the needs of the software. In order to create sounds using the piano keyboard, the user must select a part of the body displayed on screen that they wish to track.

This could be any body part that has mobility, like the hands, fingers, even a specific area of the face. The tracking ball will then be linked to this area in the video and as the user moves within the tracking box, the tracking ball will translate the movement into runs on the piano keys. When the percussive or prerecorded sounds are used, a tracking line will be viewed on the screen. The screen can be divided into anywhere from two to eight pieces by tracking lines. Sound is created by moving the tracking ball across a tracking line, the same way the ball would be moved through the tracking box. Each line can be assigned its own percussive or prerecorded sound.

A unique factor of the AUMI system is just how much creative control the user has. A music therapist using this program with a child, could have the child select which octave on the piano to play, and which scales he or she wants to use. They are able to decipher if they want to play chromatically and are able to make a variety of other decisions.

Not only can they exercise control, but they are able to create music without the assistance of another person. They are able to create a piece of music that they enjoy. Although other programs such as Soundbeam which use motion detection can bring enjoyment to children and improve motor skills and communication, they do not offer as much musical control. AUMI not only helps to improve movement, but can also help improve the musical abilities and develop the musical preferences of the child which can translate into other important areas of music therapy. AUMI is also available as an iPad App, making it easily accessible for therapy sessions as well as for home use. Although intended for creating music, AUMI can also be used as a means of communication. In the percussive option, a prerecorded sound can be assigned to each side of the line allowing the user to move the tracking ball to make a selection. This could be used to allow a non-verbal child to decide between two things if the names were recorded and put into the system or to say yes or no when asked a question.

iPad Apps

The Apple iPad, although a somewhat expensive piece of technology, has many advantages and uses in the field of music therapy. Robert Krout (2014) explores the benefits of several music-based iPad apps for children with autism, however children with other developmental delays could benefit from many of these apps as well. Although a slight disadvantage of using the iPad is that it does not promote social interaction or group play, it has often been successful in engaging children who may enjoy music but are not drawn to acoustic instruments (Krout, 2014, pg. 182).

A major benefit of using iPad apps is that for the most part, the app is either free or very affordable. Kalimba™, a free iPad app, is an African Thumb Piano. This app is very easy to use, and highly engaging due to the sounds, as well as to the animation that accompanies the sounds being created. Air Harp™, starting at $1.99 with the ability to purchase additional music at $.99 per package, features a fifteen-string harp. Children who use this app are able to work on developing and improving their fine motor skills. This is accomplished by playing the harp with finger picking, tapping or plucking movements similar to those used to play the actual instrument. A free app, Virtuoso Piano, is a virtual piano keyboard. This app features a duet mode which can be used to promote social interaction and expression between the child and the therapist or even between two children, who are trying to build social skills.

Percussions™, which costs only $6.99 in the App Store has a wide range of percussion instruments. The App allows children to play the agogo, bell tree, bongo, maracas, turn table, shaker, tambourine, timbales, triangle, vibraslap, and the woodblock. All instruments are activated by tapping, touching, or swiping across the screen, depending on the instrument and multiple instruments can be featured and played at once. Percussions also in include 16 tunes in a variety of genres for the user to improvise. . iTune tracks are already stored on the device and can be used in the app as well. Pocket Drums™ another percussion based app, costs $.99. The app is equipped with twenty-two varying drum sets that range in musical style and genre. This particular app seems to be engaging for many reasons. One reason being that the drum heads vibrate as they are struck. The on-screen movement in response to their touch has been very engaging for many children. The app is also able to record and save tracks. This allows multiple children to play and interact with each other on the same track.

Additional Technologies

Video Games

Although it may sound odd, some video games, like Guitar Hero™ or Rock Band™ can have some therapeutic benefits, as well. Gaming creates an environment where multiple children can play and interact with one another in a stress-free and in a non-aggressive atmosphere (Hadley, Steele, 2014 pg. 167). Although players receive individual scores, playing a game like Rock Band™ in a group, forces players to rely on one another and trust that each person is going to play their own part as well as learning to be dependable. Not only does the child have to rely on the other members of the group, but the other members of the group rely on the child as well.

Games like Guitar Hero™ and Rock Band™ can be particularly beneficial for children with autism who are working on social skills. If the child has the mobility to play any of the Rock Band™ instruments or the Guitar Hero™ guitars, then he or she is able to play and engage with others. These activities are not only useful for group therapy sessions but can also be used in the home, as well (Hadley, Steele, 2014 pg. 167). Guitar Hero™ and Rock Band™ do not require the presence of a therapist and the games are affordable, especially if the family already owns the gaming system required for play such as Xbox 360, Play station, or Wii. Games can be used to promote family bonding not only between parents and children, but also between siblings. Siblings may have trouble relating to or finding activities to share with a sibling who has a developmental delay. If the child has the mobility required to play any of these games, this could be an ideal opportunity.

The Axe by Harmonix™, the same video game company that created Rock Band, is another video game option. What makes The Axe different from Guitar Hero and Rock Band is that the instruments are controlled by a joy stick instead of by imitation instruments. The game comes with a variety of popular music tracks and players can select instruments to play along with the tracks. Players can choose from electric guitars, jazz guitars, pianos, saxophones, synthesizers, trumpets, and voices that are scat singing to improvise and play along with the featured tracks. The use of the joy stick, as opposed to the instruments in other game systems, may be more accommodating for a child who has limited mobility or is not able to hold the instruments to play other games.

Switch Jam/Switch Ensemble

Switch Jam and Switch Ensemble are two programs designed for use with the various switches discussed earlier in the chapter. Both programs, intended to be used with a group, can be purchased online from the website: www.switchintime.com. Switch Jam, which is the simpler of the two programs, features 10 songs in a variety of genres that children can play. In the game, children control characters in the game, who play the instruments for them. Although the game is intended for group play, one child is able to control all of the parts. Switch Jam™ makes everyone sound like a talented musician. Switch Ensemble™ is geared more towards music creation. The child is able to use his/her switch to improvise on guitars, and even sing. Switch Ensemble™ includes 90 songs and can also be used in a group setting.

Being designed to be controlled by a switch allows for children with various abilities to participate in the same activity. Games such as this can be highly motivating and can promote movement as well as social and even cognitive development. Switch Jam™ and Switch Ensemble™ also provide an opportunity for a child to practice and improve his/her abilities to use his or her switch in a fun and stress-free environment.

Alternative Communication Devices

The BIGmack and LITTLEmack switches discussed earlier in the chapter as well as Augmentative Alternative Communication devices or AACs, although intended to aid in communication for non-verbal children, can also be used in the music therapy setting. Martino and Bertolami (2014) suggest using AAC devices and the BIGmack switch with prerecorded melodies and sounds that the child can use to add dimension to group improvisations. The therapist could even record song lyrics onto the device for the child to activate at the corresponding moments in a song. There are some limitations however, because the switch can only control one sound. To accommodate multiple sounds, BIGmack switches can be used, with each different color representing a different sound. Working with AAC devices in music therapy allows a non-verbal child to either practice the skills he/she will need in order to use the AAC in daily communication or to offer the child an advantage by using technology that he/she is already familiar with and comfortable using. Working with switches in a situation such as this can also provide a base that the child can then improve upon and develop to accomplish more complex musical tasks and abilities such as using the Switch Jam or Switch Ensemble programs.

Keyboards, Drum/Rhythm Machines, and Audio Loopers

Keyboards, drum/rhythm machines, and audio loopers are all additional tools which can provide creative output for children who may not have been able to participate in other musical activities. Keyboards can provide a variety of different sounds that both imitate other instruments and those that do not. This affords the child an abundance of options. Drum/rhythm machines can work in two ways. Preprogramed rhythms can serve as the background for other sounds and music creations. Drum beats and rhythms can also be created on the machine as well. Creating a rhythm could be an activity that gets developed through multiple sessions to become the background to a larger and more intricate piece. Audio loopers take a sound that is recorded into the machines and repeat it on a loop. Whether the sound is intentionally or unintentionally created, the audio looper eliminates the need for the child to repeat the same sound multiple times (Sadnovik, 2014, pg. 251). This can be particularly beneficial if the child enjoys a specific sound, but has difficulty with the movements required to create it.

Impro-Visor

Impro-Visor™ is a computer-based improvisation program that can be downloaded online at: http://sourceforge.net/projects/impro-visor/). Originally designed to help jazz musicians compose solos, Impro-Visor now has a wider variety of uses. According to their website the program Impro-Visor, which is really "Improvising Advisor" was designed to be used to compose music ("Impro-Visor"). Although the program was designed with the intention of helping users understand how to construct solos, Impro-Visor has now been used to transcribe and transpose music, as well as to provide a track that musicians can accompany. . Already equipped with solo ideas and scale recommendations, musicians can compose original solos, hear their composition played back, and then go back and make edits or changes. Impro-Visor is also able to generate a solo which the user can then edit and change to his/her liking.

Using a program such as Impro-Visor™, or even Switch Ensemble™, which was discussed previously, can provide the child with an instant feeling of success. The nature of the Impro-Visor program is to create music successfully and help all users gain a better understanding of music composition. The program will show the child which scales and notes will sound good with the chords being played in the background. In an environment where the child is set up to succeed, there can be an increased amount of motivation, confidence, satisfaction and enjoyment.

Music Workstations

A music work station is a single piece of equipment that includes a sound module, a music sequencer, and, generally, an electronic keyboard. Workstations are designed to produce electronic music and can be used to create rhythms, beats, or full compositions using only one device. Using a workstation can provide a variety of activities for a music therapist or a child who does not want to use a computer-based instrument. When working at a workstation, the child still has control over the volume and can manipulate the sound in various ways such as with a computer-based music editing program. A benefit of the work station is that it is portable if necessary, so it can easily be used in various settings or purchased to be used in the home, if desired. Using a workstation can help improve fine motor skills and can be used as another tool in the music-making process. Having a music sequencer included in the work station allows the child to not only record and hear what he or she has created but also to edit or change the compositions. This can offer a feeling of accomplishment as well as an opportunity for growth and improvement.

FUTURE RESEARCH DIRECTIONS

Although technology is being used more regularly throughout the field of music therapy, there are still areas for research and improvement. There are often obstacles which interfere with the ability of the therapist to use technology in many therapy situations. There is a lack of awareness in regards of the benefits of technology being used for music therapy in the general public, possibly due to the lack of research published on the topic. In a research study (Magee, 2006) about why music therapists do not use technology more often, there were a variety of responses from not having training available to a lack of funds and an absence of interest. If research were conducted on a larger scale, rather than a smaller scale that relies on case studies and pilot studies, there could be greater awareness and more of a demand for funds and proper training. Although there is a plethora of research on the benefits of music and music therapy for children with developmental delays, there is very little research specifically focused on the effectiveness of the current technology being used.

The field would benefit from learning about each form of musical technology and learning how to most effectively use the technology with children with disabilities in a music therapy context. Most of the research available has mainly focused on children with autism, Down syndrome, and cerebral palsy, however, there is little research involving children with other developmental delays such as Rett syndrome or Angelman syndrome.

As new technology is being developed via iPads or tablets, music-based technology is becoming more accessible and much more affordable. However, it is still important to research and examine how exactly these technologies are beneficial, not to simply observe them in a clinical setting as a therapist. If newer and improved technologies are going to be developed, there must be an understanding of what works, and why it works.

CONCLUSION

"Music is a spirit. It heals. It's an amazing thing to be loved and appreciated" (Hayes, 2012). All kinds of people find solace and self-expression through music. Many people, including children or adults with, and without developmental delays, rely on music on a daily basis not only to express themselves but also to either embrace or change how they are feeling. Think about musicians and song writers who use their compositions and their song lyrics to communicate how they are feeling or what they are thinking. Music evokes emotions in people and affords us an opportunity to relate to one another. When a person hears a song and is able to relate to everything that song is about, then he/she knows that someone else has felt the same way and that they are not alone. Music affects us and it changes us, "[t]he identity of a person can even be considered as a 'musical form that is continually being composed to the world' (Aldridge, 1996: 23) (Blunt, 2013)."

Often times when interventions are being planned for a child with developmental delays, the main focus is doing everything possible to benefit the child. This generally involves learning skills and strategies to help the child to become successful in an educational setting and to become as self-sufficient as possible. However, what can often be forgotten is how important it is to nurture the child's interests and ensure that the child is able to find joy and excitement in what he/she is doing. If a child without a developmental delay is exposed to music, either at home or in school, then a child with a developmental delay should be able to have those very same experiences and opportunities.

As can be seen throughout the chapter, there are immense benefits to using music for therapy purposes. However, it is essential to remember that music should be a relaxing and enjoyable experience. Everyone is able to create some type of music, whether it is simply clapping a beat, generating some type of sound or rhythm on a computer or playing an acoustic instrument. Music, especially in a therapeutic situation, should not be centered upon being the best or doing everything correctly. Music should be about self-expression, experimentation, and giving all people a place where they can feel safe and good about themselves.

Music is essential to the lives of so many people. "All sound has musical (expressive) potential, and all people have sound as a fundamental experience of life. Even if we are deaf, we still experience sound as vibration; it is central to our human condition (Goddard [1996], Storr [1992, 1972], Springer and Deatsch [1998], Traux [1998])" (Ellis, Leauwen, 2000). There is no right or wrong with music. It is important to remember that all people, adults or children, with disabilities or without should be able to express themselves and should not be limited by a set of predetermined standards. If music is an important part in the life of someone without a developmental delay, then there is no reason that it should not equally important in the life of someone with such a delay.

REFERENCES

American Music Therapy Association. (n.d.). *American Music Therapy Association*. Retrieved February 24, 2014, from http://www.musictherapy.org/

Assistive Technology Products and Special Ed Curriculum for Persons with Disabilities. (n.d.). *Assistive Technology Products and Special Ed Curriculum for Persons with Disabilities*. Retrieved June 17, 2014, from http://www.ablenetinc.com/

Baxter, H. T., Berghofer, J. A., MacEwan, L., Nelson, J., Peters, K., & Roberts, P. (2007). *The individualized music therapy assessment profile: IMTAP*. Jessica Kingsley Publishers.

Berger, D. S. (2009, March). On Developing Music Therapy Goals and Objectives©. In *Voices: A World Forum for Music Therapy* (Vol. 9, No. 1).

Bunt, L. (2003). Music therapy with children: A complementary service to music education? *British Journal of Music Education*, *20*(02), 179–195. doi:10.1017/S0265051703005370

Cook, A., & Hussey, S. (1995). *Assistive technologies: principles and practice*. St Louis: Mosby Year Book.

Deep Listening Institute. (n.d.). *Deep Listening*. Retrieved March 15, 2014, from http://www.deeplistening.org/site/

Dolan, M. C. (1973). Music therapy: An explanation. *Journal of Music Therapy*, *10*(4), 172–176. doi:10.1093/jmt/10.4.172

Ellis, P., & van Leeuwen, L. (2000). *Living Sound: human interaction and children with autism. ISME commission on Music in Special Education*. Regina, Canada: Music Therapy and Music Medicine.

Green, E. J., & Drewes, A. A. (Eds.). (2013). *Integrating Expressive Arts and Play Therapy with Children and Adolescents*. John Wiley & Sons.

Harvey Mudd College. (n.d.). *HMC Computer Science*. Retrieved April 30, 2014, from http://www.cs.hmc.edu/

Kirk, R., Hunt, A., Hildred, M., Neighbour, M., & North, F. (2002). Electronic Musical Instruments-a rôle in Music Therapy? In *Dialogue and Debate-Conference Proceedings of the 10th World Congress on Music Therapy* (p. 1007).

Magee, W. L. (2006). Electronic technologies in clinical music therapy: A survey of practice and attitudes. *Technology and Disability*, *18*(3), 139–146.

Nicholas, B., Rudrasingham, V., Nash, S., Kirov, G., Own, M. J., & Wimpory, D. C. (2007). Association of Per1 and Npas2 with autistic disorder: Support for the clock genes/social timing hypothesis. *Molecular Psychiatry*, *12*(6), 581–592. doi:10.1038/sj.mp.4001953 PMID:17264841

Nisbet, P., & Poon, P. (1998). *Special Access Technology*.

Ramsey, D. W., Zigo, J., Lajoie, M., & Baker, F. (2013). *Music technology in therapeutic and health settings*. Jessica Kingsley Publishers.

Lane, S. J., & Mistrett, S. G. (1996). Play and Assistive Technology Issues for Infants and Young Children with Disabilities A Preliminary Examination. *Focus on Autism and Other Developmental Disabilities*, *11*(2), 96–104. doi:10.1177/108835769601100205

Streeter, E. (2001, April). Reactions and responses from the music therapy community to the growth of computers and technology-some preliminary thoughts. In Voices: A world forum for music therapy (Vol. 7, No. 1). doi:10.15845/voices.v7i1.467

Swingler, T. (1998). *That Was Me!*": Applications of the Soundbeam MIDI Controller as a Key to Creative Communication. Learning, Independence and Joy.

Swingler, T. (1998). The invisible keyboard in the air: An overview of the educational, therapeutic and creative applications of the EMS Soundbeam™. In *2nd European Conference for Disability, Virtual Reality & Associated Technology*.

Swingler, T., & Brockhouse, J. (2009). Getting better all the time: Using music technology for learners with special needs. *Australian Journal of Music Education*, (2), 49.

Welcome. (n.d.). *to Apollo Creative: bubble tubes, bubble walls, LED light sources, equipment for interactive lighting, interactive displays, assistive technology, and multi sensory room equipment*. Retrieved June 1, 2014, from http://www.apollocreative.co.uk/

Wigram, A. L. (1996). *The effects of vibroacoustic therapy on clinical and non-clinical populations*. (Doctoral dissertation). University of London, London, UK.

KEY TERMS AND DEFINITIONS

Alternative and Augmentative Communication Devices (AAC): Various tool and devices that are used as a means of communication that is nonverbal.

Improvisation: Creating music without preplanning or without reading music that has already been written.

Metronome: A tool used to keep the beat when playing music.

Musical Instrument Digital Interface (MIDI): Used to connect various instruments with electronic plug-in capabilities to a computer.

Sequencer: A tool or software program that can be used to record and play what has been recorded as well as to edit music.

Soundbeam: A device that creates sound using ultra sonic ranging which detects the movement of the user.

Soundbox: A box which the user can sit, stand, or lie on that allows one to experience the benefits of vibroacoustics.

Vibroacoustics: The effect that feeling the various waves created by sound has on the body.

Chapter 15
Dissemination of Assistive Technology Devices for Children with Disabilities through Realabilities

Senada Arucevic
Long Island University – Brooklyn, USA

ABSTRACT

Over the last decade, vast research has been conducted on assistive technology devices and the potential implementation of these devices in the daily lives of individuals with disabilities. Many devices are new to the public and may require further development, but it is important to disseminate information about these useful technologies, which often afford users more independence with their activities of daily living. Unfortunately individuals with disabilities often encounter stigma; research suggests that assistive technology devices may at times contribute to this ostracism. This chapter reviews a variety of technologies that have been used to improve the quality of life of individuals with varying disabilities. These devices are presented in the context of introducing a new children's television show, Realabilities, a pro-social and stop-bullying children's television program that seeks to enhance the social interaction and initiation of typical children towards children with disabilities. Directions for future research and implementation of these devices are also discussed.

BACKGROUND

Increasing awareness and accessibility of assistive technology devices and services to children with disabilities is imperative, so that children with disabilities can be equipped with the proper technology to assist them with a variety of skill sets. Assistive technology devices and services are best defined by the Assistive Technology Act of 1998, as amended (2004): "Any item, piece of equipment or product system whether acquired commercially off the shelf, modified, or customized that is used to increase, maintain, or improve the functional capabilities of individuals with disabilities" (U.S. Department of Education,

DOI: 10.4018/978-1-4666-8395-2.ch015

2006). This definition suggests that no individual with a disability is the same; therefore devices are uniquely catered to the individual. Assistive technology serves the purpose of helping and teaching and is measured based on functionality. Additionally, it can be used as a part of a rehabilitative or educational process by which technology is being used as a modality rather than as part of a person's daily life (Cook & Polgar, 2013). Examples include wheelchairs, hearing aids, screen readers for individuals who are blind, and software for individuals with learning disabilities. Working with children, parents, and other professionals is essential in selecting the most appropriate device to meet the primary needs of a child with disabilities (Isabelle, Bessey, Dragas, Blease, Shepherd faculty, & Lanefaculty, 2003).

Assistive technology devices are used as a means of helping children with disabilities achieve greater independence (Dawe, 2006). Parents and children report that despite the challenge of finding appropriate technology for their children, most of the devices increase social interaction and even appropriate interaction. Dawe (2006) found that more than 35% of assistive technology devices are purchased but not successfully adopted. Semi-structured interviews with parents and teachers of young people with cognitive disabilities were conducted in order to address the gaps in existing devices and future research. Parents and teachers identified portability, functionality, and ease of upgrade and replacement as the key factors needed to improve assistive technology devices. Hefty cumbersome devices were often abandoned; parents also recognized that these technologies will eventually "wear out" and need to be replaced (Dawe, 2006). There is an overall desire for these devices to grow along with the child.

Technology can be viewed as an equalizing agent for children with disabilities by encouraging their full participation in school and within their communities. Individuals who may experience difficulty speaking can use a portable voice synthesizer in order to ask and respond to questions (Behrmann, 1998). Technology has afforded powerful tool for teachers and families to use in order to better interact with a child with a disability. Encouraging children with disabilities to use these devices can promote social interactions with their typical peers. These relationships can enhance the school environment and promote children with disabilities' interest and success in social interaction and social initiation; furthermore it helps in developing typical children's social-emotional intelligence, understanding and sensitivity (Kamps, Kravitz, Gonzalez-Lopez, Kemmerer, Potucek, & Harrell, 1988).

LEGISLATION SUPPORTING ASSISTIVE TECHNOLOGY DEVICES AND SERVICES

During the Civil Rights Movement of the early 1950s, it was mandated that assistive technology be provided to children with special needs. *The Education for All Handicapped Children Act* (P.L. 94-142) stems from the decision made in the *Brown vs. Board of Education* case (1954) where separate education was declared not to be equal education under the 14th Amendment of the Constitution (Behrmann, 1998). With this legislation, a "free appropriate public education in the least restrictive environment" for children with disabilities was to be established. This legislation implied that they may be placed in the same classrooms as their typical peers. Inclusion continues to be debated today, and although it is encouraged in many schools, it remains a controversial issue.

The Individuals with Disabilities Education Act (IDEA) was passed in 1975 in order to dictate how states and public agencies should provide early intervention, special education and other services to children with disabilities. Adhering to the particular needs of children with disabilities would enable them to focus on their limitations and receive the necessary aid. The Rehabilitation Act of 1973 prevented individuals with disabilities from being discriminated against in the workplace. "Reasonable accommodation" entails that an employer is required to take reasonable steps to accommodate an individual's disability (U.S. Department of Education, 2004). Thus, the provision of an assistive device would be mandated by the workplace.

The Assistive Technology Act of 2004, Public Law 108-364, also known as the "Tech Act," was passed in order to increase the availability of funding for access and training with assistive technology devices and services. Additionally, the Tech Act served to increase awareness and knowledge of the benefits of assistive technology devices and services among targeted individuals. The involvement of individuals with disabilities in decisions related to the provision of assistive technology was also implemented in this law in order to encourage the participation of individuals with disabilities in the creation of these devices (U.S. Department of Education, 2006). To assess whether assistive devices and services are appropriate to the needs of the individual, researchers must obtain feedback from this individual with special needs. Changes and modifications to technologies are constantly being made in order to improve the daily lives of individuals with disabilities.

STIGMA TOWARDS CHILDREN WITH DISABILITIES

By familiarizing society with the assistive technology that individuals with disabilities might use, we help to dispel instances of stigma against children with disabilities. Children with disabilities often fear being judged by others based on their physical appearance. Assistive technology devices are tools that individuals with disabilities use, but fear of stigmatization can cause them to abandon their devices (Parette & Scherer, 2004). Children who are stigmatized often struggle with social acceptance; they tend to be self-conscious, since they feel unsure as to how "typical" individuals will identify or receive them (Goffman, 1963).

Already in 1963, Goffman was one of the first theorists to analyze stigmatized persons' feelings about themselves, their relationships to other individuals, and their position in society. He explained that there are three types of stigma: (1) stigma of character traits (2) physical stigma and (3) stigma of group identity. Stigma of character traits are character traits a person may have that cause them to be perceived as weak. Physical stigma refers to physical qualities of the body that are critiqued and stigma of group identity is rooted in race, religion, disability, etc. (Goffman, 1963). Disorders that are frequently stigmatized include: epilepsy, autism, deafness, mental retardation, alcoholism and mental illness (Gray, 1993). Children with disabilities are two to three times more likely to be bullied than their typical peers (Holmquist, 2011). Using a children's television show as a platform to introduce a variety of disabilities and assistive technologies has been effective, since children find these media to be entertaining and they can grow along with the programming. Research suggests that children imitate the behaviors of adult models and actions on television (Schunk, 1987; Friedrich & Stein, 1975). Children learn the pro-social content of television programs and generalize what they have learned to their daily lives (Friedrich & Stein, 1975).

Research on families of individuals with disabilities finds that many experience "courtesy stigma." This means that members of the family experience stigmatization because of their affiliation with the stigmatized person rather than due to a trait of their own (Gray, 1993). These families seek to maintain a "normal appearing round of family" when they encounter the public. While the literature has references to families of individuals with disabilities, there is little information that explains why individuals with disabilities feel stigmatized. Parette and Scherer (2004) explain that assistive technology is often something individuals with disabilities struggle over, deciding if they should or should not use an assistive device (ex: use of a cochlear implant). Stigma has been associated with choices that are made by families of children with disabilities not to use assistive devices due to "perceived increased visibility or attention received when children use devices in public settings" (Parette & Scherer, 2004). This causes others to behave differently around this person because the use of a device gives others the impression that what they are using is not something an ordinary individual would use (Brookes, 1998). Assistive technology should not define an individual or their disability; thus understanding the purpose of these tools is crucial.

INCLUSIVE EDUCATION

The use of assistive technologies can exacerbate a negative perception of individuals with disabilities by creating a stigma that draws attentions to the disability rather than to the strengths of the individual (Parette & Scherer, 2004). These devices may amplify perceived differences between individuals with disabilities and their typical peers. If technology were to become more familiar, these differences could be minimized. Assistive technologies are necessary for individuals with disabilities in order to partake in activities of daily living and to increase autonomy. Fortunately, these devices also afford children with disabilities more opportunities in mainstreamed classrooms. The integration of children with developmental disorders into mainstream classrooms has been encouraged and supported by acts of legislation, encouraging children with special needs to join with typical students in the classroom.

Children with disabilities are often poorly portrayed in the media, and this may cause society to harbor preconceived notions of what a child with a disability "looks" and "acts" like. Throughout the years, perceptions of individuals with disabilities have remained stagnant, and old stereotypes endure (Day, 2000). Murphy (1995) stated that, "The greatest impediment to a person participating fully in his society is not his physical flaws but rather the issue of myths, fears and misunderstandings that society attaches to them" (Hardin, 2001, p. 140). Hoover and Stenhjem (2003) describe how the continued failure of individuals with disabilities to participate in general education classes, mainstream educational clubs and organizations, and athletic programs, perpetuates a lack of understanding and interaction among students with and without disabilities. Peer interactions and relationships are critical ingredients to developing social skills during childhood (Asher & Coie, 1990). Therefore, it is essential for typical children to understand that children with disabilities may require devices like assistive technology in order to help them complete daily tasks. Such devices should not cause typical children to deem children with disabilities as "strange" or "weird" once they have been acquainted with these devices.

Children's Views of Inclusivity

Norwich and Kelly (2004) assessed the experiences of individuals with moderate learning difficulties in school. The sample size was composed of 101 boys and girls with developmental disabilities ages 10 -11 and 13 – 14. It was found that overall, 83% of the sample experienced some form of 'bullying'. About half of the pupils reported that this 'bullying' was related to their learning difficulties (Norwich & Kelly, 2004). In addition, Block and Obrusnikova (2007) reviewed and analyzed ten years (1995 - 2005) of physical education (PE) inclusion research. Of the 38 studies featured in their review, only five placed significant emphasis on the perspectives of children with disabilities. Spencer-Cavaliere and Watkinson (2010) used these data to develop a study wherein they could examine the views of children with disabilities towards inclusion in physical education. They found that many individuals with disabilities had limited participation in physical education activities, and most children reported few opportunities to meaningfully participate. Some children described complete exclusion from activities, while others mentioned assuming outside roles such as line judge; this caused the students to feel excluded, sad, and angry. The participants with disabilities viewed their friendships as a key ingredient towards feeling included and feeling like they could participate in PE activities. Children with disabilities also struggled with the ability to gain entry into a play environment. Thus, it was meaningful for the children to "be asked to play," which aided in their perception of inclusion. It is evident from these studies that inclusion is a subjective experience. and information about such experiences is best acquired from the child's perspective.

Parent's Views of Inclusivity

Inclusive education may be a preferable choice for parents with a typical child but may be frowned upon by a parent of a child with a disability, or vice-versa; these distinct opinions create an unfair debate about this form of education. Palmer, Fuller, Arora, and Nelson (2001) investigated the perspectives of parents of children with disabilities with regard to inclusivity in the classroom. Their findings indicated that parents who "(a) place a high value on socialization as an educational goal (b) have children who display relatively higher cognitive skills, fewer behavioral problems, and fewer characteristics requiring specialized services and (c) those whose children have spent more time in a general education class environment, are more likely to have positive perceptions of inclusion" (p. 468) when compared to parents who do not share similar values or do not have children with similar disabilities. There is a great concern regarding the lack of individual attention and support or the possibility of rejection or mistreatment that may result from inclusion of children with disabilities.

Parents in opposition to inclusion expressed concern about the medical needs, sensory impairments, and the lack of self-help skills that they felt would interfere with their children's placement in a general classroom. These parents also stated that inclusion would overburden or negatively impact general education teachers and typical students, thus requiring more care; parents felt that other children in the classrooms would be distracted by the special education students. and the special education students would be mistreated because of their disabilities.

Assistive technology devices can help to bridge the gap between general education teachers and typical peers by enhancing communication skills, motor skills, and improving learning techniques. These devices can also ease the concerns of parents by motivating them to help their children with a disability discover the best assistive technology that suits their particular needs.

REALABILITIES CHILDREN'S TELEVISION PROGRAM

In order to disseminate information about assistive technology, a video tool can be used which can build social skills development into its programming. *Realabilities* is a children's educational program that focuses on inspiring typical children to be more accepting of children with disabilities and to encourage more positive attitudes and behavioral intentions of typical children towards their peers with disabilities. This program features unique characters, each with a specific disability, who harness their special strengths to combat bullying in their elementary school. Uno is the character that presents with autism, Melody presents with blindness, Seemore with deafness, Rolly with paraplegia and Addy with attention-deficit/hyperactivity disorder (ADHD). Each episode presents an adventure-packed story that offers a pro-social and anti-bullying message to viewers. *Realabilities* seeks to replace often negative portrayals of individuals with disabilities on TV with positive, strong depictions of such characters. Rather than solely focusing on the limitations of individuals with disabilities, the strengths of each of the characters are highlighted and emphasized.

In order to foster a greater understanding and appreciation of typical children towards children with disabilities, it is important to familiarize them with some of the new or common technologies that children with disabilities may use to help support their learning in the classroom. The following review will introduce a variety of assistive technologies that are presented in some creative way during the show to widely disseminate the importance of assistive technologies in enhancing the learning potential and capabilities of individuals with disabilities. Each character with disabilities in the show will model the use of these technologies in various episodes to normalize the use of these tools and to demonstrate how beneficial they can be. This exposure will hopefully help limit the social and emotional barriers between typical children and children with disabilities. It will help reduce stigma placed on children with disabilities and may encourage typical children to interact with their peers with disabilities. Knowledge and sensitivity training regarding children with disabilities would be useful for parents of children with disabilities, since efforts towards social integration are critical for the healthy social-emotional development of typically developing peers and their peers with disabilities.

STRENGTHS INFORMATION AND THE AFFECT/EFFORT THEORY

The affect/effort theory (Rosenthal, 1989) suggests that expectations influence the amount of effort an individual puts forth when interacting socially with a partner. If a child is presented with a negative expectation of a social interaction partner, he/she is less involved, makes less of an effort to interact, and is less friendly towards the social interaction partner, even if the social partner does not possess significant emotional or behavioral issues (Disalvo & Oswald, 2002; Harris, Milich, Corbitt; Hoover, & Brady, 1992). Unfortunately, once typical children become aware of differences in their peers with disabilities, they may be less motivated to interact with them since they may have low expectations of the latter's social capabilities. The use of assistive technology devices and services may cause typical children to distance themselves from children with disabilities, since they do not understand the purpose of these tools. However, it is possible for typical children to overcome these negative expectancies if they are learning more about the benefits of these tools and by taking an interest in them (Darley & Oleson, 1993; Disalvo & Oswald, 2002).

If typical children are presented with positive strengths information about children with disabilities and of their accompanying assistive technology, they may have more positive expectancies of children with disabilities, and may thus take a more active social interest in them. The use of explanatory information and peer strategies information in *Realabilities* contributes to rationalizing the importance of these devices and to show how they can interact with children with disabilities who may require assistance with these devices.

AUTISM

Autism Spectrum Disorders (ASD) is the umbrella term used to define a lifelong developmental disability that impacts the ways in which a person communicates, learns, and interacts socially with others (Robins, Dautenhahn, & Dubowski, 2006, p. 481). Children with autism often fail to develop relationships with their peers, have poor social skills, and lack the ability to recognize emotion. Deficits in speech and language acquisition are also prominent; these children experience difficulty in understanding metaphors and often misinterpret speech by relying on the literal meaning of words (Ploog, Scharf, & Nelson, 2013, p. 301). Little use of eye-contact is frequently observed, and there is a strong tendency toward repetitive behaviors. Resistance to change in routine is often accompanied by tantrums due to a lack of social-communicative understanding (Ploog, Scharf, & Nelson, 2013, p. 301). The etiology of autism remains largely unknown, and there is no current cure for this disorder. However, autism research is burgeoning and many educational therapies have evolved to enhance communication and learning.

Despite the fact that individuals are characterized by these deficits, the way in which ASD manifests is unique to each individual; one individual may lack speech altogether whereas another may have superb language skills. The diagnosis of ASD would be made based upon a deficit in social and communication skills. According to the Center for Disease Control (CDC) (2014), 1 in 68 children are currently diagnosed with an ASD in the United States. Two percent of children between the ages of six and seven in 2011 – 2012 were diagnosed with autism (CDC, 2013). Additionally, autism is reported to affect more males than females: 1 in 54 boys and 1 in 252 girls (NAS, 2005; CDC, 2012). Despite great efforts to diagnose autism early and to provide early intervention, the results for a majority of children with ASD are still poor with few able to live independently when they reach adulthood (Billstedt, Gillberg, & Gillberg, 2005; Eaves & Ho, 2008; Howlin, Goode, Hutton, & Rutter, 2004). In order to increase autonomy in individuals with ASD, current therapies are targeting the use of technology to enhance social interactions, interest in others, and to improve speech articulation.

In *Realabilities,* Uno is the character who presents with autism. His special abilities relate to the strengths individuals with autism possess, particularly savant and perceptual abilities. Savant syndrome is a rare condition in which a person with a learning disability demonstrates a striking ability or skill in contrast to a background of otherwise low cognitive functioning (Pring, 2005, p. 500). Savant skills are generally limited to music performance (pitch, playing multiple instruments), art (drawing, painting), calculating, mathematics (computations of large numbers), and spatial skills (ability to measure long distances perfectly, create complex models). Usually, a single special skill exists but in some cases, several skills exist (Treffert, 2009, p. 135). Cheatham et al. (1995) identified the following as potential explanations for savant abilities: hereditary factors, eidetic memory, rote memorization, concrete versus abstract reasoning, sensory deprivation, reinforcement and cerebral dominance. While communication impairment has been one of the major challenges children with autism face, visual memory has been found to be an area of strength for children with autism. In addition, children with autism may demonstrate superior performance in pitch processing and memory (Caron, Mottron, Rainville, Chouinard, 2004, p. 467).

Whatever the origin of savant skills may be, many of these abilities require exceptional perceptual skills. Whether or not they possess savant skills, the literature suggests that a number of individuals with autism exhibit superior performance in both visual and auditory modalities while completing various cognitive tasks (Mottron, Dawson, Soulieres, Hubert & Burack, 2006). Compared to typical controls, individuals with autism demonstrated superior performance in lab situations and showed an overall superior perceptual functioning (Mottron et al., 2006). Although *Realabilities* focuses on these strengths, it is important to understand that not all individuals with ASD exhibit savant abilities. Thus, it is essential to include the therapeutic devices and services that are available to all children with ASD. The addition of assistive technologies would help to bolster the understanding and acceptance of typical children towards children with disabilities.

Multitouch Tablet Application

As previously stated, children with ASD have impaired social skills which are often the target for therapeutic regimens. Technological advancements over the last ten years have shown a great increase in the number of computer-based interventions for children with ASD (Hourcade, Bullock-Rest, & Hansen, 2012, p. 3). It has been shown that children with ASD take a strong interest in computers; there is evidence that touchscreen tablets may be easier for children with ASD to use compared to following a cursor and using a mouse on a computer (Whalen, Liden, Ingersoll, Dallaire, & Liden, 2006; Davis et al., 2009). Current research demonstrates that the use of multitouch tablet applications encourage children with ASD to partake in pro-social behavior, thus promoting more enjoyment of social activities and an increased ability to express their feelings (Hourcade et. al, 2012, p. 23).

Hourcade et al (2012) used a Dell multitouch tablet with a 12.1" screen to design simple applications that had a strong visual medium and took advantage of the children's strengths (p. 6). The four applications were entitled: (1) drawing (2) music authoring (3) untangle and (4) photogoo. For the purpose of *Realabilities,* drawing and music authoring are the applications that can most readily be applied to the show.

Drawing

The drawing application is a freehand activity that allows children with ASD to express themselves by drawing what they may feel or by sharing an idea they may have. In addition, this application is particularly useful for storytelling. Previous research finds that children with ASD lack imaginative skills, thus their ability to contribute to a story might be less imaginative compared to the storytelling of typically developing children (Boucher, 2009). Dillon & Underwood (2011) found that children with ASD and typically developing children showed no difference in engaging in the creation of stories compared to their typical counterparts (p. 177); however children with ASD demonstrated difficulty with storytelling in the reality task where they had to adhere to telling a realistic story rather than a fantasy-based story. Storytelling promotes the mastering of language skills, improves listening skills, improves attention span, and inspires curiosity and creativity (Dillon & Underwood, 2011, p. 169). The drawing application works for storytelling when used in a small group of children: one child draws something on the application and passes it onto the next child, who adds something to it. The children learn to accept each other's ideas and make them a part of a larger story (Hourcade et al., 2012, p. 9). Researchers found that the drawing application was useful in identifying children's interests and in teaching new things (19). The children enjoyed telling stories and hearing and deciphering the pieces of the stories that they had individually contributed.

The drawing application has great potential for use in *Realabilities* since Uno, the character presenting with autism, would be able to use this application when communicating with others by describing how he feels in certain situations. His teammates, peers, and teachers could zoom in or out of the images in order to determine what Uno is trying to say. Uno could also use this application to record important memos and show them to his team. For instance, in the episode, "The Real Goal," Uno utilizes his savant mathematical skills to present a game plan to his teammates via a whiteboard. This multi-touch tablet application is a unique portable device that would enable Uno to carry it along with him on his adventures, making it a convenient companion for him and his team. Uno could use this application to jot down calculations for his team, draw concept maps for any plans the team contrives, but more importantly, to express his own feelings and thoughts to others or to communicate his personal story. This tool could improve his communication and interpersonal skills and enhance his ability to articulate his thoughts.

Music Authoring

The music authoring application for the tablet transforms the screen into a harp-like device. Children tap on the screen to select a tile that elicits a sound, or musical note. The note that is being played lights up green in order to indicate which tile is being pressed. . The application has the ability to create musical songs and can be played in a group format wherein each child enters a note on the application and passes it along to the next child (Hourcade etal., 2012, p. 10). Improvisational music therapy correlates with the goals of this application, because it is an effective intervention for addressing spontaneous self-expression, emotional communication, and social engagement (Trevarthen & Aitken, 2001). Children with ASD are reported to have impaired perception of linguistic and social auditory stimuli but are reported to benefit from superior musical perception compared to their typical counterparts (Boddaert et al., 2004; Thaut, 1988). Kim, Wigram, & Gold (2009) found that children with ASD experienced joy, emotional synchronicity, and initiation of engagement when participating in improvisational music therapy compared to a toy play session (p. 405). This study emphasized the importance of social-motivational features of musical interactions between the child and the therapist as well as a greater desire for the child to direct the musical session.

Music authoring is an essential tool for use in *Realabilities* because of the strong role music plays for Melody, the character with a visual impairment. Uno and Melody have a strong friendship in the show; Melody is extroverted, Uno is timid and more reserved. They work well with each other because Melody frequently stands up for Uno, and Uno guides Melody in physical space. For instance, in the first episode, "The Real Goal," Uno instructs Melody where to kick the soccer ball in order to score a winning team goal. Uno would be able to use this music authoring application to help Melody compose music for her songs, improvise tunes to describe how he or someone else may be feeling at times, and create musical stories with the rest of the Realabilities team. Music is also an appealing medium for viewers. We would like to be able to have viewers sing along with Uno and his teammates by using the highlighted notes on the application to guide the audience. Additionally, it would be meaningful to have Uno and Melody explain the notes on the harp-like application to their teammates; it would actually resemble a music lesson. These activities may demonstrate Uno's willingness to interact with others and will help him further develop his creativity and imagination.

Mocotos: Mobile Communication Method

Many children on the autism spectrum require therapeutic devices for functional speech. It is estimated that 25 – 61% of individuals with autism fail to develop functional speech output (Weitz, Dexter, & Moore, 1997). Children with ASD often are trained using Augmentative and Alternative Communication (AAC) techniques which generally rely on images and symbols for speech development. Researchers found that digital assistive technologies in classrooms were bulky, difficult to use and had poor programming (Monibi & Hayes, 2008, p. 121). A prototype Mocoto was developed in order to improve the portability, flexibility, and quality of assistive augmentative communication devices. The Mocoto is a Nokia N800, which is the size of the average cellphone and comes preinstalled with a set of library cards that have terms and images on them. Users can add custom cards to the device by taking pictures, scanning in materials or creating digital images (Monibi & Hayes, 2008, p. 123). There is customizable data that allows the cards be grouped into different categories. Audio cues are also available on the device to initiate conversation and aid children in recalling how to identify the images on their device.

This means of communication is similar to the Picture Exchange Communication System (PECS) except that PECS is paper-based. Having this system on a mobile device is more convenient; children with ASD can carry the device with them and use it within the classroom, whereas PECS would require children to carry large binders of paper images. According to Bondy and Frost (1994), children with a limited, spontaneous vocal repertoire increased spontaneous language following the use of PECS. Additionally, anecdotal reports demonstrate the use of PECS result in decreased problematic behavior and improvement in social behavior skills (Bondy & Frost, 1994). An increase in social-communicative behaviors and a decrease in problem behaviors were also prevalent using PECS in a study examining the effectiveness of PECS (Charlop-Christy, Carpenter, Lock Le, LeBlanc, & Kellet, 2002, p. 227).

The implementation of a similar PECS on a mobile device allows for the use of a memory card where images can be added, deleted, or grouped. This device would play a significant role in Uno's daily life, because he would be able to use it to initiate and partake in conversation with his peers, family, and friends. He can pull up the image on the Mocoto when he would like to refer to something, or if he would like to inquire about something. This is a great way for Uno to interact with his teammates and it would provide support for him when speaking.

SenseCam: Recording Images

Children with autism, who are unable to speak and communicate verbally with their families or peers, are often deemed "non-verbal" (Hayes, Hirano, Marcu, Monibi, Nguyen, & Yeganyan, 2010). Video is a powerful tool for enhancing caregiver communication and collaboration as well as for encouraging social engagement (Hayes, Kientz, Truong, White, Abowd, & Pering, 2004). The SenseCam is a wearable digital camera that takes pictures of everyday life from the perspective of the person wearing the camera. There is no viewfinder or display on the camera, therefore the lens on the SenseCam is wide (fish-eye) in order to capture everything that is in the view of the individual wearing the camera. There are many electronic sensors, including a light sensor, temperature sensor and an accelerometer, that allow the SenseCam to automatically capture images at different changes in sensor readings (Hayes et al., 2010). Unlike the Motocos and PECS, this device allows children with ASD to show their caregivers, teachers, and peers realistic images rather than cartoon or abstract images. Thus, the pictures the SenseCam takes are entirely from the point of view of the child. This encourages children with ASD to share their perspective with others and allows the pictures to serve as their voice.

Children can wear the SenseCam for part of the day (ex: school trip) or for the entire day (ex: school and home), acting as a journal on behalf of the child with ASD. Caregivers can review images of the day's activities with their child at home and teachers can review images captured outside of school. The SenseCam viewing interface allows users to pause pictures, ask questions and share social stories with their child about the images. This device promotes communication and serves as a type of speech therapy that has the potential to improve linguistics in children with ASD as well as social engagement (Ozdemir, 2008). The only concern with the SenseCam is the possible violation of privacy when it's being used in the school environment, unless the parents of the children have declared permission to take and release photographs of their children. Therefore, the device may be used more in home environments and in public outings.

This piece of technology can be implemented in *Realabilities* by having Uno communicate with his teachers and teammates about interesting things his camera captures. Uno can use the SenseCam to create social stories about a trip he has taken or to highlight his adventures at school. This tool can act as Uno's journal which he can refer back to at his convenience. . *Realabilities* has an anti-bullying platform where the team members harness their special abilities to quell bullying in the school. The SenseCam can act as a source for capturing anyone who may be the victim of bullying or can help divulge where someone might be hiding. The team would be able to use Uno's camera if perhaps they were lost on a mission and needed to retrace their steps back to school or home. This tool would provide Uno the opportunity to share his thoughts through these images and contribute to helping his team solve their daily dilemmas.

ATTENTION DEFICIT HYPERACTIVITY DISORDER (ADHD)

Attention deficit hyperactivity disorder (ADHD) is a neurological disorder that occurs in early childhood, usually before the age of seven. ADHD is difficult to diagnose due to the presumptions that the signs and symptoms of ADHD are "typical" child-like behaviors. It is estimated that eleven percent of children between the ages of 4 – 17 (6.4 million) have ADHD in the United States; boys (13.2%) are more likely than girls (5.6%) to be diagnosed with the disorder. Rates of ADHD diagnosis have increased an average of 3% per year from 1997 to 2006 and 5% per year from 2003 to 2011 (Visser, Danielson, Bitsko, et al., 2014).

Children with ADHD present with hyperactivity, inattention, and impulsivity (ADHD Molecular Genetics Network, 2002). By the time typical children reach school age, they are able to sit when told, remain quiet, and follow instructions whereas many children with ADHD struggle with these skill-sets. Symptoms of inattention include making careless mistakes, being easily distracted, and having difficulty remembering things and following instructions. Hyperactive symptoms include constant fidgeting and squirming, talking excessively and moving around constantly (running and climbing). When told to sit still, children with ADHD often continue to drum their fingers and tap their feet. Signs of impulsivity are interrupting others, blurting out answers in class, saying the wrong thing at the wrong time, and acting without thinking (CDC, 2014). The causes of ADHD stem from environmental exposures such as lead, premature delivery, alcohol and substance abuse during pregnancy, and genetic factors.

Despite these characteristics, children with ADHD possess strengths that are portrayed through Addy in *Realabilities*. Addy's heightened creativity relates to studies like those by Healey and Rucklidge (2006), which suggest that children with ADHD display significantly higher levels of creativity. Adults with ADHD showed higher levels of original creative thinking and higher levels of real-world creative achievement than adults without ADHD (White & Shah, 2011). This strength can be used to maximize the therapeutic effects of assistive technology devices for children with ADHD.

Computer and Color Stimulation

Research indicates that children with ADHD possess higher levels of creativity than typically developing children (Healey & Rucklidge, 2006). However, it appears that children with this disorder underachieve academically; about 50 percent fail annual school exams by adolescence (Shaw & Lewis, 2005). In many cases, medications and classroom interventions are administered to support these children academically. Shaw and Lewis (2005) created an intervention to investigate the impact of a computer with animations in learning. Results show that children with ADHD scored the greatest number of accurate responses on computerized tasks and displayed on-task behavior on animated computerized tasks. The tasks required answering science-based questions, using on-screen pen and paper, while animated characters and speech bubbles guided the users. Motivation and effort appear to correlate with the child's ability to succeed on these tasks.

Zentall and Zentall (1983) hypothesized that children with ADHD often present with low cortical activation. Therefore, children with ADHD require more stimulation in order "to achieve and maintain an optimal level of arousal in a given context" (p. 272). Upon observing the academic performance and motor activity of children with ADHD, Zentall (1986) found that children with ADHD could be positively influenced when exposed to extra forms of stimulation. In this case, the animations of the on-screen characters would be beneficial to children with this disorder.

A laptop with animated keys and software would be a fun addition to *Realabilities* so that Addy could show how she does her homework and class activities. This will shed light on how different individuals learn and the idea that it is important to do whatever may work best for the individual. Addy's bubbly personality can reflect her laptop's design.

Weighted Vest

Children with ADHD often demonstrate an inability to focus during classroom activities. A weighted vest created for deep-pressure sensory input was designed to be used by children with ADHD to promote on-task behaviors in the classroom by dispelling inattentiveness and hyperactivity (VandenBerg, 2001; Stephenson & Carter, 2009). A weighted vest is "a vest that typically has 10% of a person's body weight evenly distributed throughout the vest" (Olson & Moulton, 2004). The vests can be composed of various materials as long as the weights are distributed evenly along the front and back of the vest. This is something that can work in favor of many children, because they can customize their vests to their own personal style. The pressure stimulation provided by the vest is thought to have calming and organizing effects on the central nervous system (Stephenson & Carter, 2009). The most common behavioral changes noted were increased attention and staying on task; on-task behavior increased from 18 – 25% (VandenBerg, 2001; Olson & Moulton, 2004).

Addy's use of this vest in future episodes of *Realabilities* can illustrate how the weighted vest helps her study for exams and concentrate on tasks in the classroom. There would be an introduction of the vest into the show wherein Addy receives a compliment on her colorful vest and its purpose would be explained to her friends. The more cognizant society is of assistive technologies or other useful innovations to aid individuals with disabilities, the less ostracized children with disabilities will be in the mainstreamed classroom.

Smart Pen

Poor handwriting performance is a life skill that has been observed in many children with ADHD. Often times, writing is illegible, there is inconsistency with letter size, and an inappropriate speed of execution is observed compared to children without ADHD (Racine, Majnemer, Shevell, & Snider, 2008). Failure of children with ADHD to attain competent handwriting skills during the school years can lead to poor academic success and low self-esteem; interventions have been essential and effective at improving handwriting for children with ADHD (Feder & Majnemer, 2007). Lapses in concentration are also evident in children with ADHD during reading and writing. A Smart Pen was created for children to detect lapses in concentration during reading; an alarm or warning is elicited from the pen when there is a substantial pause in reading to remind the child that he/she is veering off-task (DePrenger, Shao, Lu, Fleming, 2010). The purpose of this Smart Pen is to facilitate concentration as well as the independence of individuals with ADHD.

The Smart Pen would be a strong addition to *Realabilities,* since Addy can use the pen during school hours and at home. There could be scenes in the show where Addy is reading a textbook and she starts to daydream; suddenly the Smart Pen causes an alarm and she immediately gets back on task. The goal of using this tool is to ensure that it will contribute to Addy's character development and promote understanding as to why children with ADHD may use such a device.

PHYSICAL IMPAIRMENT

Rolly portrays a character with paraplegia, a form of physical impairment in *Realabilities*. Paraplegia describes the loss of movement and/or feeling in the lower half of the body due to an injury to the nervous system (Kohnle, 2011). Many individuals with paraplegia possess permanent deficits, whereas others have the possibility of regaining some level of functioning. The causes of this disorder are often due to stroke, spinal cord injury, genetic disorder, congenital, infection or a tumor within the spinal cord (Melzak, 1969; Kohlne, 2011). The major cause of paraplegia is motor vehicle accidents (46%) followed by falls (22%), violence (16%) and sports (12%) in the U.S. (CDC, 2010). Paraplegia is also associated with unexpected accidents such as high-risk sports and car accidents. Symptoms of paraplegia include loss of movement and muscle control in the legs, feet, toes and trunk, tingling in the legs and loss of bowel and bladder control (Howlett, 2012).

Paraplegia is a life-long illness that impacts activities of daily living, work, and mobility. In 2010, there were 270,000 spinal cord injuries; of these injuries, 80.6% of these injuries affected males (CDC, 2010). Wheelchairs are essential for mobility, and individuals with this disorder have to learn to make independent transfers. Individuals with paraplegia are required to strengthen the non-paralyzed muscles of their body to make these transfers and to prevent muscle atrophy (Howlett, 2012). Research indicates that respiratory, renal conditions and cardiovascular disease are comorbidities in individuals with paraplegia (Myers, Lee, Kiratli, 2006). Rolly demonstrates his superior upper-body strength by possessing the ability to effectively maneuver in his wheelchair and to beat his friends in races.

Compared to the able-bodied population, individuals with spinal cord injuries tend to be at greater risk for high cholesterol, diabetes and heart disease due to a lack of physical activity and metabolic changes (Moussavi, Ribas-Cardus, Rintala, & Rodriguez, 2001). Improved physical activity and engagement in exercise are crucial for individuals diagnosed with spinal cord injuries, and this physical activity is encouraged from the onset of the disorder.

Like the wheelchair, Electronic Aids of Daily Living (EADL) are devices that allow individuals with severe physical disabilities to control aspects of their home, school or work environment (Little, 2007); these aids allow individuals to maximize their own independence and functional ability. EADLs allow paraplegics to operate telephones, TV, stereos and lights. Such devices are prescribed to meet the specific activity goals of the individual and to achieve a goodness of fit between the person and his/her desired activity (Rigby, 2009). Unfortunately, about 30% of assistive technology devices are misused or abandoned, due to a lack of fit between the user's needs and expectations (Rigby, 2009). A study conducted in 2005 compared the functional abilities of EADL users with nonusers and determined that individuals with physical disabilities like paraplegia benefit from greater functional abilities in daily living when using an EADL, whereas those who function without an EADL depended heavily on others. The key findings demonstrate that functional abilities within the home were significantly greater when EADL were used and the psychosocial impact of using electronic aids was positive (Rigby, Ryan, Joos, Cooper, Jutai, & Steggles, 2005). Thus, assistive technology devices should be implemented for individuals with paraplegia to better improve their daily life functioning.

Paraplegic Cycling

As previously stated, individuals with paraplegia often have or may suffer from cardiovascular disease later in life. In order to be proactive and strive for improvements in general health, physical activity is encouraged (Janssen, Glaser, & Shuster, 1998). Lower limb cycling via functional electrical stimulation (FES) in individuals with paraplegia has shown an improvement in cardiopulmonary fitness and a reduction in the secondary complications that often occur with spinal cord injuries (Hunt, Stone, Negard, Schauer, Fraser, Cathcart, Ferrario, Ward, & Grant, 2004). FES is the:

"...Application of an electrical current to supplement or replace function that is lost in neurologically impaired individuals... the purpose of an FES intervention is to enable function by replacing or assisting a person's voluntary ability...stimulation is required to achieve a desired function" (Peckham & Knutson, 2005, p. 328)."

The ultimate goal of lower extremity FES systems is to allow individuals with paraplegia to walk again. Hunt et al. (2004) adapted a recumbent tricycle for paraplegic cyclists in conjunction with FES of the paralyzed muscles of the lower limbs to promote lower leg strength and ability. The alteration made in this design compared to a regular recumbent tricycle is the addition of individualized ankle braces that are fixed to the pedals of the tricycle in order to stabilize the ankles and constrain the legs. Additionally, a motor is attached behind the seat as well as to two battery packs to enable users to operate the tricycle for indoor exercise and mobile cycling (Hunt et al., 2004). The battery packs have the potential to assist the user and would be beneficial to first-time users because they will allow the bicycle to run without the individual actually having to cycle; for instance, if the user becomes tired, the battery pack enables the bicycle to continue working. This cycling device promotes the general wellbeing and enhances the physical activity of individuals with paraplegia.

Rolly's use of this device would promote his sense of independence by employing a means of transportation other than his wheelchair. This tricycle can be customized for Rolly so that it appears to be a cool device he uses on his way to school and during sports at school. In *Realabilities,* Rolly's improved use of this device can support his entry into a tricycle race within the community. Through training and practice, Rolly can demonstrate that he has the will and determination to win the race.

SmartChair Wheelchair System

It is evident that most individuals with paraplegia utilize wheelchairs. Chaves et al. (2004) sought to identify factors that related to wheelchair, impairment, and environment that affect individuals' use of wheelchairs in their homes, in the community and for transportation. The Participation Survey/Mobility (PARTS/M) questionnaire was used in order to analyze the factors that limit participation in the areas previously mentioned. Results indicate that the wheelchair was identified as limiting participation in all three settings, followed by physical impairment and the environment. Although the wheelchair is probably the most important device to individuals with paraplegia, there are many limitations such as size, maneuverability, and comfort (Chaves, Boninger, Cooper, Fitzgerald, Gray, & Cooper, 2004). These aspects are considered to be limitations to the user's autonomy.

SmartChair wheelchairs are new devices for individuals with spinal cord injuries that are undergoing remodeling and further research over the past ten years. These devices enhance the user's interaction with the wheelchair in that the user can select from a range of behaviors such as hallway navigation. Using wireless networks, the user can specify a destination on the map and obtain directions (Rao, Conn, Jung, Katupitiya, & Kientz, 2002). SmartChairs include various actions that are implemented in the software such as "go to relative position, three point turn and navigate through the doorway (p. 3586)." The device features a joystick-like interface to allow for these movements to be selected. A speech board interface also allows the occupant to communicate with others. Although continued work is being conducted on these wheelchairs, the inclusion of this device in *Realabilities* would support Rolly's ability to communicate with his teammates and move from one place to another independently. Rolly can demonstrate the speed of his wheelchair by zooming off to help those in need and using the navigation system to direct his team.

HEARING IMPAIRMENT

Hearing loss is a disability that impacts how well a person hears intensities and frequencies that are associated with speech (CDC, 2010). Intensity is the loudness of a sound measured in decibels (dB) whereas frequency is the pitch of a sound and is measured in hertz (Hz). A child is considered deaf when hearing loss is greater than 90 decibels (NICHCY, 2010). Out of 3,793 births in 2011, 8.6% of infants were reported to have experienced hearing loss (CDC, 2011). In addition, 5 out of every 1,000 (14.9%) children in U.S. are born deaf or hard-of-hearing (CDC, 2005).

Signs of hearing loss or deafness may include a child who fails to respond consistently when others call his/her name, delayed speech, increased volume on the television and the need for things to constantly be repeated. The causes of this illness can be acquired i.e. the loss occurred after birth because of illness or injury; or it can be congenital, meaning hearing loss or deafness was present at the time of birth. Common causes of acquired hearing loss include exposure to excessive noise, buildup of fluid in the eardrum, ear infections and head trauma. Congenital causes of hearing loss and deafness include a family history of the disorder, infections during pregnancy and complications during pregnancy (NICHCY, 2010). In both situations, early intervention is a key ingredient for the child's development.

It is essential to understand the effects this illness has on a child's education in order to provide the necessary interventions. Although children with hearing impairment or deafness have the same intellectual capacity as a child who is not hard of hearing, children with this disorder usually require special education services that are tailored to their individual needs (Osberger, Moeller, Eccarius, Robbins, & Johnson, 1986). Children who are hard of hearing experience difficulty with learning vocabulary and grammar where as children who are deaf fall behind their hearing peers in writing, reading, and speaking (Moeller, Osberger, & Eccarius, 1986). Children who are born deaf generally don't have the experience, cognitive skills and linguistics that are vital to achieving reading fluency (King & Quigley, 1985). The average reading score of deaf students that are 20 years old and older is a 4.5, indicating their reading level is that of a typical child between fourth and fifth grade; only 10% of deaf individuals read at or above the eighth grade level (Karchmer & Tyrbus, 1977). This indicates that interventions need to target improvement of these skills in order to enhance the reading and writing skills of individuals who are blind. Assistive technology can help facilitate early improvements in linguistics for individuals who are deaf.

In *Realabilities,* Seemore presents with hearing impairment but benefits from superior vision and insight. Seemore's special abilities derive from various studies which show that visual abilities in individuals with hearing impairments may be improved as a result of auditory deprivation and/ or because the deaf rely heavily on sign language (R.G. Bosworth and K.R. Dobkins, p. 152). Since individuals who are deaf do not have functioning auditory cells, the auditory cortex is "recruited" in order to enhance vision (Than, 2010). Since children rely mainly on sign language to communicate with the outside world, signing is said to be responsible for enhanced visual-cognitive abilities in the deaf. Other studies note that individuals with hearing impairment may benefit from enhanced peripheral vision (Bosworth & Dobkins, 1999). Seemore reveals his enhanced visual abilities throughout the show by aiding his teammates in seeing things they don't notice and teaching sign language to his peers. He also has a cochlear implant that helps him to hear and communicate more efficiently with his teammates.

Cochlear Implants

A cochlear implant is a device that helps some individuals by stimulating the auditory nerve electrically to aid in audition. There is an external piece that receives incoming sound, processes it, and transfers the signal across the skin to an implanted device. The sounds are received and decoded, causing electrodes to be stimulated in the cochlea, or inner ear (Skinner et al., 1994; Wilson et al., 1991). The use of cochlear implants promotes the development of speech perception and production in some deaf children; this brings into question when these devices should be implanted (Svirsky, Robbins, Kirk, Pisoni, & Miyamoto, 2000). Implementing use of this assistive technology in children is often criticized by the deaf community, since children are not of legal age to make their own decisions, and because they perceive their use of sign language and their hearing impairment to be a normal form of human variation (Svirsky, Robbins, Kirk, Pisoni, & Miyamoto, 2000). The implantation of these devices in deaf individuals is a controversial topic due to the deaf community's view that "there is nothing to be fixed." The deaf revolution began in the 1970's when members of the deaf community rebelled against educators who tried to teach deaf children how to speak English; it was believed that the use of sign language would be diminished, thus negatively impacting their culture (Christiansen & Leigh, 2004). Even so, it is essential to acknowledge that cochlear implants can enhance auditory acuity for some as well as language growth (Peterson, 2004).

In the field of pediatric cochlear implants, differences have been observed in performance based upon speech perception, language comprehension, clarity of speech and reading (Pisoni & Geers, 2000). While some children appear to be on their way towards acquiring spoken language, other children never reach the necessary goals for developing speech and language. Researchers assessed that perceptual processing of spoken words and working memory greatly impacted language processing (Pisoni & Geers, 2000). The definition of working memory is "the storage of information that is being processed in a range of cognitive tasks" (Baddeley, 1986, p. 34). Thus, it is suggested that working memory plays a role in mediating performance across a range of different tasks and affects phonological coding as well as rehearsal processes used to recover the representations of the spoken word. Therefore, in order to improve speech and language acquisition in children with cochlear implants, engagement in meaningful processing activities has to be encouraged in addition to having the children respond using phonology.

Seemore has a cochlear implant in *Realabilities;* with it, he has the ability to communicate with his peers and teammates. He displays the use of spoken word and sign language in each episode; the use of sign language is interpreted on-screen for viewers to understand what Seemore is signing. This encourages typical children to learn sign language and partake in a new style of communication they may have never been exposed to previously. When establishing and maintaining social relationships for children with cochlear implants, oral communication presents the greatest difficulty (Anita & Stinson, 1999). Not all children with cochlear implants have the ability to speak clearly or understand the speech of another individual, making it increasingly difficult to communicate with individuals who are not hard of hearing. According to parental reports, improvements in this device have the potential to transform the children's personality or increase their level of confidence (Bat-Chava & Deignan, 2001). The use of this device in *Realabilities* can help alleviate any stigma associated with deaf individuals. Typical children can conclude that those with cochlear implants may not be able to speak clearly, and they should not consider them strange.

Phonic and Picture Based Reading

Low literacy levels impact deaf students' ability to learn in classrooms. It is found that technology is being employed more frequently to aid deaf students in learning, through the integration of American Sign Language (ASL) and English (Trezek & Wang, 2004). Using a CD-ROM with three different story types, the efficacy of story re-telling was assessed in order to determine which story type was most effective (Gentry, Chinn, & Moutlon, 2004). Story re-telling helps children to rethink their way through a text, thus promoting comprehension of the story and encouraging the children to reflect on what they have read (Gibson, Gold, & Sgouros, 2003). The story types consisted of (1) print only (2) print and pictures (3) print and digital video of sign language and (4) print, pictures, and digital video of sign language. Researchers found that story re-telling was strongest when stories were presented to the children in the print and pictures format, contrary to their hypothesis that the addition of ASL would benefit story comprehension.

Phonics and graphemes are components of literature that aid in improving fluency, comprehension, and vocabulary in children who are hard of hearing and/or deaf. Phonics is "the understanding of phonemes (the sounds of *spoken* language) and graphemes (the letters and spellings that represent those sounds in *written* language)" (Armbruster, Lehr, & Osborn, 2001). Visual Phonics, or *See the Sound/ Visual Phonics,* is a computer-based system consisting of 46 moving hand cues and written symbols that represent the phoneme-grapheme relationship. This system aids in teaching vocabulary, word-learning strategies, and enhancing comprehension (Trezek, Wang, Woods, Gampp, & Paul, 2007).

Integration of story re-telling and Visual Phonics via a computer or tablet into *Realabilities* would demonstrate how Seemore learns and improves his speech. What makes this technological service all the more intriguing is that it can be used for typical children who may struggle with reading and writing or for children with speech disorders. A proposed episode for *Realabilities* is to have Seemore help a peer in his class who is struggling with reading by showing his peer how he uses his Visual Phonics and story re-telling methods.

American Sign Language in Virtual Space

CopyCat is an ASL game targeted towards children between the ages of 6 and 11. It uses gesture recognition technology to help the children practice their ASL skills. Ninety percent of deaf children have parents who may not know ASL and who may not have access to the language (Gallaudet, 2001). There is a critical period for language development in which learning this skill has its peak effect; if a child is exposed to language after this period, there will be a reduced effect of acquisition or no effect at all (Newport, 1990). Research indicates that this is similar in ASL acquisition (Newport, 1990; Mayberry & Eichen, 1991). CopyCat assists children with learning and practicing to sign complete phrases and provides a fun and engaging means of building these skills. The game consists of a television, a wireless mouse, colored gloves with wireless accelerometers and an IEEE1394 camera. The child wears the gloves when playing this game and uses the mouse to click on which aspect of the game he/she would like to play. There are tutorial videos available for new users, as well (Brashear, Henderson, Park, Hamilton, Lee, & Starner, 2006). Researchers report the high word accuracy of users; however, the system needs improvement when formulating and practicing the signing of sentences (Brashear, Henderson, Park, Hamilton, Lee, & Starner, 2006). CopyCat would be beneficial for *Realabilities* since Seemore would be able to introduce his friends to ASL.

VISUAL IMPAIRMENT

Individuals with visual impairment, more specifically blindness, have incorrect formation or damage to the optic nerve. The optic nerve sends images from the eyes to the brain and the brain translates these images in order to analyze what the eyes have seen. These problems with vision can develop before a child is born due to incorrect development of the optic nerve, it can be inherited or it can result from an accident like playing a sport (International Council of Opthalmology, 2002). Children who are premature are at a great risk for visual impairment due to immature circulation (Jacobson, Fernell, Broberger, Ek, & Gillber, 1998). Individuals, who are blind, rely on their other senses (touching, hearing, smelling, tasting) to enable them to see. In 2012, a total of 659,700 individuals between the ages of 4 and 20 were reported to be blind (319,100 girls and 340,600 boys) (Erickson, 2014).

Research indicates that individuals who are blind often exhibit a greater interest in music than typical children (Matawa, 2009). Melody's special musical ability derives from research that shows that music may play a more pivotal role in the lives of visually impaired children than in the lives of fully- sighted individuals. Therefore, individuals with visual impairment may exhibit a greater interest in, and/or talent for music than their sighted peers (Matawa, 2009). According to Ockelford (2009), blind children are 4,000 times more likely to have perfect pitch than their fully sighted peers. The research indicates that 48% of blind children show significant interest in everyday sounds whereas only 13% of children with sight shared this interest. More than two-thirds of blind children in the study were reported to play at least one instrument compared to 41% of children in the sighted group. This reliance on sound and interest in music helps to develop and strengthen the ability of blind children to sing, play instruments, and even to acquire exceptional pitch, sense of rhythm, and retention of melodies and lyrics.

Indoor and Outdoor Navigation System

Supplemental navigation devices for blind individuals are essential in providing information as to the individual's whereabouts. The Drishti navigation system supports the maneuvering of individuals both indoors to travel safely through their homes and outdoors to whichever destination they request (Ran, Helal, & Moore, 2004). When in new places, the system reads the layout of the room the person is traveling in, providing users with a broad picture of their environment. Additionally, this device ensures that users are aware when an obstacle is near in order to avoid any collisions or falls. Compared to walking canes and guide dogs, users have the ability to ask the device a question such as where they currently are, how far the refrigerator is from their current location, and what obstacles are in their path. This system is composed of a wearable computer, a differential GPS receiver, a wireless network, as well as an ultrasound's positioning device.

This piece of assistive technology can be implemented in *Realabilities* by having Melody use a different means of transportation than her walking cane. Although this device is new and more research is currently being conducted to decrease mechanical errors, there is great potential for supplying Melody with this tool. It would assist her in getting to places like the mall and would help her with less familiar locations.

Discussion

Realabilities seeks to disseminate knowledge about assistive technology devices to typical children in order to promote the formation of social-emotional relationships between children with disabilities and their typical peers. Ten episodes of *Realabilities* have been created thus far, and through animated interventions, Silton, Arucevic, Ruchlin, and Norkus (2013) found that typical children demonstrated enhanced cognitive attitudes and behavioral intentions. Formative research intends to be conducted at additional elementary schools on the understanding of these technological devices as well as their ultimate significance for each character. Since these technologies and devices are often associated with the stigma that individuals with disabilities encounter, it is important to expose typical children to these devices, to normalize the devices and make them more welcome both in and outside of the classroom. Assistive technology works to promote the independence of individuals with disabilities and in this show, each character will exhibit exactly how beneficial and significant their devices can be. Each individual is unique and may benefit from unique technology and *Realabilities* will help portray these realities through introducing these innovative technologies in a sensitive and effective fashion.

REFERENCES

Abraham, A., Windmann, S., Siefen, R., Daum, I., & Gunturkun, O. (2006). Creative thinking in adolescents with attention deficit hyperactivity disorder (ADHD). *Child Neuropsychology: A Journal on Normal and Abnormal Development in Childhood and Adolescence, 12* (2), 111 – 123.

Antia, S. D., & Stinson, M. S. (1999). Some conclusions on the education of deaf and hard-of-hearing students in inclusive settings. *Journal of Deaf Studies and Deaf Education, 4*(3), 246–248. doi:10.1093/deafed/4.3.246 PMID:15579892

Armburster, B. B., Lehr, F., & Osborn, J. (2001). *Put reading first: The research building blocks for teaching children to read kindergarten through grade three.* Jessup, MD: National Institute for Literacy.

Bat-Chava, Y., & Deignan, E. (2004). Peer relationships of children with cochlear implants. Oxford University Press, 6 (3), 186 – 199.

Bavelier, D., & Hirshorn, E. A. (2010). I see where you're hearing: How cross-modal plasticity may exploit homologous brain structures. *Nature Neuroscience, 13*(11), 1309–1311. doi:10.1038/nn1110-1309 PMID:20975752

Behrmann, M. (1998). *Assistive Technology for Young Children In Special Education.* Association for Supervision and Curriculum Development. Retrieved June 1, 2014, from http://www.edutopia.org/assistive-technology-young-children-special-education

Billstedt, E., Gillberg, C., & Gillberg, C. (2005). Autism after adolescence: Population-based 13- to 22-year follow-up study of 120 individuals with autism diagnosed in childhood. *Journal of Autism and Developmental Disorders, 35*(3), 351–360. doi:10.1007/s10803-005-3302-5 PMID:16119476

Boddaert, N., Chabane, N., Belin, P., Bourgeois, N., Royer, V., Barthelémy, C., & Zilbovicius, M. et al. (2004). Perception of complex sounds in autism: Abnormal auditory cortical processing in children. *The American Journal of Psychiatry, 161*(11), 2117–2120. doi:10.1176/appi.ajp.161.11.2117 PMID:15514415

Bondy, A. S., & Frost, L. (1994). The picture exchange communication system. *Focus on Autistic Behavior, 16,* 123–128. PMID:22478140

Boucher, J. (2009). *The Autistic Spectrum. Characteristics, Causes and Practical Issues.* London: Sage Publications Ltd.

Brashear, H., Henderson, V., Park, K. H., Hamilton, H., Lee, S., & Starner, T. (2006). American sign language recognition in game development for deaf children. *ASSETS, 06,* 79–84.

Brookes, N. A. (1998). *Models for understanding rehabilitation and assistive technology. Designing and using assistive technology. The human perspective.* Baltimore: Brookes.

Caron, M. J., Mottron, L., Rainville, C., & Chouinard, S. (2004). Do high functioning persons with autism present with superior spatial abilities? *Neuropsychologia, 42*(4), 467–481. doi:10.1016/j.neuropsychologia.2003.08.015 PMID:14728920

Center for Disease Control and Prevention. (2010). *Spinal cord injury (SCI): Fact sheet.* Center for Disease Control and Prevention. Retrieved June 8, 2014, from http://www.cdc.gov/traumaticbraininjury/scifacts.html

Center for Disease Control and Prevention. (2014). *Attention-deficit/hyperactivity disorder.* Center for Disease Control and Prevention. Retrieved June 8, 2014, from http://www.cdc.gov/ncbddd/adhd/facts.html

Charlop-Christy, M. H., Carpenter, M., Le, L., LeBlanc, L. A., & Kellet, K. (2002). Using the picture exchange communication system (PECS) with children with autism: Assessment of PECS acquisition, speech, social-communicative behavior, and problem behavior. *Journal of Applied Behavior Analysis, 35*(3), 213–231. doi:10.1901/jaba.2002.35-213 PMID:12365736

Chaves, E. S., Boninger, M. L., Cooper, R., Fitzgerald, S. G., Gray, D. B., & Cooper, R. A. (2004). Assessing the influence of wheelchair technology on perception of participation in spinal cord injury. *American Academy of Physical Medicine and Rehabilitation, 85*, 1854–1858. PMID:15520981

Christiansen, J. B., & Leigh, I. W. (2004). Children with cochlear implants. *Archives of Otolaryngology--Head & Neck Surgery, 130*(5), 673–677. doi:10.1001/archotol.130.5.673 PMID:15148196

Cook, A. M., & Polgar, J. M. (2013). *Cook and Hussey's Assistive Technologies: Principles and Practice*. Elsevier.

Davis, M., Dautenhahn, K., Powell, S., & Nehaniv, C. (2009). Guidelines for researchers and practitioners designing software and software trials for children with autism. *Journal of Assistive Technologies, 4*(1), 34–48.

Dawe, M. (2006). Desperately seeking simplicity: How young adults with cognitive disabilities and their families adopt assistive technologies. In *Proceedings of the SIGCHI Conference on Human Factors in Computing Systems, 22 – 27.* doi:10.1145/1124772.1124943

DePrenger, M., Shao, Y., Lu, F., & Fleming, N. (2010). Feasibility study of a smart pen for autonomous detection of concentration lapses during reading. *International Conference of the IEEE EMBS,* 1864 – 1867. doi:10.1109/IEMBS.2010.5626256

Dillon, G., & Underwood, J. (2011). Computer mediated imaginative storytelling in children with autism. *International Journal of Human-Computer Studies, 70*(2), 169–178. doi:10.1016/j.ijhcs.2011.10.002

Disability Rights Network of Pennsylvania. (2008). *Assistive technology for persons with disabilities: An overview.* Disability Rights Network of Pennsylvania. Retrieved December 15, 2013, from http://drnpa.org/File/publications/assistive-technology-for-persons-with-disabilities—an-overview.pdf

Eaves, L. C., & Ho, H. H. (2008). Young adult outcome of autism spectrum disorders. *Journal of Autism and Developmental Disorders, 38*(4), 739–747. doi:10.1007/s10803-007-0441-x PMID:17764027

Erickson, W., Lee, C., & von Schrader, S. (2014). Disability Statistics from the 2012 American Community Survey (ACS). Ithaca, NY: Cornell University Employment and Disability Institute (EDI).

Faraone, S. V.The ADHD Molecular Genetics Network. (2002). Report from the third international meeting of the attention deficit hyperactivity disorder molecular genetics network. *American Journal of Medical Genetics, 114*(3), 272–277. doi:10.1002/ajmg.10039 PMID:11920847

Feder, K. P., & Majnemer, A. (2007). Handwriting development, competency, and intervention. *Developmental Medicine and Child Neurology, 49*(4), 312–317. doi:10.1111/j.1469-8749.2007.00312.x PMID:17376144

Frierich, L. K., & Stein, A. H. (1975). Prosocial television and young children: The effects of verbal labeling and role playing on learning and behavior. *Child Development, 46*(1), 27–38. doi:10.2307/1128830

Gentry, M. M., Chinn, K. M., & Moulton, R. D. (2004). Effectiveness of multimedia reading materials when used with children who are deaf. *American Annals of the Deaf, 149*(5), 394–402. doi:10.1353/aad.2005.0012 PMID:15727058

Gibson, A., Gold, J., & Sgouros, C. (2003). The power of story retelling. *The Tutor,* Spring 2003, 1 – 11.

Goffman, E. (1963). *Stigma: Notes on the Management of Spoiled Identity.* Penguin.

Gray, D. E. (1993). Perceptions of stigma: The parents of autistic children. *Sociology of Health & Illness,* *15*(1), 102–120. doi:10.1111/1467-9566.ep11343802

Hayes, G. R., Kientz, J. A., Truong, K. N., White, D. R., Abowd, G. D., & Pering, T. (2004). Designing capture applications to support the education of children with autism. *Proceedings of the UbiComp,* *2004,* 161–178.

Holmquist, J. (2011). Bullying prevention: positive strategies. PACER Center, 1 – 6.

Hourcade, J. P., Bullock-Rest, N. E., & Hansen, T. E. (2012). Multitouch tablet application and activities to enhance the social skills of children with autism spectrum disorders. *Personal and Ubiquitous Computing,* *16*(2), 157–168. doi:10.1007/s00779-011-0383-3

Howlett, W.P. (2012). Paraplegia non traumatic. *Neurological Disorders,* 231 – 254.

Howlin, P., Goode, S., Hutton, J., & Rutter, M. (2004). Adult outcome for children with autism. *Journal of Child Psychology and Psychiatry, and Allied Disciplines,* *45*(2), 212–229. doi:10.1111/j.1469-7610.2004.00215.x PMID:14982237

Hunt, K. J., Stone, B., Negard, N. O., Schauer, T., Fraser, M. H., Cathcart, A. J., & Grant, S. et al. (2004). Control strategies for integration of electric motor assist and functional electrical stimulation in paraplegic cycling: Utility for exercise testing and mobile cycling. *IEEE Transactions on Neural Systems and Rehabilitation Engineering,* *12*(1), 89–101. doi:10.1109/TNSRE.2003.819955 PMID:15068192

International Council of Opthalmology. (2002). Visual standard: Aspects and ranges of vision loss. *International Congress of Opthalmology,* 1 – 33.

Isabelle, S., Bessey, S. F., Dragas, K. L., Blease, P., Shepherdfaculty, J. T., & Lanefaculty, S. J. (2003). Assistive technology for children with disabilities. *Occupational Therapy in Health Care,* *16*(4), 29–51. PMID:23930706

Jacobson, L., Fernell, E., Broberger, U., Ek, U., & Gillberg, C. (1998). Children with blindness due to retinopathy of prematurity: A population-based study. Perinatal data, neurological and opthalmological outcome. *Developmental Medicine and Child Neurology,* *40*(3), 155–159. doi:10.1111/j.1469-8749.1998.tb15439.x PMID:9566650

Janssen, T., Glaser, R., & Shuster, D. (1998). Clinical efficacy of electrical stimulation exercise training: Effects on health, fitness, and function. *Topics in Spinal Cord Injury Rehabilitation,* *3*(3), 33–49.

Karchmer, M., & Trybus, R. (1977). *Who are the deaf children in the 'mainstream'' programs?* Washington, DC: Gallaudet College, Office of Demographic Studies.

Kim, J., Wigram, T., & Gold, C. (2009). Emotional, motivational and interpersonal responsiveness of children with autism in improvisational music therapy. Sage Publications, 13 (4), 389 – 409.

King, C., & Quigley, S. (1985). *Reading and deafness.* San Diego, CA: College Hill.

Kohnle, D. (2011). Paraplegia. *Nucleus Medical Media, Inc,* NYU Pediatrics, 1 – 4.

Marcu, G., Dey, A. K., & Kiesler, S. (2012). Parent-driven use of wearable cameras for autism support: A field study with families. *UbiComp, 1,* 1–10.

Matawa, C. (2009). Exploring the musical interests and abilities of blind and partially sighted children and young people with retinopathy of prematurity. *British Journal of Visual Impairment, 27*(3), 252–262. doi:10.1177/0264619609106364

Mayberry, R. I., & Eichen, E. B. (1991). The long-lasting advantage of learning sign language in childhood: Another look at the critical period for language acquisition. *Journal of Memory and Language, 30*(4), 486–498. doi:10.1016/0749-596X(91)90018-F

Melzak, J. (1969). Paraplegia among children. *Lancet, 294*(7610), 45–48. doi:10.1016/S0140-6736(69)92612-9 PMID:4182806

Moeller, M. P., Osberger, M. J., & Eccarius, M. (1986). Language and learning skills of hearing-impaired students: Receptive language skills. *ASHA Monographs, 23,* 41–53. PMID:3730031

Monibi, M., & Hayes, G. R. (2008). Mocotos: Mobile communications tools for children with special needs. *IDC, 2008,* 121–124. doi:10.1145/1463689.1463736

Moore, D., Cheng, Y., McGrath, P., & Powell, N. J. (2005). Collaborative virtual environment technology for people with autism. *Focus on Autism and Other Developmental Disabilities, 20*(4), 231–243. doi:10.1177/10883576050200040501

Mottron, L., Dawson, M., Soulieres, I., Hubert, B., & Burack, J. (2006). Enhanced perceptual functioning in autism: An update, and eight principles of autistic perception. *Journal of Autism and Developmental Disorders, 36*(1), 27–43. doi:10.1007/s10803-005-0040-7 PMID:16453071

Moussavi, R. M., Ribas-Cardus, F., Rintala, D. H., & Rodriquez, G. P. (2001). Dietary and serum lipids in individuals with spinal cord injury living in the community. *Journal of Rehabilitation Research and Development, 38*(2), 225–233. PMID:11392655

Myers, J., Lee, M., & Kiratli, J. (2006). Cardiovascular disease in spinal cord injury. *American Journal of Physical Medicine & Rehabilitation, 86*(2), 1–11.

National Dissemination Center for Children with Disabilities (NICHCY). (2010). Deafness and hearing loss. *NICHCY Disability Fact Sheet,* 1 – 8.

Newport, E. L. (1990). Maturational constraints on language learning. *Cognitive Science, 14*(1), 11–28. doi:10.1207/s15516709cog1401_2

Ockelford, A. (2009). *Focus on music: Exploring the musicality of children and young people with retinopathy of prematurity.* London: British Library.

Olson, L. J., & Moulton, H. J. (2004). Use of weighted vests in pediatric occupational therapy practice. *Occupational Therapy International, 11*(1), 52–66. doi:10.1002/oti.197 PMID:15118771

Osberger, M. J., Moeller, M. P., Eccarius, M., Robbins, A. M., & Johnson, D. (1986). Language and learning skills of hearing-impaired students: Expressive language skills. *ASHA Monographs*, *23*, 54–65. PMID:3730032

Ozdemir, S. (2008). Using multimedia social stories to increase appropriate social engagement in young children with autism. *Turkish Online Journal of Educational Technology*, *7*(3), 80–88.

Parette, P., & Scherer, M. (2004). Assistive technology use and stigma. *Education and Training in Developmental Disabilities*, *39*(3), 217–226.

Peckham, P. H., & Knutson, J. S. (2005). Functional electrical stimulation for neuromuscular applications. *Annual Review of Biomedical Engineering*, *7*(1), 327–360. doi:10.1146/annurev.bioeng.6.040803.140103 PMID:16004574

Peterson, C. C. (2004). Theory-of-mind development in oral deaf children with cochlear implants or conventional hearing aids. *Journal of Child Psychology and Psychiatry, and Allied Disciplines*, *45*(6), 1096–1106. doi:10.1111/j.1469-7610.2004.t01-1-00302.x PMID:15257666

Pisoni, D. D., & Geers, A. E. (2000). Working memory in deaf children with cochlear implants: Correlations between digit span and measures of spoken language processing. *The Annals of Otology, Rhinology, and Laryngology*, *185*, 92–94. PMID:11141023

Ploog, B. O., Scahrf, A., Nelson, D., & Brooks, P. J. (2013). Use of computer-assisted technologies (CAT) to enhance social, communicative, and language development in children with autism spectrum disorders. *Journal of Autism and Developmental Disorders*, *43*(2), 301–322. doi:10.1007/s10803-012-1571-3 PMID:22706582

Pring, L. (2005). Savant talent. *Developmental Medicine and Child Neurology*, *47*(7), 500–503. doi:10.1017/S0012162205000976 PMID:15991873

Racine, M. B., Majnemer, A., Shevell, M., & Snider, L. (2008). Handwriting performance in children with attention deficit hyperactivity disorder (ADHD). *Journal of Child Neurology*, *23*(4), 399–406. doi:10.1177/0883073807309244 PMID:18401033

Ran, L., Helal, S., & Moore, S. (2004). Drishti: An integrated indoor/outdoor blind navigation system and service. *Pervasive Computing and Communications*, *2004*, 23–30.

Rao, R., Conn, K., Jung, S. H., Katupitiya, J., & Kientz, T. L. (2002). Human robot interaction: Application to smart wheelchairs. *Proceedings of the 2002 IEEE International Conference on Robotics & Automation*, 3583 – 3588. doi:10.1109/ROBOT.2002.1014265

Rigby, P., Ryan, S. E., Joos, S., Cooper, B. A., Jutai, J., & Steggles, E. (2005). Impact of electronic aids to daily living on the lives of persons with cervical spinal cord injuries. *Assistive Technology*, *17*(2), 89–97. doi:10.1080/10400435.2005.10132099 PMID:16392713

Rigby, P. J. (2009). *Assistive technology for persons with physical disabilities: Evaluation and outcomes*. Toronto Press.

Robins, B., Dautenhahn, K., & Dubowski, J. (2006). Does appearance matter in the interaction of children with autism with a humanoid robot? *Interaction Studies: Social Behaviour and Communication in Biological and Artificial Systems*, (7): 3, 479–512.

Roger, L. (2007). Electronic aids for daily living. *Journal of Rehabilitation Research and Development*, *44*(5), 7–9. PMID:17943673

Schunk, D. H. (1987). Peer models and children's behavioral change. *Review of Educational Research*, *57*(2), 149–174. doi:10.3102/00346543057002149

Skinner, M. W., Clark, G. M., Whitford, L. A., Seligman, P. M., Staller, S. J., Shipp, D. B., & Beiter, A. L. et al. (1994). Evaluation of a new spectral peak coding strategy for the Nucleus 22 channel cochlear implant system. *The American Journal of Otology*, *15*(2), 15–27. PMID:8572106

Stephenson, J., & Carter, M. (2009). The use of weighted vests with children with autism spectrum disorders and other disabilities. *Journal of Autism and Developmental Disorders*, *39*(1), 105–114. doi:10.1007/s10803-008-0605-3 PMID:18592366

Svirsky, M. A., Robbins, A. M., Kirk, K. I., Pisoni, D. B., & Miyamoto, R. T. (2000). Language development in profoundly deaf children with cochlear implants. *Psychological Science*, *11*(2), 153–158. doi:10.1111/1467-9280.00231 PMID:11273423

Thaut, M. H. (1988). Measuring musical responsiveness in autistic children: A comparative analysis of improvised musical tone sequences of autistic, normal, and mentally retarded individuals. *Journal of Autism and Developmental Disorders*, *18*(4), 561–571. doi:10.1007/BF02211874 PMID:3215882

Treffertm, D. A. (2009). The savant syndrome: An extraordinary condition. A synopsis: Past, present, future. *Philosophical Transactions of the Royal Society*, *364*, 1351–1357. PMID:19528017

Trevarthen, C., & Aitken, K. (2001). Infant intersubjectivity: Research, theory and clinical application. *Journal of Child Psychology and Psychiatry, and Allied Disciplines*, *42*(1), 3–48. doi:10.1111/1469-7610.00701 PMID:11205623

Trezek, B. J., & Wang, Y. (2004). Implications of utilizing a phonics-based reading curriculum with children who are deaf or hard of hearing. *American Annals of the Deaf*, *149*(5), 394–402. PMID:15727058

Trezek, B. J., Wang, Y., Woods, D. G., Gampp, T. L., & Paul, P. V. (2007). Using visual phonics to supplement beginning reading instruction for students who are deaf or hard of hearing. *Journal of Deaf Studies and Deaf Education*, 1–12. PMID:17515442

U.S. Department of Education. (2004). The rehabilitation act. *Laws & Guidance/Special Education & Rehabilitative Services*. Retrieved July 5, 2014, from http://www2.ed.gov/policy/speced/reg/narrative.html

U.S. Department of Education. (2006). *Assistive technology act: Annual report to Congress: Fiscal years 2004 and 2005*. Retrieved August 18, 2014, from http://www.ed.gov/about/reports/annual/rsa/atsg/2004/index.html

VandenBerg, N. L. (2001). The use of a weighted vest to increase on-task behavior in children with attention difficulties. *The American Journal of Occupational Therapy*, *55*(6), 621–628. doi:10.5014/ajot.55.6.621 PMID:12959226

Visser, S. N., Danielson, M. L., Bitsko, R. H., Holbrook, J. R., Kogan, M. D., Ghandour, R. M., & Blumberg, S. J. et al. (2014). Trends in the parent-report of health care provider-diagnosed and medicated attention-deficit/hyperactivity disorder: United States, 2003–2011. *Journal of the American Academy of Child Psychiatry, 53*(1), 34–46. doi:10.1016/j.jaac.2013.09.001 PMID:24342384

Weitz, C., Dexter, M., & Moore, J. (1997). *AAC and children with developmental disabilities. The handbook of augmentative and alternative communication*. San Diego: Singular Publishing Group.

Whalen, C., Liden, L., Ingersoll, B., Dallaire, E., & Liden, S. (2006). Behavioral improvements associated with computer-assisted instruction for children with developmental disabilities. *The Journal of Speech and Language Pathology, 1*, 11–26.

White, H. A., & Shah, P. (2011). Creative style and achievement in adults with attention deficit/hyperactivity disorder. *Personality and Individual Differences, 50*(5), 673–677. doi:10.1016/j.paid.2010.12.015

Wilson, B. S., Finley, C. C., Lawson, D. T., Wolford, R. D., Eddington, D. K., & Rabinowitz, W. M. (1991). Better speech recognition with cochlear implants. *Nature, 352*(6332), 236–238. doi:10.1038/352236a0 PMID:1857418

Zentall, S. S. (1986). Effects of color stimulation on performance and activity of hyperactive and nonhyperactive children. *Journal of Educational Psychology, 78*(2), 159–165. doi:10.1037/0022-0663.78.2.159

Zentall, S. S., & Zentall, T. R. (1983). Optimal stimulation: A model of disordered activity and performance in normal and deviant children. *Psychological Bulletin, 94*(3), 446–471. doi:10.1037/0033-2909.94.3.446 PMID:6657825

KEY TERMS AND DEFINITIONS

Assistive: Provision of aid or assistance.

Attention Deficit Hyper Activity (ADHD): A developmental disorder that affects the behavior and the ability of an individual to focus on a particular task; common childhood disorder.

Autism: A neurological disorder that presents in childhood and affects a child's social emotional and interpersonal skills.

Blind: Inability to see.

Deaf: Inability to hear or an individual may have impaired hearing abilities.

Disabilities: A condition in which an individual's physical and mental capabilities are limited due to various etiologies.

Inclusivity: Intention to include individuals in areas or in ideas in which they are normally excluded.

Technology: Use of scientific devices to enhance daily life.

Chapter 16
Using Technology to Support Social Competence

Brenda Smith Myles
Ohio Center for Autism and Low Incidence, USA

Amy Bixler Coffin
Ohio Center for Autism and Low Incidence, USA

Jan Rogers
Ohio Center for Autism and Low Incidence, USA

Wendy Szakacs
Ohio Center for Autism and Low Incidence, USA

Theresa Earles-Vollrath
University of Central Missouri, USA

ABSTRACT

Social competence includes a complex set of skills that impacts quality of life across all environments: home, school, employment, and the community. Elements that impact social competence, such as theory of mind, weak central coherence, regulation and relationship building, must be taught to individuals with disabilities, including those with autism spectrum disorder. Evidence-based interventions that incorporate low, medium and high technology have the potential to support skill development in social competence in a meaningful manner. This chapter reviews the concept known as social competence and offers a variety of practices to support its development.

INTRODUCTION

Technology is rapidly changing and has become increasingly accessible to all people. More importantly, the increased accessibility to technology can provide the needed supports and scaffolds to aid an individual with a disability to overcome barriers for access, participation, and independence (Dell, Newton, & Petroff, 2011). Assistive technologies (AT), a particular kind of technology that may be used by a person with a disability, is defined in the Technology-Related Assistance for Individuals with Disabilities Act (1988) for all individuals with disabilities and also in the Individuals with Disabilities Education Act (IDEA, 2004) relevant to children participating in educational programs. In both definitions, assistive technologies are not defined by specific devices, but rather by the intended function of the technology

DOI: 10.4018/978-1-4666-8395-2.ch016

which is to "increase, maintain, or improve the functional capabilities" of an individual with a disability. Further the definitions state that AT can be any item, equipment or product system, commercial, modified, or customized. This definition indicates the wide range of possibilities that may be considered assistive technology from very low-tech items such as paper picture supports to higher technology supports, such as dedicated communication devices. Devices, such as a screen readers for those with low vision, wheelchairs used by those with mobility challenges and alternative keyboards for those with computer access needs, are easy to recognize as AT. However, items such as smart phones, as well as tablets and laptop computers, which are used by the general population, may also be considered AT under certain circumstances; that is, when they allow a person with a disability to access a portion of life that might not otherwise be available. For example, a tablet computer that contains an application with customized social narratives may be instrumental in helping a person with autism develop and maintain relationships or seek help in an appropriate manner. A reminder app on some smart phones may be useful for an individual with a traumatic brain injury (TBI) who may have difficulties with memory. Again, AT is not defined by a specific product or device, but by the way it is used and needed by the individual with a disability.

Assistive technologies are not randomly chosen, selected only from available technologies found in the immediate environment, or identified based on a long process of trial and error, but rather should be selected using a systematic team assessment process that considers the strengths and needs of the individual, expected tasks for participation and environments where the tasks will occur. Those identified needs are then matched to features of technologies that can support the individual. Finally, trials are conducted of the possible AT solutions that contain the identified features to determine the effectiveness of the technology in meeting the identified needs of the individual. Two models are often used to help guide the AT assessment process. The first is framework called SETT that was proposed by Zabala (2002). This acronym refers to Student, Environment, Tasks, and Tools and is designed to help guide school team discussions about the need for assistive technology. Cook and Hussey (1995) suggested the HAAT model – an acronym for Human, Activity, and AT. This model is often used to plan and structure the AT assessment process for adults. Both models take into account the strength, needs and abilities of the individual, targeted tasks or activities and contexts and environments when determining the needed AT supports. While the terminology may be slightly different between the two models, the data gathered and considered is generally identical with a process that allows for a thorough problem-solving approach geared toward the selection of AT supports.

The remainder of this chapter will look specifically at how assistive technologies can support social performance. Assistive technologies can be effectively used to provide meaningful and relevant supports and scaffolds as well as support evidence-based practices (EBP) for those who experience social challenges related to their disability. Oftentimes technologies can replace or supplement person-centered supports by providing a more independent means of social functioning without the need to rely on others for assistance or at the very least reduce the need for person-centered supports.

It is important that strategies used to support social performance building fully appreciate the complexity of social interventions. Too often strategies tend to target only one element of the social process. Loomis (2008), however, approaches social competence in a more comprehensive manner. Specifically, he has identified 10 factors that should be considered when programming for social situations (see Figure 1). These factors provide the first step in the recognition that social skills are more than the sum of its parts (Koenig, De Los Reyes, Cicchetti, Scahill, & Klin, 2009). They vary across events, thus creating challenges that differ dependent on the social event. A brief review of these factors is provided in Table 1. For a more in-depth discussion, please refer to Loomis' excellent book, *Staying in the Game: Providing Social Opportunities for Children and Adolescents with Autism Spectrum Disorders and Other Developmental Disabilities.*

Figure 1.

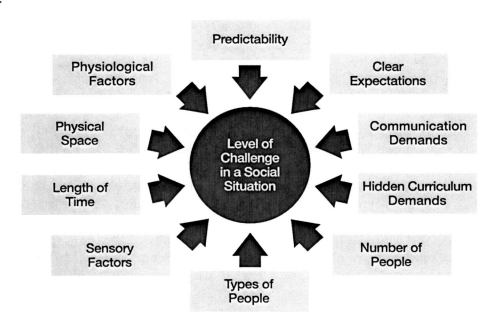

Table 1. Brief overview of Loomis' 10 factors that impact social interactions

Factor	Brief Description
Sensory Demands	All environments have sensory demands and the majority of individuals with AS have sensory challenges. A mismatch between the two can cause regulation problems.
Length of Time	Social processing can be exhausting for learners with AS. The longer a social event, the more taxing it is.
Physical Space	Crowded spaces, large open areas, noisy environments, and echoing environments can be difficult and/or exhausting for the individual with AS.
Physiological Factors	Physiological factors, including fatigue, hunger, thirst, and illness can influence social interactions.
Predictability	Individuals need to know in advance what is likely to occur.
Clear Expectations	Expectations must be clearly identified and communicated.
Communication Demands	Many individuals with ASD are visual learners. Match communication demands to the individual's learning style.
Hidden Curriculum	Unwritten rules are often difficult to understand unless they are directly taught.
Number of People	The greater the number of people, the more difficult it is to interact with them.
Types of People	Include people who are easy to communicate with, are calm, and embrace diversity.

From Loomis, J. W. (2008). *Staying in the game: Providing social opportunities for children and adolescents with autism spectrum disorders and other developmental disabilities.* Shawnee Mission, KS: AAPC Publishing. Used with permission www.aapcpublishing.net.

The following sections will identify and examine core deficits that may contribute to the social challenges that impact some individuals with disabilities. AT features that might provide an appropriate scaffold or support to allow the individual more access, participation or independence in social performance will then be matched to those core social skill deficits. Examples of available technologies that contain those features will then be presented. It should be noted, that because technology is rapidly changing, the focus should not be on the products but rather the features of the products that would support social performance. Many assistive technology features remain relatively stable over time with additional features being added to products. Therefore, it is important to gain an understanding of the features and how they match with the needs and characteristics of the individual rather than the product examples provided, which are merely a few of the many possibilities that are currently available. It is also likely that a student would need a combination of features to meet her needs, and it is this combination of features that ultimately drives the final product selection. Some technologies contain very few features and are very specific to a particular need while others are more robust with many features that may be able to be turned off and on as needed. If a student needs many different types of supports it may be best to find one product that is feature rich and supports a variety of needs rather than providing the student with many different assistive technology products with few features. This approach will limit the amount of technologies the individual will need to learn as well as physically, cognitively, and organizationally manage. All of the interventions highlighted in this chapter were carefully selected to meet the characteristics of learners, such as those on the autism spectrum, who experiences social challenges. They are largely portable, offer multiple modes of input and output, and are visual in presentation.

THEORY OF MIND

Theory of mind (ToM) is the ability to assign mental states such as beliefs, intents, desires, hopes, and opinions to oneself and others in order to understand and predict behavior. It is the ability to recognize and accept that others have differing ideas, viewpoints, values and intentions than oneself (cf., Baron-Cohen, Leslie, & Frith, 1985; Golan & Baron-Cohen, 2014). ToM allows individuals to empathize, imagine and appreciate others' hopes and dreams. It involves making the distinction between the real world and conceptual representations of the world (cf., Buron & Myles, 2014).

Theory of mind develops gradually with spontaneous social thinking emerging as early as infancy. As reported by Astington and Edward (2010), by age 2 children express awareness of the difference between thoughts and objects; distinguish between what they prefer and others' preferences; and understand when others feel happy or sad based on if they receive a desired item. Typically by age 3, children can talk about what others believe and know. At this age they begin to understand their own minds and those of others. By age 4, children usually are able to make inferences about the beliefs of others and to discriminate that sometimes a belief may be false. These discoveries were noted in the work of Wimmer and Perner (1983) and demonstrate the cognitive change in children between three and four years of age.

According to the most recent version of the Diagnostic and Statistical Manual of Mental Disorders (DSM-5; American Psychiatric Association, 2013), individuals with ASD have qualitative impairments in social communication. Deficits exist in social-emotional reciprocity, nonverbal communicative behaviors used for social interaction and the ability to develop and maintain relationships appropriate to developmental level. With that said, individuals diagnosed with ASD often struggle with skills, such as making inferences, appreciating others' interests, and interpreting the thoughts and feelings of others and making sense of their actions. In addition, they may struggle with accepting when others do not understand a particular concept. They tend to be less proficient at "mind reading" as compared to those individuals who are typically developing. It has been suggested that the theory of mind, or the ability to "mind read" is the capacity that individuals with ASD lack (Baron-Cohen et al., 1985).

Consequently, theory of mind deficits can provide a possible explanation for the social and communication impairments associated with autism spectrum disorder. An interruption in the development of ToM leads to what is called "mindblindness;" the inability to recognize the thoughts and feelings of others. For example, mindblindness can limit a person's ability to recognize sarcasm, understand when another person is becoming frustrated, or comprehend when a person is losing interest in a conversation. Baron-Cohen (1997) reported that mindblindness may explain the social differences demonstrated in individuals with ASD.

In addition, Illand (2011) reported that there is a correlation between the challenges that individuals with ASD face in relation to social and communication skills- social understanding and perspective taking- and literacy development. For instance, a student who struggles with understanding others' points of view, taking into account others' beliefs and recognizing that others have different opinions may face challenges associated with understanding characters and their intentions and interpreting the interactions between characters within a story.

An intact ToM allows an individual to infer human emotions, comprehend body language and interpret voice tone. However, individuals with ASD who demonstrate deficits in ToM struggle with such skills and frequently need additional support. Assistive technology often provides that additional support. As mentioned previously, it is extremely important that consideration is made to the features of assistive technology as they relate to the underlying deficits of ToM (Borg, Larsson, & Ostergren, 2011).

Various interventions and supports including cartooning, video modeling, the Mindreading software (Baron-Cohen, Golan, Wheelwright, and Hill, 2004),) and social autopsies may support individuals who demonstrate deficits in ToM. Interventions selected to address needs as they relate to ToM should include features such as step-by-step supports, expectations demonstrated through visual supports/video and portability. These interventions can be utilized prior to, during, or after an interaction or situation when an error related to ToM occurs.

Cartooning. This intervention uses thought bubbles, conversation bubbles, and cartoon or stick figures to illustrate people's thoughts and words during interactions in a comic-strip format (Buron & Myles, 2014). Thought and speech bubbles allow an individual to visually see a social interaction or the hidden rules, known as the hidden curriculum (Myles, Trautman & Schelvan, 2013) involved in social situations through line drawings. Cartooning involves drawing a short conversation using symbols/pictures, which represent social interactions. They present the various components of a conversation visually which allows some of the more abstract concepts of social communication to be made more "concrete" (Hutchins & Prelock, 2013; Kerr & Durkin, 2004; Rogers & Myles, 2001). Cartooning can be accomplished with paper/pencil; apps, such as Bitstrips (Bistrips, 2014), and Strip Designer (Vivid Apps, 2008). Cartooning is an EBP that falls under the category of social narratives (Centers for Medicare and Medicaid Services [CMS], 2010; National Autism Center [NAC], 2009; National Professional Development Center on Autism [NPDC], nd,).

Video modeling. Video modeling is a teaching method used to promote desired behavior and interactions as well as to support the understanding of self and others. Using this approach, the student observes a video of a peer, adult, or himself engaging in a targeted behavior (Bellini & Akullian, 2007; Burton, Anderson, Prate, & Dyches, 2013). Video modeling is also very useful when an individual has mastered individual skills, but does not know how to combine them. For example, a child may know the individual steps required to put on his coat but not know how to combine them to perform this task himself. Video modeling can be used across many areas, such as self-help skills, communication skills, social behaviors, or academic behaviors (Wilson, 2013). Videos can be homemade or commercial (i.e., Videojug [Videojug, 2014], Model Me Going Places 2 (Model Me Kids, 2010), 9th Planet [9th Planet LLC, 2013]). Video modeling is an EBP (CMS; NAC; NPDC).

Understanding emotions. Two software applications address the ToM needs of learners: the Mind Reading software and the Emotion Detective. Authored by Baron-Cohen et al. (2004), the Mind Reading software program was designed to support those individuals who have difficulties recognizing emotions in others, a challenging area for individuals with ToM deficits. *Mind Reading* is based on a taxonomic system of 412 emotions and mental states, grouped into 24 emotion groups and 6 developmental levels (from age 4 to adulthood). Each emotion group is introduced and demonstrated by a short video clip giving some clues for later analysis of the emotions presented. Each emotion is defined and demonstrated by six silent films of faces, six voice recordings, and six written examples of situations that illustrate a given emotion. The resulting library of emotional "assets" (video clips, audio clips, or brief stories) includes 7,416 units of emotion information. To facilitate generalization, the face videos and voice recordings comprise actors of both genders and of various ages and ethnicities (Golan & Baron-Cohen, 2014). The software enables the user to study emotions, learn the meaning behind certain facial expressions and tone of voice. It provides learners with 400 different emotions expressed in diverse people in both a visual and auditory format (LaCava, Golan, Baron-Cohen, & Myles, 2007). The Emotion Detective uses scenarios, graphics and real picture, to teach individuals to read social cues. Developing by InGenius Labs (2012), this app teaches (a) identifying emotions in self and others, (b) understanding nonverbal cues, (c) initiating and maintaining conversations, (d) understanding the perspectives of others, and (e) self-awareness. These software applications are considered an EBP in the categories of visual supports, technology-based treatment and antecedent based intervention (CMS; NAC; NPDC).

Social autopsy. The social autopsy, developed by Richard Lavoie, is a problem-solving strategy designed to support individuals who struggle with social interactions. It helps individuals understand social errors that are committed during social interactions and provides opportunity for choosing alternative solutions to correct those errors in the future (Bieber, 1994). The following steps are included in a social autopsy:

- Identify the error;
- Determine who was harmed by the error;
- Decide how to correct the error; and
- Develop a plan so error doesn't happen again.

Through the process, the person learns how to respond more effectively when approached with similar situations. A social autopsy can be enhanced with pictures to support comprehension. This can be considered a social-communication EBP (CMS; NAC; NPDC).

CENTRAL COHERENCE

In 1989, Frith proposed Weak Central Coherence (WCC) as a theory to explain the cognitive style of individuals with autism spectrum disorders (Frith, 1989). Central coherence is the ability to take details or pieces of information and link them together in a meaningful way, allowing us to "see the big picture"

(Loth, Gomez, & Happe, 2008). In other words, individuals with intact central coherence can focus on details as well as the whole; they can "see the forest through the trees". Individuals with ASD, however, demonstrate the opposite; they often have a "detailed-focused cognitive style" (Happe & Frith, 2006, p. 5.). Thus, they get lost in the details and tend to see all of the trees but not the forest. According to Frith (1989), WCC is a deficit *and* a strength. The strong focus on details prevents individuals with ASD from coherently linking details into a meaningful whole while simultaneously supporting areas of strength such as special talents (Frith & Happe, 1994), superior visual spatial skills (Jarrold, Butler, Cottington & Jimenez, 2000; Happe & Frith, 2006), recall of strings of random words (Frith, 1999), strong memory for details, and savant skills (Frith & Happe, 1994).

WCC is hypothesized to account for a number of common characteristics associated with individuals with ASD, such as over-selectivity, the tendency to over focus on irrelevant stimuli; difficulties with reading comprehension and using context to draw conclusions; and insistence on sameness. Weak central coherence has also been linked to difficulties generalizing concepts across different environments, people and materials, troubles with organization, problems reading facial expressions and difficulties understanding social cues that create meaning in social situations. Weak coherence is postulated to lie at the root of characteristic ASD symptoms such as insistence on sameness, attention to parts of objects, and uneven cognitive profile, including savant skills (Happe & Frith, 2006).

The following interventions can support individuals who experience challenges in this area: (a) visual supports and (b) social narratives.

Visual supports. Visual supports are tools that are used to increase the understanding of language, environmental expectations, and to provide structure and support. They facilitate understanding because they remain static or fixed in the individual's environment as compared to verbal language, which is considered transient or fleeting (Crosland & Dunlap, 2012; Koyama & Wang, 2011; Lequia, Machalicek, & Rispoli, 2012).). Visual supports can include visual schedules and first/then cards. Materials that directly support skill acquisition include: graphic organizers; study guides, outlines and content summary sheets; guided notes; models of finished products; and word banks. The Visual Schedule Planner (Good Karma Applications, 2014) application helps learner organize their day and understand which elements of their day are important.

Social narratives. Social narratives, as described in the previous section of this chapter, that directly target the understanding of salient information and less important details are also helpful for those who experience weak central coherence.

REGULATION

Emotional regulation encompasses an individual's ability to experience, recognize, express, and regulate all emotions effectively and fluidly with respect to environmental constraints (Berthoz & Hill, 2004; Laurent & Rubin, 2004). Individuals with ASD and related disorders have difficulty navigating the world of emotions, causing significant challenges in their capacity for emotional regulation. This is often evidenced by the presence of depression, anxiety, and self-esteem differences. Individuals with ASD also report experiencing more negative emotions than positive emotions, including anger, than their neurotypical counterparts. According to Quek, Sofronoff, Sheffiled, White, and Kelly (2012), 17% of young people on the autism spectrum experience clinically significant levels of anger. In their study, anxiety and depression were positively associated with anger, with depression explaining 25% of the variance in anger. Similar results were found by Matson and Nebel-Schwalm (2007) and Tantam (2000). Aggression can be defined as actions that often follow anger and include threatening, rough play; provoked lashing out; hitting, biting, or violent behavior. Aggression is a challenge experienced by approximately 50% of children through the age of 14, however, it declines significantly after age 15 (Kanne & Mazurek, 2011). Thus, Langstrom, Grann, Richkin, Sjostedt, and Murphy (2003) reported that these aggressive behaviors are evidenced in only a small percentage of adults on the autism spectrum. In fact, researchers investigating violent behavior in adults on the spectrum found that they were less likely to engage in violence than the general population, and where they did occur were associated with substance abuse, personality disorder or psychotic behavior (Langstrom et al., 2009). However, Balfe and Tantam (2010) noted quite different results in their study, a self-report by adults with HFASD, indicating that anger and aggression may be more pervasive than otherwise thought, with 84% of the individuals interviewed indicating that they anger easily and 31% stating that they often hit others.

Several interventions address the all-important area of regulation, including: (a) the Incredible 5-Point Scale (Buron & Curtis, 2012), cognitive picture rehearsal (Groden, Kantor, Woodard, & Lipsitt, 2011), photo album (Buron & Myles, 2014), Mataya and Owens' Problem Solving Program (Mataya & Owens, 2013), and the 5-Star Program (Buron, & Curtis, 2012).

The Incredible 5-Point Scale. Buron and Curtis created the Incredible 5-Point Scale to help individuals with ASD understand social and emotional concepts as well as to enhance self-understanding. The 1-5 scale system is applicable for a variety of social and self-regulation behaviors and responses to those behaviors, including feelings of anxiety, concepts of personal space and feelings of anger. The scale is unique in that it can be used as an obsessional index, a stress scale, a meltdown monitor, etc. Children and youth with ASD are taught to recognize the stages of their emotions or social challenges and methods to self-calm or "re-think" at each level. Figure 2 provides illustrations of the Incredible 5-Point Scale which is an EBP under antecedent-based interventions and visual supports.

Cognitive picture rehearsal. Cognitive Picture Rehearsal (Groden et al.) involves the repeated practice of a sequence of behaviors to teach a calm response to stressful situations. It involves imagery, where the image is supported by a visual representation of the person performing a desired behavior and the behavior resulting in a pleasant experience. The sequence is presented in a cartoon panel format illustrating a predictably stressful situation and includes a script for successfully navigating that situation. For example, if the person experiences stress when recess is cancelled due to bad weather, the drawing and script might look like the example in Figure 3.

Photo album. The photo album is based on the premise that many learners on the autism spectrum experience stress throughout their school day. The idea is to create a small photo album of approximately 6 pictures that help to make the person feel happy and calm. The photos might include a parent, a family pet, a family cabin or the person's bedroom. The photo album can be included in the person's daily routine at least once and possibly several times throughout the day. When introducing the album to the person, the educator can calmly recite a script while looking at the photos. For example, "Here is my dog, Eddie. I love my dog Eddie. Eddie helps me to feel calm and happy." A similar script can then be repeated with each of the other photographs. After an initial period of direct support from the teacher, the learner can then look at the photos independently. The words to the script can also be included at the bottom of each photo. (Buron & Myles, 2014).

Mataya and Owens' Problem Solving Program. Problem-solving skills are highly valued in home (cf. Dawson et al., 2012), community (Renzaglia, Karvonen, Drasgow, & Stoxen, 2003), school (cf. Cheng, Chiang, & Cheng, 2010), and employment settings (cf. Mat, Zhang, & Pacha, 2012) as a means

Figure 2.

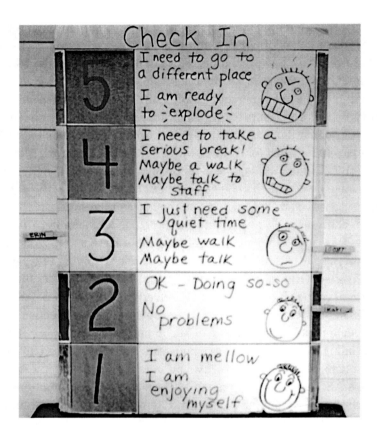

Figure 3.

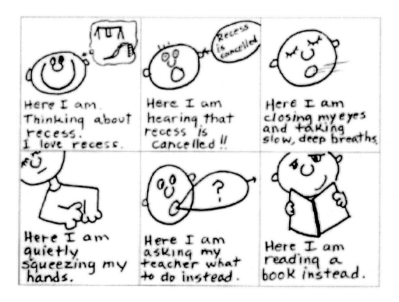

Figure 4.

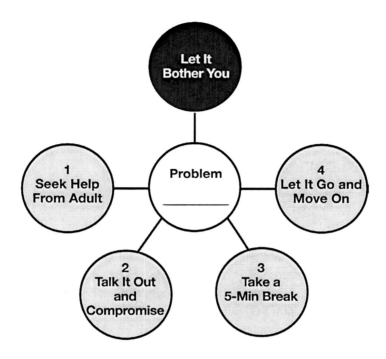

of regulating emotions and behavior. The Mataya and Owens' Problem Solving Program (Mataya & Owens) is designed to help learners understand cause and effect, problem solving and decision-making. Created for use at home, school, and community, this comprehensive and easy to use model can be used with learners across the spectrum. A rubric from the program appears in Figure 4.

The 5-Star System. Another strategy to teach self-regulation is a method called the 5-Star System (Buron, & Curtis). Shifting from one activity to another is difficult for many learners with ASD and the resulting anxiety can contribute to an inability to control emotions. 5 Stars is meant to be a visual representation of the passage of time, used as a method to help individuals better understand when it is time to stop one thing and go on to another. Its concrete, visual and systematic nature can assist the learner in maintaining self-control over a difficult situation. The 5-Star system consists of a cardboard

Figure 5.

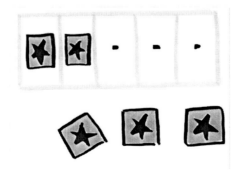

strip with 5 or 6 squares (with Velcro on each square) and 5 separate stars (also with Velcro on each star). The learner is given the cardboard strip and given a verbal prompt such as "We will be in group for 5 stars and then we can go for a walk." The adult has control of how quickly or slowly the stars are given to the learner, making it a more flexible system than a traditional timer. This is not a reward system. It is designed to be a concrete representation of the passage of time. The learner does not 'earn' or 'lose' a star. Instead of staying in a group indefinitely or for "5 minutes", the expectation is "stay in group for 5 stars" (see Figure 5).

RELATIONSHIP BUILDING

Susan Golubock, an adult diagnosed with autism at age 50, said the first question she asked of the psychiatrist who diagnosed her was, "So, how was it that after spending 30 years in a monogamous relationship I still did not understand what *having a friend* meant?" (2009). She explains that it took her twelve years of therapy and help from her family and friends to understand all she had missed and misunderstood in the area of relationships. Relationships are extremely complicated for all persons, but even more so for individuals who struggle with social competence (Bellini, 2006). This can include persons identified with ASD intellectual disabilities, non-verbal learning disability, attention deficit hyperactive disorder, gifted, and others that have social competence challenges (Myles et al., 2013).

There are many types of relationships, including those with peers, parents, siblings, family members, a romantic partner, co-workers, and community members. Initiating, building and maintaining those relationships can be a difficult process with many facets. Some of the qualities that make a relationship successful can be strengths for individuals with disabilities, such as loyalty, helpfulness, dependability, authenticity, and appreciating the differences in each other. Other qualities are often the challenges that individuals with disabilities need to overcome, such as communicating positive and negative thoughts and feelings, reciprocation, valuing each other's opinions, and remembering and taking into account a friend's preferences.

Building relationships and friendships makes a difference in the life of any human. Positive relationships give a sense of belonging, reduce stress, and are good for your health (Mayo Clinic Staff, 2014). Not having relationships and being lonely is actually dangerous to a person's health and well being. According to Marano (2003), not having social interactions can cause health issues, such as high blood pressure and heart problems, increased risk of suicide, dropping out of school, delinquency, and higher levels of stress. Further, Barnhill (2001) found a relationship between depressive symptoms and the feeling of failure due to poor social abilities in individuals with high-functioning autism. Thus, it seems that positive social relationships are key to living a happier and healthier life.

Social relationships are complicated because individuals must adapt to each setting, each different event, the persons involved, the history each person has with the other, the mood each person brings to the interaction, and the social abilities of each individual (Bellini, 2006). For some with disabilities, such as ASD, the world of relationships is a difficult and anxiety producing place (Winner, 2008). There are technology supports that can assist individuals with disabilities to learn social interaction skills and to participate more successfully in social relationships. Remember to begin with assessment of social strengths and needs, identifying the features of the technology, and matching the best features to the strengths and needs of the individual.

Multiple technology supports that can be used to teach the skills needed to develop positive social relationships. The following is a brief description of such supports; this is meant to be a starting point for exploration and are by no means totally inclusive.

Visual supports. Visual supports are an evidence-based practice that can be a picture, graphic representation, or word used to prompt an individual regarding a rule, routine, task, or social response (Smith, 2008). These supports can be on low-tech paper, on mid-tech buttons or overlays, or on high tech devices. Visual supports can be effective in increasing skills that support social relationships, including the demonstration of play skills, social interaction skills, and social initiation (CMS; NAC; NPDC,) These supports can be in the form of social rule cards (reminders of rules for the environment), step-by-step instructions (how to complete a social situation), cue cards (reminders of what to do in a social situation), written/picture scripts (possible words or phrases to use), and cartooning (draw a situation using speech and thought bubbles to enhance social understanding).

Social teaching frameworks. Teaching frameworks for learning how to approach social situations gives a person ways to enter, participate, and reflect on a variety of circumstances, people, and events. Some of those frameworks are Stop, Observe, Deliberate, Act (SODA; Bock, 2001), Situation, Options, Consequences, Choices, Strategies, Simulation (SOCCSS; Roosa cited in Myles, 2005), social behavior mapping (Buie, 2013), and social autopsies (Bieber, 1994).

1. SODA was designed to help learners approach novel situations in a strategic manner (2007a, b) by observing the environment and developing a plan of action. A description of the steps of SODA appears in Table 2.
2. SOCCSS, on the other hand, was developed to help students with social interaction problems put social and behavioral issues into a sequential form (Roosa, personal communication). The strategy helps students understand problem situations and lets them see that they have to make choices about a given event and that each choice has a consequence (see Figure 6 for a sample worksheet).

Table 2. SOCCSS steps

Situation	When a social problem arises, the teacher works with the student to identify the situation. Together they define the problem and state a goal. The stage occurs through discussion, writing, and drawings.
Options	Following identification of the situation, the student and teacher brainstorm several options. At this point, the teacher accepts all student responses and does not evaluate them. Typically, the options are listed in written or pictorial format. According to Spivak, Platt, and Shure (1976), this step is critical to problem-solving. The ability to generate multiple solutions diminishes student frustration, encourages students to see more than one perspective, and results in resiliency.
Consequences	The student and teacher work together to evaluate each of the options generated. Kaplan and Carter (1995) suggest that each of the options be evaluated using the following two criteria: (a) Efficacy – Will the solution get me what I want? and (b) Feasibility – Will I be able to do it? Each of the consequences is labeled with an E for efficacy or F for feasibility. The teacher works as a facilitator, using pointed questions to help the student develop consequences for each option, without dictating consequence.
Choices	The student then prioritizes the options and consequences and selects a solution from the list of generated options. The student- selected option is the one that has the most desirable consequences.
Strategy	The student and adult work together to develop a plan of action. Although the adult may provide guidance by asking leading questions or making suggestions, the student should ultimately develop the plan so that he has ownership.
Simulation	The student is given an opportunity to turn the abstract strategy into something more concrete either through role-play, imagery, talking with a peer about the plan, or writing or typing the plan.

Figure 6.

SOCCSS
Situation, Options, Consequences, Choices, Strategies, Simulation

Situation

Who _____   When _____

What _____   Why _____

_____

_____

Options	Consequences	Choice

Strategy – Plan of Action

Figure 7.

GETTING MY MATH DONE

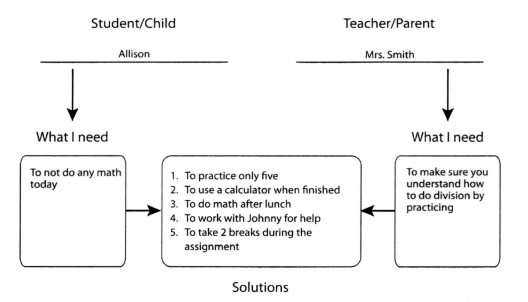

Student/Child

Allison

Teacher/Parent

Mrs. Smith

What I need

To not do any math today

1. To practice only five
2. To use a calculator when finished
3. To do math after lunch
4. To work with Johnny for help
5. To take 2 breaks during the assignment

What I need

To make sure you understand how to do division by practicing

Solutions

Table 3. Sample hidden curriculum items

People may not automatically recognize that you are upset, concerned or overwhelmed. If you are feeling one of these emotions and someone is not giving you space or helping you calm down, they might need you to tell them how you are feeling.
Sometimes your behavior can tell you how you are feeling. For example, some people will start to tap their feet or drum their fingers when they are beginning to feel upset.
People find it easiest to be around people who know how to recognize and control their emotions.
It is okay to tell someone that you are upset, overwhelmed, and confused and that you need (a) to be left alone or (b) help from someone you trust.
Even though you make plans and have routines, things will not always go as planned. Most of the time, we should try to accept the changes and realize that everything will be okay.
Almost all people need to take time for themselves throughout the day to keep calm. Some people do this by exercising, meditating, taking a walk, or going to a quiet place.
It is normal not to have the answers for all situations and it is almost always okay to ask a trusted friend or adult to help you figure out what you should do. Sometimes you will be asked to help a friend who is having difficulty.

Myles, B. S., Trautman, M. L., & Schelvan, R. L. (2013). *The hidden curriculum: Practical solutions for understanding unstated rules in social situations* (2nd ed). Shawnee Mission, KS: AAPC Publishing. Used with permission.

3.   Buie's social behavior mapping is a visual strategy that helps children make good choices with regard to their behavior by visually showing them the consequences for each action they choose at any given time. Behavior mapping helps children understand cause and effect, specifically how their behavior (cause) leads to consequences (effect). They also allow children to see (with words and pictures) how positive choices will lead to rewards, motivating them to make good choices and learn new skills. One sample of behavior mapping appears in Figure 7.

Hidden curriculum. The hidden curriculum is the set of information that is often seemingly obvious to those who are typically developing, but is not readily available to those with disabilities, without direct instruction (Myles et al., 2013). Hidden curriculum items are available in multiple publications (Endow, 2012; Myles et al., Myles & Kolar, 2013; Myles, Endow, & Mayfield, 2013). In addition, there are commercial and public access videos and virtual environment interactive animated software that show examples/non-examples of social relationship skills. Commercial products the apps, Hidden Curriculum on the Go for Kids (AAPC Publishing, 2010) and Hidden Curriculum for Adolescents and Adults (AAPC Publishing, 2010). Television shows, such as The Big Bang Theory or Parenthood, are also good sources on information on the hidden curriculum (CAUTION: Always watch any video from start to finish before using and consider the age and maturity level of the individual viewing it. Watch for inappropriate humor or language). Table 3 contains sample hidden curriculum items.

Gaining social relationship skills is a life-long journey from early childhood through adulthood. Keep the story of Susan Golubock in mind when teaching these skills. It took her 12 years starting at the age of 50 to understand how to make and keep successful relationships. This is hard work that requires insight, repetition, and the use of all the available tools. Use data to watch the skills increase and keep on teaching with all the technology accessible.

SUMMARY

Social competence includes a complex set of skills that impacts quality of life across all environments: home, school, employment, and the community. Elements that impact social competence, such as ToM, WCC, regulation, and relationship building, must be taught to individuals with disabilities, including those with ASD. Evidence-based interventions that incorporate low, medium and high technology have the potential to support skill development in social competence in a meaningful manner.

REFERENCES

AAPC Publishing, Inc. (2010). Hidden curriculum on the go for adolescents and adults. Shawnee Mission, KS: AAPC Publishing. Available from iTunes.

AAPC Publishing, Inc. (2010). Hidden curriculum on the go for kids. Shawnee Mission, KS: AAPC Publishing. Available from iTunes.

American Psychiatric Association. (2013). *Diagnostic and statistical manual of mental disorders* (5th ed.). Arlington, VA: Author.

Astington, J. W., & Edward, M. J. (2010). The development of theory of mind in early childhood. *Social Cognition in Infancy*, *5*, 1–6.

Balfe, M., & Tantam, D. (2010). A descriptive social and health profile of a community sample of adults and adolescents with Asperger syndrome. *BMC Research Notes*, *3*(1), 300–307. doi:10.1186/1756-0500-3-300 PMID:21070680

Barnhill, G. (2001). Social attributions and depression in adolescents with Asperger syndrome. *Focus on Autism and Other Developmental Disabilities*, *16*(1), 46–53. doi:10.1177/108835760101600112

Baron-Cohen, S. (1997). *Mindblindness: An essay on autism and theory of mind*. MIT Press.

Baron-Cohen, S., Leslie, A. M., & Frith, U. (1985). Does the autistic child have theory of mind? *Cognition*, *21*(1), 37–46. doi:10.1016/0010-0277(85)90022-8 PMID:2934210

Bellini, S. (2006). *Building social relationships: A systematic approach to teaching social interaction skills to children and adolescents with autism spectrum disorders and other social difficulties*. Shawnee Mission, KS: AAPC Publishing Company.

Bellini, S., & Akullian, J. (2007). A meta-analysis of video modeling and video self-modeling interventions for children and adolescents with autism spectrum disorders. *Exceptional Children*, *73*(3), 264–287. doi:10.1177/001440290707300301

Berthoz, S., & Hill, E. L. (2004). The validity of using self-reports to assess emotion regulation abilities. *European Psychiatry*, *20*(3), 291–298. doi:10.1016/j.eurpsy.2004.06.013 PMID:15935431

Bieber, J. (1994). *Learning disabilities and social skills with Richard LaVoie: Last one picked ... first one picked on* [DVD]. Washington, DC: Public Broadcasting Service.

Bitstrips, Inc. (2014). *Bitstrips*. Ontario, Canada: Author. Available from iTunes.

Bock, M. A. (2001). SODA strategy: Enhancing the social interaction skills of youngsters with Asperger Syndrome. *Intervention in School and Clinic, 36*(5), 272–278. doi:10.1177/105345120103600503

Bock, M. A. (2007a). A social behavioral learning strategy intervention for a child with Asperger Syndrome: A brief report. *Remedial and Special Education, 28*(5), 258–265. doi:10.1177/07419325070280050101

Bock, M. A. (2007b). The impact of social behavioral learning strategy training on the social interaction skills of four students with Asperger syndrome. *Focus on Autism and Other Developmental Disabilities, 22*(2), 88–95. doi:10.1177/10883576070220020901

Borg, J., Larsson, S., & Östergren, P. O. (2011). The right to assistive technology: For whom, for what, and by whom? *Disability & Society, 26*(2), 151–167. doi:10.1080/09687599.2011.543862

Buie, A. (2013). *Behavior mapping: A visual strategy for teaching appropriate behavior to individual with autism spectrum and related disabilities*. Shawnee Mission, KS: AAPC Publishing.

Buron, K., & Curtis, M. B. (2012). The Incredible 5-Point Scale: The significantly improved and expanded second edition: Assisting students in understanding social interactions and controlling their emotional responses. Shawnee Mission, KS: AAPC Publishing.

Buron, K. D., & Myles, B. S. (2014). Emotional regulation. In K. D. Buron & P. Wolfberg (Eds.), *Learners on the autism spectrum Preparing highlight qualified educators and related practitioners* (2nd ed., pp. 239–263). Shawnee Mission, KS: AAPC Publishing.

Burton, C. E., Anderson, D. H., Prater, M., & Dyches, T. T. (2013). Video self-modeling on a iPad to teach functional math skills to adolescents with autism intellectual disability. *Focus on Autism and Other Developmental Disabilities, 28*(2), 67–77. doi:10.1177/1088357613478829

Centers for Medicare and Medicaid Services. (2010). *Autism spectrum disorders: Final report on environmental scan*. Washington, DC: Author.

Cheng, Y., Chiang, H., & Cheng, L. (2010). Enhancing empathy instruction using a collaborative virtual learning environment for children with autism spectrum conditions. *Computers & Education, 55*(4), 1449–1458. doi:10.1016/j.compedu.2010.06.008

Crosland, K., & Dunlap, G. (2012). Effective strategies for the inclusion of children with autism in general education classrooms. *Behavior Modification, 36*(3), 251–269. doi:10.1177/0145445512442682 PMID:22563045

Dawson, G., Jones, E. J. H., Merkle, K., Venema, K., Lowy, R., Faja, S., & Webb, S. J. et al. (2012). Early behavioral intervention is associated with normalized brain activity in young children with autism. *Journal of the American Academy of Child and Adolescent Psychiatry, 51*(11), 1150–1159. doi:10.1016/j.jaac.2012.08.018 PMID:23101741

Dell, A. G., Newton, D., & Petroff, J. G. (2011). *Assistive technology in the classroom: Enhancing the school experiences of students with disabilities* (2nd ed.). Upper Saddle River, NJ: Pearson.

Endow, J. (2012). *Learning the hidden curriculum: The odyssey of one autistic adult.* Shawnee Mission, KS: AAPC Publishing.

Frith, U. (1989). Autism: Explaining the enigma. Blackwell, UK: Oxford.

Frith, U., & Happé, F. (1994). Autism: Beyond "theory of mind". *Cognition, 50*(1), 115–132. doi:10.1016/0010-0277(94)90024-8 PMID:8039356

Golan, O., & Baron-Cohen, S. (2014). Systemizing emotions: Using interactive multimedia as a teaching tool. In K. D. Buron & P. Wolfberg (Eds.), *Learners on the autism spectrum Preparing highlight qualified educators and related practitioners* (2nd ed.; pp. 315–335). Shawnee Mission, KS: AAPC Publishing.

Golubock, S. J. (2009). What we don't know (about relationships) CAN hurt us: The hazards of not understanding, relating to and communicating with others. *Autism Advocate, 54*(1), 55–58.

Good Karma Applications. (2014). *Visual schedule planner.* Retrieved on July 5, 2014 from http://www.goodkarmaapplications.com

Gray, C. (2000). *The original Social Story™ book: Illustrated edition.* Arlington, TX: Future Horizons.

Gresham, F. M., Van, M. B., & Cook, C. R. (2006). Social skills training for teaching replacement behaviors: Remediating acquisition deficits in at-risk students. *Behavioral Disorders, 31*, 363–377.

Groden, J., Kantor, A., Woodard, C., & Lipsitt, L. (2011). *How everyone on the autism spectrum, young and old, can become resilient, be more optimistic, enjoy humor, be kind, and increase self-efficacy: A positive psychology approach.* London: Jessica Kingsley Publishers.

Happé, F. (1999). Autism: Cognitive deficit or cognitive style? *Trends in Cognitive Sciences, 3*(6), 216–222. doi:10.1016/S1364-6613(99)01318-2 PMID:10354574

Happé, F., & Frith, U. (2006). The weak coherence account: Detail-focused cognitive style in autism spectrum disorders. *Journal of Autism and Developmental Disorders, 36*(1), 5–25. doi:10.1007/s10803-005-0039-0 PMID:16450045

Hutchins, T., & Prelock, P. (2013). Parents' perceptions of their children's social behavior: The social validity of Social Stories™ and Comic Strip Conversations™. *Journal of Positive Behavior Interventions, 15*(3), 156–168. doi:10.1177/1098300712457418

Iland, E. (2011). *Drawing a blank: Improving comprehension for readers on the autism spectrum.* Shawnee Mission, KS: AAPC Publishing.

InGenius Labs. (2012). *Emotion detective.* Perth, Australia: Author.

Jarrold, C., Butler, D. W., Cottington, E. M., & Jimenez, F. (2000). Linking theory of mind and central coherence bias in autism and in the general population. *Developmental Psychology, 36*(1), 126–138. doi:10.1037/0012-1649.36.1.126 PMID:10645750

Kanne, S. M., & Mazurek, M. O. (2011). Aggression in children and adolescents with ASD: Prevalence and risk factors. *Journal of Autism and Developmental Disorders, 41*(7), 926–937. doi:10.1007/s10803-010-1118-4 PMID:20960041

Kaplan, J. S., & Carter, J. (1995). *Beyond behavior modification: A cognitive-behavioral approach to management in the school* (3rd ed.). Austin, TX: Pro-Ed.

Kerr, S., & Durkin, K. (2004). Understanding of thought bubble as mental representations in children with autism: Implications for theory of mind. *Journal of Autism and Developmental Disorders*, *34*(6), 637–648. doi:10.1007/s10803-004-5285-z PMID:15679184

Koenig, K., De Los Reyes, A., Cicchetti, D., Scahill, L., & Klin, A. (2009). Group intervention to promote social skills in school-age children with pervasive developmental: Reconsidering disorder efficacy. *Journal of Autism and Developmental Disorders*, *39*, 1163–1172. doi:10.1007/s10803-009-0728-1 PMID:19326199

Koyama, T., & Wang, H. (2011). Use of activity schedules to promote independent performance of individuals with autism and other intellectual disabilities: A review. *Research in Developmental Disabilities*, *32*(6), 2235–2242. doi:10.1016/j.ridd.2011.05.003 PMID:21645988

LaCava, P., Golan, O., Baron-Cohen, S., & Myles, B. S. (2007). Using assistive technology to teach emotion recognition to students with Asperger Syndrome. *Remedial and Special Education*, *28*(3), 174–181. doi:10.1177/07419325070280030601

Langstrom, N., Grann, M., Richkin, V., Sjostedt, G., & Fazel, S. (2009). Risk factors for violent offending in autism spectrum disorder: A national study of hospitalized individuals. *Journal of Interpersonal Violence*, *24*(8), 1358–1370. doi:10.1177/0886260508322195 PMID:18701743

Lequia, J., Machalicek, W., & Rispoli, M. J. (2012). Effects of activity schedules on challenging behavior exhibited in children with autism spectrum disorders: A systematic review. *Research in Autism Spectrum Disorders*, *6*(1), 480–492. doi:10.1016/j.rasd.2011.07.008

Loomis, J. W. (2008). *Staying in the game: Providing social opportunities for children and adolescents with autism spectrum disorders and other developmental disabilities*. Shawnee Mission, KS: AAPC Publishing.

Loth, E., Gómez, J. C., & Happé, F. (2008). Event schemas in autism spectrum disorders: The role of theory of mind and weak central coherence. *Journal of Autism and Developmental Disorders*, *38*(3), 449–463. doi:10.1007/s10803-007-0412-2 PMID:17668309

Marano, H. E. (July 1, 2003). *Dangers of loneliness*. Retrieved June 24, 2014 from http://www.psychologytoday.com/articles/200308/the-dangers-loneliness

Mat, S. J., Zhang, D., & Pacha, J. (2012). Employability skills valued by employers as important for entry-level employees with and without disabilities. *Career Development and Transition for Exceptional Individuals*, *35*(1), 29–38. doi:10.1177/0885728811419167

Mataya, K., & Owens, P. (2013). *Successful problem-solving for high-functioning students with autism spectrum disorder*. Shawnee Mission, KS: AAPC Publishing.

Matson, J. L., & Nebel-Schwalm, M. S. (2007). Comorbid psychopathology with autism spectrum disorder in children: An overview. *Research in Developmental Disabilities*, *28*(4), 341–352. doi:10.1016/j.ridd.2005.12.004 PMID:16765022

Mayo Clinic Staff. (2014, February 15). *Friendships: Enrich your life and improve your health*. Retrieved June 24, 2014, from http://www.mayoclinic.org/healthy-living/adult-health/in-depth/friendships/art-20044860?pg=1

Model Me Kids. (2010). *Model me going places* (2nd ed.). Rockville, MD: Author. Retrieved on June 20, 2014 from http://www.modelmekids.com/autism_aspergers_faq.html

Murphy, D. (2003). Admission and cognitive details of male patients diagnosed with Asperger's syndrome detained in a special hospital: Comparison with a schizophrenia and personality disorder sample. *Journal of Forensic Psychiatry & Psychology, 14*(3), 506–524. doi:10.1080/14789940031000152736

Myles, B. S. (2005). *Children and youth with Asperger Syndrome: Strategies for success in inclusive settings*. Thousand Oaks, CA: Corwin Press.

Myles, B. S., Endow, J., & Mayfield, M. (2013). *The hidden curriculum of getting a keeping a job: Navigating the social landscape of employment*. Shawnee Mission, KS: AAPC Publishing.

Myles, B. S., Endow, J., & Mayfield, M. (2013). *The hidden curriculum of getting and keeping a job: Navigating the social landscape of employment. A guide for individuals with autism spectrum disorders and other social-cognitive challenges*. Shawnee Mission, KS: AAPC Publishing.

Myles, B. S., & Southwick, J. (2005). *Asperger Syndrome and difficult moments: Practical solutions for tantrums, rage, and melt- downs* (2nd ed.). Shawnee Mission, KS: AAPC Publishing.

Myles, B. S., Trautman, M. L., & Schelvan, R. L. (2013). *The hidden curriculum: Practical solutions for understanding unstated rules in social situations* (2nd ed.). Shawnee Mission, KS: AAPC Publishing.

Myles, H. M., & Kolar, A. (2013). *The hidden curriculum and other everyday challenges for elementary-age children with high-functioning autism*. Shawnee Mission, KS: AAPC Publishing.

National Autism Center. (2009). *National standards report: Addressing the need for evidence-based practice guidelines for autism spectrum disorders*. Randolph, MA: Author.

National Professional Development Center on Autism Spectrum Disorders. (nd). *Evidence based practice briefs*. Retrieved April 10, 2014 from http://autismpdc.fpg.unc.edu/content/briefs

Quek, L., Sofronoff, K., Sheffield, J., White, A., & Kelly, A. (2012). Co-occurring anger in young people with Asperger's syndrome. *Journal of Clinical Psychology, 68*(10), 1142–1148. doi:10.1002/jclp.21888 PMID:22806337

Renzaglia, A., Karvonen, M., Drasgow, E., & Stoxen, C. C. (2003). Promoting a lifetime of inclusion. *Focus on Autism and Other Developmental Disabilities, 18*(3), 140–149. doi:10.1177/10883576030180030201

Rogers, M. F., & Myles, B. S. (2001). Using Social Stories™ and Comic Strip Conversations™ to interpret social situations for an adolescent with Asperger Syndrome. *Intervention in School and Clinic, 36*(5), 310–313. doi:10.1177/105345120103600510

Smith, S. M., Myles, B. S., Aspy, R., Grossman, B. G., & Henry, S. A. (2010). Sustainable change in quality of life for individuals with ASD: Using a comprehensive planning process. *Focus on Exceptional Children, 43*(3), 1–24.

Spivack, G., Platt, J. J., & Shure, M. (1976). *The problem-solving approach to adjustment.* San Francisco: Jossey-Bass.

Tantam, D. (2000). Psychological disorder in adolescents and adults with Asperger syndrome. *Autism, 4*(1), 47–62. doi:10.1177/1362361300004001004

9. th Planet LLC. (2013). *9th planet.* Stillwater, MN: Author. Retrieved June 10, 2014 from http://www.9thplanet.org/products.html

VividApps. (2008). *Strip designer.* Copenhagen, Denmark: Author. Available from iTunes.

Wilson, K. P. (2013). Incorporating video modeling into a school-based intervention for students with autism spectrum disorders. *Language, Speech, and Hearing Services in Schools, 44*(1), 105–117. doi:10.1044/0161-1461(2012/11-0098) PMID:23087158

Wimmer, H., & Perner, J. (1983). Beliefs about beliefs: Representation and constraining function of wrong beliefs in young children's understanding of deception. *Cognition, 13*(1), 103–128. doi:10.1016/0010-0277(83)90004-5 PMID:6681741

Winner, M. G. (2008). *Think social: A social thinking curriculum for school-age students for teaching social thinking and related social skills to students with high-functioning autism, Asperger syndrome, PDD-NOS, ADHD, nonverbal learning disability, and for all others in the murky gray area of social thinking.* San Jose, CA: Think Social Publishing.

Compilation of References

9. ᵗʰ Planet LLC. (2013). *9ᵗʰ planet*. Stillwater, MN: Author. Retrieved June 10, 2014 from http://www.9thplanet.org/products.html

AAC TechConnect. (n.d.). *AAC TechConnect*. Retrieved April 3, 2015 from http://www.aactechconnect.com

AAPC Publishing, Inc. (2010). Hidden curriculum on the go for adolescents and adults. Shawnee Mission, KS: AAPC Publishing. Available from iTunes.

AAPC Publishing, Inc. (2010). Hidden curriculum on the go for kids. Shawnee Mission, KS: AAPC Publishing. Available from iTunes.

Abbott, C., Brown, D., Evett, L., Standen, P., & Wright, J. (2011). *Learning difference and digital technologies: A literature review of research involving children and young people using assistive technologies 2007-2010*. Retrieved from www.kcl.ac.uk/sspp/departments/education/research/crestem/steg/recentproj/assistivetech.aspx

Abirached, B., Zhang, Y., Aggarwal, J. K., Tamersoy, B., Fernandes, T., Miranda, J. C., & Orvalho, V. (2011, November). Improving communication skills of children with ASDs through interaction with virtual characters. In *Serious Games and Applications for Health (SeGAH), 2011 IEEE 1st International Conference on* (pp. 1-4). IEEE. doi:10.1109/SeGAH.2011.6165464

Ablenet. (n.d.). *Ablenet*. Retrieved April 3 from http://www.ablenetinc.com

Abraham, A., Windmann, S., Siefen, R., Daum, I., & Gunturkun, O. (2006). Creative thinking in adolescents with attention deficit hyperactivity disorder (ADHD). *Child Neuropsychology: A Journal on Normal and Abnormal Development in Childhood and Adolescence, 12*(2), 111 – 123.

Achmadi, D., Kagohara, D., van der Meer, L., O'Reilly, M. F., Lancioni, G. E., Sutherland, D., & Sigafoos, J. et al. (2012). Teaching advanced operation of an iPod-based speech-generating device to two students with autism spectrum disorders. *Research in Autism Spectrum Disorders, 6*(4), 1258–1264. doi:10.1016/j.rasd.2012.05.005

Achmadi, D., Sigafoos, J., van der Meer, L., Sutherland, D., Lancioni, G. E., O'Reilly, M. F., & Marschik, P. B. et al. (2014). Acquisition, preference, and follow-up data on the use of three AAC options by four boys with developmental disability/delay. *Journal of Developmental and Physical Disabilities, 26*(5), 565–583. doi:10.1007/s10882-014-9379-z

Adams, R., Finn, P., Moes, E., Flannery, K., & Rizzo, A. (2009). Distractibility in Attention/Deficit/ hyperactivity disorder (ADHD): The virtual reality classroom. *Child Neuropsychology, 15*(2), 120–135. doi:10.1080/09297040802169077 PMID:18608217

Alberto, P. A., Fredrick, L., Hughes, M., McIntosh, L., & Cihak, D. (2007). Components of visual literacy: Teaching logos. *Focus on Autism and Other Developmental Disabilities, 22*(4), 234–243. doi:10.1177/10883576070220040501

Alberto, P., Cihak, D., & Gama, R. (2005). Use of static picture prompts versus video modeling during simulation instruction. *Research in Developmental Disabilities, 26*(4), 327–339. doi:10.1016/j.ridd.2004.11.002 PMID:15766627

Alberto, P., & Troutman, A. (2009). *Applied behavior analysis for teachers* (8th ed.). Upper Saddle River, NJ: Prentice Hall.

Alisauskas, A., & Simkiene, G. (2013). Teachers' experiences in educating pupils having behavioural and/or emotional problems. *Specialusis Ugdymas, 28*, 62–72.

Allen, A. A., & Shane, H. (2014). Autism spectrum disorders in the era of mobile technologies: Impact on caregivers. *Developmental Neurorehabilitation, 17*(2), 110–114. doi:10.3109/17518423.2014.882425 PMID:24694311

Alliano, A., Herriger, K., Koustsoftas, A. D., & Bartlotta, T. E. (2012). A review of 21 iPad applications for augmentative and alternative communication purposes. *SIG 12 Perspectives on Augmentative and Alternative Communication, 21*(2), 60-71. doi:10.1044/aac21.2.60

Allington, R. L. (1977). If they don't read much, how they ever gonna get good? *Journal of Reading, 21*, 57–61.

Allington, R. L. (2012). *What really matters for struggling readers* (3rd ed.). Boston, MA: Pearson.

Allington, R. L., & McGill-Franzen, A. (2009). Comprehension difficulties among struggling readers. In S. E. Duffy & G. G. Duffy (Eds.), *Handbook of research on reading comprehension* (pp. 551–568). New York, NY: Routledge.

Altman, D. G. (1999). *Practical statistics for medical research*. Bristol, UK: Chapman & Hall.

American Music Therapy Association. (n.d.). *American Music Therapy Association*. Retrieved February 24, 2014, from http://www.musictherapy.org/

American Psychiatric Association. (2013). *Diagnostic and statistical manual of mental disorders* (5th ed.). Arlington, VA: American Psychiatric Publishing.

American Psychiatric Association. (2013). DSM 5. American Psychiatric Association.

American Speech-Language-Hearing Association. (1997-2014). *History of ASHA*. Retrieved 08/04/2014, 2014, from http://www.asha.org/about/history/

American Speech-Language-Hearing Association. (2001). *Roles and responsibilities of speech-language pathologists with respect to reading and writing in children and adolescents* [Guidelines]. Retrieved on April, 3, 2015 from http://www.asha.org/policy/GL2001-00062. htm#sthash.3521rREs.dpuf

American Speech-Language-Hearing Association. (2004). *Roles and responsibilities of speech-language pathologists with respect to augmentative and alternative communication: technical report* [Technical Report]. Available from www.asha.org/policy

An, H., & Alon, S. (2013). iPad implementation models in K-12 school environments: An exploratory study. In R. McBride & M. Searson (Eds.), *Proceedings of Society for Information Technology & Teacher Education International Conference 2013* (pp. 3005-3011). Chesapeake, VA: AACE.

Anderson, K., Balandin, S., & Stancliffe, R. (2014). Australian parents' experiences of speech generating device (SGD) service delivery. *Developmental Neurorehabilitation, 17*(2), 75–83. doi:10.3109/17518423.2013.857735 PMID:24304229

Announcing the AAC-RERC white paper on mobile devices and communication apps. (2001). *Augmentative and Alternative Communication, 27*(2), 131-132.

Antia, S. D., & Stinson, M. S. (1999). Some conclusions on the education of deaf and hard-of-hearing students in inclusive settings. *Journal of Deaf Studies and Deaf Education, 4*(3), 246–248. doi:10.1093/deafed/4.3.246 PMID:15579892

Armburster, B. B., Lehr, F., & Osborn, J. (2001). *Put reading first: The research building blocks for teaching children to read kindergarten through grade three*. Jessup, MD: National Institute for Literacy.

Aronin, S., & Floyd, K. K. (2013). Using an iPad in inclusive preschool classrooms to introduce STEM concepts. *Teaching Exceptional Children, 45*(4), 34–39.

Artemenko, S. (2014). App-titude: Apps that excite our youngest clients: These interactive apps feature visuals that make word-learning and talking fun for tots. *The ASHA Leader, 19*(2), 38–39. doi:10.1044/leader. APP.19022014.38

Arthur-Kelly, M., Foreman, P., Bennett, D., & Pascoe, S. (2008). Interaction, inclusion and students with profound and multiple disabilities: Towards an agenda for research and practice. *Journal of Research in Special Educational Needs, 8*(3), 161–166. doi:10.1111/j.1471-3802.2008.00114.x

Articulate Instruments, Ltd. (2013a). *EPG Products*. Retrieved 08/08/2014, 2014, from http://www.articulateinstruments.com/epg-products/

Articulate Instruments, Ltd. (2013b). *A History of EPG*. Retrieved 08/07/2014, 2014, from http://www.articulateinstruments.com/a-history-of-epg/

Arvedson, J. C. (2008). Assessment of pediatric dysphagia and feeding disorders: Clinical and instrumental approaches. *Developmental Disabilities Research Reviews*, *14*(2), 118–127. doi:10.1002/ddrr.17 PMID:18646015

ASHA, American Speech Language Hearing Association. (2014). *Augmentative and Alternative Communication (AAC)*. Retrieved 08/01/2014, 2014, from http://www.asha.org/public/speech/disorders/AAC.htm

Aslan, S., & Reigeluth, C. M. (2011). A trip to the past and future of educational computing: Understanding its evolution. *Contemporary Educational Technology*, *2*(1), 1–17.

Asselin, M. (2001). Literacy and technology. *Teacher Librarian*, *28*(3), 49–51.

Assistive Technology Act of 2004, H.R. 4278, 108th Cong. 2004.

Assistive Technology Products and Special Ed Curriculum for Persons with Disabilities. (n.d.). *Assistive Technology Products and Special Ed Curriculum for Persons with Disabilities*. Retrieved June 17, 2014, from http://www.ablenetinc.com/

Astington, J. W., & Edward, M. J. (2010). The development of theory of mind in early childhood. *Social Cognition in Infancy*, *5*, 1–6.

Attainment Company. (n.d.). *Attainment Company*. Retrieved April 3, 2015 from http://www.attainmentcompany.com/assistive-technology

Atticks, A. H. (2012). Therapy Session 2.0: From static to dynamic with the iPad. *SIG 15 Perspectives on Gerontology*, *17*(3), 84-93.

Austin, D. W., Abbott, J. A. M., & Carbis, C. (2008). The use of virtual reality hypnosis with two cases of autism spectrum disorder: A feasibility study. *Contemporary Hypnosis*, *25*(2), 102–109. doi:10.1002/ch.349

Australian Institute of Health and Welfare (AIHW). (2008). *Disability in Australia: Intellectual disability*. Canberra: AIHW.

Avaz Free Speech. (2014). *Avaz Free Speech*. Retrieved 08/12/2014, 2014, from http://avazapp.com/freespeech/

Avaz Together. (n.d.). *Avaz Together*. Retrieved April 3, 2015 from http://www.avazapp.com/features/

Ayres, K. M., Mechling, L., & Sansosti, F. J. (2013). The use of mobile technologies to assist with life skills/independence of students with moderate/severe intellectual disability and/or autism spectrum disorders: Considerations for the future of school psychology. *Psychology in the Schools*, *50*(3), 259–271. doi:10.1002/pits.21673

Bacsfalvi, P., & Bernhardt, B. M. (2011). Long-term outcomes of speech therapy for seven adolescents with visual feedback technologies: Ultrasound and electropalatography. *Clinical Linguistics & Phonetics*, *25*(11/12), 1034–1043. doi:10.3109/02699206.2011.61 8236 PMID:22106893

Badcock, J. C., & Chhabra, S. (2013). Voices to reckon with: Perceptions of voice identity in clinical and non-clinical voice hearers. *Frontiers in Human Neuroscience*, *7*. doi:10.3389/fnhum.2013.00114 PMID:23565088

Bagatell, N. (2010). From cure to community: Transforming notions of autism. *Ethos (Berkeley, Calif.)*, *38*(1), 33–55. doi:10.1111/j.1548-1352.2009.01080.x

Baharav, E., & Reiser, C. (2010). Using Telepractice in Parent Training in Early Autism. *Telemedicine Journal and e-Health*, *16*(6), 727–731. doi:10.1089/tmj.2010.0029 PMID:20583950

Baker, B. R. (2009). *MinspeakTM History*. Retrieved 08/15/2014, 2014, from http://www.minspeak.com/HistoryofMinspeak.php#.U-yIylYivuc

Balandin, S., & Iacono, T. (1999). Crews, wusses, and whoppas: Core and fringe vocabularies of Australian meal-break conversations in the workplace. *Augmentative and Alternative Communication*, *15*(2), 95–109. doi:10.1080/07434619912331278605

Balfanz, R. (2009). *Putting middle grades students on the graduation path: A policy and practice brief*. Westerville, OH: National Middle School Association.

Balfe, M., & Tantam, D. (2010). A descriptive social and health profile of a community sample of adults and adolescents with Asperger syndrome. *BMC Research Notes*, *3*(1), 300–307. doi:10.1186/1756-0500-3-300 PMID:21070680

Banajee, M., Dicarlo, C., & Burass Stricklin, S. (2003). Core vocabulary determination for toddlers. *Augmentative and Alternative Communication*, *19*(2), 67–73. doi:10.1080/0743461031000112034

Bandura, A. (1977). *Social learning theory*. Englewood Cliffs, NJ: Prentice Hall.

Barkley, R. A., Murphy, K. R., O'Connell, T., Anderson, D., & Connor, D. F. (2006). Effects of two doses of alcohol on simulator driving performance in adults with attention-deficit/hyperactivity disorder. *Neuropsychology*, *20*(1), 77–87. doi:10.1037/0894-4105.20.1.77 PMID:16460224

Barlow, D. H., Nock, M., & Hersen, M. (2009). *Single case experimental designs: Strategies for studying behavior change* (3rd ed.). New York: Allyn and Bacon.

Barnes, C. (2004). "Reflections on Doing Emancipatory Disability Research." In J. Swain, S. French, C. Barnes, C. Thomas (Eds.), Disabling Barriers--Enabling Environments (pp. 47-53). London: Sage Publications.

Barnhill, G. (2001). Social attributions and depression in adolescents with Asperger syndrome. *Focus on Autism and Other Developmental Disabilities*, *16*(1), 46–53. doi:10.1177/108835760101600112

Baron-Cohen, S. (1997). *Mindblindness: An essay on autism and theory of mind*. MIT Press.

Baron-Cohen, S., Ashwin, E., Ashwin, C., Tavassoli, T., & Chakrabarti, B. (2009). Talent in autism: Hyper-systemizing, hyper-attention to detail and sensory hyper-sensitivity. *Philosophical Transactions of the Royal Society of London. Series B, Biological Sciences*, *364*(1522), 1377–1383. doi:10.1098/rstb.2008.0337 PMID:19528020

Baron-Cohen, S., Leslie, A. M., & Frith, U. (1985). Does the autistic child have theory of mind? *Cognition*, *21*(1), 37–46. doi:10.1016/0010-0277(85)90022-8 PMID:2934210

Barreca, S., Velikonja, D., Brown, L., Williams, L., Davis, L., & Sigouin, C. S. (2003). Evaluation of the effectiveness of two clinical training procedures to elicit yes/no responses from patients with a severe acquired brain injury: A randomized single-subject design. *Brain Injury: [BI]*, *17*(12), 1065–1075. doi:10.1080/0269905031000110535 PMID:14555365

Barzilay, Z., & Hasharon, R. (2006). United States Patent No. 0259304A1.

Bat-Chava, Y., & Deignan, E. (2004). Peer relationships of children with cochlear implants. Oxford University Press, 6 (3), 186 – 199.

Bavelier, D., & Hirshorn, E. A. (2010). I see where you're hearing: How cross-modal plasticity may exploit homologous brain structures. *Nature Neuroscience*, *13*(11), 1309–1311. doi:10.1038/nn1110-1309 PMID:20975752

Baxter, H. T., Berghofer, J. A., MacEwan, L., Nelson, J., Peters, K., & Roberts, P. (2007). *The individualized music therapy assessment profile: IMTAP*. Jessica Kingsley Publishers.

Baxter, S., Enderby, P., Evans, P., & Judge, S. (2012a). Barriers and facilitators to the use of high-technology augmentative and alternative communication devices: A systematic review and qualitative synthesis. *International Journal of Communication Disorders*, *47*(2), 115–129. doi:10.1111/j.1460-6984.2011.00090.x PMID:22369053

Baxter, S., Enderby, P., Evans, P., & Judge, S. (2012b). Interventions using high-technology communication devices: A state of the art review. *Folia Phoniatrica et Logopaedica*, *64*(3), 137–144. doi:10.1159/000338250 PMID:22653226

Bean, T. W. (2000). Reading in the content areas: Social constructivist dimensions. In M. L. Kamil, P. B. Mosenthal, P. D. Pearson, & R. Barr (Eds.), *Handbook of reading research* (Vol. 3, pp. 629–654). Mahwah, NJ: Erlbaum.

Beaumont, R., & Sofronoff, K. (2008). A multi-component social skills intervention for children with Asperger syndrome: The Junior Detective Training Program. *Journal of Child Psychology and Psychiatry, and Allied Disciplines*, *49*(7), 743–753. doi:10.1111/j.1469-7610.2008.01920.x PMID:18503531

Bedesem, P. L. (2012). Using cell phone technology for self-monitoring procedures in inclusive settings. *Journal of Special Education Technology*, *27*(4), 33–46.

Begnoche, D., & Pitetti, K. H. (2007). Ef- fects of traditional treatment and partial body weight treadmill training on the motor skills of children with spastic cerebral palsy: A pilot study. *Pediatric Physical Therapy*, *19*(1), 11–19. doi:10.1097/01.pep.0000250023.06672. b6 PMID:17304093

Behrmann, M. (1998). *Assistive Technology for Young Children In Special Education*. Association for Supervision and Curriculum Development. Retrieved June 1, 2014, from http://www.edutopia.org/assistive-technology-young-children-special-education

Behrmann, M., Thomas, C., & Humphreys, K. (2006). Seeing it differently: Visual processing in autism. *Trends in Cognitive Sciences*, *10*(6), 258–264. doi:10.1016/j. tics.2006.05.001 PMID:16713326

Beirne-Smith, M., Patton, J. R., & Kim, S. H. (2006). *Mental Retardation. An introduction to intellectual disabilities*. United States of America: Pearson Prentice Hall.

Bekele, E., Crittendon, J. A., Swanson, A., Sarkar, N., & Warren, Z. E. (2013). Pilot clinical application of an adaptive robotic system for young children with autism. *Autism*, 1362361313479454. PMID:24104517

Bellini, S. (2006). *Building social relationships: A systematic approach to teaching social interaction skills to children and adolescents with autism spectrum disorders and other social difficulties*. Shawnee Mission, KS: AAPC Publishing Company.

Bellini, S. (2008). *Building social relationship: A systematic approach to teaching social interaction skills to children and adolescents with autism spectrum disorders and other social difficulties*. Shawnee Mission, KS: Autism Asperger Publishing.

Bellini, S., & Akullian, J. (2007). A meta-analysis of video modeling and video self-monitoring interventions for children and adolescents with autism spectrum disorders. *Exceptional Children*, *73*(3), 264–287. doi:10.1177/001440290707300301

Bellini, S., Peters, J. K., Benner, L., & Hopf, A. (2007). A meta-analysis of school-based social skills interventions for children with autism spectrum disorders. *Remedial and Special Education*, *28*(3), 153–162. doi:10.1177/07 419325070280030401

Bellon-Harn, M. L., & Harn, W. E. (2008). Scaffolding Strategies During Repeated Storybook Reading An Extension Using a Voice Output Communication Aid. *Focus on Autism and Other Developmental Disabilities*, *23*(2), 112–124. doi:10.1177/1088357608316606

Benford, P. (2008). *The use of Internet-based communication by people with autism*. Doctoral dissertation, University of Nottingham.

Berger, D. S. (2009, March). On Developing Music Therapy Goals and Objectives©. In *Voices: A World Forum for Music Therapy* (Vol. 9, No. 1).

Berger, J. (1995). Self-instruction: Lessons from Charlotte. *LD Forum*, *20*, 20-22.

Berg, P., Becker, T., Martian, A., Danielle, P. K., & Wingen, J. (2012). Motor control outcomes following Nintendo Wii use by a child with Down syndrome. *Pediatric Physical Therapy*, *24*(1), 78–84. doi:10.1097/ PEP.0b013e31823e05e6 PMID:22207475

Berthoz, S., & Hill, E. L. (2004). The validity of using self-reports to assess emotion regulation abilities. *European Psychiatry*, *20*(3), 291–298. doi:10.1016/j. eurpsy.2004.06.013 PMID:15935431

Beschorner, B., & Hutchinson, A. (2013). iPads as a literacy teaching tool in early childhood. *International Journal of Education in Mathematics, Science, and Technology*, *1*(1), 16–24.

Beukelman, D. R., & Mirenda, P. (1998). Augmentative and alternative communication: management of severe communication disorders in children and adults (2nd ed.). Paul H. Brooks Publishing Co., Inc.

Beukelman, D., & Mirenda, P. (1989). *Augmentative and Alternative Communication: Management of Severe Communication Impairments*. Baltimore: Brookes Publishing.

Beukelman, D., & Mirenda, P. (2013). *Augmentative and alternative communication: Supporting children and adults with complex communication needs* (4th ed.). Baltimore: Paul H. Brookes Publishing Co.

Biancarosa, G., & Snow, C. E. (2006). *Reading next — A vision for action and research in middle and high school literacy: A report to Carnegie Corporation of New York* (2nd ed.). Washington, DC: Alliance for Excellent Education.

Bidwell, M. A., & Rehfeldt, R. A. (2004). Using video modeling to teach a domestic skill with an embedded social skill to adults with severe mental retardation. *Behavioral Interventions*, *19*(4), 263–274. doi:10.1002/bin.165

Bidwell, M., Biederman, G. B., & Freedman, B. (2007). Modeling skills, signs and lettering for children with down syndrome, autism, and other severe developmental delays by video instruction in classroom setting. *Journal of Early and Intensive Behavior Intervention*, *4*(4), 736–743. doi:10.1037/h0100403

Bieber, J. (1994). *Learning disabilities and social skills with Richard LaVoie: Last one picked ... first one picked on* [DVD]. Washington, DC: Public Broadcasting Service.

Bigby, C., Patsey, F., & Ramcharan, P. (2014). Conceptualising inclusive research with people with intellectual disability. *Journal of Applied Research in Intellectual Disabilities*, *27*(1), 3–12. doi:10.1111/jar.12083 PMID:24390972

Billstedt, E., Gillberg, C., & Gillberg, C. (2005). Autism after adolescence: Population-based 13- to 22-year follow-up study of 120 individuals with autism diagnosed in childhood. *Journal of Autism and Developmental Disorders*, *35*(3), 351–360. doi:10.1007/s10803-005-3302-5 PMID:16119476

Binger, C., Kent-Walsh, J., Ewing, C., & Taylor, S. (2010). Teaching educational assistants to facilitate the multisymbol message productions of young students who require augmentative and alternative communication. *American Journal of Speech-Language Pathology*, *19*(2), 108–120. doi:10.1044/1058-0360(2009/09-0015) PMID:19948759

Binger, C., & Light, J. (2006). Demographics of preschoolers who require AAC. *Language, Speech, and Hearing Services in Schools*, *37*(3), 200–208. doi:10.1044/0161-1461(2006/022) PMID:16837443

Bitstrips, Inc. (2014). *Bitstrips*. Ontario, Canada: Author. Available from iTunes.

Blachowicz, C. L., Fisher, P. J., Ogle, D., & Watts-Taffe, S. (2006). Vocabulary: Questions from the classroom. *Reading Research Quarterly*, *41*(4), 524–539. doi:10.1598/RRQ.41.4.5

Blischak, D. M., Lombardino, L. J., & Dyson, A. T. (2003). Use of speech-generating devices: In support of natural speech. *Augmentative and Alternative Communication*, *19*(1), 29–35. doi:10.1080/0743461032000056478

Blischak, D. M., Shah, S. D., Lombardino, L. J., & Chiarella, K. (2004). Effects of phonemic awareness instruction on the encoding skills of children with severe speech impairment. *Disability and Rehabilitation*, *26*(21-22), 1295–1304. doi:10.1080/09638280412331280325 PMID:15513729

Blischak, D., Lloyd, L., & Fuller, D. (1997). Terminology issues. In L. Lloyd, D. Fuller, & H. Arvidson (Eds.), *Augmentative and alternative communication: A handbook of principles and practices* (pp. 38–42). Boston: Allyn & Bacon.

Blood, E., Johnson, J. W., Ridenour, L., Simmons, K., & Crouch, S. (2011). Using iPod Touch to teach social and self-management skills to an elementary student with emotional/behavioral disorders. *Education & Treatment of Children*, *34*(3), 299–322. doi:10.1353/etc.2011.0019

Boccanfuso, L., & O'Kane, J. M. (2011). CHARLIE: An adaptive robot design with hand and face tracking for use in autism therapy. *International Journal of Social Robotics*, *3*(4), 337–347. doi:10.1007/s12369-011-0110-2

Bock, M. A. (2001). SODA strategy: Enhancing the social interaction skills of youngsters with Asperger Syndrome. *Intervention in School and Clinic*, *36*(5), 272–278. doi:10.1177/105345120103600503

Bock, M. A. (2007a). A social behavioral learning strategy intervention for a child with Asperger Syndrome: A brief report. *Remedial and Special Education*, *28*(5), 258–265. doi:10.1177/07419325070280050101

Bock, M. A. (2007b). The impact of social behavioral learning strategy training on the social interaction skills of four students with Asperger syndrome. *Focus on Autism and Other Developmental Disabilities*, *22*(2), 88–95. doi:10.1177/10883576070220020901

Bock, S. J., Stoner, J. B., Beck, A. R., Hanley, L., & Prochnow, J. (2005). Increasing functional communication in nonspeaking preschool children: Comparison of PECS and VOCA. *Education and Training in Developmental Disabilities*, 40(3), 268–278.

Boddaert, N., Chabane, N., Belin, P., Bourgeois, N., Royer, V., Barthelémy, C., & Zilbovicius, M. et al. (2004). Perception of complex sounds in autism: Abnormal auditory cortical processing in children. *The American Journal of Psychiatry*, 161(11), 2117–2120. doi:10.1176/appi.ajp.161.11.2117 PMID:15514415

Boesch, M. C., Wendt, O., Subramanian, A., & Hsu, N. (2013). Comparative efficacy of the Picture Exchange Communication System (PECS) versus a speech-generating device: Effects on requesting skills. *Research in Autism Spectrum Disorders*, 7(3), 480–493. doi:10.1016/j.rasd.2012.12.002

Bogdashina, O. (2003). *Sensory perceptual issues in autism and Asperger Syndrome: different sensory experiences, different perceptual worlds*. London, UK: Jessica Kingsley Publishers.

Bondy, A. S., & Frost, L. (1994). The picture exchange communication system. *Focus on Autistic Behavior*, 16, 123–128. PMID:22478140

Borg, J., Larson, S., & Ostenberg, P. O. (2011). The right to assistive technology: For whom, for what, and by whom? *Disability & Society*, 26(2), 151–167. doi:10.1080/09687599.2011.543862

Boston Children's Hospital. (n. d.). *Augmentative communication program handouts and resources*. Retrieved August 13, 2014 from http://www.childrenshospital.org/centers-and-services/programs/a-_-e/augmentative-communication-program/downloads

Boucher, J. (2009). *The Autistic Spectrum. Characteristics, Causes and Practical Issues*. London: Sage Publications Ltd.

Bouck, E. C., Satsangi, R., Doughty, T. T., & Courtney, W. T. (2014). Virtual and Concrete Manipulatives: A Comparison of Approaches for Solving Mathematics Problems for Students with Autism Spectrum Disorder. *Journal of Autism and Developmental Disorders*, 44(1), 180–193. doi:10.1007/s10803-013-1863-2 PMID:23743958

Bouck, E. C., Shurr, J. C., Tom, K., Jasper, A. D., Bassette, L., Miller, B., & Flanagan, S. M. (2012). Fix it with TAPE: Repurposing technology to be assistive technology for students with high-incidence disabilities. *Preventing School Failure*, 56(2), 121–128. doi:10.1080/1045988X.2011.603396

Bowman, S. L., & Plourde, L. A. (2012). Andragogy for teen and young adult learners with intellectual disabilities: Learning, independence, and best practices. *Education*, 132(4), 789–798.

Braddock, D., Rizzolo, M. C., Thompson, M., & Bell, R. (2004). Emerging technologies and cognitive disability. *Journal of Special Education Technology*, 19(4), 49–56.

Bradshaw, J. (2013). The use of augmentative and alternative communication apps for the iPad, iPod, and iPhone: An overview of recent developments. *Tizard Learning Disability Review*, 18(1), 31–37. doi:10.1108/13595471311295996

Brady, L. (2012). iPad Apps can support evidence-based practice. *Speech Therapy for Autism: Technology, Speech Therapy and Autism*. Retrieved June 25, 2014, from http://proactivespeech.wordpress.com/author/proactivespeech/page/2/

Branch, M. (2014). Malignant side effects of nullhypothesis significance testing. *Theory & Psychology*, 24(2), 256–277. doi:10.1177/0959354314525282

Branson, D., & Demchak, M. (2009). The use of augmentative and alternative communication methods with infants and toddlers with disabilities: A research review. *Augmentative and Alternative Communication*, 25(4), 274–286. doi:10.3109/07434610903384529 PMID:19883287

Brashear, H., Henderson, V., Park, K. H., Hamilton, H., Lee, S., & Starner, T. (2006). American sign language recognition in game development for deaf children. *ASSETS*, 06, 79–84.

Brookes, N. A. (1998). *Models for understanding rehabilitation and assistive technology. Designing and using assistive technology. The human perspective*. Baltimore: Brookes.

Browder, D. M., Mims, P. J., Spooner, F., Ahlgrim-Delzell, L., & Lee, A. (2008). Teaching elementary students with multiple disabilities to participate in shared stories. *Research and Practice for Persons with Severe Disabilities, 33*(1-2), 3–12. doi:10.2511/rpsd.33.1-2.3

Browder, D. M., Spooner, F., Ahlgrim-Delzell, L., Harris, A., & Wakeman, S. (2008). A meta-analysis on teaching mathematics to students with significant cognitive disabilities. *Exceptional Children, 74*(4), 407–432.

Browder, D. M., Spooner, F., & Bingham, M. A. (2004). Current practices in alternate assessment and access to the general curriculum for students with severe disabilities in the United States of America. *Australasian Journal of Special Education, 28*(2), 17–29. doi:10.1080/1030011040280203

Browder, D. M., Wood, W. M., Test, D. W., Karvonen, M., & Algozzine, B. (2001). Reviewing resources on self-determination: A map for teachers. *Remedial and Special Education, 22*(4), 233–244. doi:10.1177/074193250102200407

Browder, D., Ahlgrim-Delzell, L., Spooner, F., Mims, P. J., & Baker, J. (2009). Using time delay to teach literacy to students with severe developmental disabilities. *Exceptional Children, 75*, 343–364.

Browder, D., Gibbs, S., Ahlgrim-Delzell, L., Courtade, G. R., Mraz, M., & Flowers, C. (2008). Literacy for students with severe developmental disabilities: What should we teach and what should we hope to achieve? *Remedial and Special Education, 30*(5), 269–282. doi:10.1177/0741932508315054

Brown, T., Prendergast, L., & Woodfin, L. (2011). Use of the iPad for students with significant intellectual disabilities. *Innovations and Perspectives.* http://www.ttacnews.vcu.edu/2011/09/use-of-the-ipad-for-students-with-significant-intellectual-disabilities/

Brown, C. (1954). *My left foot.* London: Secker & Warburg.

Brown, D. J., Standen, P. J., Proctor, T., & Sterland, D. (2001). Advanced design methodologies for the production of virtual learning environments for use by people with learning disabilities. *Presence (Cambridge, Mass.), 10*(4), 401–415. doi:10.1162/1054746011470253

Brozo, W. G., & Hargis, C. H. (2003). Taking seriously the idea of reform: One high school's efforts to make reading more responsive to all students. *Journal of Adolescent & Adult Literacy, 47*(1), 14–23. doi:10.1598/JAAL.47.1.3

Bruno-Dowling, S. (2012). *How many SLPs are really using iPads?* Retrieved June 26, 2014 http://community.advanceweb.com/blogs/sp_1/archive/2012/03/13/how-many-slps-are-really-using-ipads.aspx

Buehl, D. (2011). *Developing readers in the academic disciplines.* Newark, DE: International Reading Association.

Buggey, T., Toombs, K., Gardener, P., & Cervetti, M. (1999). Using videotaped self-modeling to train response behaviors in students with autism. *Journal of Positive Behavior Interventions, 1*, 205–214. doi:10.1177/109830079900100403

Buie, A. (2013). *Behavior mapping: A visual strategy for teaching appropriate behavior to individual with autism spectrum and related disabilities.* Shawnee Mission, KS: AAPC Publishing.

Bunnell, H. T., Pennington, C., Yarrington, D., & Gray, J. (2005). *Automatic personal synthetic voice construction.* Paper presented at the Eurospeech 2005, Lisbon, Portugal.

Bunt, L. (2003). Music therapy with children: A complementary service to music education? *British Journal of Music Education, 20*(02), 179–195. doi:10.1017/S0265051703005370

Burke, M., Kraut, R., & Williams, D. (2010). *Social use of computer-mediated communication by adults on the autism spectrum.* Paper presented at the 2010 ACM Conference on Computer Supported Cooperative Work, New York, NY.

Burke, R. V., Andersen, M. N., Bowen, S. L., Howard, M. R., & Allen, K. D. (2010). Evaluation of two instruction methods to increase employment options for young adults with autism spectrum disorders. *Research in Developmental Disabilities, 31*(6), 1223–1233. doi:10.1016/j.ridd.2010.07.023 PMID:20800988

Buron, K., & Curtis, M. B. (2012). The Incredible 5-Point Scale: The significantly improved and expanded second edition: Assisting students in understanding social interactions and controlling their emotional responses. Shawnee Mission, KS: AAPC Publishing.

Buron, K. D., & Myles, B. S. (2014). Emotional regulation. In K. D. Buron & P. Wolfberg (Eds.), *Learners on the autism spectrum Preparing highlight qualified educators and related practitioners* (2nd ed., pp. 239–263). Shawnee Mission, KS: AAPC Publishing.

Burton, C. E., Anderson, D. H., Prater, M. A., & Dyches, T. T. (2013). Video self-modeling on an iPad to teach functional math skills to adolescents with autism and intellectual disability. *Focus on Autism and Other Developmental Disabilities*, 28(2), 67–77. doi:10.1177/1088357613478829

Butler, S. R., Marsh, H. W., Sheppard, M. J., & Sheppard, J. L. (1985). Seven-year longitudinal study of the early prediction of reading achievement. *Journal of Educational Psychology*, 77(3), 349–361. doi:10.1037/0022-0663.77.3.349

Cabell, S. Q., Tortorelli, L. S., & Gerde, H. K. (2013). How do I write...? Scaffolding preschoolers' early writing skills. *The Reading Teacher*, 66(8), 650–659. doi:10.1002/trtr.1173

Calculator, S. N. (2013). Use and acceptance of AAC systems by children with Angelman Syndrome. *Journal of Applied Research in Intellectual Disabilities*, 26(6), 557–567. PMID:23606637

Campigotto, R., McEwin, R., & Epp, C. D. (2013). Especially social: Exploring the use of an iOS application in special needs classrooms. *Computers & Education*, 60(1), 74–86. doi:10.1016/j.compedu.2012.08.002

Cannella, H. I., O'Reilly, M. F., & Lancioni, G. E. (2005). Choice and preference assessment research with people with severe to profound developmental disabilities: A review of the literature. *Research in Developmental Disabilities*, 26(1), 1–15. doi:10.1016/j.ridd.2004.01.006 PMID:15590233

Cannella-Malone, H. I., Mizrachi, S. B., Sabielny, L. M., & Jimenez, E. D. (2013). Teaching physical activity to students with significant disabilities using video modeling. *Developmental Rehabilitation*, 16(3), 145–154. PMID:23477636

Cannella-Malone, H. I., Sigafoos, J., O'Reilly, M., De La Cruz, B., Edrisinha, C., & Lancioni, G. E. (2006). Comparing video prompting to video modeling for teaching daily living skills to six adults with developmental disabilities. *Education and Training in Developmental Disabilities*, 41, 344–356.

Cardon, T. (2012). Teaching caregivers to implement video modeling imitation training via iPad for their children with autism. *Research in Autism Spectrum Disorders*, 6(4), 1389–1400. doi:10.1016/j.rasd.2012.06.002

Card, R., & Dodd, B. (2006). The phonological awareness abilities of children with cerebral palsy who do not speak. *Augmentative and Alternative Communication*, 22(3), 149–159. doi:10.1080/07434610500431694 PMID:17114160

Carnahan, C. R., Basham, J. D., Christman, J., & Hollingshead, A. (2012). Overcoming challenges: Going mobile with your video models. *Teaching Exceptional Children*, 45, 50–59.

Caron, M. J., Mottron, L., Rainville, C., & Chouinard, S. (2004). Do high functioning persons with autism present with superior spatial abilities? *Neuropsychologia*, 42(4), 467–481. doi:10.1016/j.neuropsychologia.2003.08.015 PMID:14728920

CAST. (2011). *About UDL*. Retrieved from http://www.cast.org/udl/index.html

CDC, Centers for Disease Control and Prevention. (2013). *Cerebral Palsy, Data and Statistics*. Retrieved 08/04/2014, 2014, from http://www.cdc.gov/ncbddd/cp/data.html

CDC, Centers for Disease Control and Prevention. (2014). *Autism Spectrum Disorders - Data and Statistics*. Retrieved 08/04/2014, 2014, from http://www.cdc.gov/ncbddd/autism/data.html

Center for Disease Control and Prevention. (2010). *Spinal cord injury (SCI): Fact sheet*. Center for Disease Control and Prevention. Retrieved June 8, 2014, from http://www.cdc.gov/traumaticbraininjury/scifacts.html

Center for Disease Control and Prevention. (2014). *Attention-deficit/hyperactivity disorder*. Center for Disease Control and Prevention. Retrieved June 8, 2014, from http://www.cdc.gov/ncbddd/adhd/facts.html

Centers for Disease Control and Prevention. (2011). *Developmental disabilities*. Retrieved February 7, 2012, from http://www.cdc.gov/ncbddd/dd/default.htm

Centers for Disease Control and Prevention. (2014). *Developmental Disabilities Homepage*. Retrieved from: http://www.cdc.gov/ncbddd/developmentaldisabilities/specificconditions.html

Centers for Medicare and Medicaid Services. (2010). *Autism spectrum disorders: Final report on environmental scan*. Washington, DC: Author.

Chall, J. (1983). *Learning to Read: The Great Debate*. New York, NY: McGraw-Hill.

Chamak, B., Bonniau, B., Jaunay, E., & Cohen, D. (2008). What can we learn about autism from autistic persons? *Psychotherapy and Psychosomatics*, *77*(5), 271–279. doi:10.1159/000140086 PMID:18560252

Chan, J. M., Lambdin, L., Van Laarhoven, T., & Johnson, J. W. (2013). Teaching leisure skills to an adult with developmental disabilities using a video prompting intervention. *Education and Training in Autism and Developmental Disabilities*, *48*(3), 412–420.

Chantry, J., & Dunford, C. (2010). How do computer assistive technologies enhance participation in childhood occupations for children with multiple and complex disabilities? A review of the current literature. *British Journal of Occupational Therapy*, *73*(8), 351–365. doi:10.4276/030802210X12813483277107

Chapple, D. (2011). The evolution of augmentative communication and the importance of alternative access. *SIG 12 Perspectives on Augmentative and Alternative Communication, 20*(1), 34-37. doi:10.1044/aac20.1.34

Charlop-Christy, M. H., Carpenter, M., Le, L., LeBlanc, L. A., & Kellet, K. (2002). Using the picture exchange communication system (PECS) with children with autism: Assessment of PECS acquisition, speech, social-communicative behavior, and problem behavior. *Journal of Applied Behavior Analysis*, *35*(3), 213–231. doi:10.1901/jaba.2002.35-213 PMID:12365736

Charlop-Christy, M. H., Le, L., & Freeman, K. A. (2000). A comparison of video modeling with in vivo modeling for teaching children with autism. *Journal of Autism and Developmental Disorders*, *30*(6), 537–552. doi:10.1023/A:1005635326276 PMID:11261466

Chaves, E. S., Boninger, M. L., Cooper, R., Fitzgerald, S. G., Gray, D. B., & Cooper, R. A. (2004). Assessing the influence of wheelchair technology on perception of participation in spinal cord injury. *American Academy of Physical Medicine and Rehabilitation*, *85*, 1854–1858. PMID:15520981

Cheng, Y., & Chen, S. (2010). Improving social understanding of individuals of intellectual and developmental disabilities through a 3D-facial expression intervention program. *Research in Developmental Disabilities*, *31*(6), 1434–1442. doi:10.1016/j.ridd.2010.06.015 PMID:20674267

Cheng, Y., Chiang, H., Ye, J., & Cheng, L. (2010). Enhancing instruction using a collaborative virtual learning environment for children with autistic spectrum conditions. *Computers & Education*, *55*(4), 1449–1458. doi:10.1016/j.compedu.2010.06.008

Chiapparino, C., Stasolla, F., de Pace, C., & Lancioni, G. E. (2011). A touch pad and a scanning keyboard emulator to facilitate writing by a woman with extensive motor disability. *Life Span and Disdability*, *14*, 45–54.

Chi-Fishman, G., & Stone, M. (1996). A new application for electropalatography: Swallowing. *Dysphagia*, *11*(4), 239–247. doi:10.1007/BF00265208 PMID:8870350

Christakis, D. A. (2014). Interactive media use at younger than the age of 2 years: Time to rethink the *American Academy of Pediatrics Guideline? JAMA Pediatrics*, *168*(5), 399–400. doi:10.1001/jamapediatrics.2013.5081 PMID:24615347

Christiansen, J. B., & Leigh, I. W. (2004). Children with cochlear implants. *Archives of Otolaryngology--Head & Neck Surgery*, *130*(5), 673–677. doi:10.1001/archotol.130.5.673 PMID:15148196

Ciampa, K. (2014). Learning in the mobile age: An investigation of student motivation. *Journal of Computer Assisted Learning*, *30*(1), 82–96. doi:10.1111/jcal.12036

Cihak, D. F., Wright, R., & Ayres, K. M. (2010). Use of self-modeling static-picture prompts via a hand-held computer to facilitate self-monitory in the general education classroom. *Education and Training in Autism and Developmental Disabilities, 45,* 136–149.

Cihak, D., Fahrenkrog, C., Ayres, K., & Smith, C. (2010). The use of video modeling via a video iPod and a system of least prompts to improve transitional behaviors for students with autism spectrum disorders in the general education classroom. *Journal of Positive Behavior Interventions, 12*(2), 103–115. doi:10.1177/1098300709332346

Clancy, T. A., Rucklidge, J. J., & Owen, D. (2006). Road-crossing safety in virtual reality: A comparison of adolescents with and without ADHD. *Journal of Clinical Child and Adolescent Psychology, 35*(2), 203–215. doi:10.1207/s15374424jccp3502_4 PMID:16597216

Clawson, B., Selden, M., Lacks, M., Deaton, A. V., Hall, B., & Bach, R. (2008). Complex Pediatric Feeding Disorders: Using Teleconferencing Technology to Improve Access To a Treatment Program. *Pediatric Nursing, 34*(3), 213–216. PMID:18649810

Clay, M. (1993). *An observation survey of early literacy achievement.* Portsmouth, NH: Heinemann.

Cleft Lip and Cleft Palate. (n.d.). Retrieved Aug 30, 2014, from http://www.asha.org/public/speech/disorders/CleftLip/

Cochran, P. S., & Nelson, L. K. (1999). Technology applications in intervention for preschool-age children with language disorders. *Seminars in Speech and Language, 20*(3), 203–218. doi:10.1055/s-2008-1064018 PMID:10480492

Cohen, L., & Spenciner, L. J. (2005). *Teaching students with mild and moderate disabilities:Research-based practices.* Upper Saddle River, NJ: Pearson Merrill Prentice Hall.

Coleman, M. B. (2009). PowerPoint" Is Not Just for Business Presentations and College Lectures: Using" PowerPoint" to Enhance Instruction for Students with Disabilities. *Teaching Exceptional Children Plus, 6*(1), 1–13.

Collins, S., Higbee, T. S., & Salzberg, C. L. (2009). The effects of video modeling on staff implementation of a problem-solving intervention with adults with developmental disabilities. *Journal of Applied Behavior Analysis, 42*(4), 849–854. doi:10.1901/jaba.2009.42-849 PMID:20514193

Collisson, B. A., & Long, S. H. (1993). Computer-assisted language intervention: What difference does the clinician make? *Language, Speech, and Hearing Services in Schools, 24*(3), 179–180. doi:10.1044/0161-1461.2403.179

Complete Speech, L. L. C. (2010-2014). *Complete Speech Blog.* Retrieved 08/10/2014, 2014, from http://www.completespeech.com/speech/blog/P20

Complete Speech, L. L. C. (2013). *What is a SmartPalate.* Retrieved 08/08/2014, 2014, from http://www.completespeech.com/speech/smartpalate1/what_is_a_smartpalate/

Connor, C. M., Alberto, P. A., Compton, D. L., & O'Connor, R. E. (2014). *Improving Reading Outcomes for Students with or at Risk for Reading Disabilities: A Synthesis of the Contributions from the Institute of Education Sciences Research Centers (NCSER 2014-3000).* Washington, DC: National Center for Special Education Research, Institute of Education Sciences, U.S. Department of Education. This report is available on the IES website at; http://ies.ed.gov/

Conyers, C., Miltenberger, R. G., Peterson, B., Gubin, A., Jurgens, M., Selders, A., & Barenz, R. et al. (2004). An evaluation of in vivo desensitization and video modeling to increase compliance in dental procedures in persons with mental retardation. *Journal of Applied Behavior Analysis, 37*(2), 233–238. doi:10.1901/jaba.2004.37-233 PMID:15293644

Cook, A. M., Meng, M. Q. H., Gu, J. J., & Howery, K. (2002). Development of a robotic device for facilitating learning by children who have severe disabilities. *IEEE Transactions on Neural Systems and Rehabilitation Engineering: A Publication of the IEEE Engineering in Medicine and Biology Society, 10*(3), 178-187.

Cook, A. M., & Polgar, J. M. (2008). *Introduction and Framework. Cook & Hussey's Assistive Technologies: Principles and Practice.* St. Louis, MO: Mosby.

Cook, A. M., & Polgar, J. M. (2013). *Cook and Hussey's Assistive Technologies: Principles and Practice*. Elsevier.

Cook, A., Howery, K., Gu, J., & Meng, M. (2000). Robot enhanced interaction and learning for children with profound physical disabilities. *Technology and Disability, 13*(1), 1.

Cook, A., & Hussey, S. (1995). *Assistive technologies: principles and practice*. St Louis: Mosby Year Book.

Cook, B. G., Landrum, T. J., Tankersley, M., & Kauffman, J. M. (2003). Bringing research to bear on practice: Effective evidence-based instruction for students with emotional or behavioral disorders. *Education & Treatment of Children, 26*, 345–361.

Cooke, P., Laczny, A., Brown, D. J., & Francik, J. (2002). The virtual courtroom: A view of justice. Project to prepare witnesses or victims with learning disabilities to give evidence. *Disability and Rehabilitation, 24*(11), 634–642. doi:10.1080/10.1080/09638280110111414 PMID:12182804

Cooper, R. J., & Associates. Inc. (n.d.). Apps, ipads accessories, software and hardware for persons with special needs. Retrieved April 3, 2014 from http://www.rjcooper.com

Cooper-Brown, L., Copeland, S., Dailey, S., Downey, D., Petersen, M., Stimson, C., & Van Dyke, D. C. (2008). Feeding and swallowing dysfunction in genetic syndromes. *Developmental Disabilities Research Reviews, 14*(2), 147–157. doi:10.1002/ddrr.19 PMID:18646013

Copley, J., & Ziviani, J. (2004). Barriers to the use of assistive technology for children with multiple disabilities. *Occupational Therapy International, 11*(4), 229–243. doi:10.1002/oti.213 PMID:15771212

Costello, J. M., Shane, H. C., & Caron, J. (2013). *AAC, mobile devices and apps: Growing pains with evidenced based practice*. Boston Children's Hospital. Retrieved June 28, 2014 from http://www.vantatenhove.com/files/papers/AACandApps/CostelloShaneCaron-WhitePaper.pdf

Costigan, F. A., & Light, J. (2011). Functional seating for school-age children with cerebral palsy: An evidence-based tutorial. *Language, Speech, and Hearing Services in Schools, 42*(2), 223–236. doi:10.1044/0161-1461(2010/10-0001) PMID:20844273

Coughtrey, K. (2014). Connected Mind [Mind Mapping]. *Google*. Retrieved, February 4, 2014, from http://www.connected-mind.appspot.com

Couper, L., van der Meer, L., Schafer, M. C. M., McKenzie, E., McLay, L., O'Reilly, M. F., & Sutherland, D. et al. (2014). Comparing acquisition of and preference for manual signs, picture, exchange, and speech-generating devices in nine children with autism spectrum disorder. *Developmental Neurorehabilitation, 17*(2), 99–109. doi:10.3109/17518423.2013.870244 PMID:24392652

Courtade, G. R., Browder, D. M., Spooner, F., & DiBiase, W. (2010). Training teachers to use an inquiry-based task analysis to teach science to students with moderate and severe disabilities. *Education and Training in Autism and Developmental Disabilities, 45*(3), 378–399.

Courtade, G., Spooner, F., & Browder, D. M. (2007). Review of studies with students with significant cognitive disabilities which link to science standards. *Research and Practice for Persons with Severe Disabilities, 32*(1), 43–49. doi:10.2511/rpsd.32.1.43

Cox, D. J., Punja, M., Powers, K., Merkel, R. L., Burket, R., Moore, M., & Kovatchev, B. et al. (2006). Manual Transmission Enhances Attention and Driving Performance of ADHD Adolescent Males Pilot Study. *Journal of Attention Disorders, 10*(2), 212–216. doi:10.1177/1087054706288103 PMID:17085632

Crawford, M. R., & Schuster, J. W. (1993). Using microswitches to teach toy use. *Journal of Developmental and Physical Disabilities, 5*(4), 349–368. doi:10.1007/BF01046391

Cress, C. J., & Marvin, C. A. (2003). Common questions about AAC services in early intervention. *Augmentative and Alternative Communication, 19*(4), 254–272. doi:10.1080/07434610310001598242

Crosland, K., & Dunlap, G. (2012). Effective strategies for the inclusion of children with autism in general education classrooms. *Behavior Modification, 36*(3), 251–269. doi:10.1177/0145445512442682 PMID:22563045

Cubelic, C. C., & Larwin, K. H. (2014). The use of iPad technology in the kindergarten classroom: A quasi-experimental investigation of the impact on early literacy skills. *Comprehensive Journal of Educational Research, 2*(4), 47–59.

Cumming, I., Strnadová, I., Knox, M., & Parmenter, T. (2014). Mobile technology in inclusive research: Tools of empowerment? *Disability & Society*, *29*(7), 11–14. do i:10.1080/09687599.2014.886556

Cumming, T. (2007). Virtual reality as assistive technology. *Journal of Special Education Technology*, *22*(2), 55–58.

Cumming, T. (2013). Mobile Learning as a tool for students with EBD: Combining evidence based practice with new technology. *Beyond Behavior*, *23*(1), 1–6.

Da Fonte, M. A., Pufpaff, L. A., & Taber-Doughty, T. (2010). Vocabulary use during storybook reading: Implications for children with augmentative and alternative communication needs. *Psychology in the Schools*, *47*(5), 514–524.

Dahlgren Sandberg, A. (2006). Reading and spelling abilities in children with severe speech impairments and cerebral palsy at 6, 9, and 12 years of age in relation to cognitive development: A longitudinal study. *Developmental Medicine and Child Neurology*, *48*(08), 629–634. doi:10.1017/S0012162206001344 PMID:16836773

Dahlgren Sandberg, A., Smith, M., & Larsson, M. (2010). An analysis of reading and spelling abilities of children using AAC: Understanding a continuum of competence. *Augmentative and Alternative Communication*, *26*(3), 191–202. doi:10.3109/07434618.2010.5056 07 PMID:20874081

Dautenhahn, K., & Werry, I. (2004). Towards interactive robots in autism therapy: Background, motivation and challenges. *Pragmatics & Cognition*, *12*(1), 1–35. doi:10.1075/pc.12.1.03dau

Davidson, A.-L. (2012). Use of mobile technologies by young adults living with an intellectual disability: A collaborative action research study. *Journal on Developmental Disabilities*, *18*(3), 21–32.

Davies, D. K., Stock, S. E., & Wehmeyer, M. L. (2002). Enhancing independent task performance for individuals with mental retardation through use of a handheld self-directed visual and audio prompting system. *Education and Training in Mental Retardation and Developmental Disabilities*, *37*, 209–218.

Davies, D., Stock, S., & Wehmeyer, M. L. (2004). A palmtop computer-based intelligent aid for individuals with intellectual disabilities to increase independent decision-making. *Research and Practice for Persons with Severe Disabilities*, *28*(4), 182–193. doi:10.2511/rpsd.28.4.182

Davis, V. (2012). *Does electronic versus paper book experience result in differences in level of emergent literacy development in young children?* Retrieved July 25, 2014, from http://www.uwo.ca/fhs/csd/ebp/reviews/2011-12/Davis.pdf

Davis, M., Dautenhahn, K., Powell, S., & Nehaniv, C. (2009). Guidelines for researchers and practitioners designing software and software trials for children with autism. *Journal of Assistive Technologies*, *4*(1), 34–48.

Dawe, M. (2006). Desperately seeking simplicity: How young adults with cognitive disabilities and their families adopt assistive technologies. In *Proceedings of the SIGCHI Conference on Human Factors in Computing Systems*, 22 – 27. doi:10.1145/1124772.1124943

Dawson, G., Jones, E. J. H., Merkle, K., Venema, K., Lowy, R., Faja, S., & Webb, S. J. et al. (2012). Early behavioral intervention is associated with normalized brain activity in young children with autism. *Journal of the American Academy of Child and Adolescent Psychiatry*, *51*(11), 1150–1159. doi:10.1016/j.jaac.2012.08.018 PMID:23101741

Deci, E. L. (1992). *The relation of interest to the motivation of behavior: A self-determination theory perspective.* Hillsdale, NJ, England: Lawrence Erlbaum Associates, Inc.

DeCurtis, L. L., & Ferrer, D. (2011, September 20). Toddlers and technology: Teaching the techniques, *The ASHA Leader*. Retrieved June 25, 2014, from http://www.asha.org/Publications/leader/2011/110920/Toddlers-and-Technology.htm#2

Deep Listening Institute. (n.d.). *Deep Listening*. Retrieved March 15, 2014, from http://www.deeplistening.org/site/

Dell, A. G., Newton, D., & Petroff, J. G. (2011). *Assistive technology in the classroom: Enhancing the school experiences of students with disabilities* (2nd ed.). Upper Saddle River, NJ: Pearson.

Denhart, H. (2008). Deconstructing barriers: Perceptions of students labeled with learning disabilities in higher education. *Journal of Learning Disabilities*, *41*(6), 483–497. doi:10.1177/0022219408321151 PMID:18931016

DePrenger, M., Shao, Y., Lu, F., & Fleming, N. (2010). Feasibility study of a smart pen for autonomous detection of concentration lapses during reading. *International Conference of the IEEE EMBS*, 1864–1867. doi:10.1109/IEMBS.2010.5626256

Deshler, D. D., Schumaker, J. B., Lenz, B. K., Bulgren, J. A., Hock, M. F., Knight, J., & Ehren, B. J. (2001). Ensuring content-area learning by secondary students with learning disabilities. *Learning Disabilities Research & Practice*, *16*(2), 96–108. doi:10.1111/0938-8982.00011

Detrich, R. (2013, November). *Evidence or infomercial: The necessity of evaluating technological innovations.* Paper presented at the ABAI 2nd Education Conference. Innovations in Education: Apps, Games Technology & the Science of Behavior, Chicago, IL.

Deutsch, J. E., Borbely, M., Filler, J., Huhn, K., & Guarrera-Bowlby, P. (2008). Use of a low-cost, commercially available gaming console (Wii) for rehabilitation of an adolescent with cerebral palsy. *Physical Therapy*, *88*(10), 1196–1207. doi:10.2522/ptj.20080062 PMID:18689607

Didehbani, N., Kelly, K., Austin, L., & Wiechmann, A. (2011). Role of Parental Stress on Pediatric Feeding Disorders. *Children's Health Care*, *40*(2), 85–100. doi:10.1080/02739615.2011.564557

Diehl, J. J., Schmitt, L. M., Villano, M., & Crowell, C. R. (2012). The clinical use of robots for individuals with autism spectrum disorders: A critical review. *Research in Autism Spectrum Disorders*, *6*(1), 249–262. doi:10.1016/j.rasd.2011.05.006 PMID:22125579

Dillon, C. M., & Carr, J. E. (2007). Assessing indices of happiness and unhappiness in individuals with developmental disabili- ties: A review. *Behavioral Interventions*, *22*(3), 229–244. doi:10.1002/bin.240

Dillon, G., & Underwood, J. (2011). Computer mediated imaginative storytelling in children with autism. *International Journal of Human-Computer Studies*, *70*(2), 169–178. doi:10.1016/j.ijhcs.2011.10.002

Disability Rights Network of Pennsylvania. (2008). *Assistive technology for persons with disabilities: An overview.* Disability Rights Network of Pennsylvania. Retrieved December 15, 2013, from http://drnpa.org/File/publications/assistive-technology-for-persons-with-disabilities—an-overview.pdf

Dobler, E. (2012). Using iPads to promote literacy in the primary grades. *Reading Today*, *29*(3), 18–19.

Dolan, M. C. (1973). Music therapy: An explanation. *Journal of Music Therapy*, *10*(4), 172–176. doi:10.1093/jmt/10.4.172

Dolic, J., Pibernik, J., & Bota, J. (2012). Evaluation of mainstream table devices for symbol based AAC communication. *KES-AMSTA'12 Proceedings of the 6th KES international conference on Agent and Multi-Agent Systems: Technologies and Applications* (pp. 251-260). Berlin: Springer-Verlag. doi:10.1007/978-3-642-30947-2_29

Donnellan, A. M. (1984). The criterion of the least dangerous assumption. *Behavioral Disorders*, *9*(2), 141–150.

Douglas, K. H., Wojcik, B. W., & Thompson, J. R. (2012). Is there an app for that? *Journal of Special Education Technology*, *27*(2), 59–70.

Downing, J. E. (Ed.). (2005). *Teaching literacy to students with significant disabilities: Strategies for the K-12 inclusive classroom.* Thousand Oaks, CA: Sage. doi:10.4135/9781483328973

Dowrick, P. W. (1999). A review of self-modeling and related interventions. *Applied & Preventive Psychology*, *8*(1), 23–39. doi:10.1016/S0962-1849(99)80009-2

Drager, K. D. R., & Finke, E. H. (2012). Intelligibility of Children's Speech in Digitized Speech. *AAC: Augmentative & Alternative Communication*, *28*(3), 181–189. doi:10.3109/07434618.2012.704524 PMID:22946993

Drager, K. D. R., Light, J. C., Carlson, R., D'Silva, K., Larsson, B., Pitkin, L., & Stopper, G. (2004). Learning of dynamic display AAC technologies by typically developing 3-year olds: Effect of different layouts and menu approaches. *Journal of Speech, Language, and Hearing Research: JSLHR*, *47*(5), 1133–1148. doi:10.1044/1092-4388(2004/084) PMID:15603467

Drager, K. D. R., Light, J. C., & Finke, E. (2009). Using AAC technologies to build social interaction with young children with autism spectrum disorders. In P. Mirenda & T. Iacono (Eds.), *Autism spectrum disorders and AAC* (pp. 247–278). Baltimore: Paul H. Brookes Publishing Co.

Duck Duck Moose. (n.d.). *Duck Duck Moose: Award winning education apps for children*. Retrieved April 3, 2015 from http://www.duckduckmoose.com

Duffy, G. G. (2002). The case for direct explanation of strategies. In C. Block & M. P. Pressley (Eds.), *Comprehension instruction: Research-based best practices* (pp. 28–41). New York: Guilford Press.

Duker, P., Didden, R., & Sigafoos, J. (2004). *One-to-one training: Instructional procedures for learners with developmental disabilities*. Austin, TX: Pro-Ed.

Dundon, M., McLaughlin, T. F., Neyman, J., & Clark, A. (2013). The effects of a model, lead, and test procedure to teach correct requesting using two apps on an iPad with a 5 year old student with autism spectrum disorder. *Education Research International, 1*(3), 1–10.

Duquette, A., Michaud, F., & Mercier, H. (2008). Exploring the use of a mobile robot as an imitation agent with children with low-functioning autism. *Autonomous Robots, 24*(2), 147–157. doi:10.1007/s10514-007-9056-5

Durkin, D. (1978/1979). What classroom observations reveal about reading comprehension instruction. *Reading Research Quarterly, 14*(4), 481–533. doi:10.1598/RRQ.14.4.2

Eaves, L. C., & Ho, H. H. (2008). Young adult outcome of autism spectrum disorders. *Journal of Autism and Developmental Disorders, 38*(4), 739–747. doi:10.1007/s10803-007-0441-x PMID:17764027

Editorial Projects in Education Research Center. (2011). Issues A-Z: Achievement Gap. *Education Week*. Retrieved, July 24, 2014, from, http://www.edweek.org/ew/issues/achievement-gap/

Edrisinha, C., O'Reilly, M. F., Choi, H. Y., Sigafoos, J., & Lancioni, G. (2011). "Say cheese": Teaching photography to adults with developmental disabilities. *Research in Developmental Disabilities, 32*(2), 636–642. doi:10.1016/j.ridd.2010.12.006 PMID:21227636

Edyburn, D. L. (2004). Rethinking assistive technology. *Special Education Technology Practice, 5*(4), 16–23.

Edyburn, D. L. (2013). Critical issues in advancing the special education technology evidence base. *Exceptional Children, 80*(1), 7–24.

Ehri, L. C., Nunes, S. R., Stahl, S. A., & Willows, D. M. (2001). Systematic phonics instruction helps students learn to read: Evidence from the National Reading Panel's meta-analysis. *Review of Educational Research, 71*(3), 393–447. doi:10.3102/00346543071003393

Ellis, P., & van Leeuwen, L. (2000). *Living Sound: human interaction and children with autism. ISME commission on Music in Special Education*. Regina, Canada: Music Therapy and Music Medicine.

Enabling Devices. (n.d.) *Assistive technology – Products for people with disabilities*. Retrieved April 3 from https://enablingdevices.com/catalog

Endow, J. (2012). *Learning the hidden curriculum: The odyssey of one autistic adult*. Shawnee Mission, KS: AAPC Publishing.

Erickson, K., Hanser, G., Hatch, P., & Sanders, E. (2009). *Research-based practices for creating access to the general curriculum in reading and literacy for students with significant intellectual disabilities. Monograph prepared for the Council for Chief State School Officers (CCSSO) Assessing Special Education Students (ASES) State Collaborative on Assessment and Student Standards (SCASS)*. Retrieved From: http://idahotc.com/Portals/15/Docs/IAA/10-11%20Docs/Research_Based_Practices_Reading_2009.pdf

Erickson, W., Lee, C., & von Schrader, S. (2014). Disability Statistics from the 2012 American Community Survey (ACS). Ithaca, NY: Cornell University Employment and Disability Institute (EDI).

Erickson, K. A., Hatch, P., & Clendon, S. (2010). Literacy, assistive technology, and students with significant disabilities. *Focus on Exceptional Children, 42*(5), 1–16.

Erickson, K. A., Koppenhaver, D. A., Yoder, D. E., & Nance, J. (1997). Integrated communication and literacy instruction for a child with multiple disabilities. *Focus on Autism and Other Developmental Disabilities, 12*(3), 142–150. doi:10.1177/108835769701200302

Erickson, K., & Koppenhaver, D. (1995). Developing a literacy program for children with severe disabilities. *The Reading Teacher, 48*, 676–684.

Estrella, G. (1997). *1997 Edwin and Esther Prentke AAC Distinguished Lecturer.* Retrieved from: http://www.aacinstitute.org/Resources/PrentkeLecture/1997/GusEstrella.html

Ewing, G. (2000). Update from the executive director. *Incoming, 2*(7), 1. Retrieved January 12, 2005, from hp://www.mtml.ca/newslet/july00/page1.htm

Fagan, J., & Jacobs, M. (2009). Survey of ENT services in Africa: Need for a comprehensive intervention. *Global Health Action.* Feeding and Swallowing Disorders (Dysphagia) in Children. *Feeding and Swallowing Disorders (Dysphagia) in Children.* Retrieved June 7, 2014, from http://www.asha.org/public/speech/swallowing/feeding-and-swallowing-disorders-in-children/

Fager, S., Bardach, L., Russell, S., & Higginbotham, J. (2012). Access to augmentative and alternative communication: New technologies and clinical decision making. *Journal of Pediatric Rehabilitation Medicine: An Interdisciplinary Approach, 5*(1), 63–51. doi:10.3233/PRM-2012-0196 PMID:22543893

Fager, S., Bardach, L., Russell, S., & Higginbotham, J. (2012). Access to augmentative and alternative communication: New technologies and clinical decision-making. *Journal of Pediatric Rehabilitation Medicine, 5*(1), 53–61. PMID:22543893

Fallon, K. A., & Katz, L. (2008). Augmentative and alternative communication and literacy teams: Facing the challenges, forging ahead. *Seminars in Speech and Language, 29*(2), 112–119. doi:10.1055/s-2008-1079125 PMID:18645913

Fallon, K. A., Light, J., McNaughton, D., Drager, K., & Hammer, C. (2004). The effects of direct instruction on the single-word reading skills of children who require augmentative and alternative communication. *Journal of Speech, Language, and Hearing Research: JSLHR, 47*(6), 1424–1439. doi:10.1044/1092-4388(2004/106) PMID:15842020

Faraone, S. V. The ADHD Molecular Genetics Network. (2002). Report from the third international meeting of the attention deficit hyperactivity disorder molecular genetics network. *American Journal of Medical Genetics, 114*(3), 272–277. doi:10.1002/ajmg.10039 PMID:11920847

Farrall, J. (2013). AAC Apps and ASD: Giving Voice to Good Practice. *SIG 12 Perspectives on Augmentative and Alternative Communication, 22*(3), 157-163.

Feder, K. P., & Majnemer, A. (2007). Handwriting development, competency, and intervention. *Developmental Medicine and Child Neurology, 49*(4), 312–317. doi:10.1111/j.1469-8749.2007.00312.x PMID:17376144

Felce, D., & Perry, J. (1995). Quality of life: Its definition and measurement. *Research in Developmental Disabilities, 16*(1), 51–74. doi:10.1016/0891-4222(94)00028-8 PMID:7701092

Fenlon, A. G., McNabb, J., & Pidlypchak, H. (2010). So Much Potential in Reading!" Developing Meaningful Literacy Routines for Students With Multiple Disabilities. *Teaching Exceptional Children, 43*(1), 42–48.

Fernandes, T., Alves, S., Miranda, J., Queirós, C., & Orvalho, V. (2011). LIFEisGAME: A Facial Character Animation System to Help Recognize Facial Expressions. In *ENTERprise Information Systems* (pp. 423–432). Berlin, Germany: Springer. doi:10.1007/978-3-642-24352-3_44

Fernandez, B, (2011a). iTherapy: The revolution of mobile devices within the field of speech therapy. *SIG 16 Perspectives on School-Based Issues, 12*(2), 35-40. doi:10.1044/sbi12.2.35

Fernandez, B. (2011b). Is the iPad revolutionizing speech therapy? From an SLP & app developer. *ASHA Sphere.* Retrieved June 25, 2014, from http://blog.asha.org/2011/06/07/is-the-ipad-revolutionizing-speech-therapy-from-an-slp-app-developer/

Fernandez, B. (2011c). Calling all SLPs and teachers to update the iOS system on their iPads & IPods. *ASHA Sphere.* Retrieved June 25, 2014, from http://blog.asha.org/2011/04/26/calling-all-slps-and-teachers-to-update-the-ios-system-on-their-ipads-ipods/

Fernandez, E. M., & Smith Cairns, H. (2011). *Fundamentals of Psycholinguistics.* Hoboken, NJ: Wiley-Blackwell.

Ferreira, J., Rönnberg, J., Gustafson, S., & Wengelin, Å. (2007). Reading, why not? Literacy skills in children with motor and speech impairments. *Communication Disorders Quarterly*, *28*(4), 236–251. doi:10.1177/1525740107311814

Fitzgerald, G. E. (2005). Using technologies to meet the unique needs of students with emotional/behavioral disorders: Findings and directions. In D. Edyburn, K. Higgins & R. Boone (Eds.), Handbook of special education technology research and practice (pp. 335-354). Whitefish Bay, WI: Knowledge by Design, Inc.

Fletcher-Watson, S. (2014). A targeted review of computer-assisted learning for people with autism spectrum disorder: Towards a consistent methodology. *Review Journal of Autism and Developmental Disorders*, *1*(2), 87–100. doi:10.1007/s40489-013-0003-4

Flewitt, R., Kucirkova, N., & Messer, D. (2014). Touch the virtual, touching the real: iPads and enabling literacy for students experiencing disability. *Australian Journal of Language and Literacy*, *37*(2), 107–116.

Flores, M., Musgrove, K., Renner, S., Hinton, V., Strozier, S., Franklin, S., & Hil, D. (2012). A comparison of communication using the Apple iPad and a picture-based system. *Augmentative and Alternative Communication*, *28*(2), 74–84. doi:10.3109/07434618.2011.644579 PMID:22263895

Foley, B. E. (2003). Language, Literacy, and AAC: Translating Theory Into Practice. *SIG 12 Perspectives on Augmentative and Alternative Communication*, *12*(1), 5-8.

Foley, B., & Staples, A. (2006). Assistive Technology Supports for Literacy Instruction. *SIG 12 Perspectives on Augmentative and Alternative Communication*, *15*(2), 15-21.

Foley, B., & Wolter, J. A. (2010). Literacy intervention for transition-aged youth: What is and what could be. In D. McNaughton & D. Beukelman (Eds.), *Language, Literacy, and AAC Issues for Transition- Age Youth* (pp. 35–68). Baltimore, MD: Brookes.

Forts, A. M., & Luckasson, R. (2011). Reading, writing, and friendship: Adult implications of effective literacy instruction for students with intellectual disability. *Research and Practice for Persons with Severe Disabilities*, *36*(3-4), 121–125. doi:10.2511/027494811800824417

Fossett, B., & Mirenda, P. (2006). Sight word reading in children with developmental disabilities: A comparison of paired associate and picture-to-text matching instruction. *Research in Developmental Disabilities*, *27*(4), 411–429. doi:10.1016/j.ridd.2005.05.006 PMID:16112841

Fox, B. J. (2010). *Fluency contributes to comprehension.* Retrieved, 27 May 2014, http://www.education.com/reference/article/fluency-contributes-comprehension/

Franzone, E., & Collet-Klingenberg, L. (2008). Overview of video modeling. Madison, WI: The National Professional Development Center on Autism Spectrum Disorders, Waisman Center, University of Wisconsin. Retrieved from http:// autismpdc.fpg.unc.edu/sites/autismpdc .fpg.unc.edu/files/VideoModeling _Overview_l.pdf

Freeplane. (2007). Freeplane (v1.3.11) [Free mind mapping and knowledge management software]. *MediaWiki.* Retrieved, February 4, 2014, from http://www.freeplane.org./wiki/index.php/Main_Page

Fried-Oken, M., & More, L. (1992). An initial vocabulary for nonspeaking preschool children based on developmental and environmental language sources. *Augmentative and Alternative Communication*, *8*(1), 41–56. doi:10.1080/07434619212331276033

Frierich, L. K., & Stein, A. H. (1975). Prosocial television and young children: The effects of verbal labeling and role playing on learning and behavior. *Child Development*, *46*(1), 27–38. doi:10.2307/1128830

Frith, U. (1989). Autism: Explaining the enigma. Blackwell, UK: Oxford.

Frith, U., & Happé, F. (1994). Autism: Beyond "theory of mind". *Cognition*, *50*(1), 115–132. doi:10.1016/0010-0277(94)90024-8 PMID:8039356

Frost, L., & Bondy, A. (2002). *Picture Exchange Communication System training manual* (2nd ed.). Newark, DE: Pyramid Education Products.

Furman, P. (2012, June 19). Tablets' popularity is through the roof, nearly one-third of U.S. Internet users have one: survey. *New York Daily News.*

Furr, M., Larkin, E., Blakeley, R., Albert, T., Tsugawa, L., & Weber, S. (2011). Extending Multidisciplinary Management of Cleft Palate to the Developing World. *Journal of Oral and Maxillofacial Surgery*, *69*(1), 237–241-237–241.

Gallaudet Research Institute (GRI). (2011). Regional and National Summary Report of Data from the 2009-10 Annual Survey of Deaf and Hard of Hearing Children and Youth. Washington DC: Gallaudet University.

Ganz, J. B., Hong, E. R., Goodwyn, F., Kite, E., & Gilliland, W. (2013). Impact of PECS tablet computer app on receptive indentification of pictures given a verbal stimulus. *Developmental Neurorehabilitation, 18*(2), 82–87. doi:10.3109/17518423.2013.821539 PMID:23957298

Ganz, L. B., Hong, E. R., & Goodwyn, F. D. (2013). Effectiveness of the PECS Phase III app and choice between the app and traditional PECS among preschoolers with ASD. *Research in Autism Spectrum Disorders, 7*(8), 973–983. doi:10.1016/j.rasd.2013.04.003

GeekSLP. (n.d.). *GeekSLP.com: Your source of educational apps and technology information*. Retrieved April 3, 2015 from http://www.geekslp.com

Gentry, M. M., Chinn, K. M., & Moulton, R. D. (2004). Effectiveness of multimedia reading materials when used with children who are deaf. *American Annals of the Deaf, 149*(5), 394–402. doi:10.1353/aad.2005.0012 PMID:15727058

Gerber, P. J., Reiff, H. B., & Ginsberg, R. (1996). Reframing the learning disabilities experience. *Journal of Learning Disabilities, 29*(1), 98–101. doi:10.1177/002221949602900112 PMID:8648281

Gerde, H. K., Bingham, G. E., & Wasik, B. A. (2012). Writing in early childhood classrooms: Guidance for best practices. *Early Childhood Education Journal, 40*(6), 351–359. doi:10.1007/s10643-012-0531-z

Gibbon, F. E., & Lee, A. (2007). Electropalatography as a Research and Clinical Tool. *SIG 5 Perspectives on Speech Science and Orofacial Disorders, 17*, 7-13.

Gibbon, F. E., & Wood, S. E. (2010). Visual feedback therapy with electropalatography. In A. L. Williams, S. McLeod, & R. J. McCauley (Eds.), *Interventions for Speech Sound Disorders in Children* (pp. 509–536). Baltimore, MD: PH Brooks Publishing Company.

Gibson, A., Gold, J., & Sgouros, C. (2003). The power of story retelling. *The Tutor,* Spring 2003, 1 – 11.

Gibson, J., Adams, C., Lockton, E., & Green, J. (2013). Social communication disorder outside autism? A diagnostic classification approach to delineating pragmatic language impairment, high functioning autism and specific language impairment. *Journal of Child Psychology and Psychiatry, and Allied Disciplines, 54*(11), 1186–1197. doi:10.1111/jcpp.12079 PMID:23639107

Gierach, J. (2009). Assessing Students' Needs for Assistive Technology (ASNAT): A resource manual for school district teams, 5th Eds. Milton, WI: Wisconsin Assistive Technology Initiative. (nod). Retrieved From www.wati.org

Giesbrecht, E. (2013). Application of the human activity assistive technology model for occupational therapy research. *Australian Occupational Therapy Journal, 60*(4), 230–240. doi:10.1111/1440-1630.12054 PMID:23888973

Gillespie-Lynch, K., Kapp, S. K., Shane-Simpson, C., Smith, D. S., & Hutman, T. (2014). Intersections Between the Autism Spectrum and the Internet: Perceived Benefits and Preferred Functions of Computer-Mediated Communication. *Intellectual and Developmental Disabilities, 52*(6), 456–469. doi:10.1352/1934-9556-52.6.456 PMID:25409132

Gindis, B. (1995). The social/cultural implications of disability: Vygotsky's paradigm for special education. *Educational Psychologist, 30*(2), 77–81. doi:10.1207/s15326985ep3002_4

Glidden, L. M. (2008). *International Review of Research in Mental Retardation*. San Diego: Elsevier.

Goffman, E. (1963). *Stigma: Notes on the Management of Spoiled Identity*. Penguin.

Golan, O., Ashwin, E., Granader, Y., McClintock, S., Day, K., Leggett, V., & Baron-Cohen, S. (2009). Enhancing emotion recognition in children with autism spectrum conditions: An intervention using animated vehicles with real emotional faces. *Journal of Autism and Developmental Disorders, 40*(3), 269–279. doi:10.1007/s10803-009-0862-9 PMID:19763807

Golan, O., & Baron-Cohen, S. (2006). Systemizing empathy: Teaching adults with Asperger syndrome or high-functioning autism to recognize complex emotions using interactive multimedia. *Development and Psychopathology*, *18*(2), 591–617. doi:10.1017/S0954579406060305 PMID:16600069

Golan, O., & Baron-Cohen, S. (2014). Systemizing emotions: Using interactive multimedia as a teaching tool. In K. D. Buron & P. Wolfberg (Eds.), *Learners on the autism spectrum Preparing highlight qualified educators and related practitioners* (2nd ed.; pp. 315–335). Shawnee Mission, KS: AAPC Publishing.

Goldsmith, T. R., & LeBlanc, L. A. (2004). Use of Technology in Interventions for Children with Autism. *Journal of Early and Intensive Behavior Intervention*, *1*(2), 166–178. doi:10.1037/h0100287

Golomb, M. R., McDonald, B. C., Warden, S. J., Yonkman, J., Saykin, A. J., Shirley, B., . . . Nwosu, M. E. (2010). In-home virtual reality videogame telerehabilitation in adolescents with hemiplegic cerebral palsy. *Archives of Physical Medicine and Rehabilitation, 91*(1), 1-8. e1.

Golubock, S. J. (2009). What we don't know (about relationships) CAN hurt us: The hazards of not understanding, relating to and communicating with others. *Autism Advocate, 54*(1), 55–58.

Good Karma Applications. (2014). *Visual schedule planner*. Retrieved on July 5, 2014 from http://www.goodkarmaapplications.com

Good Karma Applications. (n.d.). *Good karma applications*. Retrieved April 3, 2015 from http://www.attainmentcompany.com/assistive-technology

Gosnell, J. (2011). Apps: An emerging tool for SLPs; A plethora of apps can be used to develop expressive, receptive, and other language skills. *The ASHA Leader*. Retrieved June 26, 2014 from http://www.asha.org/publications/leader/2011/111011/apps--an-emerging-tool-for-slps.htm

Gosnell, J., Costello, J., & Shane, H. (2011a). There isn't always an app for that! *Perspectives on Augmentative and Alternative Communication, 20*(1), 7–8. doi:10.1044/aac20.1.7

Gosnell, J., Costello, J., & Shane, H. (2011b). Using a clinical approach to answer 'what communication apps should we use?'. *Perspectives on Augmentative and Alternative Communication, 20*(3), 87–96. doi:10.1044/aac20.3.87

Graham, M. (2011). *Who wants lemonade?* Retrieved June 26, 2014 http://all4mychild.com/blog/?p=168

Grandin, T. (2009). How does visual thinking work in the mind of a person with autism? A personal account. *Philosophical Transactions of the Royal Society of London. Series B, Biological Sciences, 364*(1522), 1437–1442. doi:10.1098/rstb.2008.0297 PMID:19528028

Gray, C. (2000). *The original Social Story™ book: Illustrated edition*. Arlington, TX: Future Horizons.

Gray, D. E. (1993). Perceptions of stigma: The parents of autistic children. *Sociology of Health & Illness, 15*(1), 102–120. doi:10.1111/1467-9566.ep11343802

Greenbaum, B., Graham, S., & Scales, W. (1995). Adults with learning disabilities: Educational and social experiences during college. *Exceptional Children, 61*, 460–471.

Green, C. W., & Reid, D. H. (1999). A behavioral approach to identifying sources of happiness and unhappiness among individuals with profound multiple disabilities. *Behavior Modification, 23*(2), 280–293. doi:10.1177/0145445599232006 PMID:10224953

Green, E. J., & Drewes, A. A. (Eds.). (2013). *Integrating Expressive Arts and Play Therapy with Children and Adolescents*. John Wiley & Sons.

Green, J. M., Hughes, E. M., & Ryan, J. B. (2011). The use of assistive technology to improve time management skills of a young adult with an intellectual disability. *Journal of Special Education Technology, 26*(3), 13–20.

Gresham, F. M. (2002). Teaching social skills to high-risk children and youth: Preventive and remedial strategies. In M. R. Shinn, H. M. Walker & G. Stoner (Eds.), Interventions for academic and behavior problems II: Preventive and remedial approaches (pp. 403-432). Bethesda, MD: National Association of School Psychologists.

Gresham, F. M. (2002). Best practices in social skills training. In A. Thomas & J. Grimes (Eds.), *Best practices in school psychology* (4th ed.). Bethesda, MD: NASP.

Gresham, F. M., Van, M. B., & Cook, C. R. (2006). Social skills training for teaching replacement behaviors: Remediating acquisition deficits in at-risk students. *Behavioral Disorders, 31*, 363–377.

Groden, J., Kantor, A., Woodard, C., & Lipsitt, L. (2011). *How everyone on the autism spectrum, young and old, can become resilient, be more optimistic, enjoy humor, be kind, and increase self-efficacy: A positive psychology approach.* London: Jessica Kingsley Publishers.

Groom, K., Ramsey, M., & Saunders, J. (2011). Teleheal th and Humanitarian Assistance in Otolaryngology. *Otolaryngologic Clinics of North America, 44*(6), 1251–1258. doi:10.1016/j.otc.2011.08.002 PMID:22032479

Guerriere, D. N., McKeever, P., & Llewellyn-Thomas, H. et al.. (2003). Mothers' decisions about gastrostomy tube insertion in children: Factors contributing to uncertainty. *Developmental Medicine and Child Neurology, 45*(7), 470–476. doi:10.1111/j.1469-8749.2003.tb00942.x PMID:12828401

Gulchak, D. J.Daniel J. Gulchak. (2008). Using a mobile handheld computer to teach a student with an emotional and behavioral disorder to self-monitor attention. *Education & Treatment of Children, 31*(4), 567–581. doi:10.1353/etc.0.0028

Gunning, T. G. (2005). Creating literacy instruction for all students. Boston, MA: Pearson Higher Ed.

Gunning, T. G. (2012). *Creating literacy instruction for all students* (8th ed.). Boston, MA: Allyn and Bacon.

Guthrie, J. T. (2000). Contexts for engagement and motivation in reading. In M. L. Kamil, P. B. Mosenthal, P. D. Pearson, & R. Barr (Eds.), *Handbook of reading research* (Vol. 3, pp. 629–654). Mahwah, NJ: Erlbaum.

Guthrie, J. T., McRae, A., & Klauda, S. L. (2007). Contributions of concept-oriented reading instruction to knowledge about interventions for motivations in reading. *Educational Psychologist, 42*(4), 237–250. doi:10.1080/00461520701621087

Gutiérrez-Maldonado, J., Letosa-Porta, À., Rus-Calafell, M., & Peñaloza-Salazar, C. (2009). The assessment of attention deficit hyperactivity disorder in children using continous performance tasks in virtual environments. *Anuario de Psicología, 40*(2), 211–222.

Hall, L. A. (2004). Comprehending expository text: Promising strategies for struggling readers and students with reading disabilities? *Reading Research and Instruction, 44*(2), 75–95. doi:10.1080/19388070409558427

Hall, V., Conboy-Hill, S., & Taylor, D. (2011). Using virtual reality to provide health care information to people with intellectual disabilities: Acceptability, usability, and potential utility. *Journal of Medical Internet Research, 13*(4), e91. doi:10.2196/jmir.1917 PMID:22082765

Hammond, D. L., Whatley, A. D., Ayres, K. M., & Gast, D. L. (2010). Effectiveness of video modeling to teach iPod use to students with moderate intellectual disabilities. *Education and Training in Autism and Developmental Disabilities, 45*(4), 525–538.

Hannon, P. (2000). *Reflecting on literacy in education.* New York, NY: Routledge Falmer.

Hansen, D. L., & Morgan, R. L. (2008). Teaching grocery store purchasing skills to students with intellectual disabilities using a computer-based instruction program. *Education and Training in Developmental Disabilities, 43*(4), 431–442.

Hanser, G. A., & Erickson, K. A. (2007). Integrated word identification and communication instruction for students with complex communication needs preliminary results. *Focus on Autism and Other Developmental Disabilities, 22*(4), 268–278. doi:10.1177/10883576070220040901

Happé, F. (1999). Autism: Cognitive deficit or cognitive style? *Trends in Cognitive Sciences, 3*(6), 216–222. doi:10.1016/S1364-6613(99)01318-2 PMID:10354574

Happé, F., & Frith, U. (2006). The weak coherence account: Detail-focused cognitive style in autism spectrum disorders. *Journal of Autism and Developmental Disorders, 36*(1), 5–25. doi:10.1007/s10803-005-0039-0 PMID:16450045

Hardcastle, W. J. (1972). The use of electropalatography in phonetic research. *Phonetica, 25*(4), 197–215. doi:10.1159/000259382 PMID:4565321

Haring, T. G., Kennedy, C. H., Adams, M. J., & Pitts-Conway, V. (1987). Teaching generalization of purchasing skills across community settings to autistic youth using videotape modeling. *Journal of Applied Behavior Analysis*, 20(1), 89–96. doi:10.1901/jaba.1987.20-89 PMID:3583966

Harms, M. B., Martin, A., & Wallace, G. L. (2010). Facial emotion recognition in autism spectrum disorders: A review of behavioral and neuroimaging studies. *Neuropsychology Review*, 20(3), 290–322. doi:10.1007/s11065-010-9138-6 PMID:20809200

Harn, B. A., Linan-Thompson, S., & Roberts, G. (2008). Intensifying instruction does additional instructional time make a difference for the most at-risk first graders? *Journal of Learning Disabilities*, 41(2), 115–125. doi:10.1177/0022219407313586 PMID:18354932

Hart, J. E., & Whalon, K. J. (2012). Using video self-modeling via iPads to increase academic responding of an adolescent with autism spectrum disorder and intellectual disability. *Education and Training in Autism and Developmental Disabilities*, 47(4), 438–446.

Harvey Mudd College. (n.d.). *HMC Computer Science*. Retrieved April 30, 2014, from http://www.cs.hmc.edu/

Haydon, T., Hawkins, R., Denune, H., Kimener, L., McCoy, D., & Basham, J. (2012). A comparison of iPads and worksheets on math skills of high school students with emotional disturbance. *Behavioral Disorders*, 4, 232–243.

Hayes, G. R., Kientz, J. A., Truong, K. N., White, D. R., Abowd, G. D., & Pering, T. (2004). Designing capture applications to support the education of children with autism. *Proceedings of the UbiComp*, 2004, 161–178.

Hecker, L., Burns, L., Elkind, J., Elkind, K., & Katz, L. (2002). Benefits of assistive reading software for students with attention disorders. *Annals of Dyslexia*, 52(1), 244–272. doi:10.1007/s11881-002-0015-8

Helfgott, D., & Westhaver, M. (1982). *Inspiration Software (v9.0.3)*. Portland, OR: Inspire.

Hernandez, D. J. (2011). *How third-grade reading skills and poverty influence high school graduation*. Annie E. Casey Foundation.

Herrera, G., Alcantud, F., Jordan, R., Blanquer, A., Labajo, G., & De Pablo, C. (2008). Development of symbolic play through the use of virtual reality tools in children with autistic spectrum disorders: Two case studies. *Autism*, 12(2), 143–157. doi:10.1177/1362361307086657 PMID:18308764

Hershberger, D. (2011). Mobile technology and AAC apps from an AAC developer's Perspective. *SIG 12 Perspectives on Augmentative and Alternative Communication*, 20(1), 28-33. doi:10.1044/aac20.1.28

Hess, S. (2014). Digital media and student learning: Impact of electronic books on motivation and achievement. *New England Reading Association Journal*, 49(2), 35–39.

Heward, W. L. (2013). *Exceptional Children: An Introduction to Special Education*. Upper Saddle River, NJ: Pearson.

Hewlett-Packard. (n.d.). Retrieved from http://www.hackingautism.org/

Higginbotham, J. & Jacobs, S. (2011). The future of the android operating system for augmentative and alternative communication. *SIG 12 Perspectives on Augmentative and Alternative Communication*, 20(2), 52-56. doi:10.1044/aac20.2.52

Higgins, J. P. T., & Green, S. (2009). *Cochrane Handbook for Systematic Reviews of Interventions*. The Cochrane Collaboration. Available from www.cochrane-handbook.org

Hill, D., & Flores, M. (2014). Comparing the Picture Exchange Communication System and the iPad™ for Communication of Students with Autism Spectrum Disorder and Developmental Delay. *TechTrends: Linking Research & Practice to Improve Learning*, 58(3), 45–53. doi:10.1007/s11528-014-0751-8

Hoch, H., McComas, J. J., Johnson, L., Faranda, N., & Guenther, S. L. (2002). The effects of magnitude and quality of reinforcement on choice responding during play activities. *Journal of Applied Behavior Analysis*, 35(2), 171–181. doi:10.1901/jaba.2002.35-171 PMID:12102136

Hodson, H. (2014). The first family robot. *New Scientist*, 223(2978), 21. doi:10.1016/S0262-4079(14)61389-0

Holland, T., Clare, I. C. H., & Mukhopadhyay, T. (2002). Prevalence of 'criminal offending' by men and women with intellectual disability and the characteristics of 'offenders': Implications for research and service development. *Journal of Intellectual Disability Research, 46*(1), 6–20. doi:10.1046/j.1365-2788.2002.00001.x PMID:12061335

Hollauf, M., & Vollmer, T. (2006). *MindMeister* (Web 2.0) [From MeisterLabs]. Munich, Germany: MeisterLabs. Retrieved, February 4, 2014, from http://www.mindmeister.com

Holmquist, J. (2011). Bullying prevention: positive strategies. PACER Center, 1 – 6.

Holt, S., & Yuill, N. (2014). Facilitating other-awareness in low-functioning children with autism and typically-developing preschoolers using dual-control technology. *Journal of Autism and Developmental Disorders, 44*(1), 236–248. doi:10.1007/s10803-013-1868-x PMID:23756935

Hooper, C. R. (2004). Treatment of Voice Disorders in Children. *Language, Speech, and Hearing Services in Schools, 35*(4), 320–326. doi:10.1044/0161-1461(2004/031) PMID:15609635

Hopkins, I. M., Gower, M. W., Perez, T. A., Smith, D. S., Amthor, F. R., Wimsatt, C. F., & Biasini, F. J. (2011). Avatar assistant: Improving social skills in students with an ASD through a computer-based intervention. *Journal of Autism and Developmental Disorders, 41*(11), 1543–1555. doi:10.1007/s10803-011-1179-z PMID:21287255

Horner-Johnson, W., & Drum, C. E. (2006). Prevalence of maltreatment of people with intellectual disabilities: A review of recently published research. *Mental Retardation and Developmental Disabilities Research Reviews, 12*(1), 57–69. doi:10.1002/mrdd.20097 PMID:16435331

Horn, J. A., Miltenberger, R. G., Weil, T., Mowery, J., Conn, M., & Sams, L. (2008). Teaching laundry skills to individuals with developmental disabilities using video prompting. *International Journal of Behavioral and Consultation Therapy, 4*(3), 279–286. doi:10.1037/h0100857

Horovitz, M., & Matson, J. L. (2010). Communication deficits in babies and infants with autism and pervasive developmental disorder-not otherwise specified (PDD-NOS). *Developmental Neurorehabilitation, 13*(6), 390–398. doi:10.3109/17518423.2010.501431 PMID:20887201

Hourcade, J. P., Bullock-Rest, N. E., & Hansen, T. E. (2012). Multitouch tablet application and activities to enhance the social skills of children with autism spectrum disorders. *Personal and Ubiquitous Computing, 16*(2), 157–168. doi:10.1007/s00779-011-0383-3

Howlett, W.P. (2012). Paraplegia non traumatic. *Neurological Disorders,* 231 – 254.

Howlin, P., Goode, S., Hutton, J., & Rutter, M. (2004). Adult outcome for children with autism. *Journal of Child Psychology and Psychiatry, and Allied Disciplines, 45*(2), 212–229. doi:10.1111/j.1469-7610.2004.00215.x PMID:14982237

Hsu, A., & Malkin, F. (2013). Professional development workshops for student teachers: An issue of concern. *Action in Teacher Education, 35*(5-6), 354–371. doi:10.1080/01626620.2013.846165

Huffington Post (Producer). (2013). Cutting-Edge Tech Gives a Synthetic Voice to the Voiceless. *Huff Post Tech.* [Video] Retrieved from http://www.huffingtonpost.com/2013/09/13/vocalid_n_3915829.html?utm_hp_ref=tw

Hulleman, C. S., Godes, O., Hendricks, B. L., & Harackiewicz, J. M. (2010). Enhancing interest and performance with a utility value intervention. *Journal of Educational Psychology, 102*(4), 880–895. doi:10.1037/a0019506

Hunt, K. J., Stone, B., Negard, N. O., Schauer, T., Fraser, M. H., Cathcart, A. J., & Grant, S. et al. (2004). Control strategies for integration of electric motor assist and functional electrical stimulation in paraplegic cycling: Utility for exercise testing and mobile cycling. *IEEE Transactions on Neural Systems and Rehabilitation Engineering, 12*(1), 89–101. doi:10.1109/TNSRE.2003.819955 PMID:15068192

Hunt, P., Soto, G., Maier, J., Müller, E., & Goetz, L. (2002). Collaborative teaming to support students with augmentative and alternative communication needs in general education classrooms. *Augmentative and Alternative Communication, 18*(1), 20–35. doi:10.1080/aac.18.1.20.35

Hutchinson, A., Beschorner, B., & Schmidt-Crawford, D. (2012). Exploring the use of the iPad for literacy learning. *The Reading Teacher, 66*(1), 15-23. doi: 10:1002/TRTR01090

Hutchins, T., & Prelock, P. (2013). Parents' perceptions of their children's social behavior: The social validity of Social Stories™ and Comic Strip Conversations™. *Journal of Positive Behavior Interventions*, *15*(3), 156–168. doi:10.1177/1098300712457418

Hynan, A., Murray, J., & Goldbart, J. (2014). 'Happy and excited': Perceptions of using digital technology and social media by young people who use augmentative and alternative communication. *Child Language Teaching and Therapy*, *30*(2), 175–186. doi:10.1177/0265659013519258

Iacono, T. A. (2004). Accessible reading intervention: A work in progress. *Augmentative and Alternative Communication*, *20*(3), 179–190. doi:10.1080/07434610410001699744

Iacono, T., & Duncum, J. (1995). Comparison of sign alone and in combination with an electronic communication device in early language intervention: Case study. *Augmentative and Alternative Communication*, *11*(4), 249–259. doi:10.1080/07434619512331277389

IDEA Data Center. (2014). *2012 IDEA Part B Child Count and Educational Environments*. Retrieved from https://explore.data.gov/Education/2012-IDEA-Part-B-Child-Count-and-Educational-Envir/5t72-4535

Iland, E. (2011). *Drawing a blank: Improving comprehension for readers on the autism spectrum*. Shawnee Mission, KS: AAPC Publishing.

Individuals With Disabilities Education Act (IDEA), 20 U.S.C. § 1400 (2004).

Individuals with Disabilities Education Improvement Act of 2004, 20 U.S.C.§ 614 *et seq.*

Individuals With Disabilities Education Improvement Act, 20 U.S.C. (2004). Retrieved from: http://idea.ed.gov/download/statute.html

InGenius Labs. (2012). *Emotion detective*. Perth, Australia: Author.

Inspiration Software, Inc. (n.d.). *Inspiration Software, Inc.* Retrieved April 3, 2015 from http://www.inspiration.com

International Council of Opthalmology. (2002). Visual standard: Aspects and ranges of vision loss.*International Congress of Opthalmology*, 1 – 33.

International Dyslexia Association. Promoting Literacy through Research, Education and Advocacy. (2014). Retrieved June 2, 2014, from http://www.interdys.org/SignsofDyslexiaCombined.htm

IROMEC. (2015, March 31). Retrieved from http://www.iromec.org/6.0.html

Isabelle, S., Bessey, S. F., Dragas, K. L., Blease, P., Shepherdfaculty, J. T., & Lanefaculty, S. J. (2003). Assistive technology for children with disabilities. *Occupational Therapy in Health Care*, *16*(4), 29–51. PMID:23930706

iTouchiLearn Apps. (n.d.). *iTouchiLearn apps: Mobile apps for early learners*. Retrieved April 3, 2015 from http://itouchilearnapps.com

Ivancic, M. T., & Bailey, J. S. (1996). Current limits to reinforcer identification for some persons with profound multiple disabilities. *Research in Developmental Disabilities*, *17*(1), 77–92. doi:10.1016/0891-4222(95)00038-0 PMID:8750077

Jacobson, L., Fernell, E., Broberger, U., Ek, U., & Gillberg, C. (1998). Children with blindness due to retinopathy of prematurity: A population-based study. Perinatal data, neurological and opthalmological outcome. *Developmental Medicine and Child Neurology*, *40*(3), 155–159. doi:10.1111/j.1469-8749.1998.tb15439.x PMID:9566650

Jain, S., Tamersoy, B., Zhang, Y., Aggarwal, J. K., & Orvalho, V. (2012, May). An interactive game for teaching facial expressions to children with autism spectrum disorders. In *Communications Control and Signal Processing (ISCCSP), 2012 5th International Symposium* (pp. 1-4). IEEE. doi:10.1109/ISCCSP.2012.6217849

Janssen, T., Glaser, R., & Shuster, D. (1998). Clinical efficacy of electrical stimulation exercise training: Effects on health, fitness, and function. *Topics in Spinal Cord Injury Rehabilitation*, *3*(3), 33–49.

Jarrold, C., Butler, D. W., Cottington, E. M., & Jimenez, F. (2000). Linking theory of mind and central coherence bias in autism and in the general population. *Developmental Psychology*, *36*(1), 126–138. doi:10.1037/0012-1649.36.1.126 PMID:10645750

Jetter, B., & Jetter, M. (1998). MindManager (v9) [Product of Mindjet]. *Mindjet*. Retrieved, February 4, 2014, from http://www.mindjet.com/mindmanager

Jimenez, B. A., Browder, D. M., & Courtade, G. R. (2008). Teaching an algebraic equation to high school students with moderate developmental disabilities. *Education and Training in Developmental Disabilities, 43*(2), 266–274.

Johnson, J. M., Inglebret, E., Jones, C., & Ray, J. (2006). Perspectives of speech language pathologists regarding success versus abandonment of AAC. *Augmentative and Alternative Communication, 22*(2), 85–99. doi:10.1080/07434610500483588 PMID:17114167

Johnston, S. S., Davenport, L., Kanarowski, B., Rhodehouse, S., & McDonnell, A. P. (2009). Teaching sound letter correspondence and consonant-vowel-consonant combinations to young children who use augmentative and alternative communication. *Augmentative and Alternative Communication, 25*(2), 123–135. doi:10.1080/07434610902921409 PMID:19444683

Johnston, S., & Feeley, K. (2012). AAC system features. In S. Johnston, J. Reichle, K. Feeley, & E. Jones (Eds.), *AAC strategies for individuals with moderate to severe disabilities* (pp. 51–80). Baltimore: Paul H. Brookes Publishing Co.

Jones, C., Reutzel, D. R., & Fargo, J. D. (2010). Comparing two methods of writing instruction: Effects on kindergarten students' reading skills. *The Journal of Educational Research, 103*(5), 327–341. doi:10.1080/00220670903383119

Jones, R., Quigney, C., & Huws, J. (2003). First-hand accounts of sensory perceptual experiences in autism: A qualitative analysis. *Journal of Intellectual & Developmental Disability, 28*(2), 112–121. doi:10.1080/1366825031000147058

Jordan, C. J., & Caldwell-Harris, C. L. (2012). Understanding differences in neurotypical and autism spectrum special interests through internet forums. *Intellectual and Developmental Disabilities, 50*(5), 391–402. doi:10.1352/1934-9556-50.5.391 PMID:23025641

Joshi, P. (2011, November 29). Finding good apps for children with autism. *Gadgetwise: The New York Times Blog.* Available at http://gadgetwise.blogs.nytimes.com/2011/11/29/finding-good-apps-for-children-with-autism

Jreige, C., Patel, R., & Bunnell, H. T. (2009). Vocal ID: Personalizing Text-to-Speech Synthesis for Individuals with Severe Speech Impairment. *Proceedings of the 11th international ACM SIGACCESS conference on Computers and Accessibility,* 259-260.

Judge, S., & Townend, G. (2013). Perceptions of the design of voice output communication aids. *International Journal of Language & Communication Disorders, 48*(4), 366–381. doi:10.1111/1460-6984.12012 PMID:23889833

Kaboski, J. R., Diehl, J. J., Beriont, J., Crowell, C. R., Villano, M., Wier, K., & Tang, K. (2014). Brief Report: A Pilot Summer Robotics Camp to Reduce Social Anxiety and Improve Social/Vocational Skills in Adolescents with ASD. *Journal of Autism and Developmental Disorders,* 1–8. PMID:24898910

Kaderavek, J. N. (2011). *Language disorders in children: Fundamental concepts in assessment and intervention.* Boston, MA: Allyn & Bacon Publishing.

Kaderavek, J. N., & Rabidoux, P. (2004). Interactive to independent literacy: A model for designing literacy goals for children with atypical communication. *Reading & Writing Quarterly, 20*(3), 237–260. doi:10.1080/10573560490429050

Kagohara, D. M. (2011). Three students with developmental disabilities are taught to operate an iPod to access age appropriate entertainment videos. *Journal of Behavioral Education, 20*(1), 33–43. doi:10.1007/s10864-010-9115-4

Kagohara, D. M., Sigafoos, J., Achmadi, D., O'Reilly, M., & Lancioni, G. (2011). Teaching children with autism spectrum disorders to check the spelling of words. *Research in Autism Spectrum Disorders, 6*(1), 304–310. doi:10.1016/j.rasd.2011.05.012

Kagohara, D. M., Sigafoos, J., Achmadi, D., van der Meer, L., O'Reilly, M. F., & Lancioni, G. E. (2011). Teaching students with developmental disabilities to operate an iPod Touch to listen to music. *Research in Developmental Disabilities, 32*(6), 2987–2992. doi:10.1016/j.ridd.2011.04.010 PMID:21645989

Kagohara, D. M., van der Meer, L., Ramdoss, S., O'Reilly, M. F., Lancioni, G. E., Davis, T. N., & Sigafoos, J. et al. (2013). Using iPods and iPads in teaching programs for individuals with developmental disabilities: A systematic review. *Research in Developmental Disabilities, 34*(1), 147–156. doi:10.1016/j.ridd.2012.07.027 PMID:22940168

Kagohara, D., van der Meer, L., Achmadi, D., Green, V. A., O'Reilly, M. F., Lancioni, G. E., & Sigafoos, J. et al. (2012). Teaching picture naming to two adolescents with autism spectrum disorders using systematic instruction and speech-generating devices. *Research in Autism Spectrum Disorders, 6*(3), 1224–1233. doi:10.1016/j.rasd.2012.04.001

Kagohara, D., van der Meer, L., Achmadi, D., Green, V. A., O'Reilly, M. F., Mulloy, A., & Sigafoos, J. et al. (2010). Behavioral intervention promotes successful use of an iPod-based communication device by an adolescent with autism. *Clinical Case Studies, 9*(5), 328–338. doi:10.1177/1534650110379633

Kamil, M. L. (2003). *Adolescents and literacy: Reading for the 21st century*. Washington, DC: Alliance for Excellent Education.

Kandalaft, M. R., Didehbani, N., Krawczyk, D. C., Allen, T. T., & Chapman, S. B. (2013). Virtual reality social cognition training for young adults with high-functioning autism. *Journal of Autism and Developmental Disorders, 43*(1), 34–44. doi:10.1007/s10803-012-1544-6 PMID:22570145

Kanne, S. M., & Mazurek, M. O. (2011). Aggression in children and adolescents with ASD: Prevalence and risk factors. *Journal of Autism and Developmental Disorders, 41*(7), 926–937. doi:10.1007/s10803-010-1118-4 PMID:20960041

Kaplan, J. S., & Carter, J. (1995). *Beyond behavior modification: A cognitive-behavioral approach to management in the school* (3rd ed.). Austin, TX: Pro-Ed.

Karchmer, M., & Trybus, R. (1977). *Who are the deaf children in the 'mainstream'' programs?* Washington, DC: Gallaudet College, Office of Demographic Studies.

Karvonen, M., Test, D. W., Wood, W. M., Browder, D., & Algozzine, B. (2004). Putting self-determination into practice. *Exceptional Children, 71*(1), 23–41. doi:10.1177/001440290407100102

Kasari, C., Kaiser, A., Goods, K., Nietfeld, J., Mathy, P., Landa, R., & Almirall, D. et al. (2014). Communication interventions for minimally verbal children with autism: A sequential multiple assignment randomized trial. *Journal of the American Academy of Child and Adolescent Psychiatry, 53*(6), 635–646. doi:10.1016/j.jaac.2014.01.019 PMID:24839882

Kazakoff-Lane, C. (2010). Anything, anywhere, anytime: The promise of the animated tutorial sharing project for online and mobile information literacy. *Journal of Library Administration, 50*(7/8), 747–766. doi:10.1080/01930826.2010.488961

Kazdin, A. E. (2001). *Behavior modification in applied settings* (6th ed.). New York: Wadsworth.

Keegan, D. (2005). *The incorporation of mobile learning into mainstream education and training*. Retrieved from http://www.mlearn.org.za/CD/papers/keegan1.pdf

Keen, D. V. (2008). Childhood autism, feeding problems and failure to thrive in early infancy. *European Child & Adolescent Psychiatry, 17*(4), 209–216. doi:10.1007/s00787-007-0655-7 PMID:17876499

Ke, F., & Im, T. (2013). Virtual-reality-based social interaction training for children with high-functioning autism. *The Journal of Educational Research, 106*(6), 441–461. doi:10.1080/00220671.2013.832999

Kennedy, C. (2005). *Single case designs for educational research*. New York: Allyn & Bacon.

Kennedy, C. (2005). *Single-case designs for educational research*. Boston: Pearson Education Inc.

Kenney, L., & Walsh, B. (2013). Avoidant/restrictive food intake disorder (ARFID) defining ARFID. *Eating Disorders Review, 24*(3), 1.

Kent-Walsh, J., Binger, C., & Hasham, Z. (2010). Effects of parent instruction on the symbolic communication of children using augmentative and alternative communication during storybook reading. *American Journal of Speech-Language Pathology, 19*(2), 97–107. doi:10.1044/1058-0360(2010/09-0014) PMID:20181850

Kent-Walsh, J., Binger, C., & Malani, M. (2010). Teaching partners to support the communication skills of young children who use AAC: Lessons from the ImPAACT Program. *Early Childhood Services (San Diego, Calif.)*, *4*(3), 155–170.

Kern, M. L., & Friedman, H. S. (2008). Early educational milestones as predictors of lifelong academic achievement, midlife adjustment, and longevity. *Journal of Applied Developmental Psychology*, *30*(4), 419–430. doi:10.1016/j. appdev.2008.12.025 PMID:19626128

Kerr, S., & Durkin, K. (2004). Understanding of thought bubble as mental representations in children with autism: Implications for theory of mind. *Journal of Autism and Developmental Disorders*, *34*(6), 637–648. doi:10.1007/ s10803-004-5285-z PMID:15679184

Kerscher, G., & Fruchterman, J. (2002). The soundproof book: Exploration of rights conflict and access to commercial ebooks for people with disabilities. *First Monday*, *7*(6). doi:10.5210/fm.v7i6.959

Keskinen, T., Heimonen, T., Turunen, M., Rajaniemi, J.-P., & Kauppinen, S. (2012). SymbolChat: A flexible picture-based communication platform for users with intellectual disabilities. *Interacting with Computers*, *24*(5), 374–386. doi:10.1016/j.intcom.2012.06.003

Kim, J., Wigram, T., & Gold, C. (2009). Emotional, motivational and interpersonal responsiveness of children with autism in improvisational music therapy. Sage Publications, 13 (4), 389 – 409.

Kim, E. S., Berkovits, L. D., Bernier, E. P., Leyzberg, D., Shic, F., Paul, R., & Scassellati, B. (2013). Social robots as embedded reinforcers of social behavior in children with autism. *Journal of Autism and Developmental Disorders*, *43*(5), 1038–1049. doi:10.1007/s10803-012-1645-2 PMID:23111617

Kim, E. S., Paul, R., Shic, F., & Scassellati, B. (2012). Bridging the research gap: Making HRI useful to individuals with autism. *Journal of Human-Robot Interaction*, *1*(1).

King, A. M., Thomeczek, M., Voreis, G., & Scott, V. (2014). iPad use in children and young adults with Autism Spectrum Disorder: An observational study. *Child Language Teaching and Therapy*, *30*(2), 159–173. doi:10.1177/0265659013510922

King, C., & Quigley, S. (1985). *Reading and deafness*. San Diego, CA: College Hill.

King, M. L., Takeguchi, K., Barry, S. E., Rehfeldt, R. A., Boyer, V. E., & Matthews, T. L. (2014). Evaluation of the iPad in the acquisition of requesting skills for children with autism spectrum disorder. *Research in Autism Spectrum Disorders*, *8*(9), 1107–1120. doi:10.1016/j. rasd.2014.05.011

Kirk, R., Hunt, A., Hildred, M., Neighbour, M., & North, F. (2002). Electronic Musical Instruments-a rôle in Music Therapy? In *Dialogue and Debate-Conference Proceedings of the 10th World Congress on Music Therapy* (p. 1007).

Kirshner, S., Weiss, P. L., & Tirosh, E. (2011). Meal-maker: A virtual meal preparation environment for children with cerebral palsy. *European Journal of Special Needs Education*, *26*(3), 323–336. doi:10.1080/08856257.2011.593826

Kliewer, C., Biklen, D., & Kasa-Hendrickson, C. (2006). Who may be literate? Disability and resistance to the cultural denial of competence. *American Educational Research Journal*, *43*(2), 163–192. doi:10.3102/00028312043002163

Knouse, L. E., Bagwell, C. L., Barkley, R. A., & Murphy, K. R. (2005). Accuracy of self-evaluation in adults with ADHD evidence from a driving study. *Journal of Attention Disorders*, *8*(4), 221–234. doi:10.1177/1087054705280159 PMID:16110052

Koenig, K., De Los Reyes, A., Cicchetti, D., Scahill, L., & Klin, A. (2009). Group intervention to promote social skills in school-age children with pervasive developmental: Reconsidering disorder efficacy. *Journal of Autism and Developmental Disorders*, *39*, 1163–1172. doi:10.1007/ s10803-009-0728-1 PMID:19326199

Kohnle, D. (2011). Paraplegia. *Nucleus Medical Media, Inc*, NYU Pediatrics, 1 – 4.

Koppenhaver, D. (2000). Literacy in AAC: What should be written on the envelope we push? *Augmentative and Alternative Communication*, *16*(4), 270–279. doi:10.10 80/07434610012331279124

Koppenhaver, D. A., & Erickson, K. (2003). Natural emergent literacy supports for preschoolers with autism and severe communication impairments. *Topics in Language Disorders*, *23*(4), 283–293. doi:10.1097/00011363-200310000-00004

Koppenhaver, D. A., Hendrix, M. P., & Williams, A. R. (2007). Toward evidence-based literacy interventions for children with severe and multiple disabilities. *Seminars in Speech and Language*, *28*(1), 79–89. doi:10.1055/s-2007-967932 PMID:17340385

Korat, O., Shamir, A., & Arbiv, L. (2011). E-books as support for emergent writing with and without adult assistance. *Education and Information Technologies*, *16*(3), 301–318. doi:10.1007/s10639-010-9127-7

Koyama, T., & Wang, H. (2011). Use of activity schedules to promote independent performance of individuals with autism and other intellectual disabilities: A review. *Research in Developmental Disabilities*, *32*(6), 2235–2242. doi:10.1016/j.ridd.2011.05.003 PMID:21645988

Krishnaswamy, S., Shriber, L., & Srimathveeravalli, G. (2014). The design and efficacy of a robot-mediated visual motor program for children learning disabilities. *Journal of Computer Assisted Learning*, *30*(2), 121–131. doi:10.1111/jcal.12025

Kucirkova, N., Messer, D., Critten, V., & Harwood, J. (2014). Story-Making on the iPad When Children Have Complex Needs Two Case Studies. *Communication Disorders Quarterly*, 1525740114525226.

Kunda, M., & Goel, A. K. (2011). Thinking in Pictures as a Cognitive Account of Autism. *Journal of Autism and Developmental Disorders*, *41*(9), 1157–1177. doi:10.1007/s10803-010-1137-1 PMID:21103918

Kupietz, S. S. (1990). Sustained attention in normal and in reading-disabled youngsters with and without ADDH. *Journal of Abnormal Child Psychology*, *18*(4), 357–372. doi:10.1007/BF00917640 PMID:2246429

Laarhoven, T. V., Winiarski, L., Blood, E., & Chan, J. M. (2012). Maintaining vocational skills of individuals with autism and developmental disabilities through video modeling. *Education and Training in Autism and Developmental Disabilities*, *47*(4), 447–461.

LaCava, P., Golan, O., Baron-Cohen, S., & Myles, B. S. (2007). Using assistive technology to teach emotion recognition to students with Asperger Syndrome. *Remedial and Special Education*, *28*(3), 174–181. doi:10.1177/07419325070280030601

Lachapelle, Y., Wehmeyer, M. L., Haelewyck, M. C., Courbois, Y., Keith, K. D., Schalock, R., & Walsh, P. N. et al. (2005). The relationship between quality of life and self-determination: An international study. *Journal of Intellectual Disability Research*, *49*(10), 740–744. doi:10.1111/j.1365-2788.2005.00743.x PMID:16162119

Laitusis, C. (2010). Examining the impact of audio presentation on tests of reading comprehension. *Applied Measurement in Education*, *23*(2), 153–167. doi:10.1080/08957341003673815

Lamb, A., & Callison, D. (2011). Graphic inquiry for all learners. *School Library Monthly*, *28*(3), 18-22. Retrieved, February, 4, 2014 from, http://search.proquest.com/docview/1018179930?accountid=1060

Lancioni, G. E., Antonucci, M., De Pace, C., O'Reilly, M. F., Sigafoos, J., Singh, N. N., & Oliva, D. (2007). Enabling two adolescents with multiple disabilities to choose among environmental stimuli through different procedural and technological approaches. *Perceptual and Motor Skills*, *105*(2), 362–372. doi:10.2466/pms.105.2.362-372 PMID:18065057

Lancioni, G. E., Bellini, D., Oliva, D., Singh, N. N., O'Reilly, M. F., Lang, R., & Didden, R. (2011). Camera-based microswitch technology to monitor mouth, eyebrow, and eyelid responses of children with profound multiple disabilities. *Journal of Behavioral Education*, *20*(1), 4–14. doi:10.1007/s10864-010-9117-2

Lancioni, G. E., Bellini, D., Oliva, D., Singh, N. N., O'Reilly, M. F., & Sigafoos, J. (2010). Camera-based microswitch technology for eyelid and mouth responses of persons with profound multiple disabilities: Two case studies. *Research in Developmental Disabilities*, *31*(6), 1509–1514. doi:10.1016/j.ridd.2010.06.006 PMID:20598501

Lancioni, G. E., O'Reilly, M. F., Singh, N. N., Buonocunto, F., Sacco, V., Colonna, F., & Bosco, A. et al. (2009). Technology-based intervention options for post-coma persons with minimally conscious state and pervasive motor disabilities. *Developmental Neurorehabilitation, 12*(1), 24–31. doi:10.1080/17518420902776995 PMID:19283531

Lancioni, G. E., O'Reilly, M. F., Singh, N. N., Green, V. A., Oliva, D., Campodonico, F., & Buono, S. et al. (2013a). Technology-aided programs to support exercise of adaptive head responses or leg-foot and hands responses in children with multiple disabilities. *Developmental Neurorehabilitation, 16*(4), 237–244. doi:10.3109/1751 8423.2012.757661 PMID:23323848

Lancioni, G. E., O'Reilly, M. F., Singh, N. N., Sigafoos, J., Didden, R., Oliva, D., & Groeneweg, J. et al. (2009b). Persons with multiple disabilities accessing stimulation and requesting social contact via microswitch and VOCA devices: New research evaluation and social validation. *Research in Developmental Disabilities, 30*(5), 1084–1094. doi:10.1016/j.ridd.2009.03.004 PMID:19361954

Lancioni, G. E., O'Reilly, M. F., Singh, N. N., Sigafoos, J., Oliva, D., Alberti, G., & Lang, R. et al. (2013). Technology-based programs to support adaptive responding and reduce hand mouthing in two persons with multiple disabilities. *Journal of Developmental and Physical Disabilities, 25*(1), 65–77. doi:10.1007/s10882-012-9303-3

Lancioni, G. E., O'Reilly, M. F., Singh, N. N., Sigafoos, J., Oliva, D., Baccani, S., & Stasolla, F. et al. (2004b). Technological aids to promote basic developmental achievements by children with multiple disabilities: Evaluation of two cases. *Cognitive Processing, 5*(4), 232–238. doi:10.1007/s10339-004-0030-2

Lancioni, G. E., O'Reilly, M. F., Singh, N. N., Sigafoos, J., Oliva, D., & Severini, L. (2008b). Enabling two persons with multiple disabilities to access environmental stimuli and ask for social contact through microswitches and a VOCA. *Research in Developmental Disabilities, 29*(1), 21–28. doi:10.1016/j.ridd.2006.10.001 PMID:17174529

Lancioni, G. E., O'Reilly, M. F., Singh, N. N., Sigafoos, J., Oliva, D., & Severini, L. (2008c). Three persons with multiple disabilities accessing environmental stimuli and asking for social contact through microswitch and VOCA technology. *Journal of Intellectual Disability Research, 52*(4), 327–336. doi:10.1111/j.1365-2788.2007.01024.x PMID:18339095

Lancioni, G. E., O'Reilly, M. F., Singh, N. N., Sigafoos, J., Oliva, D., Smaldone, A., & Chiapparino, C. et al. (2009c). Persons with multiple disabilities access stimulation and contact the caregiver via microswitch and VOCA technology. *Life Span and Disability, 12*, 119–128.

Lancioni, G. E., O'Reilly, M. F., Singh, N. N., Sigafoos, J., Oliva, D., Smaldone, A., & Chirico, M. et al. (2011b). Technology-assisted programs for promoting leisure or communication engagement in two persons with pervasive motor or multiple disabilities. *Disability and Rehabilitation. Assistive Technology, 6*(2), 108–114. doi:10.3109/1 7483107.2010.496524 PMID:20545564

Lancioni, G. E., O'Reilly, M., Singh, N., Green, V., Chiapparino, C., De Pace, C., & Stasolla, F. et al. (2010c). Use of microswitch technology and a keyboard emulator to support literacy performance of persons with extensive neuro-motor disabilities. *Developmental Neurorehabilitation, 13*(4), 248–257. doi:10.3109/17518423.2010.4855 96 PMID:20629591

Lancioni, G. E., Olivetti Belardinelli, M., Stasolla, F., Singh, N. N., O'Reilly, M. F., Sigafoos, J., & Angelillo, M. T. (2008a). Promoting engagement, requests and choice by a man with post-coma pervasive motor impairment and minimally conscious state through a technology-based program. *Journal of Developmental and Physical Disabilities, 20*(4), 379–388. doi:10.1007/ s10882-008-9104-x

Lancioni, G. E., O'Reilly, M. F., Singh, N. N., Oliva, D., Coppa, M. M., & Montironi, G. (2005). A new microswitch to enable a boy with minimal motor behavior to control environmental stimulation with eye blinks. *Behavioral Interventions, 20*(2), 147–153. doi:10.1002/bin.185

Lancioni, G. E., O'Reilly, M. F., Singh, N. N., Sigafoos, J., Tota, A., Antonucci, M., & Oliva, D. (2006). Children with multiple disabilities and minimal motor behavior using chin movements to operate microswitches to obtain environmental stimulation. *Research in Developmental Disabilities*, 27(3), 290–298. doi:10.1016/j.ridd.2005.02.003 PMID:16005183

Lancioni, G. E., O'Reilly, M. F., Singh, N. N., Stasolla, F., Manfredi, F., & Oliva, D. (2004a). Adapting a grid into a microswitch to suit simple hand movements of a child with profound multiple disabilities. *Perceptual and Motor Skills*, 99(2), 724–728. doi:10.2466/pms.99.2.724-728 PMID:15560365

Lancioni, G. E., Sigafoos, J., O'Reilly, M. F., & Singh, N. N. (2012). *Assistive Technology, Interventions for Individuals with Severe/Profound and Multiple Disabilities*. New York: Springer.

Lancioni, G. E., Sigafoos, J., O'Reilly, M. F., & Singh, N. N. (2012). *Assistive technology: interventions for individual with severe/profound and multiple disabilities*. New York: Springer.

Lancioni, G. E., & Singh, N. N. (2014). *Assistive technologies for people with diverse abilities*. New York: Springer. doi:10.1007/978-1-4899-8029-8

Lancioni, G. E., Singh, N. N., O'Reilly, M. F., Campodonico, F., Oliva, D., & Vigo, C. M. (2005b). Promoting walker-assisted step responses by an adolescent with multiple disabilities through automatically delivered stimulation. *Journal of Visual Impairment & Blindness*, 99, 109–113.

Lancioni, G. E., Singh, N. N., O'Reilly, M. F., Campodonico, F., Piazzolla, G., Scalini, L., & Oliva, D. (2005a). Impact of favorite stimuli automatically delivered on step responses of persons with multiple disabilities during their use of walker devices. *Research in Developmental Disabilities*, 26(1), 71–76. doi:10.1016/j.ridd.2004.04.003 PMID:15590239

Lancioni, G. E., Singh, N. N., O'Reilly, M. F., Green, V. A., Oliva, D., Buonocunto, F., & Di Nuovo, S. et al. (2012b). Technology-based programs to support forms of leisure engagement and communication for persons with multiple disabilities: Two single-case studies. *Developmental Neurorehabilitation*, 15(3), 209–218. doi:10.310 9/17518423.2012.666766 PMID:22582852

Lancioni, G. E., Singh, N. N., O'Reilly, M. F., & Oliva, D. (2005). Microswitch programs for persons with multiple disabilities: An overview of the responses adopted for microswitch activation. *Cognitive Processing*, 6(3), 177–188. doi:10.1007/s10339-005-0003-0 PMID:18231820

Lancioni, G. E., Singh, N. N., O'Reilly, M. F., Oliva, D., & Basili, G. (2005). An overview of research on increasing indices of happiness of people with severe/profound intellectual and multiple disabilities. *Disability and Rehabilitation*, 27(3), 83–93. doi:10.1080/09638280400007406 PMID:15823988

Lancioni, G. E., Singh, N. N., O'Reilly, M. F., Sigafoos, J., Alberti, G., Perilli, V., & Groeneweg, J. et al. (2014a). People with multiple disabilities learn to engage in occupation and work activities with the support of technology-aided programs. *Research in Developmental Disabilities*, 35(6), 1264–1271. doi:10.1016/j.ridd.2014.03.026 PMID:24685943

Lancioni, G. E., Singh, N. N., O'Reilly, M. F., Sigafoos, J., Buonocunto, F., Sacco, V., & De Pace, C. et al. (2009a). Two persons with severe post-coma motor impairment and minimally conscious state use assistive technology to access stimulus events and social contact. *Disability and Rehabilitation. Assistive Technology*, 4(5), 367–372. doi:10.1080/17483100903038584 PMID:19565377

Lancioni, G. E., Singh, N. N., O'Reilly, M. F., Sigafoos, J., Didden, R., & Oliva, D. (2009d). A technology-based stimulation program to reduce hand mouthing by an adolescent with multiple disabilities. *Perceptual and Motor Skills*, 109(2), 478–486. doi:10.2466/pms.109.2.478-486 PMID:20038002

Lancioni, G. E., Singh, N. N., O'Reilly, M. F., Sigafoos, J., Didden, R., & Oliva, D. (2009e). Two boys with multiple disabilities increasing adaptive responding and curbing dystonic/spastic behavior via a microswitch-based program. *Research in Developmental Disabilities*, *30*(2), 378–385. doi:10.1016/j.ridd.2008.07.005 PMID:18760566

Lancioni, G. E., Singh, N. N., O'Reilly, M. F., Sigafoos, J., Oliva, D., & Basili, G. (2012). New rehabilitation opportunities for persons with multiple disabilities through the use of microswitch technology. In S. Federici & M. J. Scherer (Eds.), *Assistive technology assessment handbook* (pp. 399–419). New York: CRC Press.

Lancioni, G. E., Singh, N. N., O'Reilly, M. F., Sigafoos, J., Oliva, D., Piazzolla, G., & Manfredi, F. et al. (2007c). Automatically delivered stimulation for walker-assisted step responses: Measuring its effects in persons with multiple disabilities. *Journal of Developmental and Physical Disabilities*, *19*(1), 1–13. doi:10.1007/s10882-006-9030-8

Lancioni, G. E., Singh, N. N., O'Reilly, M. F., Sigafoos, J., Oliva, D., Scalini, L., & Di Bari, M. et al. (2007b). Promoting foot-leg movements in children with multiple disabilities through the use of support devices and technology for regulating contingent stimulation. *Cognitive Processing*, *8*(4), 279–283. doi:10.1007/s10339-007-0179-6 PMID:17680286

Lancioni, G. E., Singh, N. N., O'Reilly, M. F., Sigafoos, J., Oliva, D., Smaldone, A., & Groeneweg, J. et al. (2010a). Promoting ambulation responses among children with multiple disabilities through walkers and microswitches with contingent stimuli. *Research in Developmental Disabilities*, *31*(3), 811–816. doi:10.1016/j.ridd.2010.02.006 PMID:20207105

Lancioni, G. E., Singh, N. N., O'Reilly, M. F., Oliva, D., Smaldone, A., Tota, A., & Groeneweg, J. et al. (2006). Assessing the effects of stimulation versus microswitch-based programmes on indices of happiness of students with multiple disabilities. *Journal of Intellectual Disability Research*, *50*(10), 739–747. doi:10.1111/j.1365-2788.2006.00839.x PMID:16961703

Lancioni, G. E., Singh, N. N., O'Reilly, M. F., & Sgafoos, J. (2011). Assistive technology for behavioral interventions for persons with severe/profound multiple disabilities: A selective overview. *European Journal of Behavior Analysis*, *12*, 7–26.

Lancioni, G. E., Singh, N. N., O'Reilly, M. F., Sigaffos, J., Chiapparino, C., Stasolla, F., & Oliva, D. (2007d). Using an optic sensor and a scanning keyboard emulator to facilitate writing by persons with pervasive motor disabilities. *Journal of Developmental and Physical Disabilities*, *19*(6), 593–603. doi:10.1007/s10882-007-9073-5

Lancioni, G. E., Singh, N. N., O'Reilly, M. F., Sigafoos, J., Didden, R., Oliva, D., & Cingolani, E. (2008d). A girl with multiple disabilities increases object manipulation and reduces hand mouthing through a microswitch-based program. *Clinical Case Studies*, *7*(3), 238–249. doi:10.1177/1534650107307478

Lancioni, G. E., Singh, N. N., O'Reilly, M. F., Sigafoos, J., Green, V., Chiapparino, C., & Oliva, D. et al. (2009f). A voice detecting sensor and a scanning keyboard emuloator to support word writing by two boys with extensive motor disabilities. *Research in Developmental Disabilities*, *30*(2), 203–209. doi:10.1016/j.ridd.2008.03.001 PMID:18417320

Lancioni, G. E., Singh, N. N., O'Reilly, M. F., Sigafoos, J., Oliva, D., & Severini, L. et al.. (2007d). Microswitch technology to promote adaptive responses and reduce mouthing in two children with multiple disabilities. *Journal of Visual Impairment & Blindness*, *101*, 628–636.

Lane, K., Harris, K. R., Graham, S., Weisenbach, J. L., Brindle, M., & Morphy, P. (2008). The Effects of Self-Regulated Strategy Development on the Writing Performance of Second-Grade Students With Behavioral and Writing Difficulties. *The Journal of Special Education*, *41*(4), 234–253. doi:10.1177/0022466907310370

Lane, S. J., & Mistrett, S. G. (1996). Play and Assistive Technology Issues for Infants and Young Children with Disabilities A Preliminary Examination. *Focus on Autism and Other Developmental Disabilities*, *11*(2), 96–104. doi:10.1177/108835769601100205

Langer, J. A. (2001). Beating the odds: Teaching middle and high school students to read and write well. *American Educational Research Journal*, *38*(4), 837–880. doi:10.3102/00028312038004837

Langstrom, N., Grann, M., Richkin, V., Sjostedt, G., & Fazel, S. (2009). Risk factors for violent offending in autism spectrum disorder: A national study of hospitalized individuals. *Journal of Interpersonal Violence*, *24*(8), 1358–1370. doi:10.1177/0886260508322195 PMID:18701743

Lanyon, H. (2012). *The iPad and augmentative and alternative communication. Unpublished Graduate Research Project*. Springfield, MO: Missouri State University.

Larson, L. C. (2009). e-Reading and e-Responding: New tools for the next generation of readers. *Journal of Adolescent & Adult Literacy*, *53*(3), 255–258. doi:10.1598/JAAL.53.3.7

Lee, A., Lang, R., Davenport, K., Moore, M., Rispoli, M., van der Meer, L., . . . Chung, C. (2013). Comparison of therapist implemented and iPad-assisted interventions for children with autism. *Developmental Neurorehabilitation*. Retrieved June 25, 2014, from http://informahealthcare.com/doi/abs/10.3109/17518423.2013.830231

Lequia, J., Machalicek, W., & Rispoli, M. J. (2012). Effects of activity schedules on challenging behavior exhibited in children with autism spectrum disorders: A systematic review. *Research in Autism Spectrum Disorders*, *6*(1), 480–492. doi:10.1016/j.rasd.2011.07.008

Leu, D. J., Kinzer, C. K., Coiro, J., Castek, J., & Henry, L. A. (2013). New literacies: A dual level theory of the changing nature of literacy, instruction, and assessment. In D. E. Alvermann, N. J. Unrau, & R. B. Ruddell (Eds.), *Theoretical models and processes of reading* (6th ed.; pp. 1150–1181). Newark, DE: International Reading Association. doi:10.1598/0710.42

Leung, B., & Chau, T. (2010). A multiple camera tongue switch for a child with severe spastic quadriplegic cerebral palsy. *Disability and Rehabilitation. Assistive Technology*, *5*(1), 58–68. doi:10.3109/17483100903254561 PMID:19941441

Leyshon, R. T., & Shaw, L. E. (2008). Using the ICF as a conceptual framework to guide ergonomic intervention in occu- pational rehabilitation. *Work (Reading, Mass.)*, *31*, 47–61. PMID:18820420

Life, S.® (2003). Available from http://secondlife.com (Retrieved March 31, 2015).

Light, J., & McNaughton, D. (2012). Supporting the communication, language, and literacy development of children with complex communication needs: State of the Science and Future Research Priorities. *Assistive Technology*, *24*(1), 34–44. doi:10. 1080/10400435.2011.684717

Light, J. (1997). "Let's go star fishing": Reflections on the contexts of language learning for children who use aided AAC. *Augmentative and Alternative Communication*, *13*(3), 158–171. doi:10.1080/07434619712331277978

Light, J. (1998). Toward a definition of communication competence for individuals using augmentative and alternative communication systems. *Augmentative and Alternative Communication*, *5*(2), 137–144. doi:10.1080/07434618912331275126

Light, J. C., & McNaughton, D. (2014). Communicative competence for individuals who require augmentative and alternative communication: A new definition for a new era of communication? *Augmentative and Alternative Communication*, *30*(1), 1–18. doi:10.3109/07434618.2014.885080

Light, J., & Kelford Smith, A. (1993). Home literacy experiences of preschoolers who use AAC systems and of their nondisabled peers. *Augmentative and Alternative Communication*, *9*(1), 10–25. doi:10.1080/07434619312331276371

Light, J., & McNaughton, D. (2009). *Accessible Literacy Learning: Evidence-based reading instruction for individuals with autism, cerebral palsy, Down syndrome, and other disabilities*. San Diego, CA: Mayer-Johnson.

Light, J., & McNaughton, D. (2012a). Supporting the communication, language, and literacy development of children with complex communication needs: State of the science and future research priorities. *Assistive Technology*, *24*(1), 34–44. doi:10.1080/10400435.2011.648717 PMID:22590798

Light, J., & McNaughton, D. (2012b). The changing face of augmentative and alternative communication: Past, present, and future challenges. *Augmentative and Alternative Communication*, 28(4), 197–204. doi:10.31 09/07434618.2012.737024 PMID:23256853

Light, J., McNaughton, D., Weyer, M., & Karg, L. (2008). Evidence-based literacy instruction for individuals who require augmentative and alternative communication: A case study of a student with multiple disabilities. *Seminars in Speech and Language*, 29(2), 120–132. doi:10.1055/s-2008-1079126 PMID:18645914

Lin, M., Fulford, C. P., Ho, C. P., Iyoda, R., & Ackerman, L. K. (2012). *Possibilities and challenges in mobile learning for k-12 teachers: A pilot retrospective survey study*. Proceedings from IEEE Seventh International Conference on Wireless, Mobile, and Ubiquitous Technology in Education (pp. 132-136). Retrieved from http://doi.ieeecomputersociety.org/10.1109/WMUTE.2012.31

Lisle, K. (2011). *Identifying the negative stigma associated with having a learning disability*. (Thesis for honors in psychology). Retrieved, March 20, 2014, from, http://digitalcommons.bucknell.edu/cgi/viewcontent.cgi?article=1021&context=honors

Lohmander, A., Henriksson, C., & Havstam, C. (2010). Electropalatography in home training of retracted articulation in a Swedish child with cleft palate: Effect on articulation pattern and speech. *International Journal of Speech-Language Pathology*, 12(6), 483–496. doi:10.3109/17549501003782397 PMID:20602582

Lonigan, C. J., Allan, N. P., & Lerner, M. D. (2011). Assessment of preschool early literacy skills: Linking children's educational needs with empirically supported instructional activities. *Psychology in the Schools*, 48(5), 488–501. doi:10.1002/pits.20569 PMID:22180666

Lontis, E. R., & Struijk, L. N. (2010). Design of inductive sensors for tongue control system for computers and assistive devices. *Disability and Rehabilitation. Assistive Technology*, 5(4), 266–271. doi:10.3109/17483101003718138 PMID:20307253

Loomis, J. W. (2008). *Staying in the game: Providing social opportunities for children and adolescents with autism spectrum disorders and other developmental disabilities*. Shawnee Mission, KS: AAPC Publishing.

Lorah, E. R., Crouser, J., Gilroy, S. P., Tincani, M., & Hantula, D. (2014). Within stimulus prompting to teach symbol discrimination using an iPad® speech generating device. *Journal of Developmental and Physical Disabilities*, 26(3), 335–346. doi:10.1007/s10882-014-9369-1

Lorah, E. R., Tincani, M., Dodge, J., Gilroy, S. P., Hickey, A., & Hantula, D. (2013). Evaluating picture exchange and the iPad as a speech generating device to teach communication to young children with autism. *Journal of Developmental and Physical Disabilities*, 25(6), 637–649. doi:10.1007/s10882-013-9337-1

Lorenz, B., Green, T., & Brown, A. (2009). Using Multimedia Graphic Organizer Software in the Prewriting Activities of Primary School Students: What Are the Benefits? *Computers in the Schools*, 26(2), 115–129. doi:10.1080/07380560902906054

Lotan, M., Yalon-Chamovitz, S., & Weiss, P. L. T. (2009). Improving physical fitness of individuals with intellectual and developmental disability through a Virtual Reality Intervention Program. *Research in Developmental Disabilities*, 30(2), 229–239. doi:10.1016/j.ridd.2008.03.005 PMID:18479889

Loth, E., Gómez, J. C., & Happé, F. (2008). Event schemas in autism spectrum disorders: The role of theory of mind and weak central coherence. *Journal of Autism and Developmental Disorders*, 38(3), 449–463. doi:10.1007/s10803-007-0412-2 PMID:17668309

Lund, S. K., & Light, J. (2006). Long-term outcomes for individuals who use augmentative and alternative communication: Part I-what is a "good" outcome? *Augmentative and Alternative Communication*, 22(4), 284–299. doi:10.1080/07434610600718693 PMID:17127616

Lyons, G., & Cassebohm, M. (2012). The education of Australian school students with the most severe intellectual disabilities: Where have we been and where could we go? A discussion primer. *Australasian Journal of Special Education*, 36(1), 79–95. doi:10.1017/jse.2012.8

Macaruso, P., & Rodman, A. (2011). Efficacy of computer-assisted instruction for the development of early literacy skills in young children. *Reading Psychology*, 32(2), 172–196. doi:10.1080/02702711003608071

Machalicek, W., Sanford, A., Lang, R., Rispoli, M., Molfenter, N., & Mbesha, M. K. (2010). Literacy interventions for students with physical and developmental disabilities who use aided AAC: A systematic review. *Journal of Developmental and Physical Disabilities, 22*(3), 219–240. doi:10.1007/s10882-009-9175-3

Maclean, R. (1988). Two paradoxes of phonics. *The Reading Teacher, 41*(6), 514–517.

Macnab, I., Rojjanasrirat, W., & Sanders, A. (2012). Breastfeeding and Telehealth. *Journal of Human Lactation, 28*(4), 446–449. doi:10.1177/0890334412460512 PMID:23087193

Magee, W. L. (2006). Electronic technologies in clinical music therapy: A survey of practice and attitudes. *Technology and Disability, 18*(3), 139–146.

Malone, T. W., & Lepper, M. R. (1987). Making learning fun: A taxonomy of intrinsic motivations for learning. *Aptitude. Learning and Instruction, 3*, 223–253.

Manko, J. (2013/2014). Technology driven literacy instruction: Liberty Elementary's iPad initiative. *Reading Today, 31*(3), 35.

Marano, H. E. (July 1, 2003). *Dangers of loneliness.* Retrieved June 24, 2014 from http://www.psychologytoday.com/articles/200308/the-dangers-loneliness

Marcu, G., Dey, A. K., & Kiesler, S. (2012). Parent-driven use of wearable cameras for autism support: A field study with families. *UbiComp, 1*, 1–10.

Martin, J. E., Mithaug, D. E., & Frazier, E. S. (1992). Effects of picture referencing on PVC chair, love seat, and settee assemblies by students with mental retardation. *Research in Developmental Disabilities, 13*(3), 267–286. doi:10.1016/0891-4222(92)90029-6 PMID:1626083

Marvin, C., Beukelman, D., & Bilyeu, D. (1994). Vocabulary-use patterns in preschool children: Effects of context and time sampling. *Augmentative and Alternative Communication, 10*(4), 224–236. doi:10.1080/0743461 9412331276930

Mason, R. A., Davies, H. S., Boyles, M. B., & Goodwyn, F. (2013). Efficacy of Point of View Video Modeling: A Meta-Analysis. *Remedial and Special Education, 34*(6), 333–345. doi:10.1177/0741932513486298

Mason, R. A., Ganz, J. B., Parker, R. I., Burke, M. D., & Camargo, S. P. (2012). Moderating factors of video modeling with other as model: A meta-analysis of single-case studies. *Research in Developmental Disabilities, 33*(4), 1076–1086. doi:10.1016/j.ridd.2012.01.016 PMID:22502832

Masterson, J. J., Apel, K., & Wood, L. A. (2002). Technology and literacy: Decisions for the new millennium. In K. G. Butler & E. R. Silliman (Eds.), *Speaking, Reading, and Writing in Children with Language Learning Disabilities* (pp. 273–293). Mahwah, NJ: Lawrence Erlbaum Associates Publishers.

Matas, J., Mathy-Laikko, P., Beukelman, D., & Legresley, K. (1985). Identifying the nonspeaking population: A demographic study. *Augmentative and Alternative Communication, 1*(1), 17–31. doi:10.1080/074346185 12331273491

Matawa, C. (2009). Exploring the musical interests and abilities of blind and partially sighted children and young people with retinopathy of prematurity. *British Journal of Visual Impairment, 27*(3), 252–262. doi:10.1177/0264619609106364

Mataya, K., & Owens, P. (2013). *Successful problem-solving for high-functioning students with autism spectrum disorder.* Shawnee Mission, KS: AAPC Publishing.

Mathisen, B., Arthur-Kelly, M., Kidd, J., & Nissen, C. (2009). Using MINSPEAK: A case study of a preschool child with complex communication needs. *Disability and Rehabilitation. Assistive Technology, 4*(5), 376–383. doi:10.1080/17483100902807112 PMID:19484639

Mat, S. J., Zhang, D., & Pacha, J. (2012). Employability skills valued by employers as important for entry-level employees with and without disabilities. *Career Development and Transition for Exceptional Individuals, 35*(1), 29–38. doi:10.1177/0885728811419167

Matson, J. L., & Nebel-Schwalm, M. S. (2007). Comorbid psychopathology with autism spectrum disorder in children: An overview. *Research in Developmental Disabilities, 28*(4), 341–352. doi:10.1016/j.ridd.2005.12.004 PMID:16765022

Mayberry, R. I., & Eichen, E. B. (1991). The long-lasting advantage of learning sign language in childhood: Another look at the critical period for language acquisition. *Journal of Memory and Language, 30*(4), 486–498. doi:10.1016/0749-596X(91)90018-F

Mayo Clinic Staff. (2014, February 15). *Friendships: Enrich your life and improve your health.* Retrieved June 24, 2014, from http://www.mayoclinic.org/healthy-living/adult-health/in-depth/friendships/art-20044860?pg=1

Mazurek, M. O., & Wenstrup, C. (2013). Television, video game and social media use among children with ASD and typically developing siblings. *Journal of Autism and Developmental Disorders, 43*(6), 1258–1271. doi:10.1007/s10803-012-1659-9 PMID:23001767

McBride, D. (2011). AAC evaluations and new mobile technologies: Asking and answering the right questions. *SIG 12 Perspectives on Augmentative and Alternative Communication, 20*(1), 9-16.

McBride, D. (2011). AAC evaluations and new mobile technologies: Asking and answering the right questions. *SIG 12 Perspectives on Augmentative and Alternative Communication, 20(1),* 9-16. doi:10.1044/aac20.1.9

McCarthy, J. H., Beukelman, D. R., & Hogan, T. P. (2011). Impact of computerized "sounding out" on spelling performance of a child who use AAC: A preliminary report. *SIG 12 Perspectives on Augmentative and Alternative Communication, 20(4),* 119-124. doi:10.1044/aac20.4.119

McClanahan, B., Williams, K., Kennedy, E., & Tate, S. (2012). A breakthrough for Josh: How use of an iPad facilitated reading improvement. *TechTrends: Linking Research and Practice to Improve Learning, 56*(3), 20–28. doi:10.1007/s11528-012-0572-6

McConachie, S., Hall, M., Resnick, L., Ravi, A., Bill, V., Bintz, J., & Taylor, J. (2006). Task, text, and talk: Literacy for all subjects.[theses]. *Educational Leadership, 64*(2), 8–14.

McCullough, A. (2001). Viability and effectiveness of teletherapy for pre-school children with special needs. *International Journal of Language & Communication Disorders, 36*321–36326. PMID:11340805

McGrail, E., & Davis, A. (2011). The influence of classroom blogging on elementary student writing. *Journal of Research in Childhood Education, 25*(4), 415–437. doi:10.1080/02568543.2011.605205

McKenna, M. C. (1998). Electronic texts and the transformation of beginning reading. In D. R. Reinking, M. C. McKenna, L. D. Labbo, & R. D. Kieffer (Eds.), *Handbook of literacy and technology: Transformations in a posttypographic world* (pp. 45–59). Hillsdale, NJ: Lawrence Erlbaum.

McKenna, M. C., Reinking, D., Labbo, L. D., & Kieffer, R. D. (1999). The electronic transformation of literacy and its implications for the struggling reader. *Reading & Writing Quarterly, 15,* 111–126. doi:10.1080/105735699278233

McKenna, M. C., & Robinson, R. D. (2009). *Teaching through text: Reading and writing in the content areas.* New York, NY: Pearson.

McKeown, M., Beck, I., & Blake, R. (2009). Reading comprehension instruction: Focus on content or strategies? *Perspectives on Language and Literacy, 35*(2), 28.

McLeod, L. (2011). Game Changer. *Perspectives on AAC, 20*(1), 17–18. doi:10.1044/aac20.1.17

McNab, K. (2013). *Bridging the digital divide with iPads: Effects on early literacy.* Paper presented at the conference of the International Society for Technology in Education, San Antonio, TX.

McNaughton, D., & Light, J. (January, 2010). *Evidence-based literacy intervention for individuals with complex communication needs.* Assistive Technology Industry Association, Orlando, FL. Retrieved from: http://aac-rerc.psu.edu/_userfiles/file/ATIA%202010%20%20literacy%20HO%202%20page.pdf

McNaughton, D., & Bryen, D. N. (2007). AAC technologies to enhance participation and meaningful societal roles for adolescents and adults with developmental disabilities who require AAC. *Augmentative and Alternative Communication, 23*(3), 217–229. doi:10.1080/07434610701573856 PMID:17701741

McNaughton, D., & Light, J. C. (2013). The iPad and mobile technology revolution: Benefits and challenges for individuals who require augmentative and alternative communication. *Augmentative and Alternative Communication*, 29(2), 107–116. doi:10.3109/07434618.2013.784930 PMID:23705813

McNaughton, D., Rackensperger, T., Benedek-Wood, E., Krezman, C., Williams, M. B., & Light, J. C. (2008). "A child needs to be given a chance to succeed": Parents of individuals who use AAC describe the benefits and challenges of learning AAC technologies. *Augmentative and Alternative Communication*, 24(1), 43–55. doi:10.1080/07434610701421007 PMID:18256963

McNulty, M. A. (2003). Dyslexia and the life course. *Journal of Learning Disabilities*, 36(4), 363–381. doi:10.1177/00222194030360040701 PMID:15490908

Mechling, L. C., Ayres, K. M., Bryant, K. J., & Foster, A. L. (2014). Continuous video modeling to assist with completion of multi-step home living tasks by young adults with moderate intellectual disability. *Education and Training in Autism and Developmental Disabilities*, 49(3), 368–380.

Mechling, L. C., & Collins, T. S. (2012). Comparison of the effects of video models with and without verbal cueing on task completion by young adult s with moderate intellectual disabilities. *Education and Training in Autism and Developmental Disabilities*, 47(2), 223–235.

Mechling, L. C., Gast, D. L., & Barthold, S. (2003). Multimedia computer-based instruction to teach students with moderate intellectual disabilities to use a debit card to make purchases. *Exceptionality*, 11(4), 239–254. doi:10.1207/S15327035EX1104_4

Mechling, L. C., Gast, D. L., & Seid, N. H. (2009). Using a personal digital assistant to increase independent task completion by students with autism spectrum disorder. *Journal of Autism and Developmental Disorders*, 39(10), 1420–1434. doi:10.1007/s10803-009-0761-0 PMID:19466534

Mechling, L. C., Gast, D. L., & Seid, N. H. (2010). Evaluation of a personal digital assistant as a self-prompting device for increasing multi-step task completion by students with moderate intellectual disabilities. *Education and Training in Autism and Developmental Disabilities*, 45, 422–439.

Mechling, L. C., Pridgen, L. S., & Cronin, B. A. (2005). Computer-based video instruction to teach students with intellectual disabilities to verbally respond to questions and make purchases in fast food restaurants. *Education and Training in Developmental Disabilities*, 40, 47–59.

Mechling, L. C., & Seid, N. H. (2011). Use of a hand-held personal digital assistant (PDA) to self-prompt pedestrian travel by young adults with moderate intellectual disabilities. *Education and Training in Autism and Developmental Disabilities*, 46, 220–237.

Mechling, L., Gast, D. L., & Fields, E. A. (2008). Evaluation of a portable DVD player and system of least prompts to self-prompt cooking task completion by young adults with moderate intellectual disabilities. *The Journal of Special Education*, 42(3), 179–190. doi:10.1177/0022466907313348

Mechling, L., Gast, D., & Gustafson, M. (2009). Use of video modeling to teach extinguishing of cooking related fires to individuals with moderate intellectual disabilities. *Education and Training in Developmental Disabilities*, 44(1), 67–79.

Meder, A. (2012). *Mobile media devices and communication applications as a form of augmentative and alternative communication: An assessment of family wants, needs, and preferences.* Unpublished Master's Thesis, University of Kansas.

MediaWiki. (2014). *MediaWiki, The Free Wiki Engine.* Retrieved, February 4, 2014, from http://www.mediawiki.org/w/index.php?title=MediaWiki&oldid=740803

Melzak, J. (1969). Paraplegia among children. *Lancet*, 294(7610), 45–48. doi:10.1016/S0140-6736(69)92612-9 PMID:4182806

Melzi, G., & Caspe, M. (2005). Variations in maternal narrative styles during book reading interactions. *Narrative Inquiry*, 15(1), 101–125. doi:10.1075/ni.15.1.06mel

Millar, D. C., Light, J. C., & McNaughton, D. B. (2004). The effect of direct instruction and writer's workshop on the early writing skills of children who use augmentative and alternative communication. *AAC: Augmentative & Alternative Communication, 20*(3), 164–178. Retrieved from http://search.ebscohost.com/login.aspx?direct=true&db=rzh&AN=2005025249&site=ehost-live&scope=site

Millar, D. C., Light, J. C., & Schlosser, R. W. (2006). The impact of augmentative and alternative communication intervention on the speech production of individuals with developmental disabilities: A research review. *Journal of Speech, Language, and Hearing Research: JSLHR, 49*(2), 248–264. doi:10.1044/1092-4388(2006/021) PMID:16671842

MindGenius, Ltd. (2001). *MindGenius* (v5) [Part of Gael Group]. MindGenius, Ltd. Retrieved, February 4, 2014, from http://www.mindgenius.com

Minshew, N. J., Meyer, J., & Goldstein, G. (2002). Abstract reasoning in autism: A disassociation between concept formation and concept identification. *Neuropsychology, 16*(3), 327–334. doi:10.1037/0894-4105.16.3.327 PMID:12146680

Mintz, J., Branch, C., March, C., & Lerman, S. (2012). Key factors mediating the use of a mobile technology tool designed to develop social and life skills in children with autistic spectrum disorders. *Computers & Education, 58*(1), 53–62. doi:10.1016/j.compedu.2011.07.013

Mirenda, P. (2001). Beneath the surface. *Augmentative and Alternative Communication, 17*(1), 1–1. doi:10.1080/aac.17.1.1.1

Mirenda, P. (2003). Toward functional augmentative and alternative communication for students with autism: Manual signs, graphic symbols, and voice output communication aids. *Language, Speech, and Hearing Services in Schools, 34*(3), 203–216. doi:10.1044/0161-1461(2003/017)

Mirenda, P. (2009). Introduction to AAC for individuals with autism spectrum disorders. In P. Mirenda & T. Iacono (Eds.), *Autsim spectrum disorders and AAC* (pp. 3–22). Baltimore: Paul H. Brookes Publishing Co.

Mitchell, P., Parsons, S., & Leonard, A. (2007). Using virtual environments for teaching social understanding to 6 adolescents with autistic spectrum disorders. *Journal of Autism and Developmental Disorders, 37*(3), 589–600. doi:10.1007/s10803-006-0189-8 PMID:16900403

Mobile Education Store. (n.d.). *Mobile Education Store: Apps.* Retrieved April 3, 2015 from http://mobile-educationstore.com/category/apps

Model Me Kids. (2010). *Model me going places* (2nd ed.). Rockville, MD: Author. Retrieved on June 20, 2014 from http://www.modelmekids.com/autism_aspergers_faq.html

Moeller, M. P., Osberger, M. J., & Eccarius, M. (1986). Language and learning skills of hearing-impaired students: Receptive language skills. *ASHA Monographs, 23*, 41–53. PMID:3730031

Monibi, M., & Hayes, G. R. (2008). Mocotos: Mobile communications tools for children with special needs. *IDC, 2008*, 121–124. doi:10.1145/1463689.1463736

Moody, A. K. (2010). Using electronic books in the classroom to enhance emergent literacy s skills in young children. *Journal of Literacy and Technology, 11*(4), 22–52.

Moore, D., Cheng, Y., McGrath, P., & Powell, N. J. (2005). Collaborative virtual environment technology for people with autism. *Focus on Autism and Other Developmental Disabilities, 20*(4), 231–243. doi:10.1177/10883576050200040501

Moore, M., & Calvert, S. (2000). Brief report: Vocabulary acquisition for children with autism: Teacher or computer instruction. *Journal of Autism and Developmental Disorders, 30*(4), 359–362. doi:10.1023/A:1005535602064 PMID:11039862

Morgan, H. (2013). Multimodal children's e-books help young learners in reading. *Early Childhood Education Journal, 41*(6), 477–483. doi:10.1007/s10643-013-0575-8

Motion, S., Northstone, K., Emond, A., & Team, A. L. S. P. A. C. S. (2001). Persistent early feeding difficulties and subsequent growth and developmental outcomes. *Ambulatory Child Health, 7*(3/4), 231–237. doi:10.1046/j.1467-0658.2001.00139.x

Mottron, L., Dawson, M., Soulieres, I., Hubert, B., & Burack, J. (2006). Enhanced perceptual functioning in autism: An update, and eight principles of autistic perception. *Journal of Autism and Developmental Disorders*, *36*(1), 27–43. doi: 0.1007/s10803-005-0040-7 PMID:16453071

Moussavi, R. M., Ribas-Cardus, F., Rintala, D. H., & Rodriquez, G. P. (2001). Dietary and serum lipids in individuals with spinal cord injury living in the community. *Journal of Rehabilitation Research and Development*, *38*(2), 225–233. PMID:11392655

Mower, E., Black, M. P., Flores, E., Williams, M., & Narayanan, S. (2011). RACHEL: Design of an emotionally targeted interactive agent for children with autism. In *Multimedia and Expo (ICME), 2011 IEEE International Conference on* (pp. 1-6). IEEE.

Mullenweg, M. (2005). *Wordpress.com* (v3.9.1) [state-of-the-art semantic personal publishing platform]. San Francisco, CA: Automattic. Retrieved, February 4, 2014, from http://www.wordpress.com

Müller, J. (2011). FreeMind (v0.9.0). *MediaWiki*. Retrieved, July 29, 2014, from http://www.freemind.sourceforge.net/wiki/index.php/Main_Page

Müller, E., Schuler, A., & Yates, G. B. (2008). Social challenges and supports from the perspective of individuals with Asperger syndrome and other autism spectrum disabilities. *Autism*, *12*(2), 173–190. doi:10.1177/1362361307086664 PMID:18308766

Mumy, A. P. (2012). One-dimensional speech-language therapy: Is the iPad Alone Enough. *ASHA Sphere*. Retrieved June 25, 2014, from http://blog.asha.org/2012/06/05/one-dimensional-speech-language-therapy-is-the-ipad-alone-enough/

Murdock, L. C., Ganz, J., & Crittendon, J. (2013). Use of an iPad Play Story to Increase Play Dialogue of Preschoolers with Autism Spectrum Disorders. *Journal of Autism and Developmental Disorders*, *43*(9), 2174–2189. doi:10.1007/s10803-013-1770-6 PMID:23371509

Murphy, D. (2003). Admission and cognitive details of male patients diagnosed with Asperger's syndrome detained in a special hospital: Comparison with a schizophrenia and personality disorder sample. *Journal of Forensic Psychiatry & Psychology*, *14*(3), 506–524. doi:10.1080/1478994031000152736

Murray, D. K. C. (1997). Autism and information technology: therapy with computers. In S. Powell & R. Jordan (Eds.), *Autism and learning: a guide to good practice* (pp. 100–117). London, UK: David Fulton Publishers.

Myers, J., Lee, M., & Kiratli, J. (2006). Cardiovascular disease in spinal cord injury. *American Journal of Physical Medicine & Rehabilitation*, *86*(2), 1–11.

Myles, B. S. (2005). *Children and youth with Asperger Syndrome: Strategies for success in inclusive settings*. Thousand Oaks, CA: Corwin Press.

Myles, B. S., Endow, J., & Mayfield, M. (2013). *The hidden curriculum of getting a keeping a job: Navigating the social landscape of employment*. Shawnee Mission, KS: AAPC Publishing.

Myles, B. S., Endow, J., & Mayfield, M. (2013). *The hidden curriculum of getting and keeping a job: Navigating the social landscape of employment. A guide for individuals with autism spectrum disorders and other social-cognitive challenges*. Shawnee Mission, KS: AAPC Publishing.

Myles, B. S., & Southwick, J. (2005). *Asperger Syndrome and difficult moments: Practical solutions for tantrums, rage, and melt- downs* (2nd ed.). Shawnee Mission, KS: AAPC Publishing.

Myles, B. S., Trautman, M. L., & Schelvan, R. L. (2013). *The hidden curriculum: Practical solutions for understanding unstated rules in social situations* (2nd ed.). Shawnee Mission, KS: AAPC Publishing.

Myles, H. M., & Kolar, A. (2013). *The hidden curriculum and other everyday challenges for elementary-age children with high-functioning autism*. Shawnee Mission, KS: AAPC Publishing.

Narayanan, A. (2014b). *Systems and methods for picture based communication: Google Patents*.

Narayanan, A. (Producer). (2014a). Ajit Narayanan: A word game to communicate in any language. *TED Talks*. [Video] Retrieved from http://www.ted.com/talks/ajit_narayanan_a_word_game_to_communicate_in_any_language

Nass, C., & Gong, L. (2000). Speech interfaces from an evolutionary perspective. *Communications of the ACM*, *43*(9), 36–43. doi:10.1145/348941.348976

National Autism Center. (2009). *National standards report: Addressing the need for evidence-based practice guidelines for autism spectrum disorders.* Randolph, MA: Author.

National Autism Center. (2014). *National standards project: Addressing the need for evidence-based practice guidelines for autism spectrum disorders.* Randolph, MA: National Autism Center.

National Dissemination Center for Children with Disabilities (NICHCY). (2010). Deafness and hearing loss. *NICHCY Disability Fact Sheet, 1 – 8.*

National Early Literacy Panel. (2008). *Developing early literacy: Report of the National Early Literacy Panel.* Washington, DC: National Institute for Literacy.

National Institute of Child Health and Human Development (NICHD). NIH, DHHS. (2001). Put Reading First: The Research Building Blocks for Teaching Children to Read (N/A). Washington, DC: U.S. Government Printing Office.

National Professional Development Center on Autism Spectrum Disorders. (nd). *Evidence based practice briefs.* Retrieved April 10, 2014 from http://autismpdc.fpg.unc.edu/content/briefs

National Reading Panel. (2000). *Teaching children to read: An evidence-based assessment of the scientific research literature on reading and its implications for reading instruction* [on-line]. Retrieved From: http://www.nichd.nih.gov/publications/nrp/report.cfm

National Reading Panel. (2000). *Teaching children to read: An evidence-based assessment of the scientific research literature on reading and its implications for reading instruction.* Retrieved January 25, 2014, from http://www.nichd.nih.gov/publications/nrp/report.cfm

National Reading Panel. (2000). Teaching children to read: An evidenced-based assessment of the scientific research literature on reading and its implications for reading instruction. Retrieved June 27, 2014 from http://nationalreadingpanel.org/Publications/summary.htm

Neely, L., Rispoli, M., Camargo, S., Davis, H., & Boles, M. (2013). The effect of instructional use of an iPad on challenging behavior and academic engagement for two students with autism. *Research in Autism Spectrum Disorders, 7*(4), 509–516. doi:10.1016/j.rasd.2012.12.004

Neitzel, J., & Wolery, M. (2009). *Steps for implementation: Time delay.* Chapel Hill, NC: The National Professional Development Center on Autism Spectrum Disorders, Frank Porter Graham Child Development Institute, The University of North Carolina.

Ness, M. (2007). Reading comprehension strategies in secondary content-area classrooms. *Phi Delta Kappan, 89*(3), 229–231. doi:10.1177/003172170708900314

Ness, M. (2009). Reading comprehension strategies in secondary content area classrooms: Teacher use of and attitudes towards reading comprehension instruction. *Reading Horizons, 49*(2), 143–166.

Neumann, M. M., & Neumann, D. L. (2014). Touch screen tablets and emergent literacy. *Early Childhood Education Journal, 42*(4), 231–239. doi:10.1007/s10643-013-0608-3

Newkirk, T. (2012). *The art of slow reading: Six time-honored practices for engagement.* Portsmouth, NH: Heinemann.

Newport, E. L. (1990). Maturational constraints on language learning. *Cognitive Science, 14*(1), 11–28. doi:10.1207/s15516709cog1401_2

Nicholas, B., Rudrasingham, V., Nash, S., Kirov, G., Own, M. J., & Wimpory, D. C. (2007). Association of Per1 and Npas2 with autistic disorder: Support for the clock genes/social timing hypothesis. *Molecular Psychiatry, 12*(6), 581–592. doi:10.1038/sj.mp.4001953 PMID:17264841

NIDCD, National Institute on Deafness and Other Communication Disorders. (2010a). *Quick Statistics - Hearing Loss.* Retrieved 07/31/2014, 2014, from http://www.nidcd.nih.gov/health/statistics/Pages/quick.aspx

NIDCD, National Institute on Deafness and Other Communication Disorders. (2010b). *Quick Statistics - Statistics on Voice, Speech, and Language.* Retrieved 07/30/2014, 2014, from http://www.nidcd.nih.gov/health/statistics/vsl/Pages/stats.aspx

NIDCD, National Institute on Deafness and Other Communication Disorders. (2012). *Stuttering*. Retrieved 07/30/2014, 2014, from http://www.nidcd.nih.gov/health/voice/pages/stutter.aspx

NIDCD, National Institute on Deafness and Other Communication Disorders. (2014). *Assistive Devices for People with Hearing, Voice, Speech, or Language Disorders*. Retrieved 08/04/2014, 2014, from http://www.nidcd.nih.gov/health/hearing/pages/assistive-devices.aspx

Nielsen, J., Clemmensen, T., and Yssing, R. (2002). *Getting Access to What Goes on in People's Heads – Reflections on the Think-Aloud Technique*. NordiCHI, 2002.

Niemeijer, D., Donnellan, A. M., & Robledo, J. A. (2012). Taking the pulse of augmentative and alternative communication on iOS. *AssistiveWare*. Retrieved June 25, 2014, from http://www.assistiveware.com/taking-pulse-augmentative-and-alternative-communication-ios

Night and Day Studios. (n.d.). *Night and Day Studios*. Retrieved April 3, 2015 http://www.nightanddaystudios.com

Nikopoulos, C. K., Canavan, C., & Nikopoulou-Smyrni, P. (2009). Generalized effects of video modeling on establishing instructional stimulus control in children with autism: Results of a preliminary study. *Journal of Positive Behavior Interventions*, *11*(4), 198–207. doi:10.1177/1098300708325263

Nintendo® Wii™ (2006). Available from http://wii.com (Retrieved March 31, 2015).

Nisbet, P., & Poon, P. (1998). *Special Access Technology*.

No Child Left Behind Act of 2001, 20 U.S.C. § 6301 *et seq*.

No Child Left Behind Act of 2001, Pub. L. No. 107-110, 115 Stat. 1425 (2002). Retrieved June 26, 2014, from http://www.ed.gov/policy/elsec/leg/esea02/107-110.pdf

Nordberg, A., Carlsson, G., & Lohmander, A. (2011). Electropalatography in the description and treatment of speech disorders in five children with cerebral palsy. *Clinical Linguistics & Phonetics*, *25*(10), 831–852. doi: 10.3109/02699206.2011.573122 PMID:21591933

Norman, J., & Collins, B. (2001). Using an instructional package including video technology to teach self-help skills to elementary students with mental disabilities. *Journal of Special Education Technology*, *16*(3), 5–18.

Northup, L., & Killeen, E. (2013). A framework for using iPads to build early literacy skills. *The Reading Teacher*, *66*(7), 531–537. doi:10.1002/TRTR.1155

Novak, R. E. (2006). New Technology and Changing Demographics: Part One of a Two-Part Series on Challenges to our Professions Over the Next 10 Years, *The ASHA Leader*. Retrieved from http://www.asha.org/publications/leader/2006/060117/f060117a.htm

Oceanhouse Media. (n.d.). *Oceanhouse Media*. Retrieved April 3, 2015 from http://www.oceanhousemedia.com

Ockelford, A. (2009). *Focus on music: Exploring the musicality of children and young people with retinopathy of prematurity*. London: British Library.

Odom, S., Horner, R., Snell, M., & Blacher, J. (2007). The construct of developmental disbilities. In S. Odom, R. Horner, M. Snell, & J. Blacher (Eds.), *Handbook of developmental disabilities* (pp. 3–14). New York: The Guilford Press.

Ogilvie, C. R., & Whitby, P. (2014). Video Modeling for Individuals with Autism Spectrum Disorders. In N. Silton (Ed.), *Innovative Technologies to Benefit Children with Autism*. New York, NY: IGI Global. doi:10.4018/978-1-4666-5792-2.ch013

Ohtake, Y., Takeuchi, A., & Watanabe, K. (2014). Effects of video self-modeling on eliminating public undressing by elementary-aged students with developmental disabilities during urination. *Education and Training in Autism and Developmental Disabilities*, *49*(1), 32–44.

Oladunjoye, O. K. (2013). *iPad and computer devices in preschool: A tool for literacy development among teachers and children in preschool*. Unpublished Master's thesis, Stockholm University, Sweden. Retrieved June 27, 2014 from http://www.diva-portal.org/smash/get/diva2:640202/COVER01

Olsen, S., Fiechtl, B., & Rule, S. (2012). An Evaluation of Virtual Home Visits in Early Intervention: Feasibility of "Virtual Intervention". *The Volta Review*, *112*(3), 267–281.

Olson, L. J., & Moulton, H. J. (2004). Use of weighted vests in pediatric occupational therapy practice. *Occupational Therapy International*, *11*(1), 52–66. doi:10.1002/oti.197 PMID:15118771

Olswang, L. B., Feuerstein, J. L., Pinder, G. L., & Dowden, P. (2013). Validating dynamic assessment of triadic gaze for young children with severe disabilities. *American Journal of Speech-Language Pathology, 22*(3), 449–462. doi:10.1044/1058-0360(2012/12-0013) PMID:23813200

Ornelles, C. (2007). Providing classroom-based intervention to at-risk students to support their academic engagement and interactions with peers. *Preventing School Failure, 51*(4), 3–12. doi:10.3200/PSFL.51.4.3-12

Osberger, M. J., Moeller, M. P., Eccarius, M., Robbins, A. M., & Johnson, D. (1986). Language and learning skills of hearing-impaired students: Expressive language skills. *ASHA Monographs, 23*, 54–65. PMID:3730032

Osterling, J., Dawson, G., & McPartland, J. (2001). Autism. In C. Walker & M. Roberts (Eds.), *Handbook of clinical child psychology* (3rd ed., pp. 432–452). New York: John Wiley & Sons.

Outfit7 (n.d.). *Outfit7*. Retrieved April 3, 2015 from http://outfit7.com/apps/talking-tom-cat-1/

Ozdemir, S. (2008). Using multimedia social stories to increase appropriate social engagement in young children with autism. *Turkish Online Journal of Educational Technology, 7*(3), 80–88.

Ozkan, S. Y. (2013). Comparison of peer and self-video modeling in teaching first aid skills to children with intellectual disabilities. *Education and Training in Autism and Developmental Disabilities, 48*(1), 88–102.

Palmer, S. B., Wehmeyer, M. L., Davies, D. K., & Stock, S. E. (2012). Family members' reports of the technology use of family members with intellectual and developmental disabilities. *Journal of Intellectual Disability Research, 56*(4), 402–414. doi:10.1111/j.1365-2788.2011.01489.x PMID:21988242

Parette, H. P., Hourcade, J. J., Blum, C., Watts, E. J., Stoner, J. B., Wojcik, B. W., & Chrismore, S. B. (2013). Technology user groups and early childhood education: A preliminary study. *Early Childhood Education Journal, 41*(3), 171-179. Doi: 10:1007/s10643-012-0548-3.

Parette, P. H., & Blum, C. (2014). Using flexible participation in technology-supported, universally designed preschool activities. *Teaching Exceptional Children, 46*(3), 60–67.

Parette, P., & Scherer, M. (2004). Assistive technology use and stigma. *Education and Training in Developmental Disabilities, 39*(3), 217–226.

Park, C. J., Yelland, G. W., Taffe, J. R., & Gray, K. M. (2012). Morphological and syntactic skills in language samples of pre school aged children with autism: Atypical development? *International Journal of Speech-Language Pathology, 14*(2), 95–108. doi:10.3109/17549507.2011.645555 PMID:22390743

Parker, R. I., & Hagan-Burke, S. (2007). Median-based overlap analysis for single case data: A second study. *Behavior Modification, 31*(6), 919–936. doi:10.1177/0145445507303452 PMID:17932244

Parker, R. I., Vannest, K. J., & Brown, L. (2009). The improvement rate difference for single case research. *Exceptional Children, 75*, 135–150.

Parmenter, T. (2011). What is intellectual disability? How is it assessed and classified? *International Journal of Disability Development and Education, 58*(3), 303–319. doi:10.1080/1034912X.2011.598675

Parsons, S., & Mitchell, P. (2002). The potential of virtual reality in social skills training for people with autism spectrum disorders. *Journal of Intellectual Disability Research, 46*(5), 430–443. doi:10.1046/j.1365-2788.2002.00425.x PMID:12031025

Parsons, S., Mitchell, P., & Leonard, A. (2004). The use and understanding of virtual environments by adolescents with autistic spectrum disorders. *Journal of Autism and Developmental Disorders, 34*(4), 449–466. doi:10.1023/B:JADD.0000037421.98517.8d PMID:15449520

Parsons, T. D., Bowerly, T., Buckwalter, J. G., & Rizzo, A. A. (2007). A controlled clinical comparison of attention performance in children with ADHD in a virtual reality classroom compared to standard neuropsychological methods. *Child Neuropsychology, 13*(4), 363–381. doi:10.1080/13825580600943473 PMID:17564852

Passerino, L. M., & Santarosa, L. M. C. (2008). Autism and digital learning environments: Processes of interaction and mediation. *Computers & Education, 51*(1), 385–402. doi:10.1016/j.compedu.2007.05.015

Passig, D., & Eden, S. (2000). Improving flexible thinking in deaf and hard of hearing children with virtual reality technology. *American Annals of the Deaf, 145*(3), 286–291. doi:10.1353/aad.2012.0102 PMID:10965592

Passig, D., & Eden, S. (2001). Virtual reality as a tool for improving spatial rotation among deaf and hard-of-hearing children. *Cyberpsychology & Behavior, 4*(6), 681–686. doi:10.1089/109493101753376623 PMID:11800175

Passig, D., & Eden, S. (2003). Cognitive intervention through virtual environments among deaf and hard-of-hearing children. *European Journal of Special Needs Education, 18*(2), 173–182. doi:10.1080/0885625032000078961

Patel, R. (2002). Phonatory Control in Adults with Cerebral Palsy and Severe Dysarthria. *AAC: Augmentative & Alternative Communication, 18*(1), 2.

Patel, R. (2014). *Rupal Patel: Synthetic Voices, As Unique as Fingerprints.* YouTube.

Patel, R., & Roden, A. (2008). Intelligibility and attitudes toward a speech synthesizer vocoded using dysarthric vocalizations. *Journal of Medical Speech-Language Pathology, 16*(4), 243–249.

Pauca, V. P., & Guy, R. T. (2012, February). Mobile apps for the greater good: a socially relevant approach to software engineering. In *Proceedings of the 43rd ACM technical symposium on Computer Science Education* (pp. 535-540). ACM. doi:10.1145/2157136.2157291

Paul, P., & Wang, Y. (2012). *Literate thought -- Understanding comprehension and literacy.* Sudbury, MA: Jones & Bartlett.

Pearson, P. D., Roehler, L. R., Dole, J. A., & Duffy, G. G. (1992). Developing expertise in reading comprehension. In S. J. Samuels & A. E. Farstrup (Eds.), *What research has to say about reading instruction* (pp. 145–199). Newark, DE: International Reading Association.

Peckham, P. H., & Knutson, J. S. (2005). Functional electrical stimulation for neuromuscular applications. *Annual Review of Biomedical Engineering, 7*(1), 327–360. doi:10.1146/annurev.bioeng.6.040803.140103 PMID:16004574

Peeters, M., Verhoeven, L., de Moor, J., van Balkom, H., & van Leeuwe, J. (2009). Home literacy predictors of early reading development in children with cerebral palsy. *Research in Developmental Disabilities, 30*(3), 445–461. doi:10.1016/j.ridd.2008.04.005 PMID:18541405

Peterson, C. C. (2004). Theory-of-mind development in oral deaf children with cochlear implants or conventional hearing aids. *Journal of Child Psychology and Psychiatry, and Allied Disciplines, 45*(6), 1096–1106. doi:10.1111/j.1469-7610.2004.t01-1-00302.x PMID:15257666

Petry, K., Maes, B., & Vlaskamp, C. (2005). Domains of quality of life of people with profound multiple disabilities: The perspective of parents and direct support staff. *Journal of Applied Research in Intellectual Disabilities, 18*(1), 35–46. doi:10.1111/j.1468-3148.2004.00209.x

Piazza, C. C. (2008). Feeding disorders and behavior: What have we learned? *Developmental Disabilities Research Reviews, 14*(2), 174–181. doi:10.1002/ddrr.22 PMID:18646017

Pikulski, J. J., & Chard, D. J. (2005). Fluency: Bridge between decoding and comprehension. *The Reading Teacher, 58*(6), 510–519. doi:10.1598/RT.58.6.2

Pinger apps (n.d.). *Pinger apps.* Retrieved April 3, 2015 from https://www.pinger.com/content/apps.html

Pisoni, D. D., & Geers, A. E. (2000). Working memory in deaf children with cochlear implants: Correlations between digit span and measures of spoken language processing. *The Annals of Otology, Rhinology, and Laryngology, 185*, 92–94. PMID:11141023

Plante, E., & Beeson, P. M. (2013). *Communication & Communication Disorders: A Clinical Introduction.* Pearson Education, Inc.

Playhome Software, Ltd. (n.d.). *My playhome.* Retrieved April 3, 2015 from http://www.myplayhomeapp.com

Ploog, B. O. (2010). Stimulus overselectivity four decades later: A review of the literature and its implications for current research in autism spectrum disorder. *Journal of Autism and Developmental Disorders, 40*(11), 1332–1349. doi:10.1007/s10803-010-0990-2 PMID:20238154

Ploog, B. O., Scharf, A., Nelson, D., & Brooks, P. J. (2013). Use of computer-assisted technologies (CAT) to enhance social, communicative, and language development in children with autism spectrum disorders. *Journal of Autism and Developmental Disorders*, *43*(2), 301–322. doi:10.1007/s10803-012-1571-3 PMID:22706582

Po, S., Howard, S., Vetere, F., & Skov, M. (2004). Heuristic evaluations and mobile usability: Bridging the realism gap. In S. Brewster & M. Dunlop (Eds.), MobileHCI (LNCS), (pp. 49-60). Berlin: Springer.

Pollak, Y., Shomaly, H. B., Weiss, P. L., Rizzo, A. A., & Gross-Tsur, V. (2010). Methylphenidate effect in children with ADHD can be measured by an ecologically valid continuous performance test embedded in virtual reality. *CNS Spectrums*, *15*(2), 125–130. PMID:20414157

PrAACtical AAC. (n.d.) *PrAACtical AAC supports for language learning*. Retrieved April 3, 2015 from http://praacticalaac.org

Prazak, B., Kronreif, G., Hochgatterer, A., & Fürst, M. (2004). A toy robot for physically disabled children. *Technology and Disability*, *16*(3), 131–136.

Premack, D. (1962). Reversibility of the reinforcement relation. *Science*, *136*(3512), 255–257. doi:10.1126/science.136.3512.255 PMID:14488597

Prensky, M. (2006). *Don't bother me, mom, I'm learning*. St. Paul, MN: Paragon House.

Prentke Romich Company. (n.d.). *Lamp Words for Life*. Retrieved April 3, 2015 from https://aacapps.com

Preuß, S., Neuschaefer-Rube, C., & Birkholz, P. (2013). Prospects of EPG and OPG sensor fusion in pursuit of a 3D real-time representation of the oral cavity. *Studientexte zur Sprachkommunikation: Elektronische Sprachsignalverarbeitung*, 144-151.

Pring, L. (2005). Savant talent. *Developmental Medicine and Child Neurology*, *47*(7), 500–503. doi:10.1017/S0012162205000976 PMID:15991873

Provost, B., Lopez, B. R., & Heimerl, S. (2007). A comparison of motor delays in young children: Autism spectrum disorder, developmental delay, and developmental concerns. *Journal of Autism and Developmental Disorders*, *37*(2), 321–328. doi:10.1007/s10803-006-0170-6 PMID:16868847

Pufpaff, L. A. (2008). Barriers to participation in kindergarten literacy instruction for a student with augmentative and alternative communication needs. *Psychology in the Schools*, *45*(7), 582–599. doi:10.1002/pits.20311

Pufpaff, L. A., Blischak, D. M., & Lloyd, L. L. (2000). Effects of modified orthography on the identification of printed words. *American Journal of Mental Retardation*, *105*(1), 14–24. doi:10.1352/0895-8017(2000)105<0014:EOMOOT>2.0.CO;2 PMID:10683705

Pufpaff, L. A., & Yssel, N. (2010). Effects of a 6-week, co-taught literacy unit on preservice special educators' literacy-education knowledge. *Psychology in the Schools*, *47*(5), 493–500.

Quek, L., Sofronoff, K., Sheffield, J., White, A., & Kelly, A. (2012). Co-occurring anger in young people with Asperger's syndrome. *Journal of Clinical Psychology*, *68*(10), 1142–1148. doi:10.1002/jclp.21888 PMID:22806337

Racine, M. B., Majnemer, A., Shevell, M., & Snider, L. (2008). Handwriting performance in children with attention deficit hyperactivity disorder (ADHD). *Journal of Child Neurology*, *23*(4), 399–406. doi:10.1177/0883073807309244 PMID:18401033

Ramsey, D. W., Zigo, J., Lajoie, M., & Baker, F. (2013). *Music technology in therapeutic and health settings*. Jessica Kingsley Publishers.

Rankin-Erickson, J. L., Wood, L. A., Beukelman, D. R., & Beukelman, H. M. (2003). Early computer literacy; first graders use the "talking" computer. *Reading Improvement*, *40*(3), 132–144.

Ran, L., Helal, S., & Moore, S. (2004). Drishti: An integrated indoor/outdoor blind navigation system and service. *Pervasive Computing and Communications*, *2004*, 23–30.

Rao, R., Conn, K., Jung, S. H., Katupitiya, J., & Kientz, T. L. (2002). Human robot interaction: Application to smart wheelchairs. *Proceedings of the 2002 IEEE International Conference on Robotics & Automation*, 3583 – 3588. doi:10.1109/ROBOT.2002.1014265

Rasinski, T. V. (2004). *Assessing reading fluency*. Honolulu, HI: Pacific Resources for Education and Learning.

Rasinski, T. V. (2006). Reading fluency instruction: Moving beyond accuracy, automaticity, and prosody. *The Reading Teacher*, *59*(7), 704–706. doi:10.1598/RT.59.7.10

Rayner, C., Denholm, C., & Sigafoos, J. (2009). Video-based intervention for individuals with Autism: Key questions that remain unanswered. *Research in Autism Spectrum Disorders*, *3*(2), 291–303. doi:10.1016/j.rasd.2008.09.001

Rehfeldt, R. A., Dahman, D., Young, A., Cherry, H., & Davis, P. (2003). Teaching simple meal preparation skills to adults with moderate and severe mental retardation using video modeling. *Behavioral Interventions*, *18*(3), 209–218. doi:10.1002/bin.139

Reichle, J. (2011). Evaluating assistive technology in the education of persons with severe disabilities. *Journal of Behavioral Education*, *20*(1), 77–85. doi:10.1007/s10864-011-9121-1

Reid, D. T. (2002). The use of virtual reality to improve upper-extremity efficiency skills in children with cerebral palsy: A pilot study. *Technology and Disability*, *14*(2), 53–61.

Reid, D., & Campbell, K. (2006). The use of virtual reality with children with cerebral palsy: A pilot randomized trial. *Therapeutic Recreation Journal*, *40*(4), 255–268.

Reiter, S., & Lapidot-Lefler, N. (2007). Bullying among special education students with intellectual disabilities: Differences in social adjustment and social skills. *Intellectual and Developmental Disabilities*, *45*(3), 174–181. doi:10.1352/1934-9556(2007)45[174:BASESW]2.0.CO;2 PMID:17472426

Renzaglia, A., Karvonen, M., Drasgow, E., & Stoxen, C. C. (2003). Promoting a lifetime of inclusion. *Focus on Autism and Other Developmental Disabilities*, *18*(3), 140–149. doi:10.1177/10883576030180030201

RERC on Communication Enhancement. (2011, March 14). *Mobile devices and communication apps: An AAC-RERC white paper*. Retrieve June 27, 2014, from http://aac-rerc.psu.edu/index.php/pages/show/id/46

Richards, J., & McKenna, R. (2003). *Integrating multiple literacies in K-8 classrooms: Cases, commentaries, and practical applications*. Mahwah, NJ: Lawrence, Erlbaum.

Riffel, L., Wehmeyer, M., Turnbull, A., Lattimore, J., Davies, D., Stock, S., & Fisher, S. et al. (2005). Promoting independent performance of transition-related tasks using a palmtop PC based self-directed visual and auditory prompting system. *Journal of Special Education Technology*, *20*(2), 5–14.

Rigby, P. J. (2009). *Assistive technology for persons with physical disabilities: Evaluation and outcomes*. Toronto Press.

Rigby, P., Ryan, S. E., Joos, S., Cooper, B. A., Jutai, J., & Steggles, E. (2005). Impact of electronic aids to daily living on the lives of persons with cervical spinal cord injuries. *Assistive Technology*, *17*(2), 89–97. doi:10.1080/10400435.2005.10132099 PMID:16392713

Rispoli, M. J., Franco, J. H., van der Meer, L., Lang, R., & Carmargo, S. P. H. (2010). The use of speech generating devices in communication interventions for individuals with developmental disabilities: A review of the literature. *Developmental Neurorehabilitation*, *13*(4), 276–293. doi:10.3109/17518421003636794 PMID:20629594

Rivera, C. J. (2013). Multimedia Shared Stories: Teaching Literacy Skills to Diverse Learners. *Teaching Exceptional Children*, *45*(6), 38–45.

Rizzo, A. A., Buckwalter, J. G., Bowerly, T., Van, D. Z., Humphrey, L., Neumann, U., & Sisemore, D. et al. (2000). The virtual classroom: A virtual reality environment for the assessment and rehabilitation of attention deficits. *Cyberpsychology & Behavior*, *3*(3), 483–499. doi:10.1089/10949310050078940

Robins, B., Dautenhahn, K., & Dubowski, J. (2006). Does appearance matter in the interaction of children with autism with a humanoid robot? *Interaction Studies: Social Behaviour and Communication in Biological and Artificial Systems*, *7*(3), 509–542. doi:10.1075/is.7.3.16rob

Roche, L., Sigafoos, J., Lancioni, G. E., O'Reilly, M. F., van der Meer, L., Achmadi, D., & Marschik, P. B. et al. (2014). Comparing tangible symbols, picture exchange, and a direct selection response for enabling two boys with developmental disabilities to access preferred stimuli. *Journal of Developmental and Physical Disabilities*, *26*, 249–261. doi:10.1007/s10882-013-9361-1

Roer-Strier, D. (2002). University students with learning disabilities advocating for change. *Disability and Rehabilitation, 24*(17), 914–924. doi:10.1080/09638280210148611 PMID:12519487

Roger, L. (2007). Electronic aids for daily living. *Journal of Rehabilitation Research and Development, 44*(5), 7–9. PMID:17943673

Rogers, M. F., & Myles, B. S. (2001). Using Social Stories™ and Comic Strip Conversations™ to interpret social situations for an adolescent with Asperger Syndrome. *Intervention in School and Clinic, 36*(5), 310–313. doi:10.1177/105345120103600510

Romski, M., & Sevcik, R. A. (2005). Augmentative communication and early intervention: Myths and realities. *Infants and Young Children, 18*(3), 174–185. doi:10.1097/00001163-200507000-00002

Romski, M., Sevcik, R. A., Adamson, L. B., Cheslock, M., Smith, A., Barker, R. M., & Bakeman, R. (2010). Randomized comparison of augmented and nonaugmented language interventions for toddlers with developmental delays and their parents. *Journal of Speech, Language, and Hearing Research: JSLHR, 53*(2), 350–364. doi:10.1044/1092-4388(2009/08-0156) PMID:20360461

Rosa-Lugo, L. I., & Kent-Walsh, J. (2008). Effects of parent instruction on communicative turns of Latino children using augmentative and alternative communication during storybook reading. *Communication Disorders Quarterly, 30*(1), 49–61. doi:10.1177/1525740108320353

Rose Medical Solutions, Ltd. (2014). *Electropalatography*. Retrieved 08/08/2014, 2014, from http://www.rose-medical.com/electropalatography.html

Ross, E., & Oliver, C. (2003). The assess- ment of mood in adults who have severe or profound mental retardation. *Clinical Psychology Review, 23*(2), 225–245. doi:10.1016/S0272-7358(02)00202-7 PMID:12573671

Rostami, H. R., Arastoo, A. A., Nejad, S. J., Mahany, M. K., Malamiri, R. A., & Goharpey, S. (2012). Effects of modified constraint-induced movement therapy in virtual environment on upper-limb function in children with spastic hemiparetic cerebral palsy: A randomised controlled trial. *NeuroRehabilitation, 31*(4), 357–365. PMID:23232158

Ruben, R. J. (2000). Redefining the survival of the fittest: Communication disorders in the 21st century. *Laryngoscope, 110*(2 I), 241-245.

Ruffin, T. M. (2012). Assistive technologies for reading. *Reading Matrix: An International Online Journal, 12*(1), 98–101.

Rummel-Hudson, R. (2011). A revolution at their fingertips. *SIG 12 Perspectives on Augmentative and Alternative Communication, 20*(1), 19-23. doi:10.1044/aac20.1.19

Ruppar, A. L. (2013). Authentic literacy instruction in inclusive environments for students with severe disabilities. *Teaching Exceptional Children, 46*, 44–50.

Ryalls, J., & Behrens, S. J. (2000). *Introduction to Speech Science: From Basic Theories to Clinical Applications*. Needham Heights, MA: Allyn & Bacon.

Sailers, E. (2010). *How I became the speech guy with an iPad*. Retrieved June 26, 2014 from http://blog.asha.org/2010/09/21/how-i-became-the-speech-guy-with-an-ipad/

Sakashita, R. R., Inoue, N. N., & Kamegai, T. T. (2004). From milk to solids: A reference standard for the transitional eating process in infants and preschool children in Japan. *European Journal of Clinical Nutrition, 58*(4), 643–653. doi:10.1038/sj.ejcn.1601860 PMID:15042133

Salem, Y., Gropack, S., Coffin, D., & Godwin, E. M. (2012). Effectiveness of a low-cost virtual reality system for children with developmental delay: A preliminary randomised single-blind controlled trial. *Physiotherapy, 98*(3), 189–195. doi:10.1016/j.physio.2012.06.003 PMID:22898574

Salmon, L. G. (2014). Factors that affect emergent literacy development when engaging with electronic books. *Early Childhood Education Journal, 42*(2), 85–92. doi:10.1007/s10643-013-0589-2

Sánchez, J., & Sáenz, M. (2006). 3D sound interactive environments for blind children problem solving skills. *Behaviour & Information Technology, 25*(4), 367–378. doi:10.1080/01449290600636660

Sandlund, M., Lindh Waterworth, E., & Häger, C. (2011). Using motion interactive games to promote physical activity and enhance motor performance in children with cerebral palsy. *Developmental Neurorehabilitation*, *14*(1), 15–21. doi:10.3109/17518423.2010.533329 PMID:21241174

Sandvik, M., Smordal, O., & Osterud, S. (2012). Exploring iPads in practitioners' repertoires for language learning and literacy practices in kindergarten. *Nordic Journal of Digital Literacy*, *7*(3), 204–220.

Sansosti, F. J., Powell-Smith, K. A., & Cowan, R. J. (2010). *High functioning autism/Asperger syndrome in schools: Assessment and Intervention*. New York, NY: Guilford Press.

Saunders, M. D., Timler, G. R., Cullinan, T. B., Pilkey, S., Questad, K. A., & Saunders, R. R. (2003). Evidence of contingency awareness in people with profound multiple impairments: Response duration versus response rate indicators. *Research in Developmental Disabilities*, *24*(4), 231–245. doi:10.1016/S0891-4222(03)00040-4 PMID:12873657

Savarese, E. T., & Savarese, R. J. (2012). Literate Lungs: One Autist's Journey as a Reader. *Research and Practice for Persons with Severe Disabilities*, *37*(2), 100–110. doi:10.2511/027494812802573594

Schery, T., & O'Connor, L. C. (1992). The effectiveness of school-based computer language intervention with severely handicapped children. *Language, Speech, and Hearing Services in Schools*, *23*(1), 43–47. doi:10.1044/0161-1461.2301.43

Schery, T., & O'Connor, L. C. (1997). Language intervention: Computer training for young children with special needs. *British Journal of Educational Technology*, *28*(4), 271–279. doi:10.1111/1467-8535.00034

Schiff, N. D., Giacino, J. T., Kalmar, K., Victor, J. D., Baker, K., Gerber, M., & Rezai, A. R. et al. (2007). Behavioural improvements with thalamic stimulation after severe traumatic brain injury. *Nature*, *448*(7153), 600–603. doi:10.1038/nature06041 PMID:17671503

Schlosser, R. (1999). Social validation of interventions in augmentative and alternative communication. *Augmentative and Alternative Communication*, *15*(4), 234–247. doi:10.1080/07434619912331278775

Schlosser, R. (2003a). Roles of speech output in augmentative and alternative communication: Narrative review. *AAC: Augmentative & Alternative Communication*, *19*, 5–27.

Schlosser, R. (2003b). Comparative efficacy studies using single-subject experimental designs: How can they inform evidence-based practice? In R. Schlosser (Ed.), *The efficacy of augmentative and alternative communication: Toward evidence-based practice* (Vol. 553-595). San Diego: Academic Press.

Schlosser, R., & Blischak, D. (2001). Is there a role for speech output in interventions for persons with autism? *Focus on Autism and Other Developmental Disabilities*, *16*(3), 170–178. doi:10.1177/108835760101600305

Schlosser, R., & Sigafoos, J. (2006). Augmentative and alternative communication interventions for persons with developmental disabilities: Narrative review of comparative single-subject experimental studies. *Research in Developmental Disabilities*, *27*(1), 1–29. doi:10.1016/j.ridd.2004.04.004 PMID:16360073

Schlosser, R., & Wendt, O. (2008a). Augmentative and alternative communication intervention for children with autism. In J. Luiselli, D. Russo, W. Christian, & S. Wilczynski (Eds.), *Effective practices for children with autism: Educational and behavioral support interventions that work* (pp. 325–389). Oxford: Oxford University Press.

Schlosser, R., & Wendt, O. (2008b). Effects of augmentative and alternative communication intervention on speech production in children with autism: A systematic review. *American Journal of Speech-Language Pathology*, *17*(3), 212–230. doi:10.1044/1058-0360(2008/021) PMID:18663107

Schuchardt, K., Gebhardt, M., & Maehler, C. (2010). Working memory functions in children with different degress of intellectual disability. *Journal of Intellectual Disability Research*, *54*(4), 346–353. doi:10.1111/j.1365-2788.2010.01265.x PMID:20433572

Schunk, D. H. (1987). Peer models and children's behavioral change. *Review of Educational Research*, *57*(2), 149–174. doi:10.3102/00346543057002149

Schwarz, S. M., Corredor, J., Fisher-Medina, J., Cohen, J., & Rabinowitz, S. (2001). Diagnosis and Treatment of Feeding Disorders in Children With Developmental Disabilities. *Pediatrics*, *108*(3), 671–676. doi:10.1542/peds.108.3.671 PMID:11533334

Schweinberger, S. R., Walther, C., Zäske, R., & Kovács, G. (2011). Neural correlates of adaptation to voice identity. *British Journal of Psychology*, *102*(4), 748–764. doi:10.1111/j.2044-8295.2011.02048.x PMID:21988382

Scott, C. (2008). *iThoughts*. Retrieved February 4, 2014, from http://www.ithoughts.co.uk/_iThoughtsHD/Welcome.html

Scott, R., Collins, B., Knight, V., & Kleinert, H. (2013). Teaching adults with intellectual disability ATM use via the iPod. *Education and Training in Autism and Developmental Disabilities*, *48*(2), 190–199.

Scuito, E. W. (2013). The iPad: Using new technology for teaching reading, language, and speech for children with hearing loss. *Independent Studies and Capstones: Paper 676*. Program in Audiology and Communication Sciences, Washington University school of Medicine. St. Louis, MO. Retrieved June 26, 2014 from http://digitalcommons.wustl.edu/pacs_capstones/676/

Segal-Drori, O., Korat, O., Shamir, A., & Klein, P. S. (2010). Reading e-books and printed books with and without adult instruction: Effects on emergent reading. *Reading and Writing*, *23*(8), 913–930. doi:10.1007/s11145-009-9182-x

Semantic Compaction Systems. (2009). *AAC Core Vocabulary Communication Device - What is Minspeak*. Retrieved 08/15/2014, 2014, from http://www.minspeak.com/what.php#.U_B3w1Yivuc

Sénéchal, M., & LeFevre, J.-A. (2002). Parental involvement in the development of children's reading skill: A five-year longitudinal study. *Child Development*, *73*(2), 445–460. doi:10.1111/1467-8624.00417 PMID:11949902

Sennott, S. (2011). An introduction to the special issue on new mobile AAC technologies. *SIG 12 Perspectives on Augmentative and Alternative Communication, 20*(1), 3-6. doi:10.1044/aac20.1.3

Sennott, S., & Bowker, A. (2009). Autism, AAC, and Proloquo2Go. *SIG 12 Perspectives on Augmentative and Alternative Communication, 18*(4), 137-145.

Sennott, S., & Bowker, A. (2009). Autism, AAC, and Proloquo2Go. *Perspectives on Augmentative and Alternative Communication*, *18*(4), 137–145. doi:10.1044/aac18.4.137

Shadish, W. R. (2014). Statistical analyses of single-case designs: The shape of things to come. *Current Directions in Psychological Science*, *23*(2), 139–146. doi:10.1177/0963721414524773

Shane, H., & Costello, J. (1994, November). *Augmentative communication assessment and the feature matching process*. Mini-seminar presented at the annual convention of the American Speech-Language-Hearing Association, New Orleans, LA.

Shane, H. C., Blackstone, S., Vanderheiden, G., Williams, M., & DeRuyter, F. (2012). Using AAC technology to access the world. *Assistive Technology*, *24*(1), 3–13. doi:10.1080/10400435.2011.648716 PMID:22590795

Shane, H., Laubscher, E., Schlosser, R., Flynn, S., Sorce, J., & Abramson, J. (2012). Applying technology to visually support language and communication in individuals with autism spectrum disorders. *Journal of Autism and Developmental Disorders*, *42*(6), 1228–1235. doi:10.1007/s10803-011-1304-z PMID:21691867

Sherer, M., Pierce, K. L., Paredes, S., Kisacky, K. L., Ingersoll, B., & Schreibman, L. (2001). Enhancing conversation skills in children with autism via video technology: Which is better, "self" or "other" as a model? *Behavior Modification*, *25*(1), 140–158. doi:10.1177/0145445501251008 PMID:11151482

Shih, C. H., Chang, M. L., & Shih, C. T. (2010). A new limb movement detector enabling people with multiple disabilities to control environmental stimulation through limb swing with a gyration air mouse. *Research in Developmental Disabilities*, *31*(4), 875–880. doi:10.1016/j.ridd.2010.01.020 PMID:20381996

Shirky, C. (2008). *It's not information overload. It's filter failure*. Lecture presented at Web Expo 2.0 2008 in New York, New York. Retrieved January 31, 2014, from http://www.mascontext.com/issues/7-information-fall-10/its-not-information-overload-its-filter-failure/

Shukla-Mehta, S., Miller, T., & Callahan, K. J. (2010). Evaluating the effectiveness of video instruction on social and communication skills for children with autism spectrum disorders: A review of the literature. *Focus on Autism and Other Developmental Disabilities*, 25(1), 23–26. doi:10.1177/1088357609352901

Sigafoos, J. (1998). Choice making and personal selection strategies. In J. Luiselli & M. Cameron (Eds.), *Antecedent control: Innovative approaches to behavioral support* (pp. 187–221). Baltimore: Paul H. Brookes Publishing Co.

Sigafoos, J., & Drasgow, E. (2001). Conditional use of aided and unaided AAC: A review and clinical case demonstration. *Focus on Autism and Other Developmental Disabilities*, 16(3), 152–161. doi:10.1177/108835760101600303

Sigafoos, J., Drasgow, E., & Schlosser, R. (2003). Strategies for beginning communicators. In R. Schlosser (Ed.), *The efficacy of augmentative and alternative communication: Toward evidence-based practice* (pp. 323–346). San Diego: Academic Press.

Sigafoos, J., Green, V. A., Payne, D., Son, S. H., O'Reilly, M. F., & Lancioni, G. E. (2009). A comparison of picture exchange and speech-generating devices: Acquisition, preference, and effects on social interaction. *Augmentative and Alternative Communication*, 25(2), 99–109. doi:10.1080/07434610902739959 PMID:19444681

Sigafoos, J., Lancioni, G. E., O'Reilly, M. F., Achmadi, D., Stevens, M., Roche, L., & Green, V. A. et al. (2013). Teaching two boys with autism spectrum disorders to request the continuation of toy play using an iPad-based speech-generating device. *Research in Autism Spectrum Disorders*, 7(8), 923–930. doi:10.1016/j.rasd.2013.04.002

Sigafoos, J., O'Reilly, M., Cannella, H., Edrisinha, C., de la Cruz, B., Upadhyaya, M., & Young, D. et al. (2007). Evaluation of a video prompting and fading procedure for teaching dish-washing skills to adults with developmental disabilities. *Journal of Behavioral Education*, 16(2), 93–109. doi:10.1007/s10864-006-9004-z

Sigafoos, J., O'Reilly, M. F., Lancioni, G. E., & Sutherland, D. (2014). Augmentative and alternative communication for individuals with autism spectrum disorder and intellectual disability. *Current Developmental Disorders Reports*, 1(2), 51–57. doi:10.1007/s40474-013-0007-x

Sigafoos, J., O'Reilly, M., Cannella, H., Upadhyaya, M., Edrisinha, C., Lancioni, G., & Young, D. et al. (2005). Computer presented video prompting for teaching microwave oven use to three adults with developmental disabilities. *Journal of Behavioral Education*, 14(3), 189–201. doi:10.1007/s10864-005-6297-2

Silver Kite. (n.d.). *Silver Kite: The assistive technology solution center.* Retrieved April 3, 2015 from http://www.assistiveware.com

Simeonsson, R. J., Bjorck-Akesson, E., & Lollar, D. J. (2012). Communication, disabilities, and the ICF-CY. *Augmentative and Alternative Communication*, 28(1), 3–10. doi:10.3109/07434618.2011.653829 PMID:22364533

Simonsen, B., Fairbanks, S., Briesch, A., & Myers, D. (2008). Evidence-based practices in classroom management: Considerations for research to practice. *Education & Treatment of Children*, 31(3), 351–380. doi:10.1353/etc.0.0007

Simpson, A., Walsh, M., & Rowsell, J. (2013). The digital reading path: Research modes and multidirectionality with iPads. *Literacy*, 47(3), 123–130. doi:10.1111/lit.12009

Singh, N. N., & Solman, R. T. (1990). A stimulus control analysis of the picture-word problem in children who are mentally retarded: The blocking effect. *Journal of Applied Behavior Analysis*, 23(4), 525–532. doi:10.1901/jaba.1990.23-525 PMID:2074241

Skinner, M. W., Clark, G. M., Whitford, L. A., Seligman, P. M., Staller, S. J., Shipp, D. B., & Beiter, A. L. et al. (1994). Evaluation of a new spectral peak coding strategy for the Nucleus 22 channel cochlear implant system. *The American Journal of Otology*, 15(2), 15–27. PMID:8572106

Skoto, B. G., Koppenhaver, D. A., & Erickson, K. A. (2004). Parent reading behaviors and communication outcomes in girls with Rett Syndrome. *Exceptional Children*, 70(2), 145–166. doi:10.1177/001440290407000202

Small, L. H. (2012). *Fundamentals of Phonetics: A practical guide for students.* Upper Saddle River, NJ: Pearson Education, Inc.

Smarty Ears Apps. (n.d.). *Smarty Ears Apps.* Retrieved April 15, 2015 from http://smartyearsapps.com

Smith Myles, B., Trautman, M. L., & Schelvan, R. L. (2004). *The Hidden Curriculum: Practical solutions for understanding unstated rules in social situations.* Autism Aspergers Publishing, Co.

Smith, M. K. (1996, 2000). Curriculum theory and practice. In *The encyclopaedia of informal education.* Retrieved from www.infed.org/biblio/b-curric.htm

Smith, M. J., Ginger, E. J., Wright, K., Wright, M. A., Taylor, J. L., Humm, L. B., & Fleming, M. F. et al. (2014). Virtual Reality Job Interview Training in Adults with Autism Spectrum Disorder. *Journal of Autism and Developmental Disorders,* 1–14. PMID:24803366

Smith, M. J., Ginger, E. J., Wright, K., Wright, M. A., Taylor, J. L., Humm, L. B., & Fleming, M. F. et al. (2014). Virtual reality job interview training in adults with autism spectrum disorder. *Journal of Autism and Developmental Disorders, 44*(10), 2450–2463. Published online07May2014. doi:10.1007/s10803-014-2113-y PMID:24803366

Smith, S. M., Myles, B. S., Aspy, R., Grossman, B. G., & Henry, S. A. (2010). Sustainable change in quality of life for individuals with ASD: Using a comprehensive planning process. *Focus on Exceptional Children, 43*(3), 1–24.

Snape, J., & Maiolo, B. (2013). *Using iPads in Speech Pathology.* Independent Living Centre WA. Retrieved June 26, 2014 from http://ilc.com.au/wp-content/uploads/2013/08/ilc_tech_using_ipads_in_speech_pathology.pdf

Snow, C. E. (2001). *Improving reading outcomes: Getting beyond third grade.* Washington, DC: The Aspen Institute.

Snow, C. E., Porche, M. V., Tabors, P. O., & Harris, S. R. (2007). *Is literacy enough? Pathways to academic success for adolescents.* Baltimore, MD: Paul H. Brookes.

Software, Inc. (n.d.). Retrieved, July 29, 2014, from http://www.inspiration.com

Solman, R. T., & Wu, H. M. (1995). Pictures as feedback in single word learning. *Educational Psychology, 15*(3), 227–244. doi:10.1080/0144341950150301

Sonnenschein, S., Stapleton, L. M., & Benson, A. (2010). The relation between the type and amount of instruction and growth in children's reading competencies. *American Educational Research Journal, 47*(2), 358–389. doi:10.3102/0002831209349215

Soto, G., & Dukhovny, E. (2008). The effect of shared book reading on the acquisition of expressive vocabulary of a 7 year old who uses AAC. *Seminars in Speech and Language, 29*(2), 133–145. doi:10.1055/s-2008-1079127 PMID:18645915

Speak MODalities. (n.d.) *Speak MODalities.* Retrieved on April 3, 2015 from http://speakmod.com/products/speakall/

Spectronics. (n.d.a). *Top 10 apps for language development.* Retrieved April 3, 2015 from http://www.spectronicsinoz.com/online/resource/top-10-apps-for-language-development/

Spectronics. (n.d.b). *Apps for early literacy series.* Retrieved April 3, 2015 from http://www.spectronicsinoz.com/online/resource/apps-for-early-literacy-introduction/

Speer, L. L., Cook, A. E., McMahon, W. M., & Clark, E. (2007). Face processing in children with autism effects of stimulus contents and type. *Autism, 11*(3), 265–277. doi:10.1177/1362361307076925 PMID:17478579

Spivack, G., Platt, J. J., & Shure, M. (1976). *The problem-solving approach to adjustment.* San Francisco: Jossey-Bass.

Spooner, F., Ahlgrim-Delzell, L., Kemp-Inman, A., & Wood, L. A. (2014). Using an iPad2® With Systematic Instruction to Teach Shared Stories for Elementary-Aged Students With Autism. *Research and Practice for Persons with Severe Disabilities, 39*(1), 30–46. doi:10.1177/1540796914534631

Spooner, F., Rivera, C. J., Browder, D. M., Baker, J. N., & Salas, S. (2009). Teaching emergent literacy skills using cultural contextual story-based lessons. *Research and Practice for Persons with Severe Disabilities, 34*(3-4), 102–112. doi:10.2511/rpsd.34.3-4.102

Spriggs, A. D., Gast, D. L., & Ayres, K. M. (2007). Using picture activity schedule books to increase on-schedule and on-task behaviors. *Education and Training in Developmental Disabilities, 42,* 209–223.

Stafford, A. M., Alberto, P. M., Fredrick, L. D., Heflin, L. J., & Heller, K. W. (2002). Preference variability and the instruction of choice making with students with severe intellectual disabilities. *Education and Training in Mental Retardation and Developmental Disabilities*, 37, 70–88.

Stainthorp, R., & Hughes, D. (2004). What happens to precocious readers' performance by the age eleven? *Journal of Research in Reading*, 27(4), 357–372. doi:10.1111/j.1467-9817.2004.00239.x

Standen, P. J., & Brown, D. J. (2005). Virtual reality in the rehabilitation of people with intellectual disabilities[review]. *Cyberpsychology & Behavior*, 8(3), 272–282. doi:10.1089/cpb.2005.8.272 PMID:15971976

Standen, P. J., Brown, D., Horan, M., & Proctor, T. (2002). How tutors assist adults with learning disabilities to use virtual environments. *Disability and Rehabilitation*, 24(11), 570–577. doi:10.1080/0963828023201179244 PMID:12182796

Starfall. (n.d.). *Starfall*. Retrieved April 3, 2015 from http://www.starfall.com

Stasolla, F., & Caffò, A. O. (2013). Promoting adaptive behaviors by two girls with Rett Syndrome through a microswitch-based program. *Research in Autism Spectrum Disorders*, 7(10), 1265–1272. doi:10.1016/j.rasd.2013.07.010

Stasolla, F., Caffò, A. O., Damiani, R., Perilli, V., Di Leone, A., & Albano, V. (2015). Assistive technology-based programs to promote communication and leisure activities by three children emerged from a minimal conscious state. *Cognitive Processing*, 16(1), 69–78. doi:10.1007/s10339-014-0625-1 PMID:25077461

Stasolla, F., Caffò, A. O., Picucci, L., & Bosco, A. (2013). Assistive technology for promoting choice behaviors in three children with cerebral palsy and severe communication impairments. *Research in Developmental Disabilities*, 34(9), 2694–2700. doi:10.1016/j.ridd.2013.05.029 PMID:23770888

Stasolla, F., Damiani, R., Perilli, V., Di Leone, A., Albano, V., Stella, A., & Damato, C. (2014). Technological supports to promote choice opportunities by two boys with fragile X syndrome and severe to profound developmental disabilities. *Research in Developmental Disabilities*, 35(11), 2993–3000. doi:10.1016/j.ridd.2014.07.045 PMID:25118066

Stasolla, F., & De Pace, C. (2014). Assistive technology to promote leisure and constructive engagement by two boys emerged from a minimal conscious state. *NeuroRehabilitation*, 35, 253–259. PMID:24990021

Stasolla, F., Perilli, V., Damiani, R., Caffò, A. O., Di Leone, A., Albano, V., & Damato, C. et al. (2014). A microswitch-cluster program to enhance object manipulation and to reduce hand mouthing by three children with autism spectrum disorders and intellectual disabilities. *Research in Autism Spectrum Disorders*, 8(9), 1071–1078. doi:10.1016/j.rasd.2014.05.016

Staugler, K. (2007). Literacy Rubric: Informal Literacy Assessment Tool. https://wvde.state.wv.us/osp/supporting- literacy/documents/Literacy%20Rubric.pdf

Steele, R. & Moromoff, P. (2011). Design challenges of AAC apps, on wireless portable devices, for persons with Aphasia. *SIG 12 Perspectives on Augmentative and Alternative Communication, 20(2)*, 41-51. doi:.10.1044/aac20.2.41

Steele, S. C., & Mills, M. T. (2011). Vocabulary intervention of school-age children with language impairment: A review of evidence and good practice. *Child Language Teaching and Therapy*, 27(3), 354–370. doi:10.1177/0265659011412247 PMID:25104872

Stephenson, J. (2010). Book Reading as an Intervention Context for Children Beginning to Use Graphic Symbols for Communication. *Journal of Developmental and Physical Disabilities*, 22(3), 257–271. doi:10.1007/s10882-009-9164-6

Stephenson, J., & Carter, M. (2009). The use of weighted vests with children with autism spectrum disorders and other disabilities. *Journal of Autism and Developmental Disorders*, 39(1), 105–114. doi:10.1007/s10803-008-0605-3 PMID:18592366

Stephenson, J., & Limbrick, L. (2013). A review of the use of touch-screen mobile devices by people with developmental disabilities. *Journal of Autism and Developmental Disorders*. Published online 26 July 2013. doi:10.1007/s10803-013-1878-8 PMID:23888356

Stevenson, M. (2010). Flexible and Responsive Research: Developing Rights-Based Emancipatory Disability Research Methodology in Collaboration with Young Adults with Down Syndrome. *Australian Social Work*, *63*(1), 35–50. doi:10.1080/03124070903471041

Stewart, R. A., & O'Brien, D. G. (1989). Resistance to content area reading: A focus on pre-service teachers. *Journal of Reading*, *32*(5), 396–401.

Stichter, J. P., Laffey, J., Galyen, K., & Herzog, M. (2014). iSocial: Delivering the social competence intervention for adolescents (SCI-A) in a 3D virtual learning environment for youth with high functioning autism. *Journal of Autism and Developmental Disorders*, *44*(2), 417–430. doi:10.1007/s10803-013-1881-0 PMID:23812663

Strasberger, S. K., & Ferreri, S. J. (2013). The effects of peer assisted communication application training on the communicative and social behaviors of children with autism. *Journal of Developmental and Physical Disabilities*, *26*(5), 513–526. doi:10.1007/s10882-013-9358-9

Streeter, E. (2001, April). Reactions and responses from the music therapy community to the growth of computers and technology-some preliminary thoughts. In Voices: A world forum for music therapy (Vol. 7, No. 1). doi:10.15845/voices.v7i1.467

Strickland, D. C., Coles, C. D., & Southern, L. B. (2013). JobTIPS: A transition to employment program for individuals with autism spectrum disorders. *Journal of Autism and Developmental Disorders*, *43*(10), 2472–2483. doi:10.1007/s10803-013-1800-4 PMID:23494559

Strickland, D. C., McAllister, D., Coles, C. D., & Osborne, S. (2007). An evolution of virtual reality training designs for children with autism and fetal alcohol spectrum disorders. *Topics in Language Disorders*, *27*(3), 226–241. doi:10.1097/01.TLD.0000285357.95426.72 PMID:20072702

Strnadová, I., Cumming, T., & Marquez, E. (2014). Parents' and teachers' experiences with mobile learning for students with high support needs. *Special Education Perspectives.*, *23*(2), 43–55.

Stromer, R., Kimball, J. W., Kinney, E. M., & Taylor, B. A. (2006). Activity schedules, computer technology, and teaching children with autism spectrum disorders. *Focus on Autism and Other Developmental Disabilities*, *21*(1), 14–24. doi:10.1177/10883576060210010301

Stuart, S., Beukelman, D., & King, J. (1997). Vocabulary use during extended conversations by two cohorts of older adults. *Augmentative and Alternative Communication*, *13*(1), 40–47. doi:10.1080/07434619712331277828

Sturmey, P. (2003). Video technology and persons with Autism and other developmental disabilities: An emerging technology for PBS. *Journal of Positive Behavior Interventions*, *5*(1), 3–4. doi:10.1177/10983007030050010401

Sturm, J. (2003). Writing in AAC. *The ASHA Leader*, *8*(16), 4–5.

Sturm, J. M., & Clendon, S. A. (2004). Augmentative and alternative communication, language, and literacy: Fostering the relationship. *Topics in Language Disorders*, *24*(1), 76–91. doi:10.1097/00011363-200401000-00008

Sturm, J. M., Spadorcia, S. A., Cunningham, J. W., Cali, K. S., Staples, A., Erickson, K., & Koppenhaver, D. A. (2006). What happens to reading between first and third grade? Implications for students who use AAC. *Augmentative and Alternative Communication*, *22*(1), 21–36. doi:10.1080/07434610500243826 PMID:17114156

Sublime Speech. (n.d.). *Sublime speech: Speech therapy with a twist*. Retrieved April 3, 2015 from http://sublimespeech.com/tag/aac

Sulzby, E. (1989). Assessment of emergent writing and children's language while writing. In L. Morrow & J. Smith (Eds.), The role of assessment in early literacy instruction. Englewood Cliffs, NJ: Prentice-Hall.

Svirsky, M. A., Robbins, A. M., Kirk, K. I., Pisoni, D. B., & Miyamoto, R. T. (2000). Language development in profoundly deaf children with cochlear implants. *Psychological Science*, *11*(2), 153–158. doi:10.1111/1467-9280.00231 PMID:11273423

Swaggart, B. L. (1998). Implementing a cognitive behavior management program. *Intervention in School and Clinic*, *33*(4), 235–238. doi:10.1177/105345129803300406

Swettenham, J. (1996). Can children with autism be taught to understand false belief using computers? *Journal of Child Psychology and Psychiatry, and Allied Disciplines*, *37*(2), 157–165. doi:10.1111/j.1469-7610.1996.tb01387.x PMID:8682895

Swingler, T., & Brockhouse, J. (2009). Getting better all the time: Using music technology for learners with special needs. *Australian Journal of Music Education*, (2), 49.

Swingler, T. (1998). *That Was Me!": Applications of the Soundbeam MIDI Controller as a Key to Creative Communication*. Learning, Independence and Joy.

Swingler, T. (1998). The invisible keyboard in the air: An overview of the educational, therapeutic and creative applications of the EMS Soundbeam™. In *2nd European Conference for Disability, Virtual Reality & Associated Technology*.

Taber-Doughty, T. (2005). Considering student choice when selecting instructional strategies: A comparison of three prompting systems. *Research in Developmental Disabilities*, *26*(5), 411–432. doi:10.1016/j.ridd.2004.07.006 PMID:16168881

Taber-Doughty, T., & Brennan, S. (2008). Simultaneous and delayed video modeling: An examination of system effectiveness and student preferences. *Journal of Special Education Teaching*, *23*(1), 1–18.

Tanaka, J. W., Wolf, J. M., Klaiman, C., Koenig, K., Cockburn, J., Herlihy, L., & Schultz, R. T. et al. (2010). Using computerized games to teach face recognition skills to children with autism spectrum disorder: The Let's Face It! program. *Journal of Child Psychology and Psychiatry, and Allied Disciplines*, *51*(8), 944–952. doi:10.1111/j.1469-7610.2010.02258.x PMID:20646129

Tantam, D. (2000). Psychological disorder in adolescents and adults with Asperger syndrome. *Autism*, *4*(1), 47–62. doi:10.1177/1362361300004001004

Taylor, B. M., & Pearson, D. P. (Eds.). (2002). *Teaching reading: Effective schools, accomplished teachers*. Mahwah, NJ: Lawrence Erlbaum.

Tek, S., Mesite, L., Fein, D., & Naigles, L. (2014). Longitudinal Analyses of Expressive Language Development Reveal Two Distinct Language Profiles Among Young Children with Autism Spectrum Disorders. *Journal of Autism and Developmental Disorders*, *44*(1), 75–89. doi:10.1007/s10803-013-1853-4 PMID:23719855

Thaut, M. H. (1988). Measuring musical responsiveness in autistic children: A comparative analysis of improvised musical tone sequences of autistic, normal, and mentally retarded individuals. *Journal of Autism and Developmental Disorders*, *18*(4), 561–571. doi:10.1007/BF02211874 PMID:3215882

The Advisory Commission on Accessible Instructional Materials in Postsecondary Education for Students with Disabilities. (2011). *AIM commission report*. Retrieved, from https://www.library.cornell.edu/research/citation/apa

The Nation's Report Card. (2013). *Mathematics and Reading*. Retrieved August 13, 2014, from http://www.nationsreportcard.gov/reading_math_2013/#/

Thomas-Stonell, N., Oddson, B., Robertson, B., & Rosenbaum, P. (2009). Predicted and Observed Outcomes in Preschool Children Following Speech and Language Treatment: Parent and Clinician Perspectives. *Journal of Communication Disorders*, *42*(1), 29–42. doi:10.1016/j.jcomdis.2008.08.002 PMID:18835607

Throughton, K. E., & Hill, A. E. (2001). Relation between objectively measured feeding competence and nutrition in children with cerebral palsy. *Developmental Medicine and Child Neurology*, *43*(3), 187–190. doi:10.1111/j.1469-8749.2001.tb00185.x PMID:11263689

Tincani, M. (2004). Comparing the Picture Exchange Communication System and sign language training for children with autism. *Focus on Autism and Other Developmental Disabilities*, *19*(3), 152–163. doi:10.1177/10883576040190030301

Tobii Dynavox. (n.d.). *AAC software*. Retrieved on April 3, 2015 from http://www.tobiidynavox.com/software/#freeresources

TOCA BOCA. (n.d.). *TOCA BOCA*. Retrieved April 3, 2015 from http://tocaboca.com

Tomlinson, C. A. (2008). The goals of differentiation. *Educational Leadership, 66*(3), 26–30.

Topping, K.J., Bircham, A., & Shaw, M. (1997). Family electronic literacy: Home-school links through audiotaped books. *Reading, 31*(2), 7-12.

Torgesen, J., Houston, D., Rissman, L., & Kosanovich, M. (2007). Teaching All Students to Read in Elementary School: A Guide for Principals. *Center on Instruction.* Retrieved From: http://www.fcrr.org/Interventions/pdf/Principals%20Guide-Elementary.pdf

Treffertm, D. A. (2009). The savant syndrome: An extraordinary condition. A synopsis: Past, present, future. *Philosophical Transactions of the Royal Society, 364,* 1351–1357. PMID:19528017

Trembath, D., Balandin, S., Togher, L., & Stancliffe, R. J. (2009). Peer - mediated teaching and augmentative and alternative communication for preschool - aged children with autism. *Journal of Intellectual & Developmental Disability, 34*(2), 173–186. doi:10.1080/13668250902845210 PMID:19404838

Trevarthen, C., & Aitken, K. (2001). Infant intersubjectivity: Research, theory and clinical application. *Journal of Child Psychology and Psychiatry, and Allied Disciplines, 42*(1), 3–48. doi:10.1111/1469-7610.00701 PMID:11205623

Trezek, B. J., & Wang, Y. (2004). Implications of utilizing a phonics-based reading curriculum with children who are deaf or hard of hearing. *American Annals of the Deaf, 149*(5), 394–402. PMID:15727058

Trezek, B. J., Wang, Y., Woods, D. G., Gampp, T. L., & Paul, P. V. (2007). Using visual phonics to supplement beginning reading instruction for students who are deaf or hard of hearing. *Journal of Deaf Studies and Deaf Education,* 1–12. PMID:17515442

Truxler, J. E., & O'Keefe, B. M. (2007). The effects of phonological awareness instruction on beginning word recognition and spelling. *Augmentative and Alternative Communication, 23*(2), 164–176. doi:10.1080/07434610601151803 PMID:17487629

U.S. Department of Education. (2004). The rehabilitation act. *Laws & Guidance/Special Education & Rehabilitative Services.* Retrieved July 5, 2014, from http://www2.ed.gov/policy/speced/reg/narrative.html

U.S. Department of Education. (2006). *Assistive technology act: Annual report to Congress: Fiscal years 2004 and 2005.* Retrieved August 18, 2014, from http://www.ed.gov/about/reports/annual/rsa/atsg/2004/index.html

USC Institute for Creative Technologies. (2014). *VITA: Virtual Interactive Training Agent.* Available from http://ict.usc.edu/prototypes/vita/

Vaala, S., & Takeuchi, L. (2012). *Parent co-reading survey: Co-reading with children on iPads: Parents' perceptions and practices.* New York, NY: The Joan Ganz Cooney Center. Retrieved June 27, 2014, from http://www.joanganzcooneycenter.org/wp-content/uploads/2012/11/jgcc_ereader_parentsurvey_quickreport.pd

Vacca, R. T. (2002). Making a difference in adolescents' school lives: Visible and invisible aspects of *content area reading.* In A. E. Farstrup & S. J. Samuels (Eds.), *What research has to say about reading instruction* (3rd ed.). Newark, DE: International Reading Association. doi:10.1598/0872071774.9

van der Meer, L., & Weijers, D. (2013). Educational psychology research on children with developmental disabilities using expensive ICT devices. *Observatory for Responsible Research and Innovation in ICT.* Retrieved from http://responsible-innovation.org.uk/torrii/resource-detail/1182

van der Meer, L., Didden, R., Sutherland, D., O'Reilly, M. F., Lancioni, G. E., & Sigafoos, J. (2012). Comparing three augmentative and alternative communication modes for children with developmental disabilities. *Journal of Developmental and Physical Disabilities, 24*(5), 451–468. doi:10.1007/s10882-012-9283-3

van der Meer, L., Kagohara, D., Achmadi, D., Green, V. A., Herrington, C., Sigafoos, J., & Rispoli, M. et al. (2011). Teaching functional use of an iPod-based speech-generating device to individuals with developmental disabilities. *Journal of Special Education Technology, 26*(3), 1–11.

van der Meer, L., Kagohara, D., Achmadi, D., Green, V., Herrington, C., Sigafoos, J., & Rispoli, M. et al. (2011). Teaching functional use of an iPod-based speech-generating device to students with developmental disabilities. *Journal of Special Education Technology, 26*(3), 1–12.

van der Meer, L., Kagohara, D., Achmadi, D., O'Reilly, M. F., Lancioni, G. E., Sutherland, D., & Sigafoos, J. (2012). Speech-generating devices versus manual signing for children with developmental disabilities. *Research in Developmental Disabilities, 33*(5), 1658–1669. doi:10.1016/j.ridd.2012.04.004 PMID:22554812

van der Meer, L., Kagohara, D., Roche, L., Sutherland, D., Balandin, S., Green, V., & Sigafoos, J. et al. (2013). Teaching multi-step requesting and social communication to two children with autism spectrum disorders with three AAC options. *Augmentative and Alternative Communication, 29*(3), 222–234. doi:10.3109/07434618.2013.8158 01 PMID:23879660

van der Meer, L., Sigafoos, J., O'Reilly, M. F., & Lancioni, G. E. (2011). Assessing preferences for AAC options in communication interventions for individuals with developmental disabilities: A review of the literature. *Research in Developmental Disabilities, 32*(5), 1422–1431. doi:10.1016/j.ridd.2011.02.003 PMID:21377833

van der Meer, L., Sigafoos, J., Sutherland, D., McLay, L., Lang, R., Lancioni, G. E., & Marschik, P. B. et al. (2013). Preference-enhanced communication intervention and development of social communicative functions in a child with autism spectrum disorder. *Clinical Case Studies, 13*(3), 282–295. doi:10.1177/1534650113508221

van der Meer, L., Sutherland, D., O'Reilly, M. F., Lancioni, G. E., & Sigafoos, J. (2012). A further comparison of manual signing, picture exchange, and speech-generating devices as communication modes for children with autism spectrum disorders. *Research in Autism Spectrum Disorders, 6*(4), 1247–1257. doi:10.1016/j.rasd.2012.04.005

van der Merwe, E., & Alant, E. (2004). Associations with Minspeak™ icons. *Journal of Communication Disorders, 37*(3), 255–274. doi:10.1016/j.jcomdis.2003.10.002 PMID:15063146

Van Laarhoven, T., Johnson, J. W., Van Laarhoven-Myers, T., Grider, K. L., & Grider, K. M. (2009). The effectiveness of using a video iPod as a prompting device in employment settings. *Journal of Behavioral Education, 18*(2), 119–141. doi:10.1007/s10864-009-9077-6

Van Laarhoven, T., Kraus, E., Karpman, K., Nizzi, R., & Valentino, J. (2010). A comparison of picture and video prompts to teach daily living skills to individuals with autism. *Focus on Autism and Other Developmental Disabilities, 25*(4), 1–14. doi:10.1177/1088357610380412

Van Laarhoven, T., Zurita, L. M., Johnson, J. W., Grider, K. M., & Grider, K. L. (2009). Comparison of self, other, and subjective video models for teaching daily living skills to individuals with developmental disabilities. *Education and Training in Developmental Disabilities, 44*, 509–522.

Van Rijmenam, M. (2014). *Seven big data trends for 2014.* [Big data startup]. Retrieved, February 4, 2014, from http://www.bigdata-startups.com/big-data-trends-2014/

Van Tatenhove, G. M. (2009). Building language competence with students using AAC devices: Six challenges. *SIG 12 Perspectives on Augmentative and Alternative Communication, 18*(2), 38-47.

VandenBerg, N. L. (2001). The use of a weighted vest to increase on-task behavior in children with attention difficulties. *The American Journal of Occupational Therapy, 55*(6), 621–628. doi:10.5014/ajot.55.6.621 PMID:12959226

Vaughn, S., & Bos, C. S. (2012). *Strategies for teaching students with learning and behavior problems.* Upper Saddle River, NJ: Pearson.

Visser, S. N., Danielson, M. L., Bitsko, R. H., Holbrook, J. R., Kogan, M. D., Ghandour, R. M., & Blumberg, S. J. et al. (2014). Trends in the parent-report of health care provider-diagnosed and medicated attention-deficit/hyperactivity disorder: United States, 2003–2011. *Journal of the American Academy of Child Psychiatry, 53*(1), 34–46. doi:10.1016/j.jaac.2013.09.001 PMID:24342384

VividApps. (2008). *Strip designer.* Copenhagen, Denmark: Author. Available from iTunes.

Von Berg, S., Panorska, A., Uken, D., & Qeadan, F. (2009). DECtalk™ and VeriVox™: Intelligibility, Likeability, and Rate Preference Differences for Four Listener Groups. *AAC: Augmentative & Alternative Communication, 25*(1), 7–18. doi:10.1080/07434610902728531 PMID:19280420

Wainer, J., Dautenhahn, K., Robins, B., & Amirabdol-lahian, F. (2014). A pilot study with a novel setup for collaborative play of the humanoid robot KASPAR with children with autism. *International Journal of Social Robotics, 6*(1), 45–65. doi:10.1007/s12369-013-0195-x

Walpole, M., & McKenna, S. (2013). *The literacy coach's handbook.* New York, NY: The Guilford Press.

Walser, K., Ayres, K. M., & Foot, E. (2012). Effects of a video model to teach students with moderate intellectual disability to use features of an iPhone. *Education and Training in Autism and Developmental Disabilities, 47*(2).

Walser, K., Ayres, K. M., & Foote, E. (2012). Effects of a video model to teach students with moderate intellectual disabilities to use key features of an iPhone. *Education and Training in Autism and Developmental Disabilities, 47*, 319–331.

Ward, M., McLaughlin, T. F., & Neyman, J. (2013). Use of an iPad application as functional communication for a five-year-old preschool student with autism spectrum disorder. *International Journal of Engineering Education, 2*(4), 231–238.

Wehmeyer, M. (1996) Self-determination as an educational outcome: Why is it important to children, youth and adults with disabilities? In D. Sands & M. Wehmeyer (Eds.), Self-Determination Across the Life Span: Independence and Choice for People with Disabilities (pp. 15-34). Baltimore, MD: Brookes.

Wehmeyer, M. L., Palmer, S. B., Agran, M., Mithaug, D. E., & Martin, J. E. (2000). Promoting causal agency: The self-determined learning model of instruction. *Exceptional Children, 66*, 439–453.

Wehmeyer, M. L., Palmer, S., Smith, S. J., Davies, D., & Stock, S. (2008). The efficacy of technology use by people with intellectual disability: A single-subject design meta-analysis. *Journal of Special Education Technology, 23*(3), 21–30.

Wehmeyer, M. L., Sands, D. J., Doll, B., & Palmer, S. (1997). The development of self-determination and implications for educational interventions with students with disabilities. *International Journal of Disability Development and Education, 44*(4), 305–328. doi:10.1080/0156655970440403

Wehmeyer, M. L., & Schwartz, M. (1998). The relationship between self-determina-tion, quality of life, and life satisfaction for adults with mental retardation. *Education and Training in Mental Retardation and Developmental Disabilities, 33*, 3–12.

Weitz, C., Dexter, M., & Moore, J. (1997). *AAC and children with developmental disabilities. The handbook of augmentative and alternative communication.* San Diego: Singular Publishing Group.

Welcome. (n.d.). *to Apollo Creative: bubble tubes, bubble walls, LED light sources, equipment for interactive lighting, interactive displays, assistive technology, and multi sensory room equipment.* Retrieved June 1, 2014, from http://www.apollocreative.co.uk/

Wendt, O. (2009). Research on the use of manual signs and graphic symbols in autism spectrum disorders: A systematic review. In P. Mirenda & T. Iacono (Eds.), *Autism spectrum disorders and AAC* (pp. 83–140). Baltimore: Paul H. Brookes Publishing Co.

West, D. M. (2012). *Digital schools: How technology can transform education.* Washington, D.C.: Brookings Institution Press.

Westervelt, E. (June 11, 2014). *iPads allow kids with challenges to play in high school's band.* Retrieved June 27, 2014, from http://www.wbur.org/npr/320882414/ipads-allow-kids-with-challenges-to-play-in-high-schools-band

Whalen, C., Liden, L., Ingersoll, B., Dallaire, E., & Liden, S. (2006). Behavioral improvements associated with computer-assisted instruction for children with developmental disabilities. *The Journal of Speech and Language Pathology, 1*, 11–26.

White, H. A., & Shah, P. (2011). Creative style and achievement in adults with attention deficit/hyperactivity disorder. *Personality and Individual Differences, 50*(5), 673–677. doi:10.1016/j.paid.2010.12.015

Wiederholt, J. L., & Bryant, B. R. (2001). *Gray oral reading test-IV examiner's manual.* Austin, TX: Pro-Ed.

Wiegand, K., & Patel, R. (2014). *Towards More Intelligent and Personalized AAC.* Paper presented at the CHI 2014, Toronto, Canada. http://homepage.cs.uiowa.edu/~hourcade/workshops/complexcommunication-needs/papers/wiegand.pdf

Wigram, A. L. (1996). *The effects of vibroacoustic therapy on clinical and non-clinical populations.* (Doctoral dissertation). University of London, London, UK.

Wild, M. (2009). Using computer-aided instruction to support the systematic practice of phonological skills in beginning readers. *Journal of Research in Reading, 32*(4), 413–432. doi:10.1111/j.1467-9817.2009.01405.x

Williams, E. (2004). *Blogspot.com* [Blogger]. Retrieved February 4, 2014, from http://www.blogger.com

Williams, K. E., Riegel, K., & Kerwin, M. (2009). Feeding Disorder of Infancy or Early Childhood: How Often Is It Seen in Feeding Programs? *Children's Health Care, 38*(2), 123–136. doi:10.1080/02739610902813302

Wilson, B. S., Finley, C. C., Lawson, D. T., Wolford, R. D., Eddington, D. K., & Rabinowitz, W. M. (1991). Better speech recognition with cochlear implants. *Nature, 352*(6332), 236–238. doi:10.1038/352236a0 PMID:1857418

Wilson, K. P. (2013). Incorporating video modeling into a school-based intervention for students with autism spectrum disorders. *Language, Speech, and Hearing Services in Schools, 44*(1), 105–117. doi:10.1044/0161-1461(2012/11-0098) PMID:23087158

Wimmer, H., & Perner, J. (1983). Beliefs about beliefs: Representation and constraining function of wrong beliefs in young children's understanding of deception. *Cognition, 13*(1), 103–128. doi:10.1016/0010-0277(83)90004-5 PMID:6681741

Winner, M. G. (2008). *Think social: A social thinking curriculum for school-age students for teaching social thinking and related social skills to students with high-functioning autism, Asperger syndrome, PDD-NOS, ADHD, nonverbal learning disability, and for all others in the murky gray area of social thinking.* San Jose, CA: Think Social Publishing.

Wolowiec Fisher, K., & Shogren, K. A. (2012). Integrating Augmentative and Alternative Communication and Peer Support for Students with Disabilities: A Social-Ecological Perspective. *Journal of Special Education Technology, 27*(2), 23–39.

Wood Jackson, C., Wahlquist, J., & Marquis, C. (2011). Visual supports for shared reading with young children: The effect of static overlay design. *Augmentative and Alternative Communication, 27*(2), 91–102. doi:10.3109/07434618.2011.576700 PMID:21592004

Wood, L., & Masterson, J. J. (1999). The use of technology to facilitate language skills in school-age children. *Seminars in Speech and Language, 20*(3), 219–232. doi:10.1055/s-2008-1064019 PMID:10480493

Write:OutLoud. (1993). Wauconda, IL: Don Johnston Developmental Equipment.

XMind, Ltd. (2008). *XMind 2013* (v3.4.1) [The world's most popular mind mapping tool]. Hong Kong, People's Republic of China: XMind, Ltd. Retrieved February 4, 2014, from http://www.xmind.net

Yakubova, G., & Taber-Doughty, T. T. (2013). Brief report: Learning via the electronic interactive whiteboard for two students with autism and a student with moderate intellectual disability. *Journal of Autism and Developmental Disorders, 43*(6), 1465–1472. doi:10.1007/s10803-012-1682-x PMID:23080208

Zekovic, B., & Renwick, R. (2003). Quality of life for children and adolescents with developmental disabilities: Review of conceptual and methodological issues relevant to public policy. *Disability & Society, 18*(1), 19–34. doi:10.1080/713662199

Zentall, S. S. (1986). Effects of color stimulation on performance and activity of hyperactive and nonhyperactive children. *Journal of Educational Psychology, 78*(2), 159–165. doi:10.1037/0022-0663.78.2.159

Zentall, S. S., & Zentall, T. R. (1983). Optimal stimulation: A model of disordered activity and performance in normal and deviant children. *Psychological Bulletin*, *94*(3), 446–471. doi:10.1037/0033-2909.94.3.446 PMID:6657825

Zipse, L., Norton, A., Marchina, S., & Schlaug, G. (2012). When right is all that is left: Plasticity of right-hemisphere tracts in a young aphasic patient. *Annals of the New York Academy of Sciences*, *1252*(1), 237–245. doi:10.1111/j.1749-6632.2012.06454.x PMID:22524365

Zirpoli, T. J., & Melloy, K. J. (2007). *Behavior management: Applications for teachers* (5th ed.). Upper Saddle River, NJ: Prentice-Hall.

Zwiers, J. (2008). Building academic language: Essential practices for content classrooms, grades 5-12. San Francisco, CA: Jossey-Bass.

About the Contributors

Nava R. Silton, a developmental psychologist, received her B.S. from Cornell University in 2002 and her M.A. and Ph.D. from Fordham University in 2009. Silton has worked at Nickelodeon, Sesame Street Workshop, and Mediakidz. She has taught undergraduate and graduate psychology courses at Fordham University, Hunter College, Touro College and is now relishing her time at Marymount Manhattan College. She was a Postdoctoral Templeton Fellow at the Spears Research Institute from 2009-2010, and has consulted on projects conducted by the Autism Seaver Center, by Sesame Street Workshop, and Netflix. Silton's primary research interests include determining how to: (1) Enhance typical children's sensitivity to children with disabilities, (2) Teach social-emotional and cognitive skills to children with disabilities, and (3) Harness Assistive Technology to meet the needs of individuals with disabilities. Nava published her most recent peer-reviewed articles and texts in the area of increasing typical children's knowledge and sensitivity towards individuals with disabilities and in evaluating Assistive Technology for individuals with disabilities. Nava published her first book: *Innovative Technologies to Benefit Children with Autism* in March 2014 and is now preparing her third book: *Exploring the Benefits of Creativity in Business, Media and the Arts* (June 2016). She is currently testing her television show and graphic novel series, *Realabilities* in the schools. Much of her work focuses on disability awareness via programming and on promoting a stop bullying platform in the schools. Additionally, Nava is a Psychology point person for Fox 5 News and NBC News. Silton is also a weekly coach for Special Olympics Gymnastics, helps run Jewish learning and visiting the sick programs, and chairs a variety of fundraising initiatives in Manhattan. Nava is married to Dr. Ariel Brandwein, a Pediatric ICU fellow at LIJ Medical Center, and is the proud mother of two wonderful little guys, Judah and Jonah Brandwein.

* * *

Joséphine Ancelle graduated as class valedictorian with her B.A. in Speech-Language Pathology and Audiology and with a minor in Language Sciences from Marymount Manhattan College in the spring of 2014. She currently is completing her M.S. in Communication Sciences and Disorders with a bilingual extension certification at Teachers College, Columbia University. Her research interests include bilingual language acquisition, the use of music as a tool for speech and language treatment, and language processing.

Senada Arucevic is a nursing student at the Harriet Rothkopf Heilbrunn School of Nursing at Long Island University in Brooklyn, NY. She is pursuing a second Bachelors Degree in nursing due to her desire to work with children in a medical context. Arucevic discovered her passion through a compelling internship in the Pediatric Intensive Care Unit at the Steven and Alexandra Cohen Children's Medical Center of the North Shore LIJ Health System. Her previous degree in biology and psychology was achieved at Marymount Manhattan College where she also conducted research with Dr. Nava Silton for four years on the behavioral intentions and cognitive attitudes of typical children towards children with disabilities. Arucevic joined Silton on the Realabilities project in 2011, has contributed to the development of each of the characters and has written two of the episodes as well as edited others. She was an integral part of the research team that tested the efficacy of the show in different elementary schools throughout New York and New Jersey. Arucevic hopes to continue conducting research with Dr. Silton and plans on attending graduate school to become a Doctor of Nursing Practice (DNP).

Jody Marie Bartz is an Assistant Professor of Practice at Northern Arizona University in Flagstaff, Arizona where she teaches courses in Early Childhood Special Education and Severe Disabilities. Additionally, she is the TASH@NAU Faculty Advisor. She completed her Ph.D. in Disability and Psycho-educational Studies with a major emphasis in Early Childhood Special Education and a minor in Family Studies and Human Development at the University of Arizona in Tucson, Arizona. As a former special educator and the aunt of two nephews with autism, Jody is known as a strong advocate and is passionate about ensuring inclusive educational opportunities, especially for children with significant support needs. Her research agenda includes studying the effects of family involvement as well as the impact of educational, community, medical, and familial collaboration on outcomes for children with special health care needs and disabilities.

Peña L. Bedesem is an Assistant Professor at Kent State University. Her research interests include the use of evidence-based practices and technology to support students with learning and behavior problems.

Michael Ben-Avie, Ph.D., was the data analyst for Connecticut General Assembly Special Act 08-5: An Act Concerning the Teaching of Children with Autism and Other Developmental Disabilities (2008-2009). He is a senior researcher with the Center of Excellence on Autism Spectrum Disorders and conducted research on a federal grant addressing "Handheld Technology to Improve Educational Outcomes for Students with Autism Spectrum Disorders" (2010-2013). He worked as a job coach at a school that serves students with Autism Spectrum Disorders and other Developmental Disorders. As Principal Investigator and Co-P.I., he conducted outcome evaluations of federal grants, including grants from the U.S. Department of Health and Human Services' Center for Substance Abuse Treatment, U.S. Department of Education, the Substance Abuse and Mental Health Services Administration's Center for Mental Health Services, and a collaboration among the U.S. Departments of Education, Health and Human Services, and Justice. Dr. Ben-Avie is a nationally-recognized expert on public education as co-editor of six books on educational change and youth development with James. P. Comer, M.D., Associate Dean of the Yale School of Medicine. He is chair of the Tag Institute for Social Development.

Michelle Blumstein recently graduated from Marymount Manhattan College. While there she studied Early Childhood Education, with a special interest in students with disabilities and Psychology, more generally. She started playing instruments and appreciating music at a young age and music has been her passion ever since. Finding a way to incorporate that passion into something that can help and benefit others is realizing a dream for Michelle. She truly believes that music has the ability to heal, not only on an emotional level, but on a physical level, as well. There are various ways that music can benefit all people, not only through creating music, but through listening to music as well. Music is one of the greatest gifts we can give as well as receive and Blumstein contends that everyone should have the opportunity to love and enjoy it.

Patricia Brooks is Professor of Psychology at the College of Staten Island, City University of New York (CUNY), where she directs the Language Learning Laboratory. She completed her PhD studies in Experimental Psychology at New York University and post-doctoral fellowships at Carnegie Mellon University and Emory University, before joining the CUNY faculty in 1997. Dr. Brooks serves as Deputy Executive Officer of the PhD Program in Psychology at The Graduate Center, CUNY, and as Faculty Advisor of the Graduate Student Teaching Association of the American Psychological Association. Her research interests are in two broad areas: (1) individual differences in language learning and development and (2) effective teaching and learning. Dr. Brooks has authored or co-authored over 75 scientific papers and book chapters. With Vera Kempe, she co-authored the textbook Language Development (Wiley-Blackwell, 2012), and co-edited the Encyclopedia of Language Development (Sage, 2014).

Amy Bixler Coffin, M.S., is Program Director of the Autism Center at OCALI. A special educator for 24 years, Coffin has served as an intervention specialist, low-incidence supervisor, director of special education, and autism program director. She currently coordinates and provides regional and statewide professional development for districts, families, and organizations. Coffin has presented at state, national, and international conferences, contributed to several articles and book chapters, and has authored a book on supporting individuals with ASD in the community.

Terry Cumming is a Senior Lecturer in Special Education and the Deputy Head of School (Learning and Teaching) at the School of Education at the University of New South Wales. Her research interests include: students with emotional and behavioural disorders, social skills training, positive behavioural interventions, the use of technology in the classroom, and life transitions for people with disabilities. As part of the School of Education's Special Education Research Group, Terry's research is focused on life transitions for people with disabilities, positive behaviour support, and using iPads to support individuals with disabilities.

Janis Doneski-Nicol is the program director of the Northern Arizona University (NAU) Institute for Human Development Assistive Technology Center. She manages grants, contracts, fee for service activities and the NAU Graduate Certificate in Assistive Technology. Ms. Nicol has diverse experiences in the field of assistive technology as a cross categorical special education teacher, speech-language pathologist, and part-time faculty member. She is credentialed as an Assistive Technology Professional through the Rehabilitation Engineering and Assistive Technology Society of North America and is a member of the American Speech Language and Hearing Association (ASHA). She maintains membership in the ASHA Augmentative and Alternative Communication and Telepractice Special Interest Groups.

Ms. Nicol is also a doctoral candidate at NAU in the College of Education Curriculum and Instruction Doctoral Program with a research focus. Ms. Nicol has been providing assistive technology services and systems to adults and children with disabilities for over twenty years. She also provides web-based distance training, observations, and coaching to optimize access and inclusion of persons with disabilities. Ms. Nicol's teaching and research interests focus on the use of assistive technology tools and strategies to enhance language, literacy, learning, and communication. Her primary interest area is in literacy, complex communication needs and augmentative and alternative communication.

Cathi Draper Rodríguez, Ph.D., NCSP, is an Associate Professor and the Chair of the School of Education at California State University, Monterey Bay. Dr. Draper Rodriguez teaches curriculum, assessment, and introduction to research in the Special Education and Masters programs. Since earning her doctorate from the University of Nevada, Las Vegas, she has focused her research on using technology with English learners with and without disabilities and the diagnosis of disabilities in English learners, assessment in education and multicultural education. Dr. Draper Rodriguez is a Nationally Certified School Psychologist. Her previous work experience includes serving as a bilingual school psychologist in a public school setting and as an early interventionist providing services to young Latina mothers.

Diane Weaver Dunne is the executive director of the Connecticut Radio Information System. She holds a master's degree in Communication from the University of Hartford and a bachelor's degree in journalism from Syracuse University. She was an adjunct professor in communication at the University of Hartford for several years. Diane was the news editor for Education World, and the managing/interim editor at the Hartford Business Journal.

Theresa L. Earles-Vollrath, Ph.D. is a Professor of Special Education at the University of Central Missouri. Over the past 25 years, Dr. Vollrath has performed numerous jobs and activities related to educating children and youth with autism spectrum disorders. She is a consultant, presents on topics relating to ASD, has co-authored a state grant that funded an autism assessment center and has authored or co-authored numerous articles, books, and book chapters.

Naomi Gaggi is an undergraduate student at Macaulay Honors College at the College of Staten Island, City University of New York (CUNY). She is anticipating her Bachelor of Science in Psychology, with a concentration in neuroscience, in May of 2017. Her recent undergraduate work was mentored by Dr. Patricia J. Brooks and Dr. Kristen Gillespie-Lynch. Her work focused on social behaviors of college-aged students with Autism Spectrum Disorder and other disabilities. She is currently working on a study concerning college-aged adults with Autism Spectrum Disorder and social media, supervised by Christina Shane-Simpson. Naomi plans on obtaining her Ph.D. in Neuropsychology and holding a job as a professor.

Kristen Gillespie-Lynch is Assistant Professor of Psychology at the College of Staten Island. She received a PhD in Developmental Psychology from UCLA. Building upon her experiences teaching people with ASD, she investigates strengths and weaknesses associated with ASD across the lifespan. Her work includes the first study to examine relations between early childhood attention sharing and adult outcomes in autism, evaluations of eye-tracking measures as potential risk markers of autism, and assessment of potential benefits of computer-mediated communication for people who are and are not on the spectrum. In collaboration with a colleague on the spectrum, she developed a survey to examine conceptions of autism among people with and without ASD. Their findings suggested that people on the spectrum and those aware of the neurodiversity (or autism rights movement) are less interested in curing autism than their counterparts. However, participants who were and were not on the spectrum were equally interested in developing supports to increase the quality of life of people on the spectrum. Given that supports for adults on the spectrum are currently limited, she now directs and evaluates a mentorship program for college students with ASD.

Emily Hotez is a doctoral student in developmental psychology at the Graduate Center of CUNY. Throughout the course of her research, Emily has developed, implemented, and evaluated intervention and education programs for individuals across the lifespan. Emily's dissertation research investigates the role of parenting-related cognitions and emotions in the context of a parent-mediated intervention for children with autism spectrum disorder. She recently collaborated on a project that aimed to improve developmental screening practices among pediatricians and early childhood providers serving New York City. In addition to her graduate studies, Emily currently serves as a research analyst at the CUNY Institute for State and Local Governance. She has taught introductory psychology, health psychology, and basic and applied child development courses at Hunter College. Emily received her bachelor's degree in psychology from the George Washington University in 2011 and her master's degree in developmental psychology from the Graduate Center of CUNY in 2014.

Chris Kelly is the CRISKids for Schools Coordinator at CRIS Radio. As the coordinator, he recruits schools, trains teachers and students in the use of the technology, works with area partners to expand service to niche groups, convenes focus groups of teachers to integrate experiences into updated versions, develops and distributes surveys seeking student feedback and presents at conferences and seminars.

Taylor Luke attends The University of Texas at Austin, where she is pursuing a Master of Arts degree in Speech-Language Pathology. Taylor received her Bachelor of Arts degree in Speech-Language Pathology and Audiology with a minor in Psychology from Marymount Manhattan College, where she graduated magna cum laude. In the course of her undergraduate career, she served as a research assistant under Ann D. Jablon, Ph.D., CCC-SLP and Linda Z. Solomon, Ph.D., during which she discovered an interest and excitement for academia. Inspired by the teachings of Dr. Maria Montessori, Taylor has an affinity toward the developing minds of the pediatric population. Through her internship opportunities, she has discovered the power and potential of technology in the field of treating developmental disorders. In the future, Taylor would like to provide traditional speech-language and feeding services to the pediatric population while continuing to investigate how technology can serve as an effective modality for treatment.

Toby Mehl-Schneider, M.S. CCC-SLP, is a speech-language pathologist in New York City. She received a Bachelor of Arts, cum laude, in speech-language pathology and audiology and a Master of Science in speech-language pathology from Brooklyn College, The City University of New York. Toby is currently a doctoral student in the Department of Speech-Language-Hearing Sciences at The Graduate Center, The City University of New York in New York City. Toby Mehl-Schneider served as the lead researcher for the analysis, translation and standardization of the Preschool Language Scale (PLS-4) Hebrew Edition, adapting the PLS-4 English assessment materials to reflect the appropriate cultural and linguistic aspects of the Hebrew language. Her research for this standardization project as well as her research in other language-based areas have been presented at various national and international conferences. Toby has been providing therapeutic intervention to school-age children with varied speech and language disorders, including many with AAC needs, in the New York City Department of Education for nine years.

Brenda Smith Myles, Ph.D., a consultant with the Ohio Center for Autism and Low Incidence (OCALI) and the Ziggurat Group, is the recipient of the Autism Society of America's Outstanding Professional Award, the Princeton Fellowship Award, The Global and Regional Asperger Syndrome (GRASP) Divine Neurotypical Award, American Academy of Pediatrics Autism Champion, and two-time recipient of the Council for Exceptional Children, Division on Developmental Disabilities Burton Blatt Humanitarian Award. She served as the editor of Intervention in School and Clinic, the third largest journal in special education and has been a member of the editorial board of several journals, including Focus on Autism and Other Developmental Disabilities, Remedial and Special Education, and Autism: The International Journal of Research. Brenda has made over 1000 presentations all over the world and written more than 250 articles and books on ASD. In addition, she served as the co-chair of the National ASD Teacher Standards Committee, was on the National Institute of Mental Health's Interagency Autism Coordinating Committee's Strategic Planning Consortium and collaborated with the National Professional Center on Autism Spectrum Disorders, National Autism Center, and the Centers for Medicare and Medicaid Services who identified evidenced based practices for individuals with autism spectrum disorders and served as Project Director for the Texas Autism Resource Guide for Teachers (TARGET). Myles is also on the executive boards of several organizations, including the Scientific Council of the Organization for Autism Research (SCORE), College Internship Program, Early Autism Risk Longitudinal Investigation Network, and ASTEP – Asperger Syndrome Training and Education Program. Further, in the latest survey conducted by the University of Texas, she was acknowledged as the second most productive applied researcher in ASD in the world.

Christine Ogilvie was a middle school teacher in Massachusetts and Vermont before making the jump into higher education. A PhD graduate of the University of Central Florida in Orlando, FL, Dr. Ogilvie has established a notable presence in the area of Autism Spectrum Disorders. Her specific focus is working with adolescents with High Functioning Autism and Asperger Syndrome in the area of social skills instruction. As an avid supporter of video modeling and simulation technology for social skills instruction, Dr. Ogilvie continues to pursue an active research agenda in order to impact a larger number of adolescents on the Autism Spectrum, their teachers, families and the community at large.

Viviana Perilli, psychologist and PhD in psychology of cognitive, emotional and communicative processes, is a research assistant at the No-Profit Organization Lega del filo d'Oro site in Lesmo, Italy. She graduated in Clinical Psychology of Development and Relationships (2008) and earned her PhD (2013) at the University of Bari, Italy. During the PhD she started the first researches on cognitive rehabilitation of dementia, in particular on the process of intervention aimed at supporting the residual abilities in patients with Alzheimer's disease by the use of assistive technologies. Currently she is involved in research projects that focus on cognitive-behavioral interventions for persons affected by psycho-sensorial disabilities, extensive motor disabilities and developmental disabilities. The author works with assistive technologies for promoting communication opportunities, adequate physical exercise or ambulation, self management of instruction cues and leisure activities.

Bertram Ploog, as an undergraduate at the U. of California, San Diego, was mentored by Drs. George Reynolds, Edmund Fantino, and Ben Williams, who got him interested in experimental behavior analysis. In graduate school, with Dr. Laura Schreibman as his advisor, he first focused on applied behavior analysis. His Ph.D. dissertation, under Dr. Ben Williams's guidance, was an investigation of errorless learning in pigeons (theoretically relevant for an educational setting and applied behavior analysis, especially for autism). He spent his postdoctoral fellowship at Hunter College, in Dr. Phil Zeigler's lab, where he learned novel techniques relevant for neuroscientific research. A current research focus is on behavioral animal models to study abnormal attention patterns in children with autism. He is also directly studying attention processes (incl. language) in these children. He is now affiliated with three CUNY PhD training areas/subprograms (Animal Behavior & Comparative Psychology and Behavior Analysis in Psychology and Neuroscience in Biology). He has taught primarily behavior analysis and statistics courses.

Lisa Proctor received her Ph.D. from the University of Nebraska-Lincoln in 1998. She is a professor in the department of Communication Sciences and Disorders at Missouri State University. Her teaching and research interests include language and literacy development of children with complex communication needs.

Régine Randall is an assistant professor and coordinator of the graduate reading program in the department of Special Education and Reading at Southern Connecticut State University. She earned a Ph.D. from the University of Connecticut in Curriculum and Instruction with an emphasis on reading education. Régine has a wide array of professional and creative interests including adolescent literacy, content area reading and writing, assessment and intervention, teacher education, the special education needs of emergent bilinguals and the use of mixed media in K-12 classrooms. Prior to accepting a position at Southern Connecticut, Régine worked as a high school reading consultant as well as a research associate at the Yale Center for Learning Research.

Jan Rogers is currently the Program Director of the OCALI Assistive Technology Center. She is an occupational therapist and is also a RESNA certified ATP who has worked in a variety of agencies serving the needs of individuals with disabilities. She has taught assistive technology courses at The Ohio State University and currently teaches in the on-line AT certification and Master's program at Bowling Green State University. Additionally, she is a frequent presenter at local, state and national conferences on the topic of assistive technology.

Rebecca Ruchlin is currently pursuing a master's degree in speech-language pathology at Monmouth University. She holds a Bachelor of Arts degree in Speech-Language Pathology and Audiology from Marymount Manhattan College, where she graduated cum laude. Rebecca was a research assistant for Dr. Nava Silton for three years, working on a children's television show entitled Realabilities, encouraging typically developing children to be accepting and supportive of their disabled peers. She is currently working on a project at Monmouth University, evaluating the language abilities of individuals with autism, and the impact it has on empathy. Rebecca would like to work with children with autism, and other developmental disabilities. Her interest in that particular population derives from her own experiences with having a brother who has autism. He has been a source of inspiration for her since his diagnosis over 16 years ago.

Frank J. Sansosti, Ph.D., NCSP is an Associate Professor and Coordinator of School Psychology at Kent State University. He has extensive experience working with individuals with autism spectrum disorders (ASD) and behavioral disorders in both school and clinic settings. As a practitioner he provided coaching and technical assistance for early intervention and best practice approaches for students with disabilities in inclusive settings and coordinated efforts between parents, teachers, administrators, and district level personnel. Currently, Dr. Sansosti's primary research and professional interests focus on the development and implementation of behavioral and social skills interventions for individuals with ASD and best practice approaches for the inclusion of students with low-incidence disabilities. In addition, Dr. Sansosti has been active in conducting professional workshops for educators working with students with severe disabilities at local, regional, national, and international venues and he serves as a consultant to multiple school districts/agencies.

Christina Shane-Simpson is a doctoral student in Developmental Psychology at The Graduate Center, CUNY. Christina uses mixed methods to explore the dynamic interactions that occur between humans through computer-mediated environments. She currently studies college students' activity choices on social networking sites as they relate to compulsive tendencies, self-esteem and autistic traits. She is also designing technology-based interventions to assist students with autism and other disabilities to effectively navigate social networking sites for both entertainment and educational purposes. Her interests in integrating technology within the formal and informal classroom environment have led Christina to pursue a Certificate in Interactive Technology and Pedagogy from The Graduate Center, while she currently teaches Human Development at Hunter College. Christina also joined New Knowledge Organization, Ltd. as a Graduate Research Fellow to supplement her graduate work and further advance her research on the human-technology relationship.

Fabrizio Stasolla, PhD, is assistant professor at University of Bari. His topic concerns the assistive technologies for children with multiple disabilities, developmental disabilities, autism spectrum disorders, Rett and Down syndromes and cerebral palsy. He is interested in cognitive-behavioral deals with cognitive-behavioral interventions and alternative augmentative communication strategies for non verbal individuals. He teaches psychology of disabilities and rehabilitation to educational sciences students. The author works on PECS, VOCA, literacy process, ambulation responses, self-monitoring and self management of instruction cues to promote on-task behavior by students with learning disabilities. He is ad-hoc reviewer for Autism - open access, Journal of Autism and Developmental Disorders, Journal of Behavioral Education, Life Span and Disability, Research in Autism Spectrum Disorders, and Research in Developmental Disabilities. Moreover, he is a member of editorial board of the International Journal of Behavioral Research & Psychology (ISSN 2332-3000, SCI DOC Publishers).

Iva Strnadová is an Associate Professor in Special Education at the University of New South Wales in Sydney, Australia. She is also an Honorary Senior Lecturer at the University of Sydney, Faculty of Education and Social Work, Australia. Her research aims to contribute to better understanding and the improvement of life experiences of people with disabilities. Iva's previous research and ongoing research interests include the well-being of people with developmental disabilities (intellectual disabilities and autism) and their families over the life span, transitions for people with disabilities, mobile learning for people with developmental disabilities and women with intellectual disabilities.

Deborah Sturm is an Associate Professor of Computer Science at the College of Staten Island, City University of New York (CUNY) where she teaches undergraduate and graduate courses. She designed and teaches two gaming electives and introduced an area concentration in game development. Dr. Sturm is the faculty coordinator for the Faculty Interest Group in Gaming and Pedagogy under the auspices of the Faculty Center for Professional Development and is a member of the CUNY Games Network Advisory Board. She was a Project Director and Co-PI on a NSF-STEM grant, "Science and Technology Expansion via Applied Mathematics (STEAM)," a comprehensive, NSF-funded program to expand and support undergraduate education in science, technology, engineering and mathematics. Through this and other grants, she collaborates with members of the Psychology Department to design and develop research apps for children on the Autism spectrum.

Wendy Szakacs has been working with persons with disabilities for twenty-four years, while specializing in autism for the past seventeen years. She is presently employed as the Ohio Center for Autism and Low Incidence (OCALI) Regional Consultant for Autism and Low Incidence for Northeast /eastern Ohio. She develops evidence-based materials, provides technical assistance and professional development leading projects in social competence, bullying, behavior and communication. Szakacs began her career as an activities instructor for adults with disabilities at a county workshop setting. Next, she taught high school level students with orthopedic handicaps. She then taught students with multiple disabilities for several years before founding a unit for students with autism spectrum disorder. Mrs. Szakacs also was the educational consultant for a county autism consultation team that served students on the autism spectrum in twenty districts. Mrs. Szakacs has a B. S. degree in special education and a Master's degree in special education with a focus on autism, both from Youngstown State University. She has presented at local, state, and national conferences on various topics about autism spectrum disorder, including comprehensive program planning, structured teaching, social competence, and behavior.

Larah van der Meer, Ph.D. is an Assistant Professor in the School of Education at Victoria University of Wellington, New Zealand. She received the Vice Chancellor's Strategic Research Scholarship to complete her doctoral studies in Education at Victoria University of Wellington. This research focused on enhancing communication intervention for children with autism spectrum disorders. She completed a Postgraduate Diploma in Special Education from Massey University, New Zealand and worked as a behavior therapist for children with autism spectrum disorders. Dr van der Meer is currently involved in research projects investigating the use of iPods and iPads as AAC devices to support the communicative functioning of children and adults with various developmental and intellectual disabilities. She has co-authored various peer-reviewed research articles and presented her research at international and local conferences.

Krista Vince Garland, originally from Orlando, Florida, earned her Ph.D. in exceptional education at the University of Central Florida. Her research interests include the use of technology and simulation in teacher preparation, autism spectrum disorders, severe/profound disabilities, behavior management and single subject research. Dr. Vince Garland has taught a wide range of students with exceptionalities from kindergarten through eighth grades, across a continuum of educational settings, including facilitation, resource, and self-contained classrooms. Dr. Vince Garland frequently consults and presents at national professional conferences. She is actively involved in several professional organizations, including the Council for Exceptional Children, where she is a member of the Teacher Education Division professional development committee, the Technology and Media Division committee, and the Educators with Disabilities Caucus. She is also an active member of the Division of Autism and Developmental Disabilities, Council of Children with Behavioral Disorders, Autism Research Institute and Best Buddies.

Ye Wang, an associate professor and the Program Coordinator for Education of the d/Deaf and Hard of Hearing (EDHH) Program in the Department of Health and Behavior Studies, Teachers College, Columbia University, earned both of her M.A. and Ph.D. in School of Teaching & Learning from The Ohio State University. Her primary research interest is the language and literacy development of students who are d/Deaf or hard of hearing. Her other research and scholarly interests include multiple literacies, technology and literacy instruction, inclusive education, research methodology and early intervention.

Peggy Schaefer Whitby, Ph.D. is an associate professor at the University of Arkansas. Dr. Whitby is the program coordinator for the M.Ed. in special education with an emphasis in autism and behavior analysis. Her research interests are in the area of high-functioning autism and academic achievement. Dr. Schaefer Whitby has multiple publications in peer-reviewed journals including Education and Training in Autism and Developmental Disabilities, Beyond Behavior, Intervention in School and Clinic, and Focus on Autism and Other Developmental Disabilities.

Index

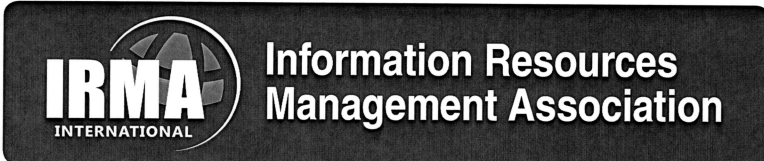

Become an IRMA Member

Members of the **Information Resources Management Association (IRMA)** understand the importance of community within their field of study. The Information Resources Management Association is an ideal venue through which professionals, students, and academicians can convene and share the latest industry innovations and scholarly research that is changing the field of information science and technology. Become a member today and enjoy the benefits of membership as well as the opportunity to collaborate and network with fellow experts in the field.

IRMA Membership Benefits:

- **One FREE Journal Subscription**

- **30% Off Additional Journal Subscriptions**

- **20% Off Book Purchases**

- Updates on the latest events and research on Information Resources Management through the IRMA-L listserv.

- Updates on new open access and downloadable content added to Research IRM.

- A copy of the Information Technology Management Newsletter twice a year.

- A certificate of membership.

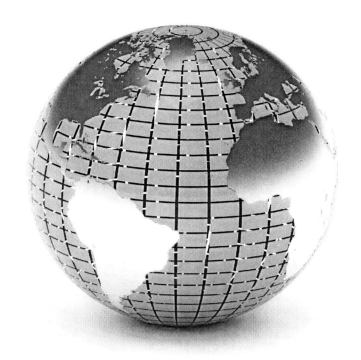

IRMA Membership $195

Scan code to visit irma-international.org and begin by selecting your free journal subscription.

Membership is good for one full year.

CPSIA information can be obtained
at www.ICGtesting.com
Printed in the USA
LVOW09*1740291117
558023LV00021B/354/P

0 1341 1717236 8